ANESTHESIA FOR OBSTETRICS

ANESTHESIA FOR OBSTETRICS

Sol M. Shnider, M.D.

Professor of Anesthesia,
Obstetrics, Gynecology and Reproductive Sciences
Vice Chairman, Department of Anesthesia
University of California, San Francisco
School of Medicine
San Francisco, California

Gershon Levinson, M.D.

Assistant Professor of Anesthesia,
Obstetrics, Gynecology and Reproductive Sciences
University of California, San Francisco
School of Medicine
San Francisco, California

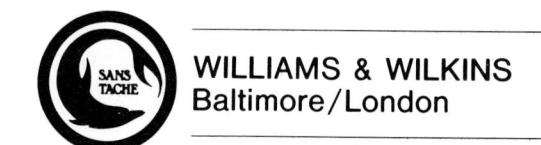

WILLIAMS & WILKINS
Baltimore/London

Copyright ©, 1979
The Williams & Wilkins Company
428 E. Preston Street
Baltimore, Md. 21202, U.S.A.

All rights reserved. This book is protected by copyright. No part of this book may be reproduced in any form or by any means, including photocopying, or utilized by any information storage and retrieval system without written permission from the copyright owner.
Made in the United States of America

Library of Congress Cataloging in Publication Data

Reprinted 1980

Main entry under title:

Anesthesia for obstetrics.

   Includes index.
   1. Anesthesia in obstetrics. I. Shnider, Sol M., 1929–   II. Levinson, Gershon.
[DNLM: 1. Anesthesia, Obstetrical. W0450 S559]
RG732.A55   617'.9682   78-25652
ISBN 0-683-07747-3

Composed and printed at the
Waverly Press, Inc.
Mt. Royal and Guilford Aves.
Baltimore, Md. 21202, U.S.A.

Dedication

To
Jeannie, Charles, Suzanne, Denys and Uncle
for their patience, love and friendship

PREFACE

Anesthesia for Obstetrics is a textbook covering all aspects of obstetric anesthesia. Physiologic, pharmacologic and clinical aspects have been integrated to provide a sound basis for the safe practice of obstetric anesthesia.

The editors—together with 17 distinguished authorities in the fields of anesthesiology, obstetrics, neonatology and law—have provided an up-to-date review of anesthesia for vaginal delivery and cesarean section, anesthesia for complicated obstetrics, anesthetic complications and evaluation and resuscitation of the fetus and neonate. We have oriented this textbook to practitioners and students of anesthesia. The comprehensive and concise coverage and authoritative nature of this publication should make the book appeal to all health care providers of pregnant women. Skillful application of the information in this volume will help provide optimum care for the mother and her newborn.

We wish to express our gratitude to all of our contributors as well as to the many publishers of scientific journals and books who permitted us to reproduce their previously published figures.

We are deeply appreciative of the efforts of Anita Edgecombe in the preparation of the manuscript and of Karen Olson and Doctors E. I. Eger, II, W. K. Hamilton, P. L. Wilkinson and R. K. Creasy, who provided valuable advice in the editing of this book. We also thank Merrilyn Jones and Judy Johnson for help in proofreading and preparing the index and Mary Briscoe for her original illustrations.

CONTRIBUTORS

Diane R. Biehl, M.D.
Assistant Professor
Department of Perinatology
St. Boniface Hospital
Winnipeg, Manitoba, Canada

Philip R. Bromage, M.B., B.S. (Lond), F.F.A.R.C.S., FRCP(c)
Professor of Anesthesiology, Obstetrics and Gynecology
Duke University Medical Center
Durham, North Carolina

Sheila E. Cohen, M.B., Ch.B., F.F.A.R.C.S
Assistant Professor
Department of Anesthesiology
Stanford University
Palo Alto, California

Ermelando V. Cosmi, M.D., L.D.
Professor of Anesthesiology, Obstetrics and Gynecology
University of Rome
School of Medicine
Rome, Italy

Marrs Craddick, LL.B., J.D.
Attorney-at-Law
Walnut Creek, California

Jay S. DeVore, M.D.
Assistant Professor
Department of Anesthesiology
University of California, Irvine
Irvine, California

George A. Gregory, M.D.
Professor of Anesthesia and Pediatrics
Department of Anesthesia
University of California, San Francisco
San Francisco, California

Brett B. Gutsche, M.D.
Associate Professor
Department of Anesthesiology
University of Pennsylvania
Philadelphia, Pennsylvania

David Karp, M.A.
Medical Malpractice Consultant
San Rafael, California

Russell K. Laros, Jr., M.D.
Professor and Vice Chairman
Department of Obstetrics, Gynecology and Reproductive Sciences
University of California, San Francisco
San Francisco, California

Gershon Levinson, M.D.
Assistant Professor of Anesthesia, Obstetrics, Gynecology and Reproductive Sciences
University of California, San Francisco
School of Medicine
San Francisco, California

Dennis Thomas Mangano, Ph.D., M.D.
Assistant Professor
Department of Anesthesia (V. A. Hospital)
University of California, San Francisco
San Francisco, California

Julian T. Parer, M.D., Ph.D.
Associate Professor
Department of Obstetrics, Gynecology and Reproductive Sciences
University of California, San Francisco
San Francisco, California

Roderic H. Phibbs, M.D.
Associate Professor
Department of Pediatrics and Cardiovascular Research Institute
University of California, San Francisco
San Francisco, California

David H. Ralston, M.D.
Assistant Professor
Anesthesia Research Center
Department of Anesthesiology
School of Medicine
University of Washington
Seattle, Washington

Sol M. Shnider, M.D.
Professor of Anesthesia, Obstetrics, Gynecology and Reproductive Sciences
Vice Chairman, Department of Anesthesia
University of California, San Francisco
School of Medicine
San Francisco, California

Richard G. Wright, M.D.
Chief Resident
Toronto General Hospital
Toronto, Ontario, Canada

Contents

Preface ix

SECTION ONE / Obstetric Physiology and Pharmacology

1: Maternal Physiologic Alterations During Pregnancy
   Brett B. Gutsche, M.D. 3
2: Utero-Placental Circulation and Respiratory Gas Exchange
   Julian T. Parer, M.D., Ph.D. 12
3: Obstetric Anesthesia and Uterine Blood Flow
   Ermelando V. Cosmi, M.D., L.D. and Sol M. Shnider, M.D. 23
4: Effects of Anesthesia on Uterine Activity and Labor
   Jay S. DeVore, M.D. 42
5: Perinatal Pharmacology
   David H. Ralston, M.D. 53

SECTION TWO / Anesthesia for Vaginal Delivery

6: Psychological Anesthesia for Obstetrics
   Jay S. DeVore, M.D. 65
7: Systemic Medication for Labor and Delivery
   Gershon Levinson, M.D. and Sol M. Shnider, M.D. 75
8: Regional Anesthesia for Labor and Delivery
   Sol M. Shnider, M.D., Gershon Levinson, M.D., and David H. Ralston, M.D. 93
9: Choice of Local Anesthetics in Obstetrics
   Philip R. Bromage, M.B., B.S. (Lond.), F.F.A.R.C.S., F.R.C.P. (c) ... 109
10: Inhalation Analgesia and Anesthesia for Vaginal Delivery
    Sheila E. Cohen, M.B., Ch.B., F.F.A.R.C.S. 121

SECTION THREE / Complicated Obstetrics

11: Pre-term Labor
    Part 1: Pharmacologic Therapy for Pre-term Labor 141
    Part 2: Anesthetic Considerations in Pre-term Labor
         Ermelando V. Cosmi, M.D., L.D. 155
12: Anesthesia for Abnormal Positions, Presentations and Multiple Births
    Gershon Levinson, M.D. and Sol M. Shnider, M.D. 170
13: Anesthesia for the Pregnant Cardiac Patient
    Dennis Thomas Mangano, Ph.D., M.D. 180

14: Anesthetic Considerations for Preeclampsia-Eclampsia
Brett B. Gutsche, M.D. **224**

15: Coagulation Disorders in the Obstetric and Surgical Patient
Russell K. Laros, Jr., M.D. **235**

16: Antepartum and Postpartum Hemorrhage
Diane R. Biehl, M.D. **243**

17: Anesthesia for Cesarean Section
Sol M. Shnider, M.D. and Gershon Levinson, M.D. **254**

SECTION FOUR/Anesthetic Complications

18: Hypotension and Regional Anesthesia in Obstetrics
Richard G. Wright, M.D. and Sol M. Shnider, M.D. **279**

19: Pulmonary Aspiration of Gastric Contents in the Obstetric Patient
Brett B. Gutsche, M.D. **288**

20: Neurologic Complications of Regional Anesthesia for Obstetrics
Philip R. Bromage, M.B., B.S. (Lond.), F.F.A.R.C.C., F.R.C.P. (c) ... **301**

21: Anesthesia for Operations during Pregnancy
Gershon Levinson, M.D. and Sol M. Shnider, M.D. **312**

22: Obstetrical Anesthesia and Lawsuits
David Karp, M.A. and Marrs Craddick, LL.B., J.D. **331**

SECTION FIVE/Fetus and Newborn

23: Evaluation of the Fetus
Russell K. Laros, Jr., M.D. **343**

24: Diagnosis and Management of Fetal Asphyxia
Julian T. Parer, M.D., Ph.D. **357**

25: Evaluation of the Neonate
Sheila E. Cohen, M.B., Ch.B., F.F.A.R.C.S. **370**

26: Resuscitation of the Newborn
Gershon Levinson, M.D. and Sol M. Shnider, M.D. **385**

27: Unusual Causes of Neonatal Respiratory Failure in the Delivery Room
George A. Gregory, M.D. **402**

28: Retrolental Fibroplasia: Anesthetic Implications
Roderic H. Phibbs, M.D. **411**

APPENDICES

Appendix A: Fetal and Neonatal Effects of Maternally Administered Drugs (Table)
Richard G. Wright, M.D. and Sol M. Shnider, M.D. **421**

Appendix B: The University of California, San Francisco Hospital and Clinics: Anesthesia Record—Obstetrics **434**

Appendix C: The University of California, San Francisco Obstetric Anesthesia Code Sheet **436**

Index **443**

SECTION ONE

OBSTETRIC PHYSIOLOGY AND PHARMACOLOGY

CHAPTER 1

Maternal Physiologic Alterations During Pregnancy

Brett B. Gutsche, M.D.

Pregnancy, labor and delivery are associated with major physiologic changes. Many of these changes have been long recognized and have been reviewed in detail.[1-3] However, some of these alterations—their onset, duration and magnitude—are still not fully understood.

This chapter will review some of the more important physiologic alterations that occur during normal pregnancy, particularly those related to the pulmonary and cardiovascular system. The implications of these changes on the anesthetic management of the parturient will be discussed. Familiarity with these changes and implications contribute to the safest possible administration of anesthesia to the parturient.

RESPIRATORY CHANGES DURING PREGNANCY

The respiratory changes which occur during pregnancy are of special significance to the anesthetist (Table 1.1). Capillary engorgement of the mucosa takes place throughout the respiratory tract, causing swelling of the naso- and oral pharynx, larynx and trachea.[1] As a result of this capillary engorgement, the parturient frequently shows symptoms of an upper respiratory infection with nasal congestion and laryngitis. These changes may be markedly exacerbated by a mild upper respiratory infection or the edema accompanying toxemia of pregnancy.

Manipulation of the upper airway requires extreme care. Suctioning, the placement of airways and careless laryngoscopy may result in bleeding and trauma. Upper airway obstruction may occur early in anesthetic induction. When endotracheal intubation is performed, a 6.5 to 7.0-mm cuffed endotracheal tube is recommended because the area of the false cords is usually swollen. Attempts to intubate the parturient with an 8-mm cuffed tube, normally suitable for the adult female, may result in trauma and inability to place the endotracheal catheter.

Lung volumes and capacities of the gravid patient at term compared to the non-gravid female are shown in Figure 1.1. Minute ventilation at term is increased about 50 per cent.[4] Recent work[5] indicates this increase in minute ventilation is primarily the result of an increased tidal volume with little change, or at most a slight increase, in respiratory rate. As a result of this increased alveolar ventilation at term, maternal $PaCO_2$ is usually decreased to about 32 torr, but little maternal alkalosis results because of a compensatory decrease in serum bicarbonate of about 4 mEq/L (from 26 to 22 mEq/L). During labor, particularly in the latter first stage

Table 1.1
Changes in the Respiratory System[4-10]

Variable	Direction of Change	Average Change
Minute ventilation	↑	50%
Alveolar ventilation	↑	70%
Tidal volume	↑	40%
Respiratory rate	↑	15%
Dead space	no change	
Airway resistance	↓	36%
Total pulmonary resistance	↓	50%
Total compliance	↓	30%
Lung compliance (alone)	no change	
Chest wall compliance (alone)	↓	45%
Arterial PCO_2	↓	10 torr
Serum bicarbonate	↓	4 mEq/L
Arterial pH	no change	
Arterial PO_2	↑	10 torr
Total lung capacity	↓	0-5%
Inspiratory lung capacity	↑	5%
Functional residual capacity	↓	20%
Expiratory reserve volume	↓	20%
Residual volume	↓	20%
Vital capacity	no change	
Closing volume	no change or ↓	
Oxygen consumption	↑	20%

and second stage as pain becomes severe, maternal minute ventilation may be increased as much as 300 per cent compared to the non-pregnant state, with the development of marked maternal hypocarbia ($PaCO_2$ 20 torr or less) and alkalemia (pH greater than 7.55). Fisher and Prys-Roberts[7] demonstrated that effective epidural analgesia alone can markedly diminish this hyperventilation, which indicates that the hyperventilation is in part due to the pain of labor.

Lung volumes and lung capacities are not greatly changed by pregnancy. Changes are primarily limited to the functional residual capacity. Vital capacity, taken in the same position, remains essentially unchanged throughout pregnancy. A significant decrease in vital capacity during pregnancy may indicate pulmonary or cardiovascular dysfunction. Earlier data[1,8] have indicated total lung capacity at term is decreased about 5 per cent due to a 4-cm elevation of the diaphragm caused by the gravid uterus. A recent study disputes this decrease in total lung capacity and indicates that there is an increase in transverse and anterior posterior diameter of the chest which compensates for the elevation of the diaphragm. Contrary to previous reports, the diaphragm is not splinted at term, but moves freely. However, abdominal breathing is decreased in favor of thoracic breathing as pregnancy progresses.

Functional residual capacity is decreased 15 to 20 per cent in the gravida at term (Figure 1.1). It is well established that a large proportion of this decrease is due to a decrease in the expiratory reserve volume secondary to the increase in tidal volume.

Measurements of closing volume (lung volume during expiration at which airways begin to close in the dependent zones of the lungs) indicate that in the supine position one-third of parturients will develop airway closure during normal tidal ventilation.[10] Thus, one would expect the parturient to be more susceptible to atelectasis and to develop an increased oxygen alveolar-arterial ($P_{A-a}O_2$) gradient more readily. However, this concept has recently been challenged.[9]

Oxygen uptake in pregnancy is markedly increased both at rest (greater than 20 per cent)[10] and during exercise[11] at term as compared to the non-pregnant state. This is due to an increase in maternal metabolism as well as increased work required in breathing. Oxygen consumption, which is increased even more in labor, can be sig-

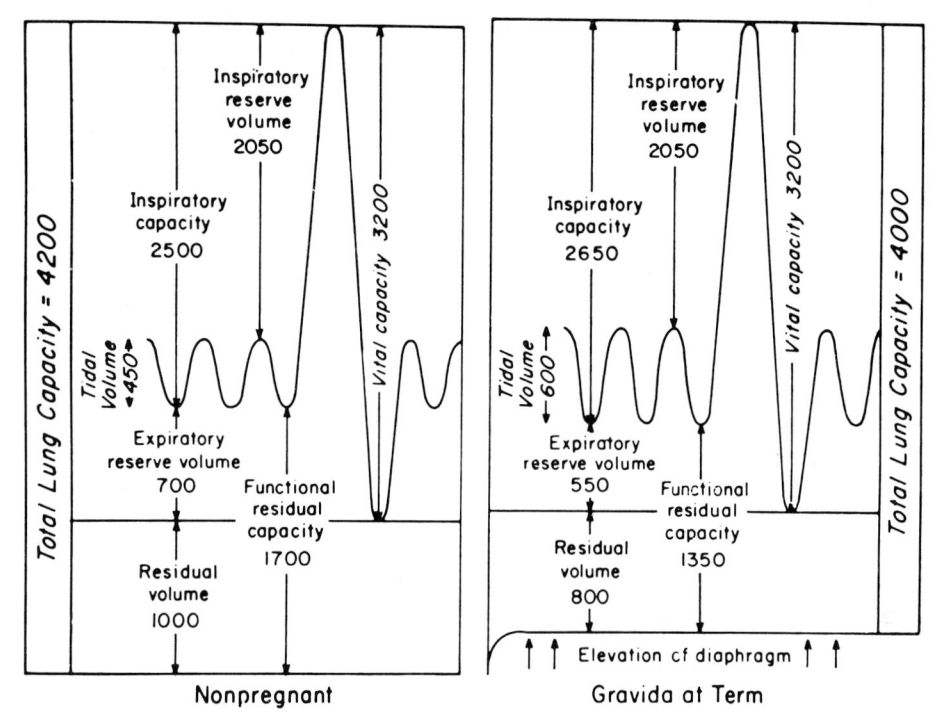

MATERNAL PHYSIOLOGIC ALTERATIONS DURING PREGNANCY

Figure 1.1. Pulmonary volumes and capacities during pregnancy, labor and postpartum period. (Reprinted by permission from Bonica JJ: *Principles and Practice of Obstetric Analgesia and Anesthesia.* F. A. Davis Co., Philadelphia, 1967.)

nificantly decreased with regional analgesia.[12] Flow volume loops, timed forced expiratory volume and other flow characteristics during pregnancy are little changed from the non-pregnant state.[9]

Changes of respiratory function during pregnancy have great significance to the anesthetist. The decrease in functional residual capacity combined with the increased minute ventilation increases the rapidity of induction with inhalation anesthetics. In addition, the anesthetic requirements of inhalation drugs are decreased in pregnancy.[13] The above factors combine to make the parturient very sensitive to inhalation anesthetic agents. Low concentrations of inhalation gases administered for analgesia may produce general anesthesia with loss of protective airway reflexes. Higher doses, safe in the non-pregnant patient, may produce overdosage with severe cardiopulmonary depression in the parturient.

The decrease in functional residual capacity lowers the oxygen reserve. Endotracheal intubation in the parturient breathing air, in contrast to the non-parturient, is associated with a more precipitous decrease of PaO_2 after only a short period of apnea.[14] The tendency for rapid development of hypoxia is aggravated by the increased oxygen consumption during labor. Rapid development of hypoxia may be avoided by administration of 100 per cent oxygen before induction of anesthesia.

CARDIOVASCULAR CHANGES DURING PREGNANCY

Numerous changes take place in the cardiovascular system during pregnancy which provide for the needs of the fetus and prepare the mother for delivery (Table 1.2). Maternal blood volume markedly increases during pregnancy[15, 16] (Figure 1.2). Plasma volume increases from 40 to 70 ml/kg and red blood cell volume from 25 to 30 ml/kg. The increase in maternal blood volume begins in the first trimester, has its maximum rate of increase in the second trimester and continues to rise at a slower rate early in the third trimester. Contrary to earlier studies, maternal blood volume decreases only slightly, if at all, in the third trimester.[16] Near term there is about a 35 to 40 per cent increase or an expansion of the blood volume of more than 1000 ml. Much of this increased blood volume perfuses the gravid uterus, and with contractions 300 to 500 ml may be forced from the uterus into the maternal vascular system. An average blood loss of 400 to 600 ml occurs in a normal vaginal delivery. With the uncomplicated vaginal delivery of twins or at cesarean section, approximately 1,000 ml of maternal blood are lost. The normal non-pregnant blood volume is not reached until 7 to 14 days postpartum.

Red blood cell mass increases with pregnancy, but at a slower rate than plasma volume and blood volume, thus accounting for the relative anemia of pregnancy. At term, in the normal parturient, the red blood cell mass is increased about 20 per cent or approximately 350 ml. Although it is normal to see a fall in hematocrit or hemoglobin during pregnancy, hematocrits of less than 33 per cent or hemoglo-

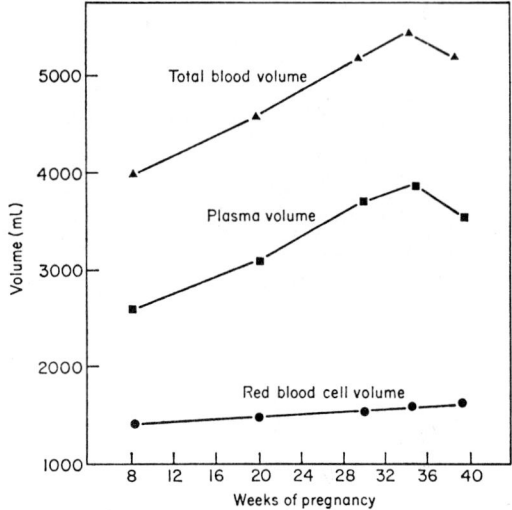

Figure 1.2. Changes in total blood volume, plasma volume and red blood cell volume in normal pregnancy. Note the continued increase in red blood cell volume with minimal decrease in total blood volume and plasma volume late in the third trimester. (Reprinted by permission from Moir DD, Carty MJ: *Obstetric Anesthesia and Analgesia*. Williams & Wilkins Co., Baltimore, 1977.)

Table 1.2
Changes in Cardiovascular System[15-21]

Variable	Direction of Change	Average Change
Blood volume	↑	35%
Plasma volume	↑	45%
Red blood cell volume	↑	20%
Cardiac output	↑	40%
Stroke volume	↑	30%
Heart rate	↑	15%
Total peripheral resistance	↓	15%
Mean arterial blood pressure	↓	15 torr
Systolic blood pressure	↓	0-5 torr
Diastolic blood pressure	↓	10-20 torr
Central venous pressure	no change	
Femoral (uterine?) venous pressure	↑	15 torr

bins of less than 11 gm represent maternal anemia, usually secondary to iron deficiency.

It should be obvious that the normal parturient is well prepared to lose considerable blood at the time of delivery and rarely will require transfusion unless blood in excess of 1,500 ml is lost. Not only does the parturient have an increased blood volume, but, at the time of delivery, the uterus will contract, giving in excess of 500 ml of blood to the vascular system. The contracted uterus also effectively decreases the vascular space by the same volume. However, the gravida with hypertension, whether essential hypertension or that secondary to toxemia of pregnancy, may actually have a diminished blood volume at term (see chapter 14).

During the first trimester of pregnancy, cardiac output is elevated approximately 30 to 40 per cent. Additional slight elevation occurs during the second trimester. Earlier studies indicated that cardiac output then fell toward non-pregnant values during the third trimester. These earlier studies, however, were done with the gravid patient supine. Lees et al.[17, 18] and Ueland et al.[19] showed that the marked decrease in cardiac output after 28 weeks which occurred in the supine position was due primarily to obstruction of the inferior vena cava and did not occur in the lateral position (Figure 1.3). Ueland showed, however, that cardiac output was reduced, but to a lesser extent, in the sitting and lateral positions when the patient approached term.[19]

During labor, cardiac output rises 15 per cent during the latent phase, 30 per cent during the active phase and 45 per cent during the expulsive stage, compared with pre-labor values.[20] This rise in cardiac output is due to an increase in both heart rate and stroke volume. Each uterine contraction increases cardiac output an additional 10 to 25 per cent.[21] The greatest increase occurs immediately after delivery when the cardiac output is an average of 80 per cent above pre-labor values. Cardiac output then gradually declines to non-pregnant levels by 2 weeks after delivery.

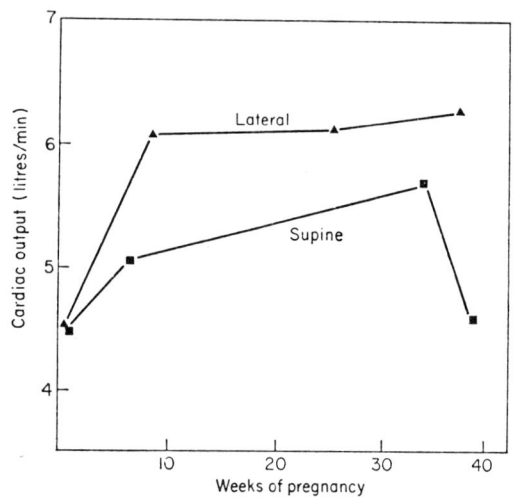

Figure 1.3. Cardiac output in pregnancy in the supine and lateral position. Note the marked increased cardiac output in the early first trimester which is maintained throughout pregnancy when measured in the lateral position. (Reprinted by permission from Moir DD, Carty MJ: *Obstetric Anesthesia and Analgesia*. Williams & Wilkins Co., Baltimore, 1977. From data by Lees MM, Taylor SH, Scott DB, et al.: A study of cardiac output at rest throughout pregnancy. J Obstet Gynaecol Br Commonw 74:319, 1967.)

Blood pressure is not elevated during normal pregnancy, indicating a decrease in peripheral vascular resistance. During labor each uterine contraction is associated with an increase in blood pressure. Up to 10 per cent of pregnant patients near term develop signs of shock—including hypotension, pallor, sweating, nausea, vomiting and changes in cerebration—when they assume the supine position. Howard and co-workers[22] described the syndrome and named it the "supine hypotension syndrome." By injection of radiopaque dye in a femoral vein, Kerr and co-workers[23] showed that the inferior vena cava was totally obstructed by the gravid uterus in the supine position. Blood from below the obstructed inferior vena cava returned in part to the heart via the paravertebral (epidural) veins emptying into the azygos system. Turning the gravid patient to the side partially relieved the obstruction of the vena cava. The maternal symptoms of the supine hypotensive syndrome were attributed to lack of venous return to the heart. Compression of the inferior vena cava is most common late in pregnancy before the presenting fetal part becomes fixed in the pelvis. This compression tends to produce pooling of venous blood and increased venous pressure in the lower torso which may explain the tendency toward phlebitis and the development of venous varicosities in pregnancy. The increase in uterine venous pressure may affect the well-being of the fetus through a resultant decrease in uterine blood flow. Blood flow to the uterus is directly related to the perfusion pressure, that is uterine artery minus uterine venous pressure. In the supine position, even without arterial hypotension, uterine perfusion pressure falls due to the increased uterine venous pressure.

Bieniarz and co-workers[24] took serial x-rays of the aorta after injection of radiopaque dye in the femoral arteries and found the aorta to be partially occluded when the gravid patient was supine. Compression of the aorta is not associated with maternal symptoms but causes arterial hypotension in the lower extremities and uterine arteries, which can further decrease uterine blood flow and result in fetal asphyxia and fetal distress.[25]

It is imperative that the anesthetist appreciate the importance of the aortocaval compression syndrome and realize that anesthesia may augment its symptoms. Drugs causing vasodilation, such as halothane and thiopental, or techniques causing sympathetic block, such as subarachnoid or epidural anesthesia, will further decrease venous return to the heart in the presence of vena caval obstruction. Furthermore, a sympathectomy removes the parturient's ability to compensate by vasoconstriction for the decreased venous return. Thus arterial hypotension is much more common and severe during spinal and epidural anesthesia in pregnancy compared to the non-pregnant state.[26]

Obviously prevention of aortocaval compression is preferred to treatment. The gravida at term should never be allowed to assume the supine position. Currently, with the widespread use of continuous fetal heart rate monitoring, abnormal patterns indicating utero-placental insufficiency have been frequently found in patients in the supine position. This is especially true if they are receiving a sympathetic blockade or general anesthesia. Prevention of aortocaval compression consists of left uterine displacement (LUD). LUD can be accomplished by manual displacement of the uterus in which the uterus is lifted and displaced to the left. Alternatively, the patient may be positioned on her left side either by tipping the operating or delivery table 15° to the left or by using sheets or a foam rubber wedge to elevate the right buttock and back about 10 to 15-cm. Stationary left uterine displacers such as the one designed by Kennedy,[27] which mounts to the side of the operating table, or that designed by Colon-Morales,[28] which is placed under the patient's right hip, are effective and commercially available.* Placing the patient in the Trendelenburg position without LUD is not an appropriate means of prophylaxis and may actually worsen the condition by shifting the uterus further back onto the vena cava and aorta. If hypotension develops in the gravid patient near term, one

---

* The Kennedy displacer is available from the H. E. Richards Company, Box 345, Toledo, Ohio 43601. The Colon-Morales device is available from Resuscitation Laboratory, P.O. Box 3051, Bridgeport, Connecticut 06605.

CENTRAL NERVOUS SYSTEM CHANGES DURING PREGNANCY

Anesthesia requirement for inhalation agents is decreased up to 40 per cent during pregnancy.[13] The mechanism for this decrease in anesthesia requirement is uncertain, but hormonal changes during pregnancy may be responsible. For example, progesterone levels increase 10- to 20-fold during late pregnancy.[29] Progesterone has a sedative activity[30] and in large doses induces loss of consciousness in man.[31] The decrease in anesthetic requirement is important clinically. Concentrations of inhalation agents which would not produce loss of consciousness in the surgical patient may be perilously close to anesthetizing concentrations in the parturient, thereby subjecting her to the dangers of vomiting and aspiration.

Circulatory changes within the vertebral column will have profound effects on subarachnoid and epidural techniques of regional analgesia. Due to increased intraabdominal pressure, epidural veins become engorged, making inadvertent intravascular injection during lumbar epidural or caudal epidural block common. This engorgement decreases the size of the epidural space. In addition, each spinal nerve root as it passes out its intravertebral foramen is accompanied by an epidural vein which will be swollen, thus decreasing the size of the opening. The decrease in size of the epidural space and the blocking of the intravertebral foramina explains the one-third decrease in the amount of local anesthetic required to produce a given level of epidural block in the parturient as compared to the non-pregnant patient.[32]

Engorgement of the epidural veins, in addition to decreasing the volume of the epidural space, may also decrease the volume of cerebrospinal fluid (CSF) contained within the subarachnoid space of the vertebral column. This would explain the 30 to 50 per cent reduction of local anesthetic required for subarachnoid block in the parturient as compared to the non-gravid patient.

Although the CSF pressure is not elevated in pregnancy, painful uterine contractions with maternal Valsalva maneuvers result in a rise in CSF pressure. A markedly increased level of anesthetic block can result if local anesthetic is injected into the subarachnoid space during a contraction. This rise in CSF pressure may reach 70 cm H_2O during contractions with maternal bearing down during the second stage of labor.[33]

GASTROINTESTINAL CHANGES DURING PREGNANCY

Pregnancy is associated with a shift in the position of the stomach due to the gravid uterus which changes the angle of the gastroesophageal junction. This frequently results in incompetence of the gastroesophageal pinchcock mechanism, which allows gastric reflux and production of esophagitis. It makes the parturient prone to silent regurgitation and aspiration during general anesthesia or impaired consciousness from any cause. Gastric motility and emptying time are slowed in pregnancy, further increasing the parturient's risk of pulmonary aspiration. The enlarged uterus displaces the pylorus upwards and backwards and retards gastric motility. The hormone gastrin produced by the placenta raises the acid, chloride and enzyme content of the stomach to levels above normal.[34] Recent investigations by Roberts and Shirley[35, 36] indicated that approximately 25 per cent of parturients undergoing elective cesarean section after an overnight fast still have greater than 25 ml of gastric juice with a pH less than 2.5; they are, therefore, at high risk for pulmonary aspiration with the development of the acid aspiration syndrome.

RENAL CHANGES DURING PREGNANCY

Renal plasma flow (RPF) and glomerular filtration rate (GFR) increase rapidly during the first trimester of pregnancy, reaching 50 per cent above non-pregnant values by the fourth month of gestation.[37] During the third trimester RPF and GFR slowly return toward normal. The high RPF and GFR result in an increase in creatinine clearance. The upper limits of normal for BUN and serum creatinine are lower in the pregnant woman. There is a 40 per cent reduction in BUN to 8 or 9 mg per cent and creatinine to 0.46 mg per cent during a normal pregnancy. Tubular reabsorption of electrolytes and water increases in proportion to the GFR; therefore, no loss or accumulation of electrolytes occurs.

Renal calyces, pelves and ureters dilate after the third month of gestation. The dilation is due first to progesterone, which induces atony of the calyces and ureters.[38] Later the ureters are compressed at the pelvic brim by the enlarging uterus, further contributing to the dilation.

HEPATIC CHANGES DURING PREGNANCY

Elevated SGOT, LDH, alkaline phosphatase and cholesterol levels are common during pregnancy and labor, and 80 per cent of parturients have abnormal Bromsulfalein excretion tests.[39] These abnormal liver function tests do not necessarily indicate hepatic disease. Serum bilirubin and hepatic blood flow are unaltered. Total protein concentration decreases as does the albumin to globulin ratio.[40] Although plasma cholinesterase activity is reduced during pregnancy and the immediate postpartum period,[41] succinylcholine and chloroprocaine are usually metabolized easily.

References

1. Bonica JJ: *Principles and Practice of Obstetric Analgesia and Anesthesia.* F. A. Davis, Philadelphia, 1967, pp 13–39.
2. Marx GF, Orkin LR: *Physiology of Obstetric Anesthesia.* Charles C Thomas, Springfield, Ill., 1967.
3. Moir DD, Carty MJ: *Obstetric Anesthesia and Analgesia.* Williams & Wilkins, Baltimore, 1977, pp 8–35.
4. Prowse CM, Gaensler EA: Respiratory and acid base changes during pregnancy. Anesthesiology 26:381, 1965.
5. Pernoll ML, Metcalf J, Kovach PA, et al.: Ventilation during rest and exercise in pregnancy and postpartum. Resp Physiol 25:295, 1975.
6. Gee JBL, Packer BS, Millen JE, et al.: Pulmonary mechanics during pregnancy. J Clin Invest 46:945, 1967.
7. Fisher A, Prys-Roberts C: Maternal pulmonary gas exchange. A study during normal labor and extradural blockade. Anaesthesia 23:350, 1968.
8. Cugell DW, Frank NR, Gaensler EA, et al.: Pulmonary function in pregnancy. I. Serial observations in normal women. Am Rev Tuberc 67:538, 1953.
9. Baldwin GR, Moorthi DS, Whelton JA, et al.: New lung functions and pregnancy. Am J Obstet Gynecol 127:235, 1977.
10. Bevan DR, Holdcroft A, Loh L, et al.: Closing volume and pregnancy. Br Med J 1:13, 1974.
11. Pernoll ML, Metcalf J, Schlenker TL, et al.: Oxygen consumption at rest and during exercise in pregnancy. Resp Physiol 25:285, 1975.
12. Sangoul F, Fox GS, Houle GL: Effect of regional analgesia on maternal oxygen consumption during the first stage of labor. Am J Obstet Gynecol 121:1080, 1975.
13. Palahniuk RJ, Shnider SM, Eger EI II: Pregnancy decreases the requirements for inhaled anesthetic agents. Anesthesiology 41:82, 1974.
14. Archer GW Jr, Marx GF: Arterial oxygen tension during apnoea in parturient women. Br J Anaesth 46:358, 1974.
15. Pritchard JA: Changes in blood volume during pregnancy and delivery. Anesthesiology 26:393, 1965.
16. Ueland K: Maternal cardiovascular dynamics. VII. Intrapartum blood volume changes. Am J Obstet Gynecol 126:671, 1976.
17. Lees MM, Taylor SH, Scott DB, et al.: A study of cardiac output at rest throughout pregnancy. J Obstet Gynaecol Br Commonw 74:319, 1967.
18. Lees MM, Scott DB, Kerr MG, et al.: The circulatory effects of recumbant postural change in late pregnancy. Clin Sci 32:453, 1967.
19. Ueland K, Novy MJ, Peterson EN, et al.: Maternal cardiovascular dynamics. IV. The influence of gestational age on the maternal cardiovascular response to posture and exercise. Am J Obstet Gynecol 104:856, 1969.
20. Ueland K, Hansen JM: Maternal cardiovascular

dynamics. III. Labor and delivery under local and caudal analgesia. Am J Obstet Gynecol 103:8, 1969.
21. Ueland K, Hansen JM: Maternal cardiovascular dynamics. II. Posture and uterine contractions. Am J Obstet Gynecol 103:1, 1969.
22. Howard BK, Goodson JH, Mengert WF: Supine hypotension syndrome in late pregnancy. Obstet Gynecol 1:371, 1953.
23. Kerr MG, Scott DB, Samule E: Studies of the inferior vena cava in late pregnancy. Br Med J 1: 532, 1964.
24. Bieniarz J, Crottogini JJ, Curachet E: Aortocaval compression by the uterus in late human pregnancy. Am J Obstet Gynecol 100:203, 1968.
25. Marx GF: Aortocaval compression: Incidence and prevention. Bull NY Acad Med 50:443, 1974.
26. Assali NS, Prystosky H: Studies on autonomic blockade. I. Comparison between the effects of tetraethyl ammonium chloride (TEAC) and high selective spinal anesthesia on the blood pressure of normal and toxemic pregnancy. J Clin Invest 29:1354, 1950.
27. Kennedy RL: An instrument to relieve inferior vena cava occlusion. Am J Obstet Gynecol 107: 331, 1970.
28. Colon-Morales MA: A self-supporting device for continuous left uterine displacement during cesarean section. Anesth Analg 49:223, 1970.
29. Yannone ME, McCurdy JR, Goldfein A: Plasma progesterone levels in normal pregnancy, labor and the puerperium. II. Clinical data. Am J Obstet Gynecol 101:1058, 1968.
30. Selye H: Studies concerning the anesthetic action of steroid hormones. J Pharmacol Exp Ther 73: 127, 1941.
31. Merryman W: Progesterone "anesthesia" in human subjects. J Clin Endocrinol Metab 14:1567, 1954.
32. Bromage PL: Continuous lumbar epidural analgesia for obstetrics. Can Med Assoc J 85:1136, 1961.
33. Marx GF, Oka Y, Orkin LR: Cerebrospinal fluid pressures during labor. Am J Obstet Gynecol 84: 213, 1967.
34. Attia RR, Eberd AM, Fischer JE: Gastrin: Placental, maternal and plasma cord levels, its possible role in maternal residual gastric acidity. In *Abstracts of Scientific Papers*, Annual Meeting, American Society of Anesthesiologists, San Francisco, 1976, p 547.
35. Roberts RB, Shirley MB: Reducing the risk of acid aspiration during cesarean section. Anesth Analg 53:859, 1974.
36. Roberts RB, Shirley MB: The obstetrician's role in reducing the risk of aspiration pneumonitis with particular reference to the use of oral antacids. Am J Obstet Gynecol 124:611, 1976.
37. Dignam WJ, Titus P, Assali NS: Renal function in human pregnancy. I. Changes in glomerular filtration rate and renal plasma flow. Proc Soc Exp Biol Med 97:512, 1958.
38. Van Wagenen G, Jenkins RH: An experimental examination of factors causing ureteral dilation of pregnancy. J Urol 42:1010, 1939.
39. Smith BE, Moya F, Shnider SM: The effects of anesthesia on liver function during labor. Anesth Analg 41:24, 1962.
40. McNair RD, Jaynes RV: Alterations in liver function during normal pregnancy. Am J Obstet Gynecol 80:500, 1960.
41. Shnider SM: Serum cholinesterase activity during pregnancy, labor and puerperium. Anesthesiology 26:335, 1965.

CHAPTER 2

Utero-Placental Circulation and Respiratory Gas Exchange

Julian T. Parer, M.D., Ph.D.

The placenta is a union of maternal and fetal tissues for purposes of physiologic exchange. Because most stillbirths and depressed fetuses are the result of intrauterine asphyxia, the factors responsible for adequacy of placental function, particularly respiratory gas exchange, assume great importance.

PLACENTAL ANATOMY AND CIRCULATION

The human placenta is described as a villous hemochorial type. The villi are projections of fetal tissue surrounded by chorion which are exposed to circulating maternal blood. The chorion is the outermost fetal tissue layer. At term the human placenta weighs about 500 gm and is disc shaped with a diameter of approximately 20 cm and a thickness of 3 cm. The fetal to placental weight ratio is normally approximately six to one at term. Prior to this the placenta is relatively heavier and the ratio is less, e.g. three to one at 30 weeks' gestation.

Circulation of blood through the placenta is illustrated in Figure 2.1. The maternal blood is carried initially in the uterine arteries, and these ultimately divide into spiral arteries in the basal plate. Blood is spurted, probably under arterial pressure, from these arteries into the intervillous space. It traverses upward toward the chorionic plate, passing fetal villi in its passage, and finally drains back to veins in the basal plate. It is likely that throughout this passage past the villi the maternal blood is exchanging substances with fetal blood within the villi.

The fetal circulation within the placenta is quite different. Blood is carried into the placenta by two umbilical arteries which successively divide into smaller vessels within the fetal villi. Ultimately, capillaries traverse the tips of the fetal villi and it is at this point that exchange occurs with maternal blood within the intervillous space. The blood is finally collected into a single umbilical vein in the umbilical cord, and this carries the nutrient-rich and waste-poor blood to the fetus.

Fetal and maternal blood are separated by three microscopic tissue layers in the human placenta. The first layer is the fetal trophoblast which consists of cytotrophoblast and syncytiotrophoblast. The syncytiotrophoblast is the most metabolically

---

Supported by Grant HD09980 from the National Institutes of Health, United States Public Health Service.

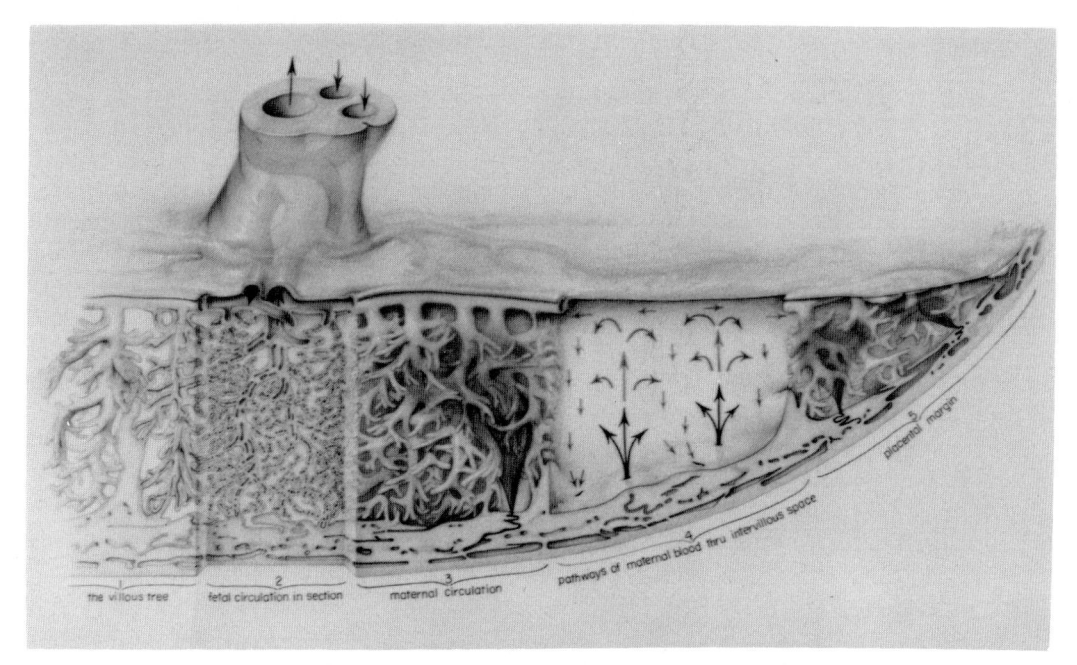

UTERO-PLACENTAL CIRCULATION AND RESPIRATORY GAS EXCHANGE

Figure 2.1. The circulation of blood in the primate placenta. Fetal circulation is shown in the *two panels at left* and the umbilical cord (*above*). The *right panels* show the maternal blood spurting from spiral arteries in the basal area through the intervillous space. The blood passes fetal villi, exchanges substances with fetal blood within the villi and ultimately drains into veins in the basal area. (Drawing by Ranice W. Crosby for Dr. Elizabeth M. Ramsey. Reproduced by courtesy of the Carnegie Institution of Washington.)

active part of the placenta, where much of the endocrine function of the placenta occurs. The other tissue layers are fetal connective tissue, which serves to support the villi, and the endothelium of fetal capillaries (Figure 2.2).

The quantitative relationship of fetal and maternal blood flow and relative concentrations of substances at any one point in the human placenta are quite complex. The relative rates of blood flow in various areas of the placenta are quite variable, and there is a continually changing concentration of nutrients and waste materials in various areas of the placenta as exchange occurs.[1]

MECHANISMS OF EXCHANGE

Substances are exchanged across the placenta membrane by five mechanisms:[2]

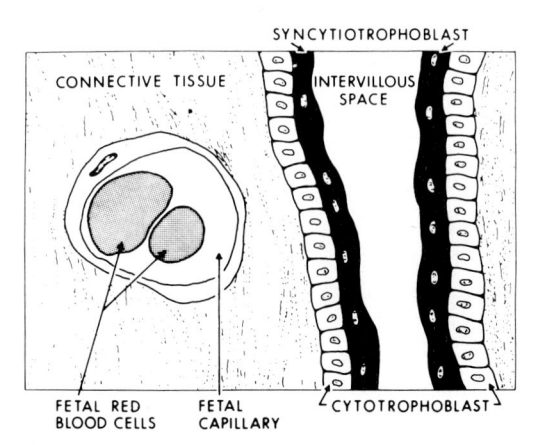

Figure 2.2. Drawing from an electron micrograph of cross-section through parts of two fetal villi, showing tissue layers which separate fetal and maternal blood in the human placenta. The cytotrophoblastic layer is much less distinct in the third trimester than is depicted here. (Reproduced by courtesy of Berkeley Bio-Engineering Inc., California.)

1. Diffusion

This is a physicochemical process in which no energy is required and substances pass from one area to another on the basis of a concentration gradient. The respiratory gases, oxygen and carbon dioxide, the fatty acids and the smaller ions, e.g. Na^+ and Cl^-, are transported by this mechanism.[2]

Facilitated diffusion describes the mechanism of passage of glucose and some other carbohydrates. With this mechanism substances still pass down a concentration gradient, but the rate of passage is greater than can be explained by the gradient alone. Possibly carrier molecules are involved, and there may be need for energy expenditure.

2. Active Transport

This mechanism allows for the passage of substances in a direction against the concentration gradient. Energy is required, there are carrier molecules involved and active transport is subject to inhibition by certain metabolites. The amino acids, water soluble vitamins and some of the larger ions, e.g. Ca^{++} and Fe^{++}, are transported by this mechanism.

3. Bulk Flow

This describes the passage of substances due to a hydrostatic or osmotic gradient. Water is transported by this mechanism and may also carry some solutes with it under the influence of this mechanism.

4. Pinocytosis

Some large molecules such as the immune globulins appear to be transported by being enclosed in small vesicles consisting of cell membranes. These are pinched off on one side of the placenta and traverse to the other side where their contents are released.

5. Breaks

The delicate filmy villi may at times break off within the intervillous space, and the contents may be extruded into the maternal circulation. It is also thought that maternal intravascular contents may be taken up by the fetal circulation at times. The most important result of this is seen when fetal Rh-positive red cells are deposited in the vascular system of an Rh-negative mother, resulting in isoimmunization and subsequent erythroblastosis fetalis.

DIFFUSION

When limitations of placental transfer occur in the human, they usually are first recognized as limitations of those substances which are exchanged by diffusion. For example, an acute decrease in placental function limits passage of oxygen to and carbon dioxide from the fetus, resulting in fetal asphyxia. A more chronic decrease in placental function may result in limitation of substances necessary for growth, for example carbohydrates, thus giving rise to a fetus which is growth-retarded. Hence, the process of diffusion will be examined in some detail.

Fick's diffusion equation describes the physicochemical process:

$$\text{Rate of transfer} = \frac{\text{concentration gradient} \times \text{area} \times \text{permeability}}{\text{membrane thickness}}$$

Each of the factors determining rate of passage of substances by diffusion will be considered in turn.

Concentration Gradient

The concentration gradient of a substance across the placenta is equal to the difference between the mean maternal blood concentration and the mean fetal blood concentration within each of the

UTERO-PLACENTAL CIRCULATION AND RESPIRATORY GAS EXCHANGE

exchanging areas. As noted above, however, it is most unlikely that this gradient is constant throughout the placenta because of its peculiar circulatory anatomy. It probably varies from place to place and also from time to time in any particular area. However, by considering a simplified exchanging membrane with blood flowing in from each side, each of the factors which would affect the concentration gradient can be conceptually discussed (Figure 2.3). These factors are:

1. *Concentration of substance in maternal arterial blood.*
2. *Concentration of substance in fetal arterial blood.*
3. *Maternal intervillous space blood flow.*
4. *Fetal placental blood flow.*
5. *Diffusing capacity of the placenta for the substance.*
6. *Ratio of maternal to fetal blood flow in exchanging areas.* This is analogous to ventilation perfusion ratios as applied to the lung. Inequalities in ratio give rise to decreased efficiency of transfer. Exchange of substances is optimal if the flows are evenly matched.
7. *Binding of substances to molecules and dissociation rates.* Depending on the rate of dissociation, this reaction time could limit the transfer of a substance. This does not appear to be limiting with regard to the dissociation of oxygen and hemoglobin.
8. *Geometry of exchanging surfaces*

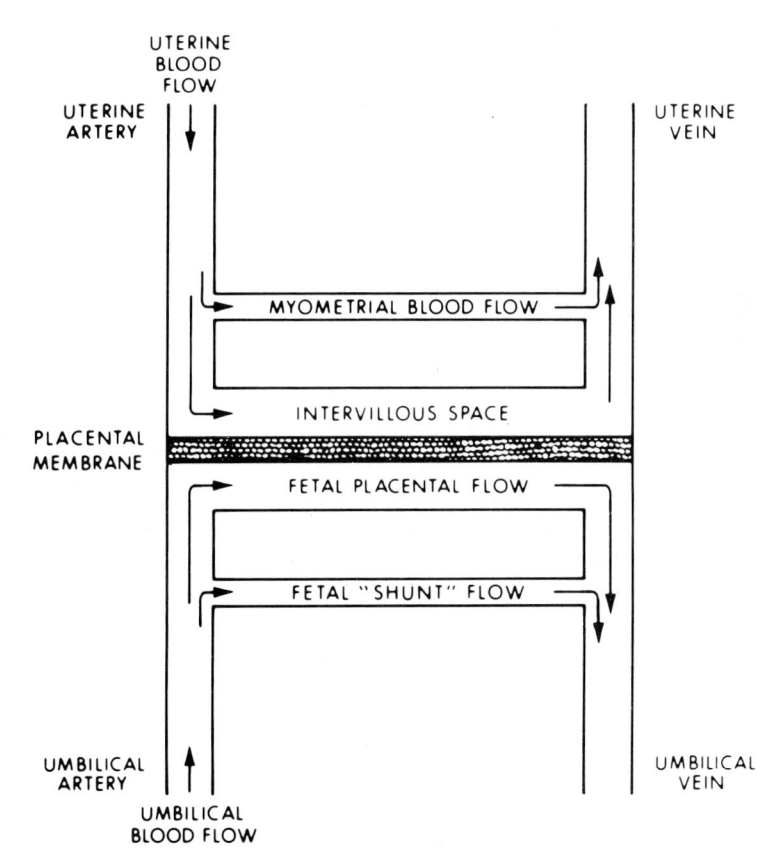

Figure 2.3. Simplified diagram of pattern of circulation through the placenta. (Reproduced by courtesy of Berkeley Bio-Engineering Inc., California.)

with respect to blood flow. If blood flows are traveling in the same direction during exchange the system is called concurrent. If the bloods are traveling in opposite directions the system is called countercurrent. This latter system is the most efficient from the exchange point of view. As can be seen in Figure 2.1, in the human placenta it is unlikely that either of these simplified concepts holds. The human pattern has been described as the multivillous stream system.[1] The evaluation of the mean concentration gradient of any nutrient in this system becomes extremely complex.

9. *The metabolism of the substance.* If a substance is consumed within the placenta its rate of passage across the placenta will not be reflected by the concentration gradient. For example, oxygen is consumed in considerable quantities by the trophoblast and the rate of passage appears to be relatively inefficient when based on oxygen tension gradients alone.

Area of the Placenta

The villous surface area of the human term placenta[3] is approximately 11 m^2. In comparison the lung has an alveolar surface area of 70 m^2. The area of actual exchange, the vasculosyncytial membrane, that is the area where fetal capillaries approach closely enough to the surface to exchange materials with maternal blood, is 1.8 m^2.

Placental area is decreased in a number of clinical situations. An acute decrease occurs with abruptio placentae. With part of the placenta separated, the fetus does not necessarily expire through asphyxia. Its ability to survive depends on the placental reserve which existed before the episode of abruption. Some placentas, particularly those in cases of maternal hypertension or those which have infarcted fibrotic areas, have a reduced area available for exchange and, hence, lowered reserve. Thus, the placenta of a mother with long-term hypertension is likely to be smaller than expected, as is the fetus. The infarctions are thought to be caused by maternal arteriolar deficiencies giving rise to devitalization of certain cotyledonary areas, resulting in fibrosis of the villi. Additionally, in certain cases of intrauterine infection or congenital defects the placentas are decreased in size and area. Large placentas are found in certain diabetics and in erythroblastosis fetalis. In the former case it is not sure whether the increased area improves the transfer of nutrients to the fetus. In the latter case most of the increased placental mass is thought to be hydropic in origin and, hence, is unlikely to improve the exchange characteristics of the placenta.

Permeability of the Placental Membrane

The permeability of a membrane to a substance depends on characteristics both of the membrane and of the substance which is exchanging. The units for permeability can be found by a transposition of Fick's diffusion equation. There are three major determinants of permeability:

1. *Molecular size.* A molecular weight of 1,000 is a rough dividing line between those substances which cross the placenta by diffusion and those which are relatively impermeable by diffusion. Below a molecular weight of 1,000 the rate of passage of the molecule is related to its weight unless other properties (see below) prevent or hasten rate of passage. A common clinical example is found in cases in which it is necessary to anticoagulate a pregnant woman. If one uses heparin with a molecular weight above 6,000 one does not concomitantly heparinize the fetus. However, with the use of warfarin (Coumadin) with a molecular weight of 330 the fetus will also be anticoagulated. This is considered undesirable, particularly in the intrapar-

tum period, when fetal bleeding may occur. Also, warfarin may have some teratogenic effects in the first trimester.

2. *Lipid solubility.* A lipid-soluble substance traverses the placenta more rapidly than one which is not lipid-soluble.

3. *Electrical charge.* This deters the passage of a substance across the placenta. For example, succinylcholine, commonly used during balanced anesthesia, is highly ionized and is poorly diffusable across the placenta despite its molecular weight of 361. Thiopental, with a molecular weight of 264, is lipid-soluble, relatively unionized and moves very rapidly into the fetal circulation.

Substances are classified into those in which the rate of passage is either "permeability-limited" or "flow-limited."[4] A substance which is poorly permeable is limited in its rate of passage across the placenta by permeability and not by rates of blood flow. Hence, increasing the rate of blood flow will not improve its rate of passage much at all. The majority of biologic molecules are limited in their rate of passage across the placenta by resistance to diffusion. However, substances which are highly permeable are limited by the rates of blood flow. Oxygen and carbon dioxide are examples of this. Decreasing the rates of blood flow decreases the rate of exchange considerably.

Diffusion Distance.

The average distance for diffusion across the placenta[3] has been measured as approximately 3.5 μ. This contrasts with the much smaller distance from alveolus to pulmonary capillary in the lung, 0.5 μ. The diffusion distance decreases as the placenta matures, but it is not clear whether this improves its characteristics for exchange. The distance is increased in several conditions such as erythroblastosis fetalis and congenital syphilis. This increased distance is probably due to villous edema and presumably decreases the organ's efficiency for exchange. Fibrous or calcific deposits on the placental vasculature, such as are found in diabetes mellitus or preeclampsia, presumably increase diffusion distance.

UTERINE BLOOD FLOW

Because uterine blood flow is one of the prime determinants of passage of a number of critical substances across the placenta, its characteristics and factors affecting it will be discussed. A detailed discussion of the effects of obstetrical anesthesia on uterine blood flow will be found in the next chapter.

Uterine blood flow in the term human is approximately 700 ml per minute. This represents about 10 per cent of the cardiac output. Approximately 70 to 90 per cent of the uterine blood flow passes through the intervillous space, and the remainder largely supplies the myometrium.

The uterine vascular bed is thought to be almost maximally dilated under normal conditions with little capacity to dilate further.[5] It is not autoregulated, so flow is proportional to the mean perfusion pressure. However, it is capable of marked vasoconstriction by α-adrenergic action. It is not responsive to changes in respiratory gas tensions. The uterine blood flow is determined by the following relationship:

$$\text{Uterine blood flow} = \frac{\text{uterine arterial} - \text{uterine venous pressure}}{\text{uterine vascular resistance}}$$

Hence, any factor affecting either of the three values on the right-hand side of the above relationship will alter uterine blood flow. A number of causes of decreased uterine blood flow are shown in Table 2.1.

Uterine contractions decrease uterine blood flow due to increased uterine venous

Table 2.1
Factors Causing Decreased Uterine Blood Flow

Uterine contractions
Hypertonus
   Abruptio placenta
   Tetanic contraction
   Overstimulation with oxytocin
Hypotension
   Sympathetic block
   Hypovolemic shock
   Supine hypotensive syndrome
Hypertension
   Essential
   Preeclampsia
Vasoconstriction, endogenous
   Sympathetic discharge
   Adrenal medullary activity
Vasoconstrictors, exogenous
   Most sympathomimetics (α-adrenergic effects)
   Exception is ephedrine (primarily β-adrenergic effect)

pressure brought about by increased intramural pressure of the uterus. There may also be a decrease in uterine arterial pressure with contractions. Uterine hypertonus causes a decreased uterine blood flow through the same mechanism.

In sheep it has been shown that if uterine arterial perfusion pressure is altered without changing the resistance of the uterine vascular bed, there is a direct relationship between uterine blood flow and the pressure.[6] Hence, hypotension through any of the mechanisms noted in Table 2.1 will cause a decrease in blood flow.

In the case of maternal arterial hypertension it is likely that there is a concomitant increased vascular resistance which is shared by the uterine vascular bed. This, therefore, results in a decrease in uterine blood flow. Either endogenous or exogenous vasoconstriction results in decreased blood flow because of increased uterine vascular resistance.

There are few useful means of increasing uterine blood flow in cases in which it is known to be less than optimal. The most important clinical considerations are the avoidance of or correction of factors responsible for an acute decrease in blood flow, e.g. excessive uterine activity or maternal hypotension.

Clinically it has been known for many years that maternal bed rest may improve the outcome in suspected fetal growth retardation. There is now some evidence that bed rest does improve fetal growth, as evidenced by increasing estriol excretion.[7]

Some of the betamimetic agents which are used as uterine relaxants for premature labor may increase uterine blood flow, but this effect is still under investigation. There are a number of experimental means of increasing uterine blood flow, sometimes transiently, but these have no place clinically. Examples of such treatments include estrogens, acetylcholine, nitroglycerine, cyanide, ischemia and hypoxia, the latter either mild acute or chronic.[5]

UMBILICAL BLOOD FLOW

The umbilical blood flow is approximately 250 ml per minute at delivery.[8] However, this measurement may be affected by the acute events occurring at the time of delivery. It is 600 ml per minute in the chronically instrumented term sheep fetus, which is about the same size as the human fetus at term.[9] The umbilical blood flow is approximately 40 per cent of the combined ventricular output[10] and about 20 per cent of this blood flow is "shunted," that is, it does not exchange with maternal blood.[1] It is either carried through actual vascular shunts within the fetal side of the placenta or else it does not approach closely enough to maternal blood for exchange with it.

Umbilical blood flow is unaffected by acute moderate hypoxia but is decreased by severe hypoxia.[11] Innervation of the umbilical cord is still questionable, but umbilical blood flow decreases with the administration of catecholamines. It is decreased by acute cord occlusion. There are no known means of increasing umbilical flow in cases where it is thought to be decreased chronically. However, certain fetal heart rate patterns, namely variable decelerations, have been ascribed to transient umbilical cord compression in the fetus during labor. Manipulation of maternal position either to the lateral or Trendelenburg position can sometimes abolish these patterns, the implication being that cord compression has been relieved.

OXYGEN TRANSFER TO THE FETUS

As mentioned previously, it is likely that most stillbirths and cases of fetal depression are the result of inadequate exchange of the respiratory gases. Oxygen has the lowest storage to utilization ratio of all nutrients in the fetus. From animal experimentation it can be calculated that in a term fetus the quantity of oxygen is approximately 42 ml and the normal oxygen consumption is approximately 21 ml per minute.[11] This means that, in theory, the fetus has a 2-minute supply of oxygen. Fetuses do not, however, consume the total quantity of oxygen in their body within 2 minutes, nor do they expire after this time. In fact, irreversible brain damage does not occur until about 10 minutes have elapsed.[12] This is because the fetus has a number of important compensatory mechanisms which enable it to survive on a lesser quantity of oxygen for longer periods. The clinical situations where there is total cessation of oxygen delivery are rare. These include sudden total abruption of the placenta or complete umbilical cord compression, generally after prolapse of the cord.

It is known from animal experimentation that the compensations which occur in the hypoxic fetus are: (1) redistribution of blood flow to vital organs including heart, brain and placenta; (2) decreased total oxygen consumption; for example, with moderate hypoxia the fetal oxygen consumption drops to 50 per cent of the normal level; and (3) dependence of certain vascular beds on anaerobic metabolism. These compensatory mechanisms appear to be initiated with mild hypoxia and have been noted to occur even without severe acidosis or fetal heart rate changes.[11]

It is of value to examine the factors which determine oxygen transfer from mother to fetus (Table 2.2). Because the transfer of oxygen to the fetus is dependent on rates of blood flow and not limitations of diffusion, the respective blood flow on each side of the placenta assumes major importance for maintenance of fetal oxygenation. Animal work suggests that in the normal placenta there is a "safety factor" of approximately 50 per cent in the uterine blood flow. That is, the uterine blood flow will drop to half its normal value before fetal acidosis becomes evident.[13] This only applies to the normal situation with normal placental reserve and is unlikely to be so in pathologic situations, such as the infant of the hypertensive mother. In such situations the placen-

Table 2.2
Factors Affecting Oxygen Transfer from Mother to Fetus

Intervillous blood flow
Fetal placental blood flow
Oxygen tension in maternal arterial blood
Oxygen tension in fetal arterial blood
Oxygen affinity of maternal blood
Oxygen affinity of fetal blood
Hemoglobin concentration or oxygen capacity of maternal blood
Hemoglobin concentration or oxygen capacity of fetal blood
Maternal and fetal blood pH and PCO_2 (Bohr effect)
Placental diffusing capacity
Placental vascular geometry
Ratio of maternal to fetal blood flow in exchanging areas
Shunting around exchange sites
Placental oxygen consumption

tal function may be adequate for oxygenation but not for fetal growth, and a growth-retarded infant may result from such a pregnancy. Furthermore, with superimposition of uterine contractions on such a fetus, there may be transient inadequacy of uterine blood flow during the uterine contractions; this may be recognized by responses of the fetal heart rate, namely late decelerations.

Additional important determinants of fetal oxygenation include oxygen tension in maternal arterial and fetal arterial blood. In general, maternal arterial oxygen tension depends on adequate ventilation and pulmonary integrity. Disruptions of this function are relatively rare in obstetrics although they can occur with pulmonary disease, such as asthma, or congestive heart failure or in mothers with congenital cardiac defects. The oxygen affinity and oxygen capacity of maternal and fetal bloods are also important determinants of fetal oxygen transfer. At a given oxygen tension the quantity of oxygen carried by blood depends on the oxygen capacity, which is dependent on the hemoglobin concentration and the oxygen affinity. The oxygen affinity of fetal blood is greater than that of maternal blood. That is, the oxygen dissociation curve of the fetus is to the left of that of the mother. In addition, the hemoglobin concentration of fetal blood is approximately 15 gm/100 ml in the term fetus, whereas that of the mother is approximately 12 gm/100 ml. Both of these factors, an increased oxygen affinity and higher oxygen capacity, confer advantages to the fetus for oxygen uptake across the placenta. Probable values of the oxygen content and oxygen tension in umbilical vessels and maternal uterine artery and vein are illustrated in Figure 2.4.

Because most measurements have been made in the human fetus during or after labor, the values of oxygen saturation, oxygen tension and pH are generally depressed compared with those of the mother. In fact, investigations on chronically instrumented animals have shown that the oxygen saturation and content of fetal blood and acid-base status is very close to that of maternal blood. Only the PO_2 is lower. The arteriovenous oxygen differences across each side of the placenta are also illustrated in Figure 2.4. Notice that the quantity of oxygen delivered or taken up by each 100 ml of circulating blood in the placenta is approximately equal in the mother and fetus. This further suggests approximate equality of blood flows on each side of the placenta. A number of additional miscellaneous factors determine the rate of oxygen transfer across the placenta; they are listed in Table 2.2 as the last six determinants. They appear to be relatively minor compared with the major factors already outlined.

CARBON DIOXIDE AND ACID-BASE BALANCE

Carbon dioxide crosses the placenta even more readily than does oxygen. In general the determinants for oxygen transfer also apply to carbon dioxide transfer across the placenta. It is limited by rate of blood flow and not by resistance to diffusion. The carbon dioxide tension in fetal blood in the undisturbed state is close to 40 mm Hg.[1] It is well known that the maternal arterial carbon dioxide tension is approximately 34 mm Hg, and the mother is in a state of compensated respiratory alkalosis. The pH of fetal blood under undisturbed conditions is probably close to 7.4, and the bicarbonate concentration is close to that in maternal blood.

Bicarbonate and the fixed acids cross the placenta much more slowly than does carbon dioxide, i.e. equilibration takes a matter of hours rather than seconds. There is a situation analogous to "respiratory acidosis" which occurs in the fetus when blood flow, either uterine or umbilical, is acutely compromised. In such cases, the

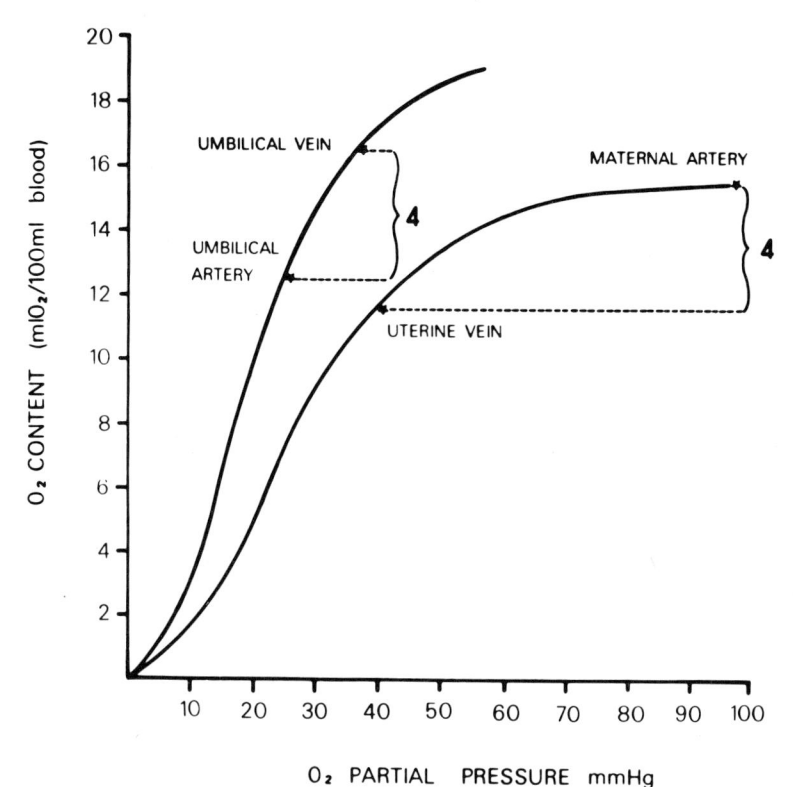

UTERO-PLACENTAL CIRCULATION AND RESPIRATORY GAS EXCHANGE

Figure 2.4. Oxygen contents and tensions, and arteriovenous oxygen concentration differences (*brackets*), on fetal and maternal side of the placenta. These are probable values in the undisturbed human, although use has been made of data from many sources including experimental animals. (Reproduced by courtesy of Berkeley Bio-Engineering Inc., California.)

pH drops and CO_2 tension is elevated, but the metabolic acid-base status remains unchanged. This occurs during severe or profound fetal decelerations called variable decelerations in association with certain uterine contractions, especially during the second stage of labor. These acid-base changes are generally rapidly resolved with cessation of the contraction and the bradycardia. However, as noted earlier, if there is significant oxygen lack which is unrelieved the fetus will decrease its oxygen consumption, redistribute blood flow and depend partly on anaerobic metabolism to supply its energy needs, albeit with decreased efficiency. Under these conditions lactate (an end product of anaerobic metabolism) is produced, resulting in a metabolic acidosis. The acidosis may also be aggravated by a combined respiratory acidosis because of retained carbon dioxide. Unlike carbon dioxide, lactate is lost rather slowly from the fetus.

CLINICAL IMPLICATIONS

Fetal compromise results from a disruption of normal placental exchange mechanisms. With a knowledge of the components involved in exchange of nutrients and waste materials across the placenta, potential problems can be recognized and corrections can be made.

The most important components of placental exchange are the rates of blood flow on each side of the placenta and the area available for exchange. Uterine blood flow will decline in the presence of factors causing decreased perfusion pressure or increased uterine vascular resistance. Common clinical occurrences are hypotension, hypertension, endogenous or exogenous vasoconstriction and, possibly, severe psychological stress. The uterine vascular bed is not autoregulated and has little capacity to dilate further. During labor it is most likely that the rate of uterine blood flow is the limiting factor in cases of fetal compromise because of the intermittent decline in uterine blood flow with each uterine contraction. In addition, transient or persistent umbilical cord compression may cause fetal asphyxia.

References

1. Metcalfe J, Bartels H, Moll W: Gas exchange in the pregnant uterus. Physiol Rev 47:782, 1967.
2. Longo LD: Placental transfer mechanisms—an overview. In *Obstetrics and Gynecology Annual*, RM Wynn, ed. Appleton-Century-Crofts, New York, 1972, pp 103–138.
3. Aherne W, Dunnill MS: Morphometry of the human placenta. Br Med Bull 22:5, 1966.
4. Meschia G: Physiology of transplacental diffusion. In *Obstetrics and Gynecology Annual*, RM Wynn, ed. Appleton-Century-Crofts, New York, 1976, pp 21–38.
5. Assali NS, Brinkman CR III: The uterine circulation and its control. In *Respiratory Gas Exchange and Blood Flow in the Placenta*, LD Longo and H Bartels, eds. US Department of Health, Education and Welfare, Washington DC, 1972, pp 121–141.
6. Greiss F Jr: Concepts of uterine blood flow. In *Obstetrics and Gynecology Annual*, RM Wynn, ed. Appleton-Century-Crofts, New York, 1973, pp 55–83.
7. Beischer NA, Drew JH, Kenny JM, et al.: The effect of rest and intravenous infusion of hypertonic dextrose on subnormal estriol excretion in pregnancy. In *Clinics In Perinatology*, A Milunsky, ed. W. B. Saunders, Philadelphia, 1974, pp 253–272.
8. Stembera ZK, Hodr J, Janda J: Umbilical blood flow in healthy newborn infants during the first minutes after birth. Am J Obstet Gynecol 91:568, 1965.
9. Berman W Jr, Goodlin RC, Heymann MA, et al.: Measurement of umbilical blood flow in fetal lambs in utero. J Appl Physiol 39:1056, 1975.
10. Rudolph AM, Heymann MA: Control of the fetal circulation. In *The Mammalian Fetus*, ESE Hafez, ed. Charles C Thomas, Springfield, Ill., 1975 pp 5–19.
11. Parer JT: Fetal oxygen uptake and umbilical circulation during maternal hypoxia in the chronic sheep. In *Fetal and Newborn Cardiovascular Physiology*. LD Longo, ed. Garland Publishing, New York, 1978.
12. Myers RE: Two patterns of perinatal brain damage and their conditions of occurrence. Am J Obstet Gynecol 112:246, 1972.
13. Parer JT, Behrman RE: The influence of uterine blood flow on the acid-base status of the rhesus monkey. Am J Obstet Gynecol 107:1241, 1970.

CHAPTER 3

Obstetric Anesthesia and Uterine Blood Flow

Ermelando V. Cosmi, M.D., L.D.*
Sol M. Shnider, M.D.

The integrity of the utero-placental circulation is of paramount importance to maternal and fetal homeostasis and neonatal survival. Obstetric anesthesia and analagesia may directly affect uterine blood flow or may alter the response of the utero-placental circulation to noxious stimuli and to various pharmacologic agents.

As has been stated in the previous chapter, uterine blood flow varies directly with the perfusion pressure, i.e. uterine arterial minus uterine venous pressure, and inversely with uterine vascular resistance.

Obstetric anesthesia may affect uterine blood flow by (1) changing the perfusion pressure, that is, altering the uterine arterial or venous pressure; or (2) changing uterine vascular resistance either directly through changes in vascular tone or indirectly by altering uterine contractions or uterine muscle tone.

Direct measurement of uterine blood flow is not usually possible because of the relative inaccessibility of the human utero-placental circulation. Changes in uterine blood flow are usually assessed from fetal and neonatal acid-base and heart rate status. Direct information on the effects of anesthesia on utero-placental circulation has been derived mainly from animal experiments, recognizing that because of species differences extrapolation of these data to the human pregnancy must be done with caution.

The development of chronic maternal-fetal animal preparations has allowed precise measurement of changes in uterine and placental blood flow and of the effect of these changes on fetal cardiovascular and acid-base status (Figure 3.1). Uterine blood flow can be measured directly by placing an electromagnetic flow probe on a branch of the uterine artery[1] or indirectly using a steady state diffusion technique (Fick principle) with either antipyrine,[2] tritiated water[3] or nitrous oxide.[4] Distribution of blood flow within the uterus to the placenta, myometrium and endometrium can be measured by the injection of radioactive microspheres into the maternal left ventricle.[5] Details of these techniques may be found in review articles by Schenk and Race[6] and Lewis.[7] This chapter will review the effects of commonly used anesthetic agents, techniques and adjuvants and of anesthetic complications on uterine blood flow.

INTRAVENOUS INDUCTION AGENTS

Barbiturates

Cosmi and co-workers[8-11] reported that clinical doses of thiopental or thiamylal

---
* Supported in part by Consiglio Nazionale delle Richerche (Italia), Grant Number 77.01560.65 and by the National Science Foundation (United States).

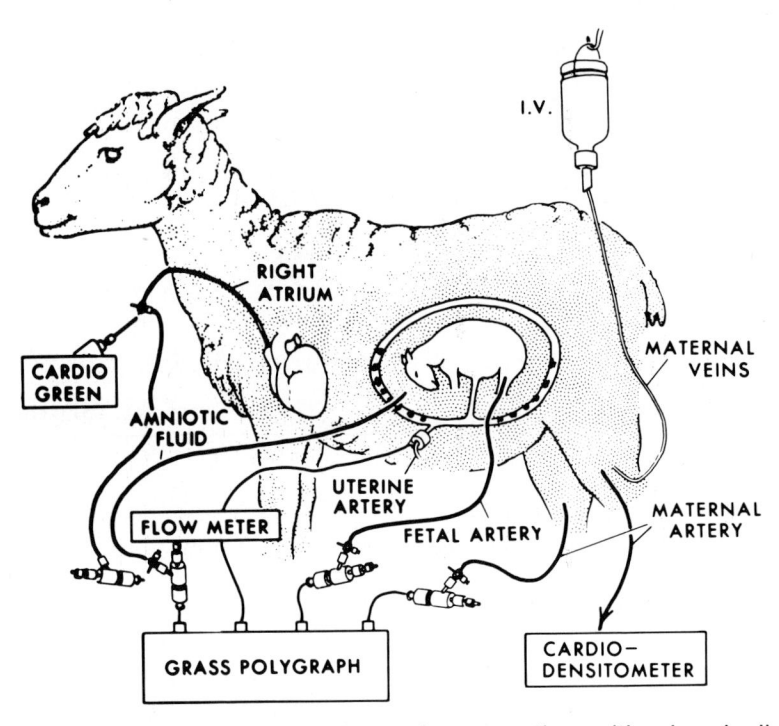

Figure 3.1. Diagram of sheep experimental preparation with chronically implanted maternal and fetal intravascular catheters and an electromagnetic flow probe around a branch of uterine artery. (Reprinted by permission from Ralston DH, Shnider SM, deLorimier AA: Effects of equipotent ephedrine, metaraminol, mephentermine and methoxamine on uterine blood flow in the pregnant ewe. Anesthesiology 40:354, 1974.)

injected intravenously to the ewe reduced maternal systolic and diastolic pressure and uterine blood flow; however, uterine contractions were not affected. These changes usually appeared 20 to 30 seconds after injection and lasted from 3 to 8 minutes. They were accompanied by an increase of fetal heart rate, blood pressure and umbilical blood flow. These changes usually were without consequences to the healthy fetus. On the other hand, they enhanced fetal hypoxia and acidosis when the fetal condition was already compromised.

Methohexital produced similar effects on maternal blood pressure and uterine blood flow. These effects were, however, of smaller magnitude and shorter duration and were not associated with significant changes in maternal and fetal PaO_2 and acid-base status (Figure 3.2). Thus, it seems that the fall in arterial pressure was the cause of the fall in uterine blood flow. These findings suggest that, although the effects of clinical doses of ultra short-acting barbiturates on the mother and the fetus are minimal and transient, an already compromised fetus may not be able to tolerate them. Ultra short-acting barbiturates are most commonly used for induction of anesthesia and are usually followed by endotracheal intubation and nitrous oxide maintenance. Palahniuk and Cumming[12] studied this sequence and reported that uterine blood flow fell 20 per cent after induction of anesthesia without a significant fall in maternal arterial blood pressure. Fetal oxygen saturation and pH also fell. They postulated that the increase in uterine vascular resistance was due to maternal catecholamine release during light anesthesia.

Diazepam

In pregnant sheep diazepam in doses as high as 0.5 mg/kg did not alter maternal and fetal cardiovascular function and utero-placental blood flow.[13] However, larger doses produced an 8 to 12 per cent decrease in arterial pressure with an equivalent decrease in uterine blood flow. Fetal oxygenation was not affected. Cosmi[11, 14] also observed that the bolus injection of diazepam to the ewe in doses of 0.18 mg/kg has no deleterious effects on maternal and fetal blood pressure or acid-base status.

Ketamine

Ketamine usually increases arterial blood pressure. Studies by Greiss and Van Wilkes[15] and Ralston et al.[16] have shown that drugs which cause increases in maternal arterial blood pressure as a result of vasoconstriction may lead to a decrease in uterine blood flow with consequent fetal hypoxia and acidosis. Levinson and co-workers[17] administered 5 mg/kg of ketamine to a group of pregnant ewes near term. They found a 15 per cent increase in mean maternal blood pressure and a 10 per cent increase in uterine blood flow. Eng and co-workers[18] reported similar results in monkeys. Cosmi evaluated the effects of ketamine in pregnant sheep not in

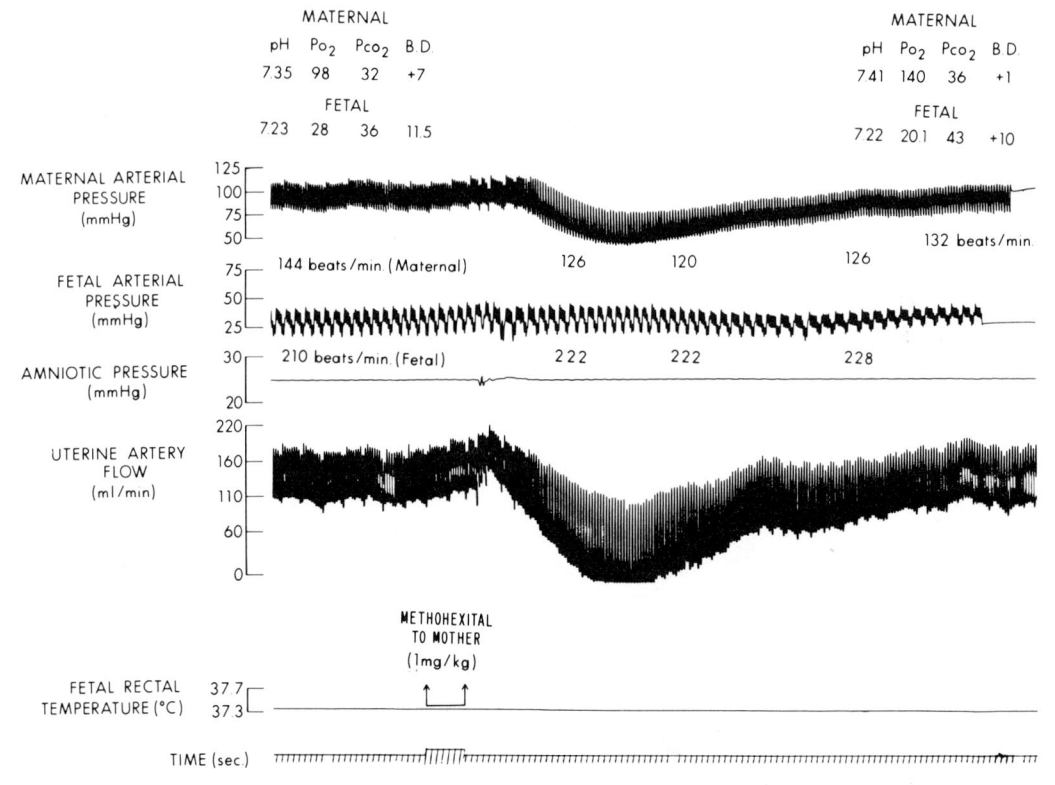

Figure 3.2. Methohexital, 1 mg/kg, administered intravenously to the ewe. Fetus is moderately acidotic. Note transient reduction in maternal blood pressure and uterine blood flow. (Reprinted by permission from Cosmi EV: Drugs, anesthetics and the fetus. In *Reviews in Perinatal Medicine*, EM Scarpelli and EV Cosmi, eds, vol 1. University Park Press, Baltimore, 1976, p 191.)

labor and during labor. In the ewes not in labor (condition resembling that of elective cesarean section), the drug was administered intravenously in doses of 1.8 to 2.2 mg/kg. Anesthesia was maintained with nitrous oxide and oxygen, and the ventilation was controlled. Under these conditions ketamine produced increases in mean maternal blood pressure and heart rate and in uterine blood flow without significant changes in fetal cardiovascular and acid-base status.[11, 19]

However, when ketamine in doses of 0.9 to 5 mg/kg was given to the ewes in labor, they observed a marked increase of maternal ventilation as well as increases in uterine tone and in frequency and intensity of uterine contractions and a slight decrease of uterine blood flow. These changes were dose-related and accompanied by fetal tachycardia and acidosis. Galloon[20] has also reported a dose-related increase in uterine muscle tone after ketamine administration in the human parturient.

Therefore, there is a variability in the maternal circulatory response to ketamine related in part to the presence or absence of labor. Despite this, it would appear that in low doses ketamine does not adversely affect uterine blood flow. Several studies report normal neonatal clinical and acid-base conditions after the administration of ketamine in doses up to 1 mg/kg for vaginal and abdominal delivery.[19, 21-24]

INHALATION AGENTS

The effect of inhalation analgesia-anesthesia on the utero-placental circulation and on the fetus is still a controversial matter. Some authors[25, 26] report fetal asphyxia, whereas others[27, 28] indicate that well conducted inhalation anesthesia produces no effects on the fetus and the uteroplacental circulation.

Halothane

Halothane has a unique and specific place in obstetric anesthesia because of its potent uterine relaxant properties. Hence, it is the agent of choice when uterine relaxation is required, e.g. for version and extraction, breech delivery, retained placenta, tetanic contractions and surgical manipulations.[29-31] Recent attempts to improve fetal oxygenation by increasing maternal inspired oxygen concentration[32] have stimulated interest in the use of halothane with lower concentrations of nitrous oxide for cesarean section.[33] In addition, its use has also been recommended to improve fetal oxygenation in case of fetal distress caused by uterine tetany.[34]

Several investigators have studied the effect of halothane on uterine blood flow. Palahniuk and Shnider[35] found that in the pregnant ewe during light and moderately deep anesthesia (1.0 and 1.5 MAC) maternal blood pressure was slightly depressed (less than 20 per cent from control), but uterine vasodilation occurred and uteroplacental blood flow was maintained. Fetal hypoxemia or metabolic acidosis did not occur (Figure 10.1). Deep levels of anesthesia (2.0 MAC) produced greater reductions in maternal blood pressure and cardiac output. Despite uterine vasodilation, uterine blood flow decreased and the fetuses became hypoxic and acidotic. Similar results have been reported by Cosmi[11] and Carenza and Cosmi[36] in pregnant sheep and by Eng et al.[37] in pregnant monkeys. Furthermore, Cosmi has reported that in humans light to moderate planes of halothane anesthesia, i.e. 0.5 to 1 vol per cent, did not alter either maternal cardiovascular function or fetal acid-base status. In contrast, deep planes, i.e. 1.5 vol per cent or greater, produced maternal hypotension and fetal acidosis.[25]

Thus, it seems that low concentrations of halothane do not adversely affect uteroplacental circulation and, in fact, produce uterine vasodilation. Increasing concentrations produce progressive decreases in the uterine blood flow due to maternal hypotension.

Isoflurane

Studies by Palahniuk and Shnider[35] indicate that isoflurane is essentially indistinguishable from halothane in its effects on maternal and fetal cardiovascular and acid-base status. Light planes of anesthesia do not decrease uterine blood flow, but deep planes do.

Methoxyflurane

Smith and co-workers[38] reported that, in contrast to halothane, light anesthesia (1.0 and 1.5 MAC) with methoxyflurane did not produce uterine vasodilation. Slight to moderate falls in maternal arterial pressure produced comparable falls in uterine blood flow. No serious fetal deterioration was seen. Deep levels of methoxyflurane anesthesia (2.0 MAC) produced marked falls in maternal blood pressure, cardiac output and uterine blood flow. Fetal hypoxemia and acidosis developed.

Enflurane

Cosmi[11] and Carenza and Cosmi[36] have studied the effect of enflurane in pregnant sheep and found that light to moderate planes of anesthesia, i.e. 0.4 to 0.8 vol per cent, did not alter maternal and fetal cardiovascular performance, utero-placental blood flow, and fetal acid-base status. However, deep anesthesia, i.e. concentrations of 1 vol per cent or greater, produced maternal and fetal bradycardia, a decrease of uterine artery blood flow and fetal acidosis, especially when the fetal condition had already deteriorated (Figure 3.3). These changes were dose-related.

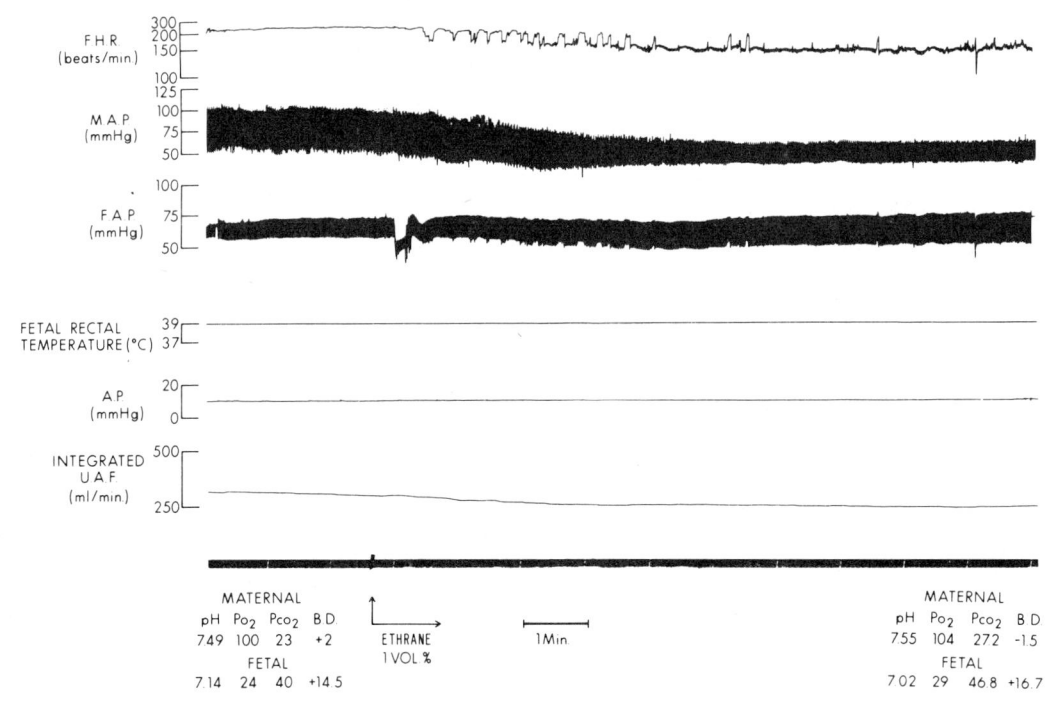

Figure 3.3. Ethrane, 1 vol%, administered to the ewe with an acidotic fetus. *F.H.R.*, fetal heart rate; *M.A.P.*, maternal arterial pressure; *F.A.P.*, fetal arterial pressure; *A.P.*, intra-amniotic pressure; *U.A.F.* uterine artery blood flow. (Reprinted by permission from Cosmi EV: Drugs, anesthetics and the fetus. In *Reviews in Perinatal Medicine*, EM Scarpelli and EV Cosmi, eds, vol 1. University Park Press, Baltimore, 1976, p 191.)

Fluroxene

Eng et al.[39] studied the effect of fluroxene in the pregnant primate and found that inhalation of 4 vol per cent of fluroxene combined with nitrous oxide and oxygen did not affect utero-placental circulation or fetal and maternal cardiovascular and acid-base status. In contrast, at 8 vol per cent, fluroxene produced a decrease of maternal blood pressure and uterine artery blood flow, fetal hypoxia and acidosis.

LOCAL ANESTHETICS

Gibbs and Noel[40] and Cibils[41] demonstrated a vasoconstricting effect of both lidocaine and mepivacaine using an *in vitro* preparation of human uterine artery segments obtained from cesarean hysterectomy specimens. The concentrations of local anesthetics ranged from 400 to 1,000 µg/ml, concentrations well above levels achieved during clinical use. Uterine vasoconstriction was not seen with lower concentrations nor in uterine arteries taken from non-pregnant hysterectomy specimens indicating that the response was dose-related and occurs only during pregnancy. Pre-treatment of the strips with phenoxybenzamine (an α-adrenergic blocker) did not abolish the vasoconstrictive response.

Greiss et al.,[42] injecting 20-, 40- and 80-mg boluses of either lidocaine or mepivacaine into the dorsal aorta of eight anesthetized pregnant ewes, found a dose-related transient (2 to 3 minutes) decrease in uterine blood flow and a simultaneous increase in intrauterine pressure (Figure 3.4). Uterine arterial blood levels were not measured. These investigators also infused lidocaine, mepivacaine, bupivacaine and procaine directly into the uterine artery of non-pregnant ewes (Figure 3.5). The following uterine arterial concentrations re-

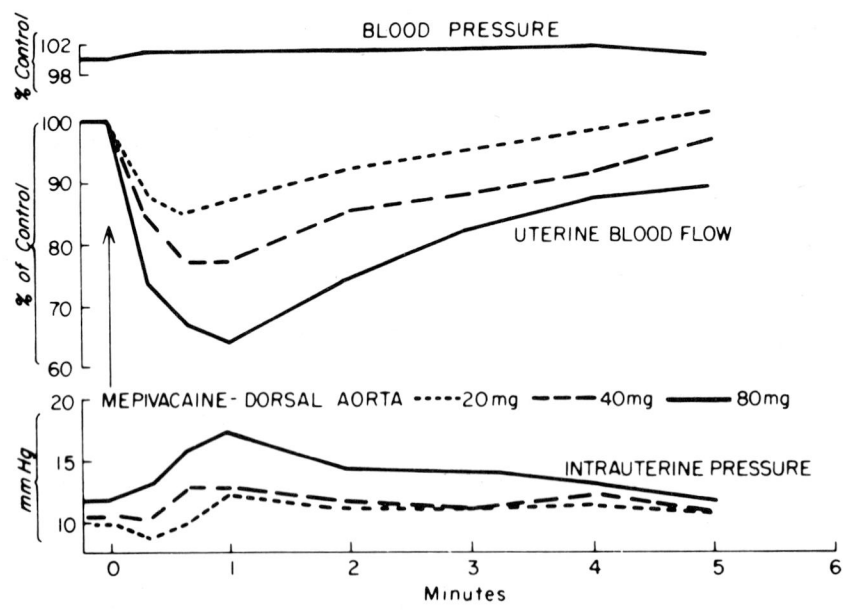

Figure 3.4. Effects of increasing intra-aortic doses of mepivacaine on uterine blood flow and intrauterine pressure in pregnant ewes near term. Note the progressive decrease in uterine blood flow with similar inverse changes in intrauterine pressure. (Reprinted by permission from Greiss FC Jr, Still JG, Anderson SG: Effects of local anesthetic agents on the uterine vasculatures and myometrium. Am J Obstet Gynecol 124:889, 1976.)

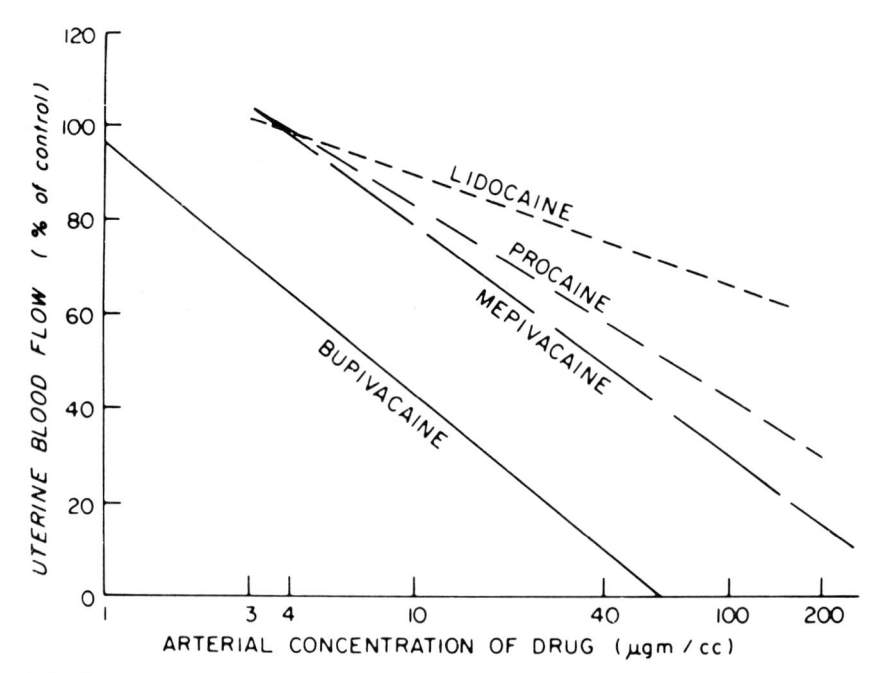

Figure 3.5. Dose response curves with four local anesthetics in non-pregnant ewes illustrating comparative responses. (Reprinted by permission from Greiss FC Jr, Still JG, Anderson SG: Effects of local anesthetic agents on the uterine vasculatures and myometrium. Am J Obstet Gynecol 124:889, 1976.)

duced mean uterine blood flow by 40 per cent: bupivacaine 5 μg/ml, mepivacaine 40 μg/ml, procaine 40 μg/ml and lidocaine 200 μg/ml. Such enormously high concentrations could not occur during epidural anesthesia in the absence of an intravenous injection.

Subsequent studies in the pregnant ewe by Fishburne et al.[43] and Pue et al.[44] produced similar findings of uterine vasoconstriction occurring only at very high blood levels which might be found in the uterine vasculature during paracervical blocks (close proximity of the injected drugs to the uterine arteries) or during systemic toxic reactions. Morishima et al.[45] found that during lidocaine-induced maternal convulsions in the pregnant ewe, uterine blood flow was reduced 55 to 71 per cent of control values.

The lack of uterine vasoconstriction with low blood levels of lidocaine was demonstrated by Biehl et al.[46] These investigators infused the local anesthetic intravenously to produce blood levels (2 to 4 μg/ml) in the pregnant ewe comparable to those usually found in the human parturient undergoing epidural anesthesia during the first and second stages of labor. They found that a 2-hour exposure to these low concentrations of lidocaine did not significantly decrease uterine blood flow or increase intra-amniotic pressure.

REGIONAL ANESTHESIA

The most frequent complication of spinal, lumbar epidural and caudal anesthesia is systemic hypotension. The decrease in mean arterial blood pressure reduces uterine blood flow proportionately.[47, 48] On the other hand, epidural anesthesia uncomplicated by arterial hypotension is associated with no alterations in uterine blood flow.[49]

Brotanek et al.[50] found that epidural anesthesia with mepivacaine did not change uterine blood flow in pregnant women in labor provided the blood pressure did not fall. These studies, performed with a heated thermistor probe, allowed only a qualitative estimate of the changes in flow. No fetal cardiovascular or acid-base data were obtained.

Wallis et al.[49] measured uterine blood flow and percentage of uterine blood flow distributed to the placenta during lumbar epidural anesthesia in the pregnant ewe. Chloroprocaine with and without epinephrine was used. Blood pressure was maintained by intravenous fluid infusion. Except for a transient 14 per cent decrease in uterine blood flow in the ewes receiving chloroprocaine with epinephrine, uterine blood flow remained near control values and was sufficient at all times to maintain stable fetal acid-base and blood gas values (Figure 3.6). Percentage of uterine blood flow distributed to the placenta in the absence of uterine contractions was not altered by epidural anesthesia or by addition of epinephrine to the anesthetic solution.

Jouppila et al.[51] recently measured placental blood flow in human parturients during the first stage of labor using a Xe-

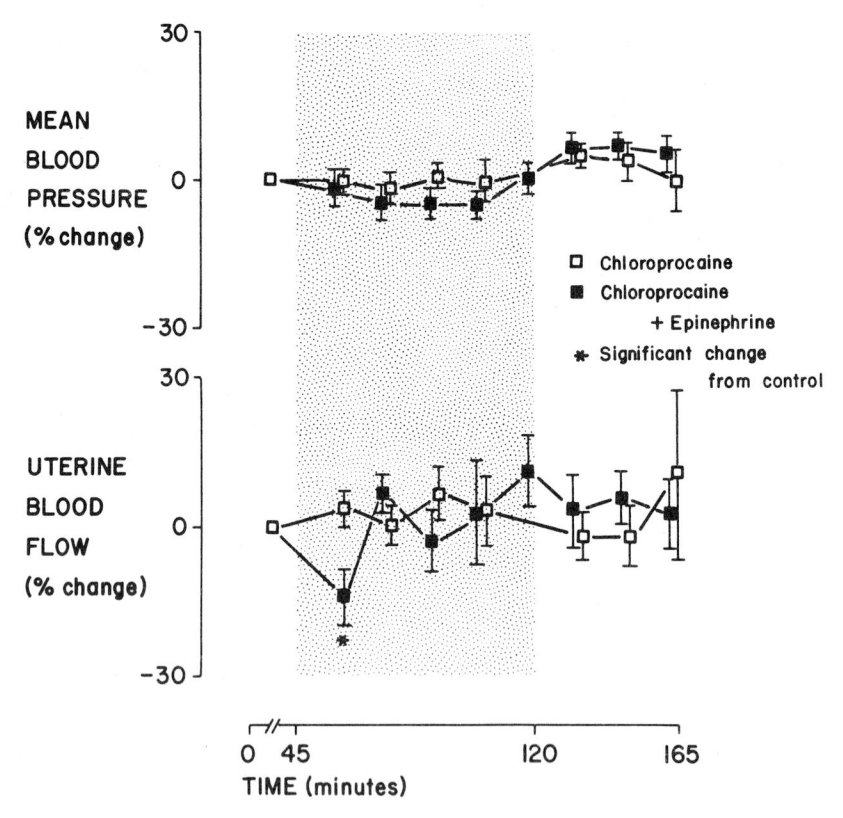

Figure 3.6. Effects of epidural anesthesia (denoted by *shaded area*) on mean maternal blood pressure and uterine blood flow. All values subsequent to each control value are given as mean percentage changes with standard errors. (Reprinted by permission from Wallis KL, Shnider SM, Hicks JS, et al.: Epidural anesthesia in the normotensive pregnant ewe: Effects on uterine blood flow and fetal acid-base status. Anesthesiology 44:481, 1976.)

non-133 clearance technique. This relatively new technique consists of injecting 2 mCi of radioactive Xenon-133 in physiologic saline into the maternal antecubital vein. Because Xenon is freely diffusable it is cleared completely from the circulation during passage through the lungs. However, when the patient holds her breath for 20 seconds after the injection, the radioisotope enters the systemic circulation and reaches the uterus. The clearance of the isotope is measured with a scintillation detector over the placenta, and the rate of clearance reflects blood flow and can be calculated with the appropriate equations. Epidural anesthesia produced with 10 ml of 0.5 per cent bupivacaine with or without epinephrine did not change placental blood flow significantly.

CATECHOLAMINES AND STRESS

Adrenergic stimulation produced by either exogenous or endogenous catecholamines can constrict uterine vessels and reduce uterine blood flow. Exogenous catecholamines (primarily epinephrine) are administered with local anesthetics to produce vasoconstriction at the site of injection. Endogenous catecholamines (primarily norepinephrine) are released during anxiety and pain. Vasopressors are frequently used to prevent or treat spinal or epidural hypotension.

Epinephrine

Epinephrine has significant effects on both α- and β-adrenergic receptors. High epinephrine blood levels achieved by inadvertent intravascular injection of epinephrine-containing local anesthetics produce α-adrenergic effects including hypertension, increased total peripheral resistance, uterine vasoconstriction, increased uterine activity and decreased uterine blood flow. In ewes given 0.10 to 1.00 μg/kg/min of epinephrine, maternal pressure rose 65 per cent above control and uterine blood flow fell 55 to 75 per cent.[52]

Low blood levels of epinephrine, such as occur from systemic absorption during caudal or epidural block, have been shown to produce a generalized β-adrenergic response that becomes maximal 15 minutes after epidural injection.[53] Although total peripheral resistance decreases, uterine vascular resistance increases. Rosenfeld and colleagues[54] infused 50 to 100 μg of epinephrine intravenously over a 5-minute period into pregnant ewes. Although the systemic blood pressure did not change, they found reductions of blood flow to the uterus, pancreas and skin overlying the mammary gland, with increased flows to skeletal muscle, spleen and fat. They postulated that reproductive tissues in the pregnant ewe may be more sensitive to α-adrenergic stimulation than are other tissues.

The addition of epinephrine to local anesthetics when administered for epidural anesthesia has also been reported to increase the incidence of hypotension.[55] However, Levinson et al.[56] found that with prophylactic ephedrine, fluid administration and left uterine displacement, there was no difference in the incidence of hypotension during epidural anesthesia whether epinephrine was included or not. Furthermore, the addition of epinephrine did not adversely affect neonatal acid-base status or Apgar score, implying that transient fluctuations in uterine blood flow were inconsequential in healthy fetuses.

Stress

Myers[57] reported that maternal stress and anxiety in the pregnant rhesus monkey produced fetal asphyxia, likely due to uterine vasoconstriction as a consequence of maternal catecholamine release. Shnider et al.[58] found that stress sufficient to produce maternal hypertension resulted in a precipitous fall in uterine blood flow and increase in plasma norepinephrine in pregnant ewes. Similarly, Martin and Gingerick[59] found a marked reduction in uterine blood flow in response to severe stress in the pregnant rhesus monkey.

Vasopressors

Vasopressors with predominant α-adrenergic activity reduce uterine blood flow and may adversely affect the fetus.[60, 61] Methoxamine, phenylephrine, angiotensin or norepinephrine treatment of spinal hypotension in animals diminishes uterine blood flow and leads to fetal asphyxia.[61-63] Ephedrine, mephentermine and metaraminol restore uterine blood flow toward normal[64-66] (Figure 3.7).

Prophylactic vasopressor administration has also been studied. Eng et al.[61] reported that methoxamine infusion in pregnant primates decreased uterine blood flow and produced fetal asphyxia. Infusion of ephedrine, a predominantly β-adrenergic stimulating drug had no discernible effect on uterine blood flow or fetal acid-base status during the infusion. In normotensive pregnant ewes, Ralston et al.[16] found that infusion of methoxamine or metaraminol decreased uterine blood flow at all dose levels. On the other hand, doses of ephedrine which raised blood pressure to even 50 per cent above control had no detrimental effect on uterine blood flow or fetal acid-base status (Figure 3.8). Therefore, it seems that drugs such as

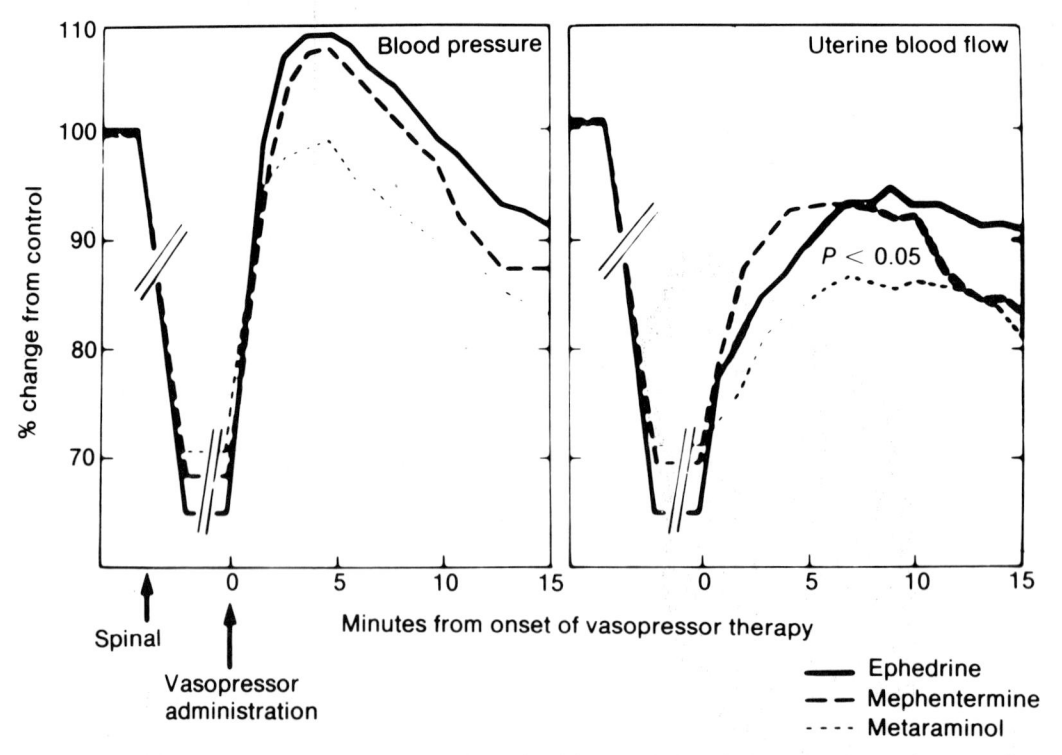

Figure 3.7. Average response patterns to ephedrine and slow infusions of mephentermine and metaraminol after hypotension induced by spinal anesthesia. After 4 minutes uterine blood flow was significantly higher with ephedrine and mephentermine than with metaraminol therapy. (Reprinted by permission from James FM III, Greiss FC Jr, Kemp RA: An evaluation of vasopressor therapy for maternal hypotension during spinal anesthesia. Anesthesiology 33:25, 1970.)

OBSTETRIC ANESTHESIA AND UTERINE BLOOD FLOW

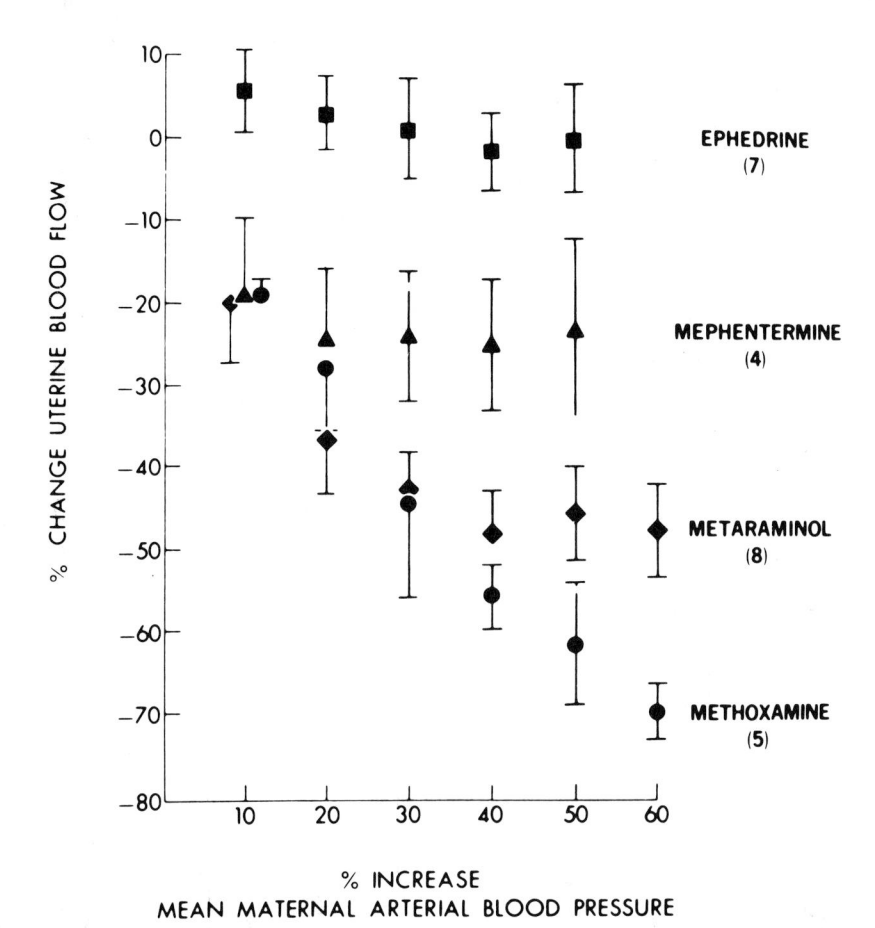

Figure 3.8. Mean changes in uterine blood flow at equal elevations of mean arterial blood pressure after vasopressor administration. (Reprinted by permission from Ralston DH, Shnider SM, deLorimier AA: Effects of equipotent ephedrine, metaraminol, mephentermine and methoxamine on uterine blood flow in the pregnant ewe. Anesthesiology 40: 354, 1974.)

ephedrine or mephentermine, which support maternal blood pressure primarily by central adrenergic stimulation (positive inotropic and chronotropic activity) have minimal effects on uterine blood flow in the normotensive mother and restore uterine blood flow when used to treat spinal or epidural hypotension.

Dopamine, a catecholamine which stimulates dopaminergic and α- and β-adrenergic receptors has been studied in normotensive and hypotensive pregnant sheep. In normotensive animals doses which increase maternal blood pressure and cardiac output decrease uterine blood flow.[67] When used to treat spinal hypotension, dopamine corrected maternal blood pressure but resulted in a further fall in uterine blood flow.[68] This was due to a significant increase in uterine vascular resistance despite minimal changes in total peripheral resistance. A similar vasoconstrictive effect on uterine blood vessels has been reported with β-adrenergic drugs such as isoxsuprine,[69] ritodrine[70] and, as previously described, low-dose epinephrine.[54] The effects of dopamine on the uterine vessels likely represent an increased

ANTIHYPERTENSIVE AGENTS

Hypertensive disorders of pregnancy frequently require therapy. Ideally, drugs used to treat maternal hypertension should reduce blood pressure and uterine vascular resistance so that uterine blood flow is either unchanged or increased.

Hydralazine, a slow-acting antihypertensive drug, is used widely in the treatment of gestational hypertension. The effects of hydralazine on uterine blood flow in the hypertensive pregnant ewe have been studied by Brinkman and Assali.[71] These investigators induced severe hypertension and reduction in uterine blood flow by placing a modified Goldblatt clamp around one renal artery and removing the contralateral kidney. Hydralazine, in this preparation, reduced blood pressure while increasing uterine blood flow. Similarly, in a study by Ring et al.[72] during phenylephrine-induced hypertension, hydralazine slowly lowered the blood pressure while significantly increasing uterine blood flow.

Nitroprusside, a rapidly acting antihypertensive has recently become popular in the management of non-obstetric hypertensive emergencies. Similar to hydralazine, the drug causes a decrease in total peripheral resistance and an increase in coronary and mesenteric blood flow.[73–75] Ring et al.[72] reported that, although nitroprusside decreased total peripheral resistance, it failed to correct the fall in uterine blood flow (Figure 3.9). Thus, although both nitroprusside and hydralazine produced selective vasodilation in various vascular beds, apparently only hydralazine dilates the uterine vasculature in the presence of an alpha agonist.

An additional disadvantage to nitroprusside is its rapid placental transfer. Naulty

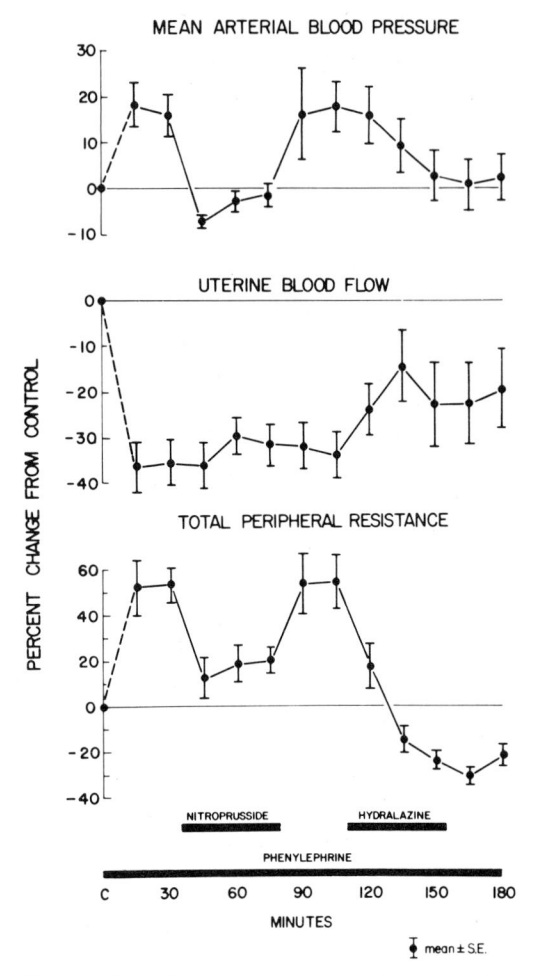

Figure 3.9. Per cent change from control of maternal mean arterial blood pressure, uterine blood flow and total peripheral resistance during phenylephrine-induced hypertension and correction of hypertension with nitroprusside and hydralazine. Hydralazine, but not nitroprusside, resulted in a significant increase in uterine blood flow (p < .05). (Reprinted by permission from Ring G, Krames E, Shnider SM, et al.: Comparison of nitroprusside and hydralazine in hypertensive pregnant ewes. Obstet Gynecol 50:598, 1977.)

et al.[76] have recently reported that, in pregnant ewes receiving an infusion of nitroprusside for 1 hour, maternal arterial and umbilical venous levels of nitroprusside were identical. Furthermore, in some animals fetal cyanide toxicity and death occurred. Presuming the applicability of these experimental data in sheep to the hypertensive human parturient, it would appear that nitroprusside will find little place in the treatment of gestational hypertension.

Magnesium Sulfate

Since its first use in obstetrics reported in 1925 by Lazard[77] and Dorsett,[78] magnesium sulfate has been used parenterally as an adjunct in the management of certain hypertensive diseases of pregnancy, especially preeclampsia and eclampsia.

Although the effects on the central and peripheral nervous system and on neuromuscular transmission have been well documented, its action on the maternal and fetal cardiovascular systems and utero-placental circulation has only recently been investigated in pregnant normotensive and hypertensive ewes.[79, 80] Magnesium sulfate was administered to the mother in amounts sufficient to produce a constant serum concentration of between 5 and 12 mEq/L in a study by Dandavino et al.[79] and between 5 and 7 mEq/L in study by Krames et al.[80] Dandavino and co-workers found that magnesium sulfate produced a fall in the systemic arterial blood pressure both in hypertensive and normotensive animals. However, this effect was transient, lasting less than 10 minutes. The utero-placental blood flow increased by about 10 per cent. Administration of high doses of magnesium sulfate (a 4-gm bolus injection followed by a 2- to 4-gm per hour infusion) produced an initial and transitory decrease of maternal arterial pressure which was greater in the hypertensive than in the normotensive animals. However, 5 to 10 minutes after the start of the infusion, the mean arterial pressure in both groups had returned to control values. The utero-placental blood flow increased an average of 13.5 per cent in the normotensive and 7.7 per cent in the hypertensive animals. Krames et al. found that magnesium sulfate produced a decrease in mean arterial blood pressure of 7 per cent with a 7 per cent rise in uterine vascular conductance, thereby resulting in no change in uterine blood flow.

The results of these two studies suggest that magnesium sulfate has only a mild and transient effect on maternal arterial pressure and uterine blood flow.

RESPIRATORY GASES

Contrary to earlier beliefs, **moderate** hypoxia, hypercapnia and hypocapnia do not affect utero-placental blood flow.[81, 82] On the other hand, marked changes in respiratory gases decrease placental perfusion. Dilts et al.[83] measured uterine blood flow in pregnant sheep during severe maternal hypoxia induced by ventilating the lungs with 6 per cent or 12 per cent oxygen gas mixtures. When the lungs were ventilated with a gas mixture containing 6 per cent oxygen, there was an increase in cardiac output and a decrease in maternal systemic vascular resistance. Utero-placental vascular resistance increased, and uterine blood flow decreased markedly (Figure 3.10). Milder hypoxia induced with 12 per cent oxygen produced changes which were qualitatively smaller. They attributed these hemodynamic changes to the enhanced output of catecholamines induced by hypoxia. When the mother was made hypoxic by reducing arterial PO_2 to 40 torr, the fetus also became hypoxic.

Effects of maternal **hypercapnia** on the utero-placental circulation are variable. Increase,[84] decrease[85] and no changes[2, 86] have been reported. Walker et al.,[87] using chronic unanesthetized sheep preparations, found that by increasing the arterial PCO_2 to 60 torr, uterine blood flow in-

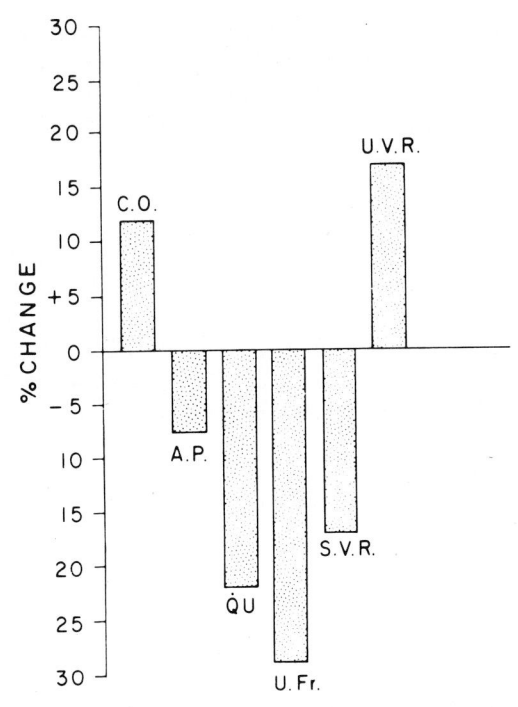

Figure 3.10. Per cent change in systemic and utero-placental hemodynamics during experimental hypoxia induced by ventilating the ewe with a gas mixture containing 6 per cent oxygen. Note the increase in cardiac output (*C.O.*) and in the uterine vascular resistance (*U.V.R.*) and the marked fall in uterine blood flow (*QU*), uterine fraction of cardiac output (*U. Fr.*), systemic vascular resistance (*S.V.R.*) and arterial pressure (*A.P.*). (Reprinted by permission from Dilts PV Jr, Brinkman CR III, Kirschbaum TH, et al.: Uterine and systemic hemodynamic interrelationships and their response to hypoxia. Am J Obstet Gynecol 103:138, 1969.)

creased. Mean arterial pressure rose while uterine vascular resistance was unchanged. However, at $PaCO_2$ levels above 60 torr, uterine vascular resistance increased progressively and uterine blood flow fell, despite further increases in mean arterial pressure (Figure 3.11).

Maternal **hypocapnia** is a frequent phenomenon in pregnant women. It may occur spontaneously as a result of painful uterine contractions, anxiety and apprehension during labor or improperly performed Lamaze technique. Controlled ventilation during anesthesia may also inadvertently produce severe maternal alkalemia. Controversy still exists regarding its effects on the fetus and the utero-placental circulation. Some investigators have reported that marked hyperventilation ($PaCO_2$ of 17 mm Hg or less) causes utero-placental vasoconstriction, decreases utero-placental blood flow and induces fetal hypoxia, acidosis and neonatal depression.[88, 89] Others have denied that maternal hyperventilation, even of marked degree, is harmful to the fetus. They found minimal changes in the acid-base status of the fetus and no significant effect on utero-placental blood flow.[90, 91] Levinson et al.[85] studied changes in uterine blood flow and fetal oxygenation in unanesthetized pregnant ewes during mechanical hyperventilation. In order to evaluate separately the effects of maternal hypocapnia and positive pressure ventilation, CO_2 was added to the inspired air during mechanical hyperventilation to produce normocapnia and hypercapnia. Uterine blood flow decreased approximately 25 per cent during all hyperventilation periods (Figure 3.12). Because the reduction in uterine blood flow was unrelated to changes in maternal $PaCO_2$ (range 17 to 64 torr) or pH (range 7.74 to 7.24), the decrease probably was caused by the mechanical effect of positive pressure ventilation.

Metabolic alkalosis may also be detrimental to the fetus as a result of decreased utero-placental blood flow and displacement of maternal oxygen-hemoglobin dissociation curve to the left, resulting in increased affinity of maternal hemoglobin for oxygen and decreased release at the placenta.[89, 92–94] In the pregnant ewe Cosmi[11, 14] found that maternal metabolic alkalosis induced by intravenous infusion of tri-hydroxymethylaminomethane (THAM) caused maternal bradycardia and hypotension, decreased uterine blood flow and induced fetal hypoxia and acidosis. Ralston et al.[93] produced maternal alkalemia with the infusion of sodium bicarbonate in normal pregnant ewes and found a 16 per cent reduction in uterine blood flow with a concomitant decrease in fetal oxygenation and pH. On the other hand, in Cosmi's study, the infusion of small doses of sodium bicarbonate, e.g. 100 mEq over

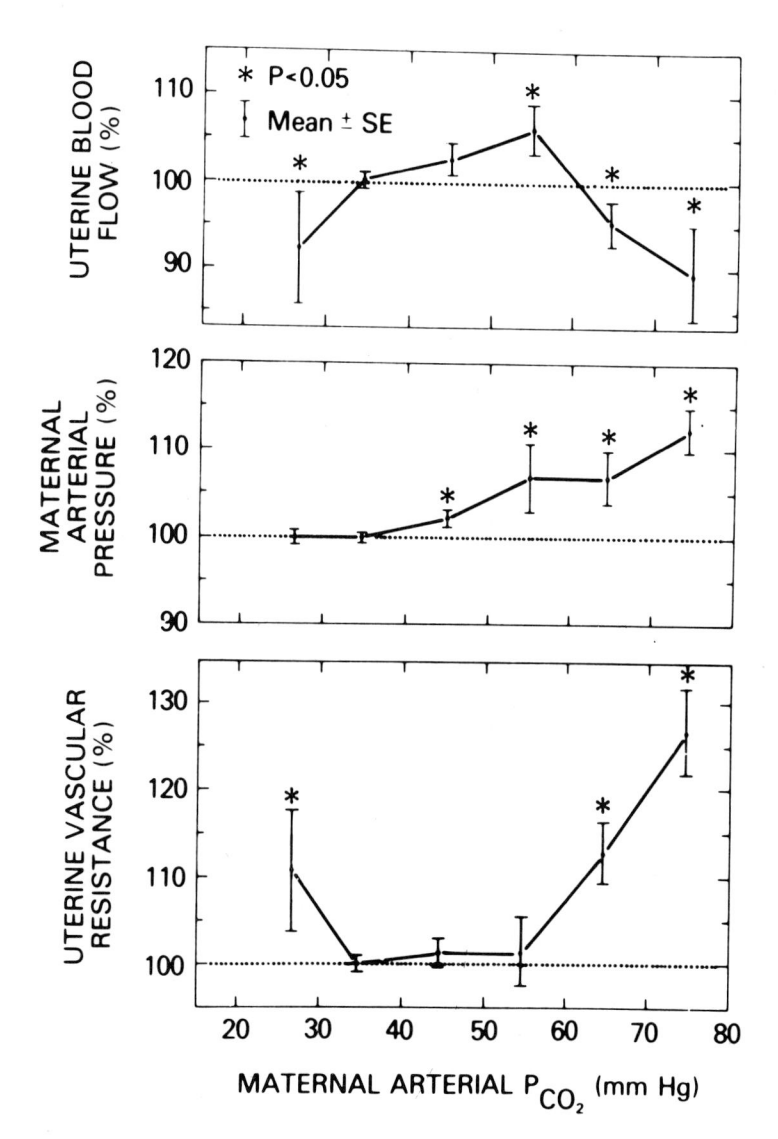

Figure 3.11. Per cent change of uterine blood flow, maternal arterial pressure and uterine vascular resistance during progressive increases of arterial P_{CO_2} induced in conscious pregnant ewes by adding CO_2 to inspired gas mixture. (Reprinted by permission from Walker AM, Oakes GK, Ehrenkranz R, et al.: Effects of hypercapnia on uterine and umbilical circulations in conscious pregnant sheep. J Appl Physiol 41:727, 1976.)

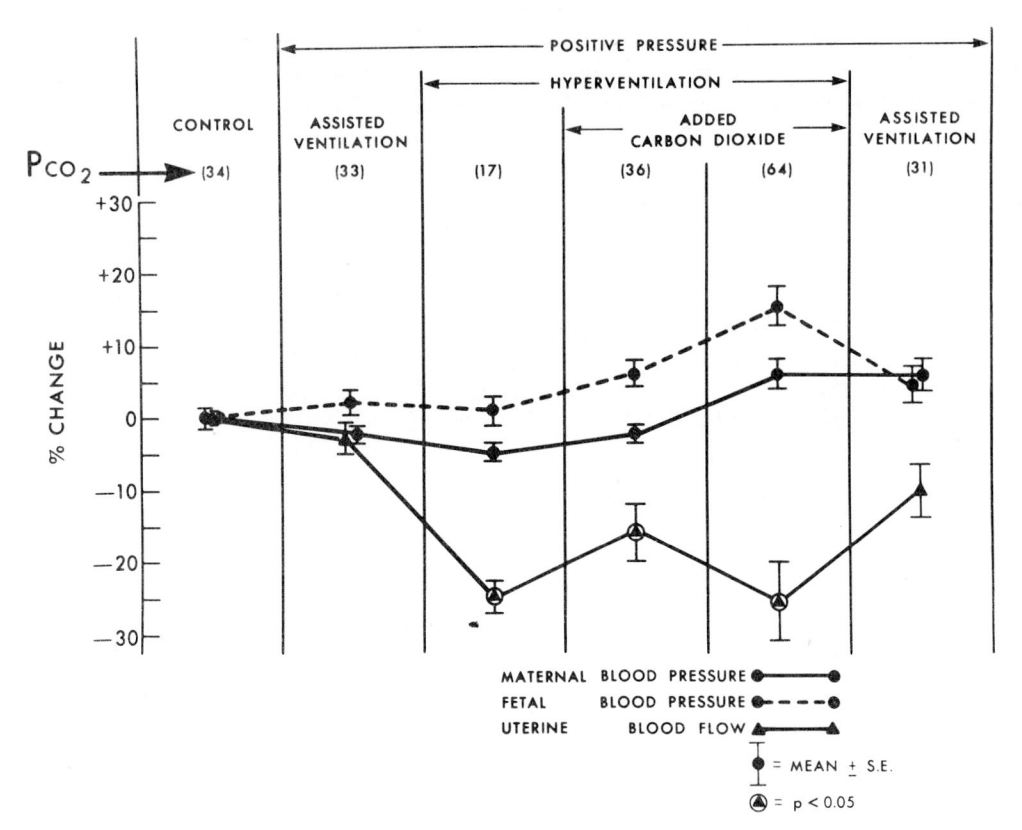

Figure 3.12. Changes from control values in mean maternal and fetal arterial blood pressure and uterine blood flow during five periods of positive pressure ventilation. Mean maternal PaCO$_2$ during each period is indicated at the top of the figure. (Reprinted by permission from Levinson, G, Shnider SM, deLorimier AA, et al.: Effects of maternal hyperventilation on uterine blood flow and fetal oxygenation and acid-base status. Anesthesiology 40:340, 1974.)

12 minutes, to the acidotic ewe did not alter uterine blood flow.[11]

SUMMARY

Intravenous induction agents, inhalation and local anesthetics, endogenous and exogenous catecholamines and vasopressors, antihypertensive agents and magnesium sulfate, respiratory gases and metabolic alkalosis can all alter uterine blood flow. Their net effects on uterine blood flow ultimately depend on how these agents alter uterine perfusion pressure relative to uterine vascular resistance.

References

1. Greiss FC: The uterine vascular bed: Effect of adrenergic drug stimulation. Obstet Gynecol 21: 295, 1963.
2. Huckabee WE: Uterine blood flow. Am J Obstet Gynecol 84:1623, 1962.
3. Parer JT, Lannoy CW, Behrman RE: Uterine blood flow and oxygen consumption in rhesus monkeys with retained placentas. Am J Obstet Gynecol 100:806, 1968.
4. Assali NS, Rauramo L, Peltonen T: Measurement of uterine blood flow and uterine metabolism VIII. Am J Obstet Gynecol 79:86, 1960.
5. Makowski EL, Meschia G, Droegemueller W, et al.: Distribution of uterine blood flow in the pregnant sheep. Am J Obstet Gynecol 101:409, 1968.
6. Schenk WG Jr, Race D: Methods of measurement of blood flow: A current appraisal. J Surg Res 6: 361, 1966.

7. Lewis BV: Uterine blood flow. Obstet Gynecol Surv 24:1211, 1969.
8. Cosmi EV, Condorelli S, Scarpelli EM: Fetal asphyxia induced by sodium thiopental, thiamylal and methohexital. 4th European Congress of Perinatal Medicine, Praha, 1974, Abstract No. IV, 3/12.
9. Cosmi EV, Condorelli S, Scarpelli EM: Effects of barbiturates on maternal and fetal cardiovascular dynamics and on acid-base status and fetal breathing. *Proceedings of the 6th World Congress of Anaesthesiology*, Mexico City, 1976. Excerpta Medica, The Hague, 1977, p 25.
10. Scarpelli EM, Condorelli S, Cosmi EV: Cutaneous stimulation and generation of breathing in the fetus. Pediatr Res 11:24, 1977.
11. Cosmi EV: Drugs, anesthetics and the fetus. In *Reviews in Perinatal Medicine*, EM Scarpelli and EV Cosmi, eds, vol 1. University Park Press, Baltimore, 1976, p 19.
12. Palahniuk RJ, Cumming M: Foetal deterioration following thiopentone-nitrous oxide anaesthesia in the pregnant ewe. Can Anaesth Soc J 24:361, 1977.
13. Mofid M, Brinkman CR III, Assali NS: Effects of diazepam on uteroplacental and fetal hemodynamics and metabolism. Obstet Gynecol 41:364, 1973.
14. Cosmi EV: Fetal homeostasis. In *Pulmonary Physiology of the Fetus, Newborn and Child*, EM Scarpelli and PAM Auld, eds. Lea & Febiger, Philadelphia, 1975, p 61.
15. Greiss FC, van Wilkes D: Effects of sympathomimetic drugs and angiotensin on the uterine vascular bed. Obstet Gynecol 23:925, 1964.
16. Ralston DH; Shnider SM, deLorimier AA: Effects of equipotent ephedrine, metaraminol, mephentermine and methoxamine on uterine blood flow in the pregnant ewe. Anesthesiology 40:354, 1974.
17. Levinson G, Shnider SM, Gildea JE, et al.: Maternal and foetal cardiovascular and acid-base changes during ketamine anaesthesia in pregnant ewes. Br J Anaesth 54:1111, 1973.
18. Eng M, Berges PU, Bonica JJ: The effects of ketamine on uterine blood flow in the monkey. In *Abstracts of Scientific Papers*, Annual Meeting, Society for Gynecological Investigation, Atlanta, 1973, abstract 75, p. 48.
19. Cosmi EV: Effetti della ketamina sulla madre e sul feto. Studio sperimentale e clinico. Minerva Anestesiol 43:379, 1977.
20. Galloon S: Ketamine for obstetric delivery. Anesthesiology 44:522, 1976.
21. Chodoff P, Stella JG: Use of Cl-581-A phencyclidine derivative for obstetrical anesthesia. Anesth Analg 45:527, 1966.
22. Meer FM, Downing JW, Coleman AJ: An intravenous method of anaesthesia for caesarean section. Part II, Ketamine. Br J Anaesth 45:191, 1973.
23. Akamatsu TJ, Bonica JJ, Rehmet R, et al.: Experiences with the use of ketamine for parturition. I. Primary anesthetic for vaginal delivery. Anesth Analg 53:284, 1974.
24. Hodgkinson R, Marx GF, Kim SS, et al.: Neonatal neurobehavioral tests following vaginal delivery under ketamine, thiopental and extradural anesthesia. Anesth Analg 56:548, 1977.
25. Cosmi EV, Marx GF: The effect of anesthesia on the acid-base status of the fetus. Anesthesiology 30:238, 1969.
26. Brann AW Jr, Myers RE, DiGiacomo R: The effect of halothane-induced maternal hypotension in the fetus. In *Medical Primatology 1970*, Proceedings of the 2nd Conference on Experimental Medicine and Surgery in Primates, New York, 1969. S. Karger, Basel, 1971, p 637.
27. Moir DD: Anaesthesia for caesarean section. An evaluation of a method using low concentrations of halothane and 50 per cent of oxygen. Br J Anaesth 42:136, 1970.
28. Bonica JJ: Halothane in obstetrics. In *The Anesthesiologist, Mother and Newborn*, SM Shnider and F Moya, eds. Williams & Wilkins, Baltimore, 1974.
29. Allard E, Guimond C: L'halothane en obstetrique. Can Anaesth Soc J 11:83, 1964.
30. Stoelting VK: Fluothane in obstetric anesthesia. Anesth Analg (Cleve) 43:243, 1964.
31. Crawford JS: The place of halothane in obstetrics. Br J Anaesth 34:386, 1962.
32. Marx GF, Mateo CV: Effects of different oxygen concentrations during general anesthesia for elective cesarean section. Can Anaesth Soc J 18:587, 1971.
33. Galbert MW, Gardner AE: Use of halothane in a balanced technique for cesarean section. Anesth Analg (Cleve) 51:701, 1972.
34. Phillips JM, Evans JA: Acute anesthetic and obstetric management of patients with severe abruptio-placenta. Anesth Analg 49:998, 1970.
35. Palahniuk RJ, Shnider SM: Maternal and fetal cardiovascular and acid-base changes during halothane and isoflurane anaesthesia in the pregnant ewe. Anesthesiology 41:462, 1974.
36. Carenza L, Cosmi EV: Analgo-anetesia in travaglio e nel parto: Valutazione des metodi e dei farmaci. In *58th Congress of the Italian Society of Obstetrics and Gynecology 1977*. Mattioli Publ. Fidenza, Italy, 1977, p 286.
37. Eng M, Bonica JJ, Akamatsu TJ, et al.: Maternal and fetal responses to halothane in pregnant monkeys. Acta Anaesth Scand 19:154, 1975.
38. Smith JB, Manning FA, Palahniuk RJ: Maternal and foetal effects of methoxyflurane anaesthesia in the pregnant ewe. Can Anaesth Soc J 22:449, 1975.
39. Eng M, Berges PU, Der Yuen D, et al.: A comparison of the effects of the inhalation of 4% and 8% fluoroxene in the pregnant primate. Acta Anaesth Scand 20:183, 1976.
40. Gibbs CP, Noel SC: Human uterine artery responses to lidocaine. Am J Obstet Gynecol 126:313, 1976.
41. Cibils LA: Response of human uterine arteries to local anesthetics. Am J Obstet Gynecol 126:202, 1976.

42. Greiss FC Jr, Still JG, Anderson SG: Effects of local anesthetic agents on the uterine vasculatures and myometrium. Am J Obstet Gynecol 124:889, 1976.
43. Fishburne JI, Hopkinson RB, Greiss FC Jr: Responses of gravid uterine vasculature to arterial levels of local anesthetic agents. In *Abstracts of Scientific Papers*, Annual Meeting, Society for Obstetric Anesthesia and Perinatology, Seattle, 1977, p 37.
44. Pue AF, Plumer MH, Resnik R, et al.: Effects of local anesthetics on uterine blood flow in pregnant sheep. In *Abstracts of Scientific Papers*, Annual Meeting, Society for Obstetric Anesthesia and Perinatology, Seattle, 1977, p 47.
45. Morishima HO, Gutsche BB, Keenaghan JB, et al.: The effect of lidocaine-induced maternal convulsions on the fetal lamb. In *Abstracts of Scientific Papers*, Annual Meeting, American Society of Anesthesiologists, New Orleans, 1977, p 293.
46. Biehl D, Shnider SM, Levinson G, et al.: The direct effects of circulating lidocaine on uterine blood flow and foetal well-being in the pregnant ewe. Can Anaesth Soc J 24:445, 1977.
47. Greiss FC Jr, Crandell DL: Therapy for hypotension induced by spinal anesthesia during pregnancy. JAMA 191:793, 1965.
48. Greiss FC Jr: Pressure-flow relationship in the gravid uterine vascular bed. Am J Obstet Gynecol 96:41, 1966.
49. Wallis KL, Shnider SM, Hicks JS, et al.: Epidural anesthesia in the normotensive pregnant ewe: Effects on uterine blood flow and fetal acid-base status. Anesthesiology 44:481, 1976.
50. Brotanek V, Vasicka A, Santiago A: The influence of epidural anesthesia on uterine blood flow. Obstet Gynecol 42:276, 1973.
51. Jouppila R, Jouppila P, Hollmen A, et al.: Effect of segmental extradural analgesia on placental blood flow during normal labour. Br J Anaesth 50:563, 1978.
52. Barton MD, Killam AP, Meschia G: Response of ovine uterine blood flow to epinephrine and norepinephrine. Proc Soc Exp Biol Med 145:996, 1974.
53. Bonica JJ, Akamatsu TJ, Berges PU, et al.: Circulatory effects of peridural block. II. Effects of epinephrine. Anesthesiology 34:514, 1972.
54. Rosenfeld CR, Barton MD, Meschia G: Effects of epinephrine on distribution of blood flow in the pregnant ewe. Am J Obstet Gynecol 124:156, 1976.
55. Akamatsu TJ: Cesarean section under epidural anesthesia with epinephrine. Anesthesiol Rev 1:28, 1974.
56. Levinson G, Shnider SM, Krames E, et al.: Epidural anesthesia for cesarean section: Effects of epinephrine in the local anesthetic solution. In *Abstracts of Scientific Papers*, Annual Meeting, American Society of Anesthesiologists, Chicago, 1975, p 285.
57. Myers RE: Maternal psychological stress and fetal asphyxia: A study in the monkey. Am J Obstet Gynecol 122:47, 1975.
58. Shnider SM, Wright RG, Levinson G, et al.: Uterine blood flow and plasma norepinephrine changes during maternal stress in the pregnant ewe. 50: 30, 1979.
59. Martin CB Jr, Gingerick B: Uteroplacental physiology. J Obstet Gynecol Nurs (Suppl) 5:16, 1976.
60. Adamsons K, Mueller-Heubach E, Myers RE: Production of fetal asphyxia in the rhesus monkey by administration of catecholamines to the mother. Am J Obstet Gynecol 109:248, 1971.
61. Eng M, Berges PU, Ueland K, et al.: The effects of methoxamine and ephedrine in normotensive pregnant primates. Anesthesiology 35:354, 1971.
62. Shnider SM, deLorimier AA, Asling JH, et al.: Vasopressors in obstetrics. II. Fetal hazards of methoxamine administration during obstetric spinal anesthesia. Am J Obstet Gynecol 106:680, 1970.
63. Greiss FC Jr, Gobble FL Jr: Effect of sympathetic nerve stimulation on the uterine vascular bed. Am J Obstet Gynecol 97:962, 1967.
64. James FM III, Greiss FC Jr, Kemp RA: An evaluation of vasopressor therapy for maternal hypotension during spinal anesthesia. Anesthesiology 33:25, 1970.
65. Eng M, Berges PU, Parer JT, et al.: Spinal anesthesia and ephedrine in pregnant monkeys. Am J Obstet Gynecol 115:1095, 1973.
66. Shnider SM, deLorimier AA, Steffenson JL: Vasopressors in obstetrics. III. Fetal effects of metaraminol infusion during obstetric spinal hypotension. Am J Obstet Gynecol 108:1017, 1970.
67. Callender K, Levinson G, Shnider SM, et al.: Dopamine administration in the normotensive pregnant ewe. Obstet Gynecol 51:586, 1978.
68. Rolbin SH, Levinson G, Shnider SM, et al.: Dopamine treatment of spinal hypotension decreases uterine blood flow in the pregnant ewe. Anesthesiology 51:36, 1978.
69. Ehrenkranz RA, Hamilton LA, Bennan SC, et al.: Effects of salbutamol and isoxsuprine on uterine and umbilical blood flow in pregnant sheep. Obstet Gynecol 128:287, 1977.
70. Ehrenkranz RA, Walker AM, Oakes GK, et al: Effect of ritodrine infusion on uterine and umbilical blood flow in pregnant sheep. Obstet Gynecol 126:343, 1976.
71. Brinkman CR III, Assali NS: Uteroplacental hemodynamic response to antihypertensive drugs in hypertensive pregnant sheep. In *Hypertension in Pregnancy*, MD Lindheimer, AI Katz and FP Zuspan, eds. John Wiley & Sons, New York, 1976, pp 363–375.
72. Ring G, Krames E, Shnider SM, et al.: Comparison of nitroprusside and hydralazine in hypertensive pregnant ewes. Obstet Gynecol 50:598, 1977.
73. Schlant RC, Tsagaris TS, Robertson RJ Jr: Studies on the acute cardiovascular effects of intravenous sodium nitroprusside. Am J Cardiol 9:51, 1972.
74. Styles MB, Coleman AJ, Leary WP: Some hemodynamic effects of sodium nitroprusside. Anesthesiology 38:173, 1973.
75. Ross G, Cole PV: Cardiovascular actions of sodium nitroprusside in dogs. Anaesthesia 28:400, 1973.
76. Naulty JS, Cefalo R, Rodkey FL: Placental transfer

and fetal toxicity of sodium nitroprusside. In *Abstracts of Scientific Papers*, Annual Meeting, American Society of Anesthesiologists, San Francisco, 1976, p 543.
77. Lazard EM: Preliminary report on intravenous use of magnesium sulfate in puerperial eclampsia. Am J Obstet Gynecol 9:178, 1925.
78. Dorsett L: Intramuscular injection of magnesium sulfate for the control of convulsions in eclampsia. Am J Obstet Gynecol 11:227, 1926.
79. Dandavino A, Woods JR Jr, Murayama K, et al.: Circulatory effects of magnesium sulfate in normotensive and renal hypertensive pregnant sheep. Am J Obstet Gynecol 127:769, 1977.
80. Krames E, Ring G, Wallis KL, et al.: The effect of magnesium sulfate on uterine blood flow and fetal well-being in the pregnant ewe. In *Abstracts of Scientific Papers*, Annual Meeting American Society of Anesthesiologists, Chicago, 1975, p 287.
81. Greiss FC Jr, Anderson SG, King LC: Uterine vascular bed: Effects of acute hypoxia. Am J Obstet Gynecol 113:1057, 1972.
82. Makowski EL, Hertz RH, Meschia G: Effect of acute maternal hypoxia and hyperoxia on the blood flow to the pregnant uterus. Am J Obstet Gynecol 115:624, 1973.
83. Dilts PV Jr, Brinkman CR III, Kirschbaum TH, et al.: Uterine and systemic hemodynamic interrelationships and their response to hypoxia. Am J Obstet Gynecol 103:138, 1969.
84. Assali NS, Holm LW, Sehgal N: Hemodynamic changes in fetal lamb in utero in response to asphyxia, hypoxia and hypercapnia. Circ Res 11:423, 1962.
85. Levinson G, Shnider SM, deLorimier AA, et al.: Effects of maternal hyperventilation on uterine blood flow and fetal oxygenation and acid-base status. Anesthesiology 40:340, 1974.
86. Wolkoff AS, McGee JA, Flowers CE, et al.: Alterations in uterine blood flow in the pregnant ewe. I. Associated changes in blood gases. Obstet Gynecol 23:636, 1964.
87. Walker AM, Oakes GK, Ehrenkranz R, et al.: Effects of hypercapnia on uterine and umbilical circulations in conscious pregnant sheep. J Appl Physiol 41:727, 1976.
88. Morishima HO, Daniel SS, Adamsons K Jr, et al.: Effects of positive pressure ventilation of the mother upon the acid-base state of the fetus. Am J Obstet Gynecol 93:269, 1965.
89. Motoyama EK, Rivard G, Acheson F, et al.: Adverse effect of maternal hyperventilation on the foetus. Lancet 1:286, 1966.
90. Lumley J, Renou P, Newman W, et al.: Hyperventilation in obstetrics. Am J Obstet Gynecol 103:847, 1969.
91. Parer JT, Eng M, Aoba H, et al.: Uterine blood flow and oxygen uptake during maternal hyperventilation in monkeys at cesarean section. Anesthesiology 32:130, 1970.
92. Johnson GH, Brinkman CR III, Assali NS: Effects of acid and base infusion on umbilical hemodynamics. Am J Obstet Gynecol 112:1122, 1972.
93. Ralston DH, Shnider SM, deLorimier AA: Uterine blood flow and fetal acid-base changes after bicarbonate administration to the pregnant ewe. Anesthesiology 40:348, 1974.
94. Buss DD, Bisgard EG, Rawlings CA, et al.: Uteroplacental blood flow during alkalosis in the sheep. Am J Physiol 228:1497, 1975.

CHAPTER 4

Effects of Anesthesia on Uterine Activity and Labor

Jay S. DeVore, M.D.

The conduct of an obstetric anesthetic and the progress and management of labor are inextricably bound together. Much controversy exists regarding the degree to which anesthesia affects uterine activity and labor. Much of the dialogue between obstetricians and obstetric anesthetists centers on this topic.

DEFINITIONS

Uterine activity is defined in terms of the frequency of contraction of the uterus and the pressure generated by these contractions. Uterine activity can be monitored indirectly by a tocodynamometer applied to the maternal abdomen or directly by inserting a plastic catheter transcervically into the amniotic sac and attaching the distal end to a strain gauge. The tocodynamometer is triggered by the changing shape of the uterus during a contraction, and, when it is externally applied, the data are only quantitative in respect to the frequency of contractions. The intra-amniotic catheter will also measure the intrauterine pressure during contractions as well as resting uterine tone, that is the lowest pressure recorded between contractions.

Several other systems have been devised for assessing uterine activity. One of the earliest and most commonly used was devised by Caldeyro-Barcia.[1] This system takes the number of contractions in a 10-minute period and multiplies this by the peak amplitude in millimeters of mercury of these contractions. The result is stated in Montevideo units. Another method measures the area under the uterine pressure curve and yields a result which is expressed in torr-minutes or uterine activity units.[2] Another system simply records the mean peak amplitude of contractions over a 10-minute period. All of these methods have been used in assessing the effect of drugs on uterine activity.

Progress of labor refers to increasing cervical dilation, effacement and the descent in the pelvis of the presenting fetal part with time as originally described by Friedman[3] (Figure 4.1).

Abnormal progress of labor can be classified as *slow latent phase, active phase arrest, slow slope active phase, slow descent and arrest of descent*. Diagnostic features for abnormal progress of labor are listed in Table 4.1. During the latent phase, excessive sedation or anesthesia is the commonest cause for prolongation, primarily due to decreased uterine activity. During the active phase or second stage of labor, cephalopelvic disproportion and malposition and malpresentation are the most common etiologic factors.

Uterine relaxation is defined as diminution or cessation of uterine contractions and a decrease in resting uterine tone.

INHALATION AGENTS

Many inhalation anesthetics have a direct and dose-related effect on uterine ac-

EFFECTS OF ANESTHESIA ON UTERINE ACTIVITY AND LABOR

tivity. Naftalin et al.[4,5] using in vitro preparations of both rat and human myometrium, demonstrated a dose-related reduction in both resting tone and peak developed tension with halothane (Figure 4.2). Similar findings have been reported by Munson et al.[6] for diethyl ether, halothane, enflurane and isoflurane in pregnant and non-pregnant human myometrial strips. Equipotent doses of the halogenated agents halothane, enflurane and isoflurane produce equal uterine relaxation.[7] Methoxyflurane is also capable of producing marked uterine muscle depression in high concentrations.[8] Nitrous oxide and cyclopropane have little or no effect on the uterus.[6]

The most reliable way of rapidly producing uterine relaxation is with general anesthesia. Diethyl ether was the traditional agent for relaxing the uterus either for therapy of a tetanic contraction or for

MEAN LABOR CURVE

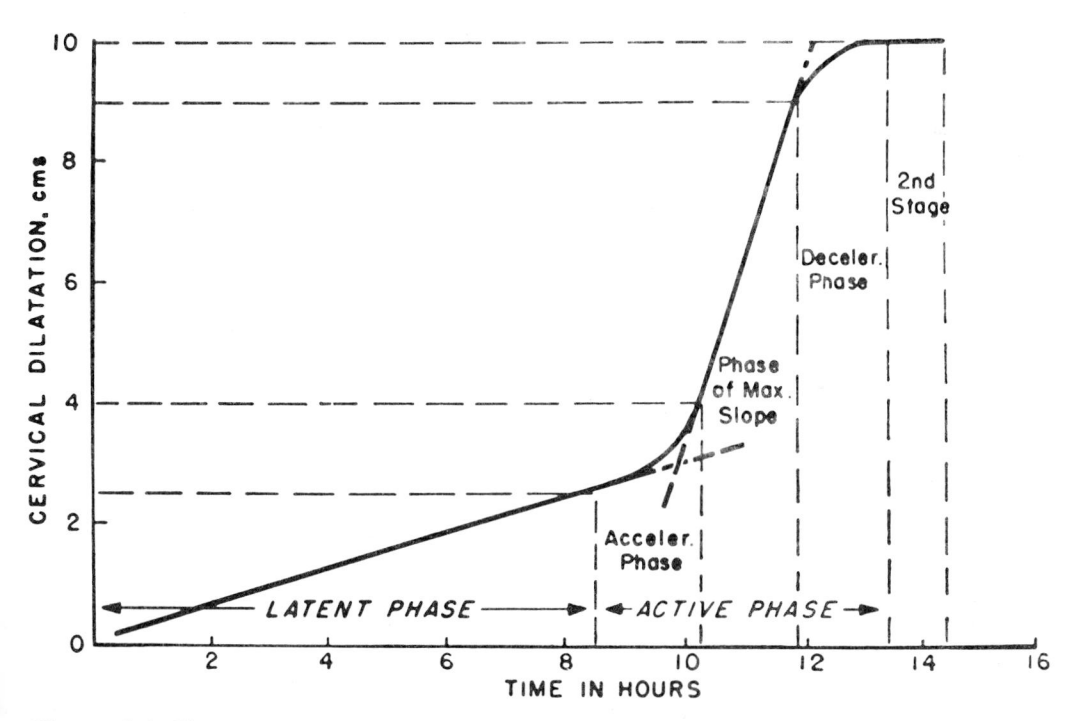

Figure 4.1. The mean labor curve (cervical dilation versus time) based on a graphicostatistical analysis of 500 primigravidas at term. (Reprinted by permission from Friedman EA: Primigravid labor. A graphicostatistical analysis. Obstet Gynecol 6:567, 1955.)

Table 4.1
Prolonged Labor: Diagnostic Features

	Slow Latent Phase	Slow Slope Active Phase	Active Phase Arrest	Slow Descent of Fetus	Arrest of Descent
Nulliparas	> 20 hrs	< 1.2 cm/hr	No cervical dilation for 2 hr	< 1 cm/hr	No descent for 1 hr
Multiparas	> 14 hrs	< 1.5 cm/hr		< 2 cm/hr	

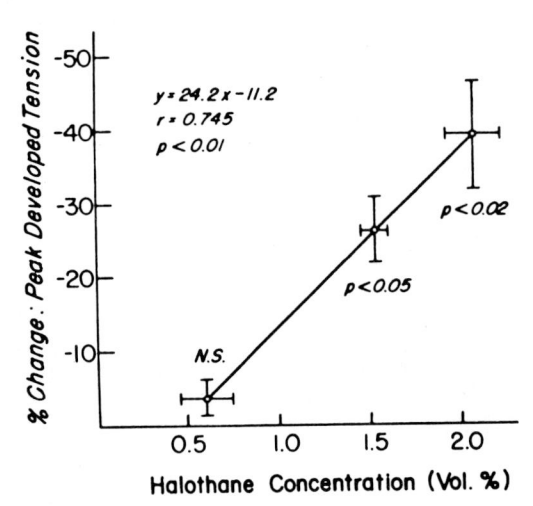

Figure 4.2. Effect of halothane on isometric developed tension in pregnant rat myometrium. *Brackets* include standard errors of the mean. P values refer to changes in developed tension from control. (Reprinted by permission from Naftalin NJ, Phear WPC, Goldberg AH: Halothane and isometric contractions of isolated pregnant rat myometrium. Anesthesiology 42:458, 1975.)

intrauterine manipulations. Due to flammability and slowness of onset, diethyl ether has largely been abandoned in favor of halothane. Inspired concentrations of halothane above 1 per cent will relax the uterus. Although drugs that relax the uterus may increase blood loss after delivery, if the agent is blown off rapidly and an oxytocic agent is administered, the uterus will contract and bleeding from the placental bed will stop.

The response of the uterus to oxytocic agents during halothane or enflurane anesthesia is related to the dose of the anesthetic.[9] At high concentrations, halothane (1.6 volume per cent) and enflurane (3 volume per cent) will block the uterine response to oxytocin. Halothane (1 volume per cent) and enflurane (2 volume per cent), while relaxing the uterus, will not block the response to 10 milliunits of oxytocin.

Inhalation analgesia with low-dose methoxyflurane, enflurane or isoflurane is not associated with decreased tone or activity, prolongation of labor or increased postpartum blood loss. Similarly, investigators[10-12] have found no additional maternal bleeding during anesthesia for cesarean section with low doses of halothane or enflurane. Marx and co-workers,[9] studying parturients in the immediate postpartum period, found that 0.5 volume per cent of halothane or 1 volume per cent of enflurane did not decrease uterine tone or contractility and did not alter the uterine response to oxytocin.

PARENTERAL AGENTS

DeVoe et al.[13] reported that meperidine (100 mg) administered intravenously during the active phase of labor produced either no change or an increase in uterine activity in 42 of 45 patients. However, 38 of the patients were receiving oxytocin stimulation, and there were no controls; therefore, the increase may have been due to the natural course of labor. Similarly, Filler et al.[14] noted increases in Montevideo units after meperidine, pentazocine or low spinal anesthesia. Both of the above studies concluded that the decrease in pain provided by the analgesia decreased maternal epinephrine secretion and its β-adrenergic agonism, thereby improving uterine contractility.

On the other hand, Petrie et al.[15] using uterine activity units, reported that total uterine activity in unmedicated labor increases with the passage of time. They observed the effect of several systemic analgesics and hypnotics by comparing the total uterine activity units in a 30-minute control period with a 30-minute period after intravenous administration of the drug. They also compared the slope of the increase of uterine activity in the pre- and post-injection periods. (Figure 4.3). They found that with the narcotics meperidine,

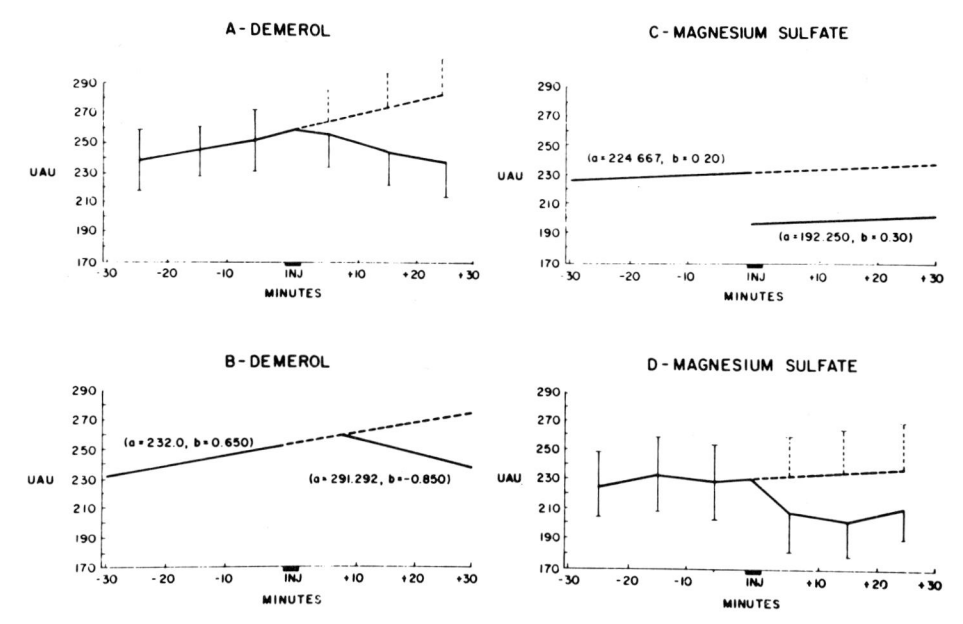

Figure 4.3. Results of administration of Demerol and magnesium sulfate. A and D, mean uterine activity (UAU ± SE) per 10-minute segment of labor in the pre-injection and post-injection periods is contrasted with the expected (----) UAU for the study period. B and C, regression line for the pre-injection period is contrasted with the observed post-injection values. (Reprinted by permission from Petrie RH, Wu R, Miller FC, et al.: The effect of drugs on uterine activity. Obstet Gynecol 48:431, 1976.)

morphine and alphaprodine the total number of uterine activity units pre- and post-injection was not significantly different, but the post-injection slope changed from the expected positive to negative. The same was true for the tranquilizing agents hydroxyzine and promethazine. The implication of these results is that the agents studied would somewhat slow the course of labor, although the authors were careful to point out that their studies did not include direct measurement of the progress of labor as previously defined.

The anesthetic agent ketamine has received considerable attention in obstetrics. Ketamine in doses of .27 to 2.2 mg/kg increases uterine tone.[16] In doses below 1.1 mg/kg this increase is less than 10 per cent, whereas 2.2 mg/kg produces an increase of nearly 40 per cent. Marx et al.[17] studying postpartum uterine pressures with different doses of ketamine, failed to demonstrate an increase in uterine tone, although uterine activity increased briefly.

REGIONAL ANESTHESIA

Regional anesthesia may affect uterine activity and the course of labor either directly or indirectly. First, there is the direct effect of local anesthetics on the uterus. In the concentrations generally achieved in the clinical situation, there seems to be no direct effect of local anesthetics on uterine contractility.[18] However, high concentrations such as might be achieved by an inadvertent intravascular injection or paracervical block (dose of local anesthetic injected in close proximity to uterine arteries) may increase uterine tone.[19] When Greiss et al.[20] injected local anesthetics directly into the uterine artery of pregnant ewes, a dose-related increase in uterine tone was noted. In vitro studies of uterine

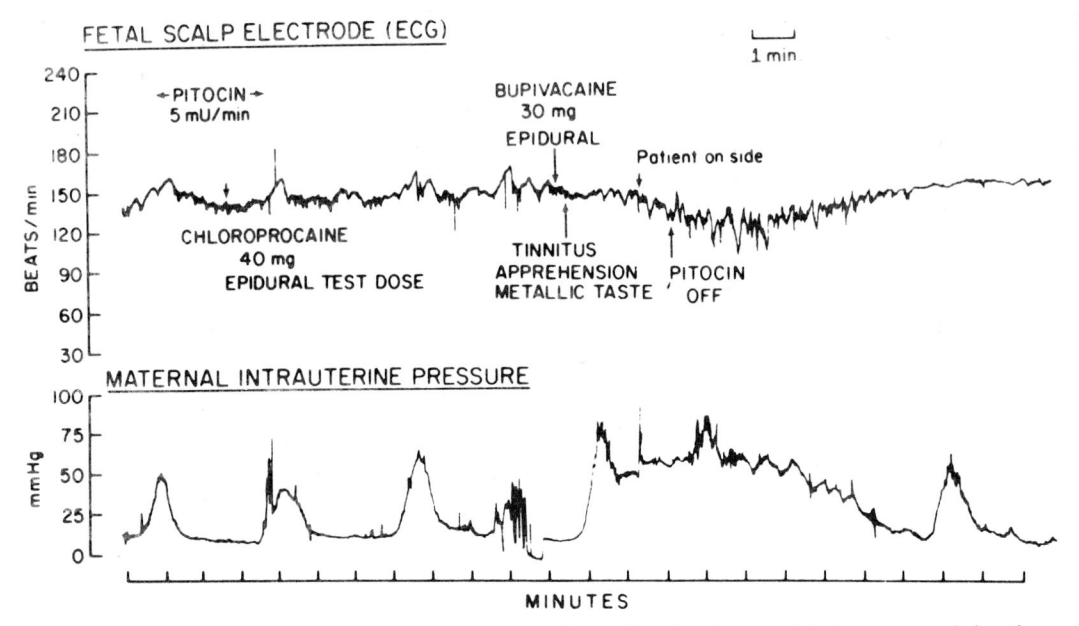

Figure 4.4. Tetanic uterine contraction occurring after inadvertant intravenous injection of bupivacaine. (Reprinted by permission from Greiss FC, Still JG, Anderson SG: Effects of local anesthetic agents on the uterine vasculatures and myometrium. Am J Obstet Gynecol 124:889, 1976.)

muscle strips demonstrate that local anesthetics increase tone but decrease the rate and strength of contractions.[21] This effect is antagonized by calcium.[22] Jenssen[23] showed that paracervical block increases the rate of contraction and decreases the rate of relaxation. Very high concentrations can lead to tetanic contractions (Figure 4.4).

There may be considerable indirect effects of conduction anesthesia on the course of labor through changes in uterine activity or maternal expulsive efforts. It has generally been taught that conduction anesthesia administered too early in the course of labor will significantly slow labor whereas the same technique applied when labor is well established will have little or no effect.[24] In fact, some believe that properly administered regional anesthesia can shorten prolonged labor.[25] This, of course, is extremely difficult to evaluate because labor is so variable and many labors will slow even without the administration of anesthesia.

There have been many studies attempting to assess the effects of regional anesthesia on the course of labor, and the data are not at all conclusive. Lowensohn et al.[26] observed a significant depression of uterine activity lasting approximately 30 minutes after lidocaine injection through lumbar epidural catheters (Figure 4.5). They did not make a similar observation after propitocaine. (Propitocaine is seldom used due to its unfortunate tendency to cause methemoglobinemia.) The same phenomenon was observed with lidocaine by Zador and Nilsson.[27] On the other hand, Crawford[28] and Schellenberg,[29] both investigating lumbar epidural anesthesia with bupivacaine, and Tyack et al.[30] investigating caudal epidural anesthesia with bupivacaine, noticed no decrease in uterine activity after injection. This implies that bupivacaine has less effect on the uterus than does lidocaine; however, there are other variables to be considered. The most important seems to be avoidance of vena caval compression. This is well demon-

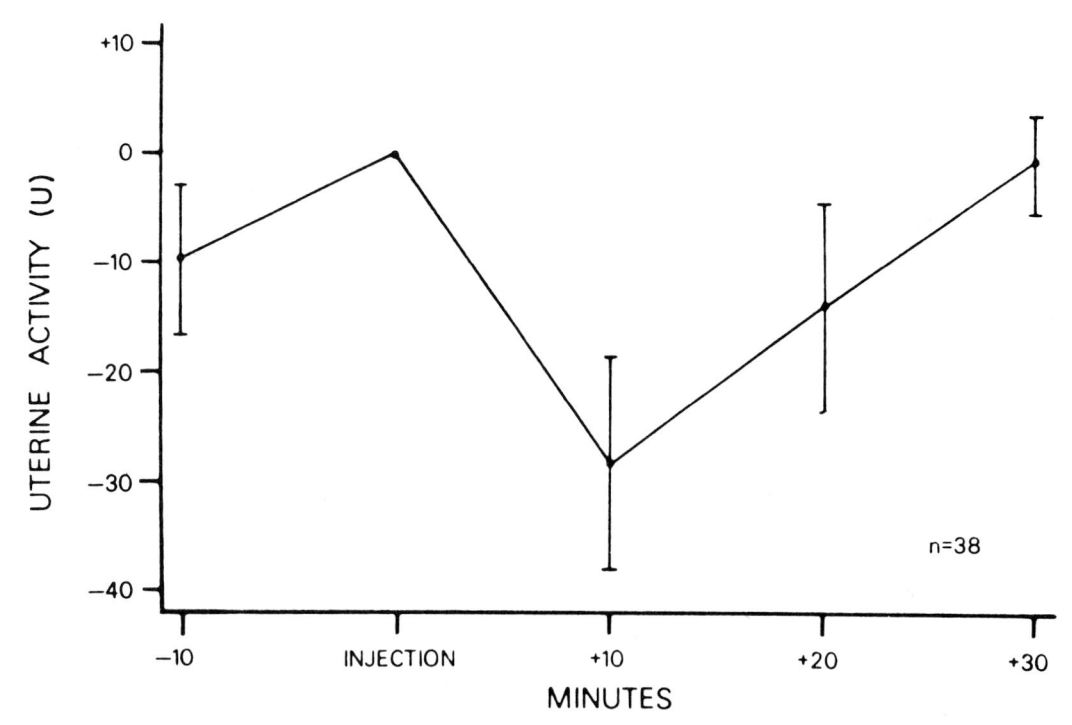

Figure 4.5. Uterine activity in patients receiving lidocaine (+2 SE). (Reprinted by permission from Lowensohn RI, Paul R, Fales S, et al.: Intrapartum epidural anesthesia: An evaluation of effects on uterine activity. Obstet Gynecol 44:388, 1974.)

strated in a study by Craft et al.[31], who showed that uterine activity did not decrease after lidocaine if the patient is kept on her side (Table 4.2). This seems to indicate that decreased uterine perfusion can occur in the absence of demonstrable systemic hypotension.

To summarize, during the active phase of the first stage of labor a T10 sensory level produced by either spinal[32-35] or lumbar epidural[36-38] block has no significant effect on uterine activity or progress of labor provided fetal malposition or malpresentation is absent and hypotension is avoided. A small, transient (10 to 20 minutes) decrease in uterine activity after spinal,[32, 35, 37] caudal[14, 39] and epidural block[26, 30, 32, 37, 40] has been reported. On the other hand, other authors report enhanced and more effective uterine contractility after epidural[41-44] or caudal[35, 36, 45, 46] anesthesia. In fact, these techniques have been used effectively to manage parturients with incoordinate uterine activity during labor,[37, 44, 47-50] multiple gestation[51] or breech presentation.[52, 53]

Regional anesthesia, by removing the parturient's reflex urge to bear down or by decreasing muscle function, may prolong the second stage of labor. Johnson et al.[32] compared the effects of pudendal, spinal, and epidural anesthesia on uterine activity and maternal expulsive efforts during the second stage of labor. High subarachnoid block decreased voluntary effort and prolonged the second stage. Uterine contraction intensity, however, was unchanged. Epidural anesthesia with a T10 to S5 block reduced the intensity of uterine contraction and voluntary effort, but the second stage was not prolonged. Sensory analgesia, causing interruption of Ferguson's reflex (oxytocin release in response to cervical dilation) may cause uterine inhibi-

Table 4.2
Effect of Local Analgesic on Cervical Dilation and Uterine Forces*

Drug	Measurement	
	First 20 min	Second 20 min
	cervical dilation, cm†	
1.5% lidocaine with 1/200,000 epinephrine	+0.7 ± 0.6	+1.6 ± 0.4 (p < .001)
1.5% lidocaine (plain)	+0.8 ± 0.3 (p < 0.05)	+2.0 ± 0.4 (p < .001)
	Uterine forces, M.U‡	
1.5% lidocaine with 1/200,000 epinephrine	−47.8 ± 17.6 (p < .02)	+1.9 ± 19.6
1.5% lidocaine (plain)	+6.2 ± 18.1	+30.8 ± 26

* Reprinted by permission from Craft JB, Epstein BS, Coakley CS: Effect of lidocaine with epinephrine versus lidocaine (plain) on induced labor. Anesth Analg. 51:243, 1972.
† All changes are related to the baseline period and are tabulated for the first period and then for the total of both periods.
‡ All changes are related to the baseline period and are tabulated for *each* 20-min period.

tion.[54] However, this reflex has not been demonstrated in humans.

Although major regional anesthesia may prolong labor, there is no evidence that this harms the fetus. In fact, less fetal acidosis develops during a prolonged first or second stage of labor in parturients during epidural anesthesia than in non-anesthetized mothers.[27, 55-59] An increased incidence of mid-forceps deliveries may occur in parturients with conduction anesthesia.[32, 42, 60, 61] Relaxation of the pelvic musculature interferes with flexion and internal rotation of the fetus. Withholding the perineal dose of epidural anesthesia until descent and rotation of the fetus has occurred, or using a lower concentration of anesthetic to preserve skeletal muscle tone, should reduce this problem.[37, 62] Furthermore, parturients who are properly instructed can deliver spontaneously with epidural anesthesia.[32, 37, 62, 63]

VASOPRESSORS

A major side effect of regional anesthesia in obstetrics is hypotension. Occasionally, vasopressors must be used to restore blood pressure. The effect of these agents on uterine blood flow has been discussed in the previous chapter. These agents may also have direct effects on uterine muscle. It has been demonstrated that there are α- and β-adrenergic receptors in uterine muscle. Alpha stimulation leads to uterine hypertonus, whereas β stimulation causes a decrease in uterine tone and contractility. Methoxamine has been used in the past to counteract the hypotension of regional anesthesia. Its use in obstetrics should be avoided primarily because of its direct constricting effect on the uterine artery, and also because its α-stimulating effect has been reported to cause tetanic uterine contractions[38] (Figure 4.6). Ephedrine, the vasopressor of choice in obstetrics, seems to have little effect on uterine activity.

Epinephrine is sometimes added to local anesthetics to prolong their duration and decrease their circulating blood level. The β-stimulating effect of this small dose of epinephrine may affect uterine activity and the course of labor.

Gunther and Bauman[64] and Gunther and Bellville[65] showed that the first stage of

EFFECTS OF ANESTHESIA ON UTERINE ACTIVITY AND LABOR

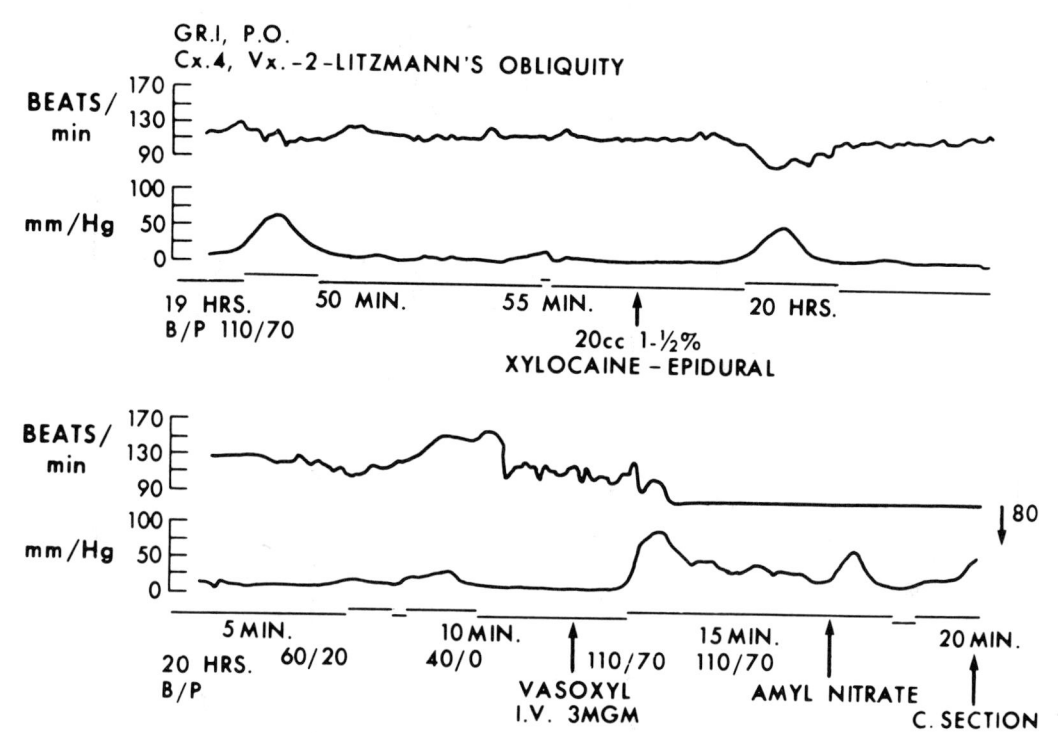

Figure 4.6. Three milligrams of methoxamine were administered to treat maternal hypotension following epidural anesthesia. The *upper tracing* (fetal heart rate) shows a severe fetal bradycardia; the *lower tracing* (intra-amniotic pressure) shows the tetanic uterine contraction which resulted from methoxamine. (Reprinted by permission from Vasicka A, Hutchinson HT, Eng M, et al.: Spinal and epidural anesthesia, fetal and uterine response to acute hypo- and hypertension. Am J Obstet Gynecol 90:800, 1964.)

labor was prolonged in parturients receiving lidocaine or mepivacaine with epinephrine compared to those receiving lidocaine or mepivacaine without epinephrine during continuous caudal anesthesia. In addition, almost twice as many parturients required oxytocin augmentation when solutions containing epinephrine were used.[65] The doses of epinephrine ranged between 100 and 125 μg. Craft et al.[31] compared lidocaine with and without epinephrine for lumbar epidural anesthesia and found that, although patients receiving the epinephrine-containing solution had a slight decrease in uterine activity, the over-all progress of labor was not significantly affected. Zador and Nilsson,[27] using 0.5 and 1 per cent lidocaine with and without epinephrine in lumbar epidural anesthesia, noted a transitory decrease in intensity of contractions after each injection; however, the decrease was more pronounced when the epinephrine-containing solution was used. Whether or not the influence of epinephrine in the local anesthetic solution on the course of labor is clinically significant is still open to question. Beyond this, however, is the question of the need for epinephrine. Bupivacaine, now commonly used in obstetrics, is long-acting and has low toxicity compared to other amides. Furthermore, epinephrine seems to have little effect on its duration[66-68] or maternal blood level. Chloroprocaine has also become popular, and adding epinephrine to it also seems to be illogical. One of the advantages of chloroprocaine is its short duration of action, and one would not want to prolong it with the addition of epinephrine. Its very rapid metabolism in the plasma negates the need for epinephrine to decrease its toxicity.

SUMMARY

The course of labor is quite unpredictable because it is influenced by many factors. Maternal pain, catecholamines, oxytoxic agents, size of the baby, parity of the mother, spinal reflexes and extrauterine forces can all shorten or prolong labor. Anesthetic techniques can and do affect uterine activity and the progress of labor, but judicious management by both anesthetist and obstetrician can result in maternal comfort without significantly prolonging labor or increasing the risk to mother or baby.

References

1. Alvarez H, Caldeyro-Barcia R: Contractility of the human uterus recorded by new methods. Surg Gynecol Obstet 91:1, 1950.
2. Hon EH, Paul RH: Quantitation of uterine activity. Obstet Gynecol 42:368, 1973.
3. Friedman EA: The functional divisions of labor. Am J Obstet Gynecol 109:274, 1971.
4. Naftalin NJ, Phear WPC, Goldberg AH: Halothane and isometric contractions of isolated pregnant rat myometrium. Anesthesiology 42:458, 1975.
5. Naftalin NJ, McKay DM, Phear WPC, et al.: The effects of halothane on pregnant and nonpregnant human myometrium. Anesthesiology 46:15, 1977.
6. Munson ES, Maier WR, Caton D: Effects of halothane, cyclopropane and nitrous oxide on isolated human uterine muscle. J Obstet Gynaecol Br Commonw 76:27, 1969.
7. Munson ES, Embro WJ: Enflurane, isoflurane, and halothane and isolated human uterine muscle. Anesthesiology 46:11, 1977.
8. Munson ES: Uterine activity and anesthesia. In *Obstetrical Anesthesia: Current Concepts and Practice*, SM Shnider, ed. Williams & Wilkins, Baltimore, 1969, p 29.
9. Marx GF, Kim YI, Lin CC, et al.: Postpartum uterine pressures under halothane or enflurane anesthesia. Obstet Gynecol 51:695, 1978.
10. Moir DD: Anaesthesia for caesarean section. An evaluation of a method using low concentrations of halothane and 50 per cent oxygen. Br J Anaesth 42:136, 1970.
11. Galbert MW, Gardner AE: Use of halothane in a balanced technique for cesarean section. Anesth Analg 51:701, 1972.
12. Coleman AJ, Downing JW: Enflurane anesthesia for cesarean section. Anesthesiology 43:354, 1975.
13. DeVoe SJ, DeVoe K Jr, Rigsby WC, et al.: Effect of meperidine on uterine contractility. Am J Obstet Gynecol 105:1004, 1969.
14. Filler WW Jr, Hall WC, Filler NW: Analgesia in obstetrics. Am J Obstet Gynecol 98:832, 1967.
15. Petrie RH, Wu R, Miller FC, et al.: The effect of drugs on uterine activity. Obstet Gynecol 48:431, 1976.
16. Galloon S: Ketamine and the pregnant uterus. Can Anaesth Soc J 20:141, 1973.
17. Marx GF, Hwang HS, Chandra P: Post-partum uterine pressures with different doses of ketamine. In *Abstracts of Scientific Papers*, Annual Meeting, American Society of Anesthesiologists, New Orleans, 1977, p 301.
18. Epstein BS, Banerjee S, Chamberlain G, et al.: The effect of the concentration of local anesthetic during epidural anesthesia on the forces of labor. Anesthesiology 29:187, 1968.
19. Evans JA, Chastain GM, Philips JM: The use of local anesthetic agents in obstetrics. South Med J 62:519, 1969.
20. Greiss FC, Still JG, Anderson SG: Effects of local anesthetic agents on the uterine vasculatures and myometrium. Am J Obstet Gynecol 124:889, 1976.
21. McGaughey HS Jr, Corey EL, Eastwood D, et al.: Effects of synthetic anesthetics on the spontaneous motility of human uterine muscles in vitro. Obstet Gynecol 19:233, 1962.
22. Feinstein MB: Inhibition of contraction and Ca^{++} exchangeability in rat uterus by local anesthetics. J Pharmacol Exp Ther 152:516, 1966.
23. Jenssen H: The shape of the amniotic pressure curve before and after paracervical block during labour. Acta Obstet Gynecol Scand (Suppl) 42:1, 1975.
24. Friedman EA, Sachtleben MR: Caudal anesthesia. The factors that influence its effect on labor. Obstet Gynecol 13:442, 1959.
25. Bonica JJ: Lumbar epidural versus caudal anesthesia. In *Obstetrical Anesthesia: Current Concepts and Practice*, SM Shnider, ed. Williams & Wilkins, Baltimore, 1969, p 73.
26. Lowensohn RI, Paul R, Fales S, et al.: Intrapartum epidural anesthesia: An evaluation of effects on uterine activity. Obstet Gynecol 44:388, 1974.
27. Zador G, Nilsson B: Low dose intermittent epidural anaesthesia with lidocaine for vaginal delivery. II. Influence on labour and foetal acid-base status. Acta Obstet Gynecol Scand (Suppl) 34:17, 1974.
28. Crawford JS: Patient management during extradural anaesthesia for obstetrics. Br J Anaesth 47:

273, 1975.
29. Schellenberg JS: Uterine activity during lumbar epidural analgesia with bupivacaine. Am J Obstet Gynecol 127:26, 1977.
30. Tyack AJ, Parsons RJ, Millar DR, et al.: Uterine activity and plasma bupivacaine levels after caudal epidural analgesia. J Obstet Gynaecol Br Commonw 80:896, 1973.
31. Craft JB, Epstein BS, Coakley CS: Effect of lidocaine with epinephrine versus lidocaine (plain) on induced labor. Anesth Analg 51:243, 1972.
32. Johnson WL, Winter WW, Eng M, et al.: Effect of pudendal, spinal and peridural block anesthesia on the second stage of labor. Am J Obstet Gynecol 113:166, 1972.
33. Malpas P: The pattern of the contractions of the pregnant uterus under spinal anaesthesia: The attendant changes in the reactivity of the myometrium. J Obstet Gynaecol Br Emp 51:112, 1944.
34. Phillips OC, Nelson AT, Lyons WB, et al.: Spinal anesthesia for vaginal delivery. Obstet Gynecol 13:437, 1959.
35. Reynolds SRM, Harris JS, Kaiser IH: *Clinical Measurement of Uterine Forces in Pregnancy and Labor.* Charles C Thomas, Springfield, Ill., 1954, p 232.
36. Alvarez H, Poseiro JJ, Pose SV, et al.: Effects of the anesthetic blockage of the spinal cord on the contractility of the pregnant human uterus. XXI International Congress of Physiological Sciences, Buenos Aires, 1959, p 14.
37. Berges PU: Regional anesthesia for obstetrics. In *Clinical Anesthesia,* JJ Bonica, F. A. Davis, Philadelphia, 1971, p 141.
38. Vasicka A, Kretchmer H: Effect of conduction and inhalation anesthesia on uterine contractions. Am J Obstet Gynecol 82:600, 1961.
39. Alfonsi PL, Massi GB: Effetti delgi anesthetici sulla contrattilita uterina. Riv Obstet Ginecol 18: 37, 1963.
40. Matadial L, Cibils LA: The effect of epidural anesthesia on uterine activity and blood pressure. Am J Obstet Gynecol 125:846, 1976.
41. Akamatsu TJ: Advances in obstetric anesthesiology during the period 1960–1970. In *Clinical Anesthesia: A Decade of Clinical Progress,* LW Fabian, ed. F. A. Davis, Philadelphia, 1971, p 222.
42. Cowles GT: Experiences with lumbar epidural block. Obstet Gynecol 26:734, 1965.
43. Moir DD, Willocks J: Management of incoordinate uterine action under continuous epidural analgesia. Br Med J 3:396, 1967.
44. Ruppert H: The influence of extradural spinal anesthesia on the motility of the gravid uterus. In *Proceedings of the First World Congress of Anesthesiologists.* Burgess, Minneapolis, 1956.
45. Cibils LA, Spackman TJ: Caudal analgesia in first-stage labor: Effect on uterine activity and the cardiovascular system. Am J Obstet Gynecol 84: 1042, 1962.
46. Hunter CA: Uterine motility studies during labor: Observations on bilateral sympathetic nerve block in the normal and abnormal first stage of labor. Am J Obstet Gynecol 85: 681, 1963.
47. Climie GR: The place of continuous lumbar epidural analgesia in the management of abnormally prolonged labour. Med J Aust 2:447, 1964.
48. Mercer WH, Simons EG, Philpott RH: The use of lumbar epidural analgesia during the first stage of labour in high risk pregnancies. S Afr Med J 48:774, 1974.
49. Moir DD: Continuous epidural analgesia in incoordinate uterine action. Acta Anaesthesiol Scand (Suppl) 23:144, 1966.
50. Moir DD, Willocks J: Management of incoordinate uterine action under continuous epidural analgesia. Br Med J 3:396, 1967.
51. Crawford JS: An appraisal of lumbar epidural blockade in labour in patients with multiple pregnancy. Br J Obstet Gynaecol 82:929, 1975.
52. Crawford JS: An appraisal of lumbar epidural blockade in patients with a singleton fetus presenting by the breech. J Obstet Gynaecol Br Commonw 81:867, 1974.
53. Donnai P, Nicholas AD: Epidural analgesia, fetal monitoring and the condition of the baby at birth with breech presentation. Br J Obstet Gynaecol 82:360, 1975.
54. Caldeyro-Barcia R, Alvarez H: Juicio critico y resultados de la induccion y conduccion del parto. III. Congr. Lat. Amer. Obst. Y. Ginec. Mexico 1958, p 131.
55. Belfrage P, Raabe N, Thalme B, et al.: Lumbar epidural analgesia with bupivacaine in labor. Determinations of drug concentration and pH in fetal scalp blood and continuous fetal heart rate monitoring. Am J Obstet Gynecol 121:360, 1975.
56. Pearson JF, Davies P: The effect of continuous lumbar epidural analgesia on the acid-base status of maternal arterial blood during the first stage of labour. J Obstet Gynaecol Br Commonw 80: 218, 1973.
57. Thalme B, Raabe N, Belfrage P: Lumbar epidural analgesia in labour. I. Acid-base balance and clinical condition of mother, fetus, and newborn child. Acta Obstet Gynecol Scand 53:27, 1974.
58. Thalme B, Raabe N, Belfrage P: Lumbar epidural analgesia in labour. II. Effects on glucose, lactate, sodium, chloride, total protein, haematocrit and haemoglobin in maternal, fetal, and neonatal blood. Acta Obstet Gynecol Scand 53:113, 1974.
59. Zador G, Willdeck-Lund G, Nillson BA: Continuous drip lumbar epidural anaesthesia in labour. II. Influence on labour and foetal acid-base status. Acta Obstet Gynecol Scand (Suppl) 34:41, 1974.
60. Hoult IJ: Lumbar epidural analgesia in labour: Relation to fetal malposition and instrumental delivery. Br Med J 6052:14, 1977.
61. Shnider SM: Experience with regional anesthesia for vaginal delivery. In *The Anesthesiologist, Mother and Newborn,* SM Shnider and F Moya, eds. Williams & Wilkins, Baltimore, 1974, p 38.
62. Van Derick G, Geerinckx K, Van Steenberge AL, et al.: Bupivacaine 0.125% in epidural block analgesia during childbirth: Clinical evaluation. Br J Anaesth 46:838, 1974.

63. Noble AD, deVere RD: Epidural analgesia in labour (Correspondence). Br Med J 2:296, 1970.
64. Gunther RE, Bauman J: Obstetrical caudal anesthesia. I. A randomized study comparing 1% lidocaine plus epinephrine. Anesthesiology 31:5, 1969.
65. Gunther RE, Bellville JW: Obstetrical caudal anesthesia. II. A randomized study comparing 1 per cent mepivacaine with 1 per cent mepivacaine plus epinephrine. Anesthesiology 37:288, 1972.
66. Covino BG, Vassallo HG: *Local Anesthetics: Mechanisms of Action and Clinical Use.* Grune & Stratton, New York, 1976, p 104.
67. Lund PC, Cwik JC, Gannon RT: Extradural anaesthesia: Choice of local anaesthetic agents. Br J Anaesth 47:313, 1975.
68. Mather LE, Tucker GT, Murphy TM, et al.: The effects of adding adrenaline to etidocaine and lignocaine in extradural anaesthesia. II. Pharmacokinetics. Br J Anaesth 48:989, 1976.

CHAPTER 5

Perinatal Pharmacology

David H. Ralston, M.D.

Perinatal pharmacology is concerned with the classic pharmacologic processes of drug absorption, distribution, biotransformation and excretion, not in one individual but in two—the mother and the fetus.[1-4] The perinatal period begins with the pre-implantation blastocyst and extends to the neonate at 28 days of age. The discovery of vaginal adenosis in young women whose mothers were exposed to diethylstilbesterol during pregnancy[5] demonstrates the long-term effect that drugs administered during the perinatal period are capable of producing. This chapter will focus on the period of parturition and the effect of anesthetic drugs on the fetus and neonate. The basic concepts of placental drug transfer (absorption),[6] fetal and neonatal disposition of anesthetic drugs (distribution, biotransformation, excretion)[7,8] and the clinical implications of anesthetic drug effects on the newborn[9] will be examined. Because local anesthetics are among the most commonly used group of drugs in obstetrics and are currently being studied extensively throughout the world, their pharmacology will be used to illustrate principles of perinatal pharmacology.

DETERMINANTS OF PLACENTAL TRANSFER

To achieve a physiologic effect, a critical concentration of "free" drug, i.e. non-ionized and non-protein-bound, must arrive at and react with a given tissue receptor site[6-8,10] (Figure 5.1). To reach the fetus, maternally administered drug must first traverse the placenta, a process determined by maternal, placental and fetal factors (Figure 5.2).

Maternal Factors

Drug delivery to the placental exchange site depends on the fraction of total uterine blood flow which perfuses the intervillous space. Total uterine blood flow in humans at term has been estimated at approximately 150 ml/min/kg of total weight of gravid uterus.[11] In the sheep, total uterine blood flow is 250 to 350 ml/min/kg,[12] and approximately 80 per cent perfuses the intervillous space[13] (Figure 5.3). A similar distribution probably exists in humans.

Little information is available on how changes in maternal hemodynamics alter delivery of drug to the placenta. To illustrate the complexity of this process, assume that a drug is injected as a bolus into venous blood of a woman in active labor. During the peak of a uterine contraction, uterine arterial flow ceases; hence, the drug would theoretically be unable to reach the placenta, at least during the first maternal circulation time. However, if the drug arrived at the onset or decline of a uterine contraction when only uterine venous outflow was impeded, the drug could be sequestered in the intervillous space and potentially cross the placenta to a greater extent. The supine position with its attendant vena caval or aortic obstruc-

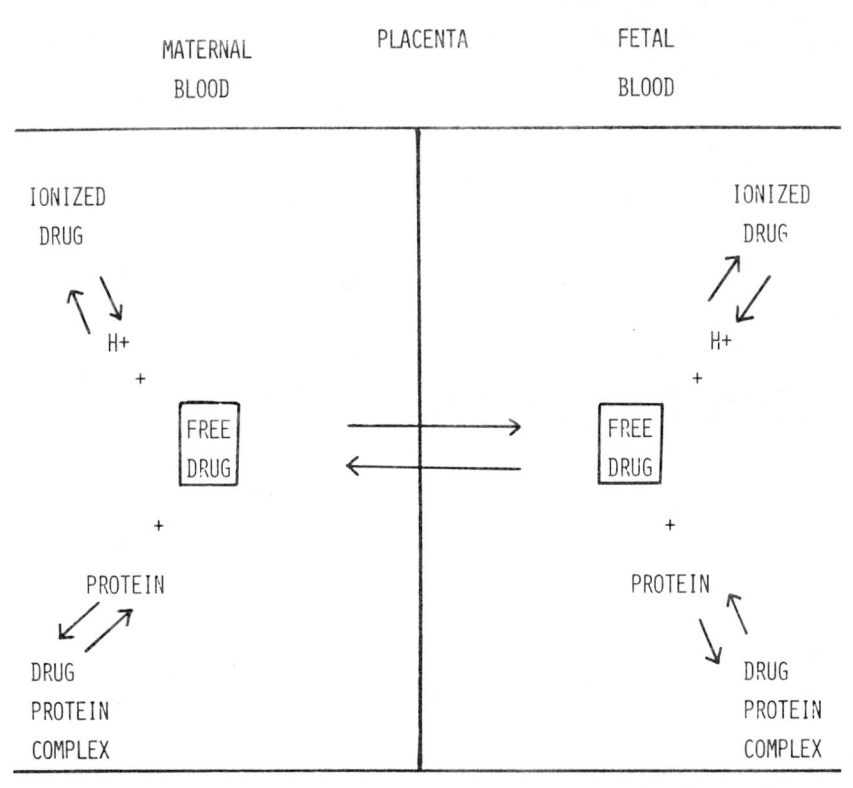

Figure 5.1. Drug in blood or tissue exists in several forms: ionized, protein-bound, or as the non-ionized, non-protein-bound free form. It is this lipid-soluble, free form of the drug which readily passes biological membranes such as the placenta.

tion could also alter drug delivery to the placenta. Maternal hypotension or hypertension may also affect delivery of drug to the placenta to an unknown extent.

The uterine artery concentration of "free drug" (Cm) which arrives at the intervillous space is itself dependent on several factors (Table 5.1).

Increasing the total dose of drug, irrespective of the route of administration, increases the maternal arterial blood concentration.[14] Fetal drug blood concentration increases as well.

Injection of local anesthetic into the highly vascular caudal epidural space results in higher peak maternal blood levels than occur after lumbar epidural administration,[15] whereas maternal concentrations of local anesthetics are similar after injection into the lumbar epidural, pudendal or paracervical areas.[16]

Epinephrine reduces the peak maternal local anesthetic concentration by 30 to 50 per cent with lidocaine or mepivacaine but has little effect on peak levels of bupivacaine or etidocaine[14, 17] (Figure 5.4).

Maternal metabolism and elimination

Table 5.1
Factors Which Determine the Concentration of Free Drug in Uterine Arterial Blood

Total dose
Route of administration
Presence of epinephrine in anesthetic solution
Maternal metabolism and excretion
Maternal protein binding
Maternal pH and pKa of drug

PERINATAL PHARMACOLOGY

Delivery   **Transfer (Diffusion)**   **Uptake**

Maternal Shunt — Uterine Artery — C_m — C_f — Umbilical Artery — Fetal Shunt — Uterine Vein — Umbilical Vein

Maternal
A. Blood flow to IVS
B. Uterine artery concentrations of "free drug" (C_m)

Placental
$$C/t = K \cdot A \frac{C_m - C_f}{X}$$
(Fick's Law of Passive Diffusion)

Fetal
A. Blood flow to IVS
B. Umbilical artery concentration of "free drug" (C_f)

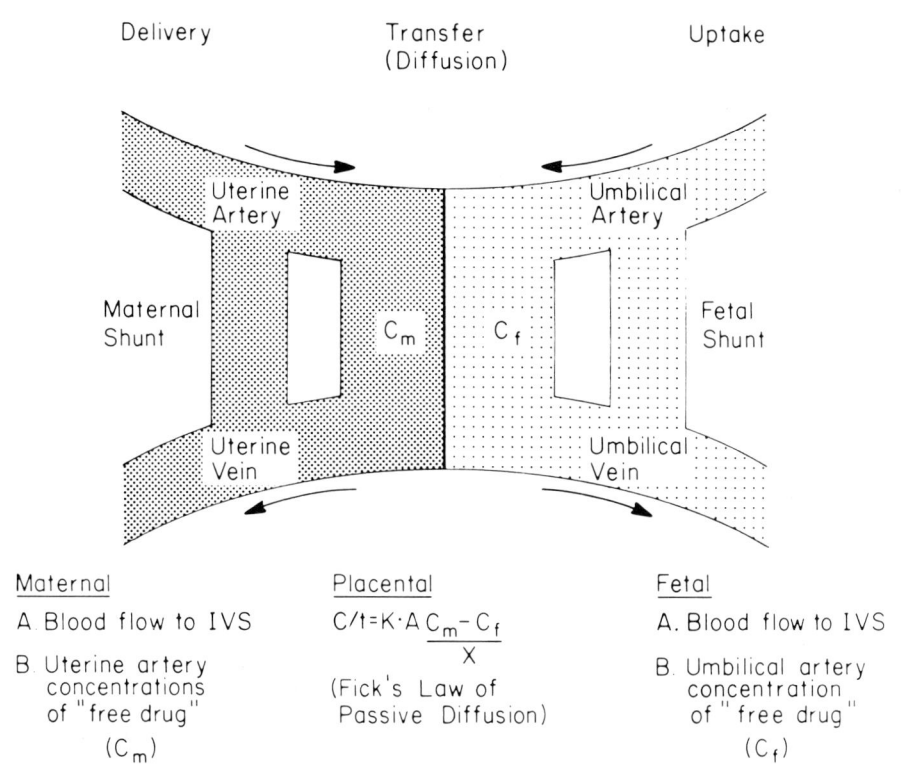

Figure 5.2. A schematic diagram of the placental exchange site and the maternal, placental and fetal factors which influence drug transfer and fetal drug uptake. *IVS*, intervillous space; *c/t*, rate of diffusion; *K*, diffusion constant of drug and membrane; *A*, surface available for transfer; *Cm*, drug concentration in maternal blood; *Cf*, drug concentration in fetal blood; *X*, thickness of membrane.

reduce drug concentrations at the intervillous space. In human volunteers, the elimination half-lives for the commonly administered local anesthetics range from 1½ hours for lidocaine to 3½ hours for bupivacaine.[18] Detailed pharmacokinetic studies in pregnant females have not been possible, although available data suggest an elimination half-life of 60 to 90 minutes for lidocaine after intravenous bolus administration of 3.0 mg/kg.[16] When bupivacaine is administered epidurally for cesarean section, the drug disappears from maternal blood in two phases, an initial rapid elimination with a half-life of 47 minutes and a slow elimination with a half-life of 9 hours.[19]

Maternal protein binding of local anesthetic varies with the individual drug and its concentration (Figure 5.5). At the usually encountered clinical concentrations, the percentage of binding for lidocaine or mepivacaine is 50 to 70 per cent and for bupivacaine and etidocaine is 95 per cent.[18, 20] The higher degree of protein binding with bupivacaine and etidocaine may impede placental transfer by reducing the concentration of free drug available for diffusion (Figure 5.1). In fact, several authors[9,21] have attributed the lower umbilical cord to maternal vessel concentration ratios of bupivacaine and etidocaine to high maternal serum protein binding. However, the rate of drug-protein dissocia-

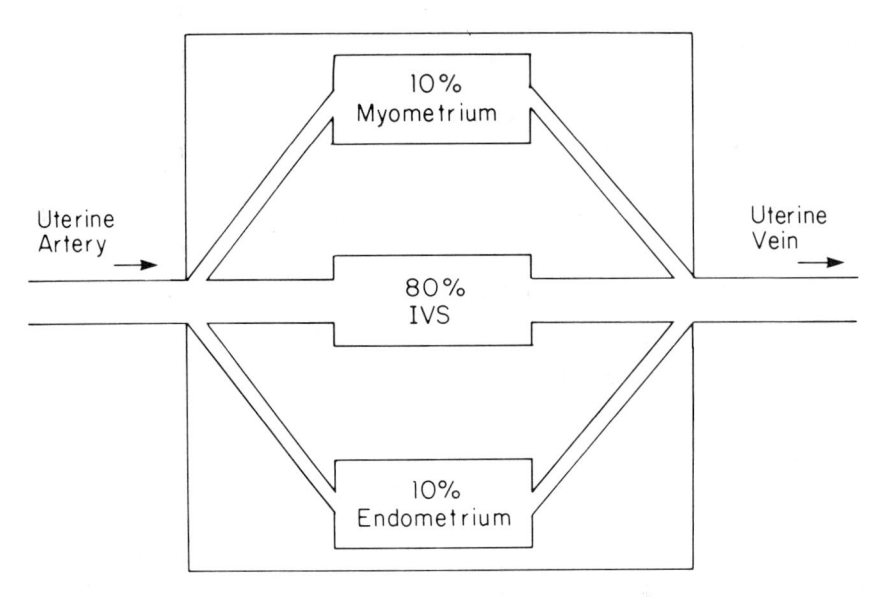

Figure 5.3. The distribution of uterine blood flow in the pregnant sheep. A similar distribution may occur in the human. (Modified from Makowski EL, Meschia G, Droegemueller W, et al.: Distribution of uterine blood flow in the pregnant sheep. Am J Obstet Gynecol 101: 409, 1968.)

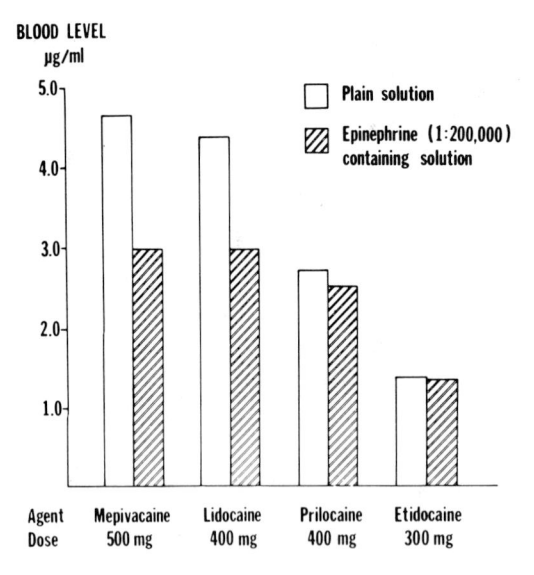

Figure 5.4. The peak concentration of various local anesthetics after epidural administration with and without epinephrine. (Reprinted by permission from Covino BG, Vassallo HG: *Local Anesthetics: Mechanisms of Action and Clinical Use.* Grune & Stratton, New York, 1976, p 104.)

tion is also important in assessing the significance of local anesthetic protein binding. Tucker[20] suggested that protein binding of local anesthetic does not significantly impede diffusion of drug across the placenta, because the dissociation of drug from protein is essentially instantaneous. Supporting the thesis that a high degree of local anesthetic protein binding may not impede placental transfer is the work of Morishima et al.,[22] who measured blood and tissue local anesthetic levels in pregnant guinea pigs after maternal intravenous administration of lidocaine or etidocaine. Despite the higher percentage of protein binding of etidocaine compared to lidocaine, these investigators found similar fetal tissue levels for both drugs, implying a similar degree of placental transfer.

The pKa of a drug is the pH at which 50 per cent of drug is ionized and 50 per cent is non-ionized. Because most local anesthetics and narcotics are weak bases, with pKa's above the maternal pH, a significant

PERINATAL PHARMACOLOGY

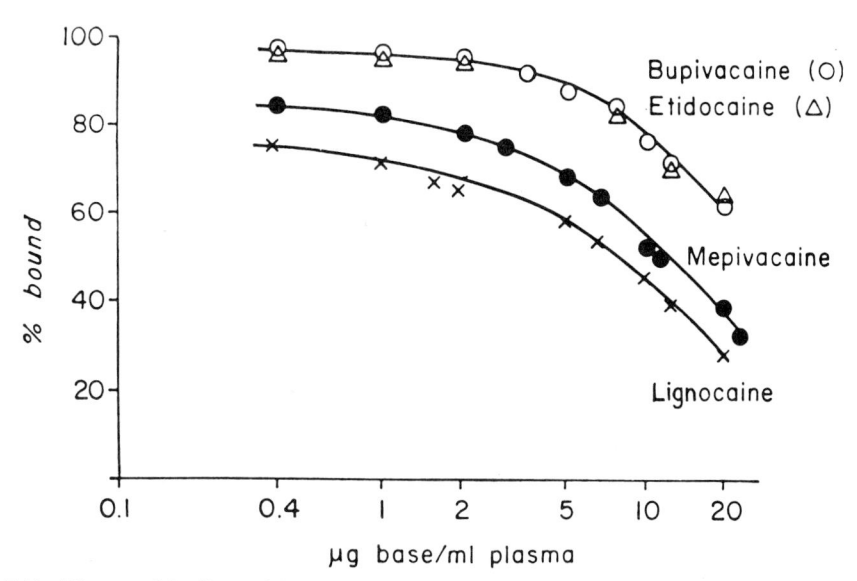

Figure 5.5. Plasma binding of four anilide local anesthetics at plasma concentrations of 0.4 to 20 μg/ml. (Reprinted by permission from Tucker GT, Mather LE: Pharmacokinetics of local anesthetic agents. Br J Anaesth 47: 213, 1975.)

quantity of these drugs exist as the lipid-soluble, non-ionized form in maternal blood.

Placental Factors

Once a given drug has reached the intervillous space, the quantity transferred per unit time is described by Fick's equation of passive diffusion[23] (Figure 5.2). Expressed mathematically,

$$Q/t = K \cdot A \frac{Cm - Cf}{X}$$

where K is a diffusion constant determined by drug physicochemical properties such as molecular weight, lipid solubility, degree of ionization and spatial configuration. This equation states that the amount of transfer is proportional to the free-drug concentration difference between maternal and fetal blood and the surface area available for diffusion and is inversely related to the thickness of the membrane. At equilibrium the concentration of free drug on both sides of the membrane is equal. Therefore, placental drug transfer is facilitated by a high concentration of non-ionized, lipid-soluble, non-protein-bound drug. High molecular weight, poor lipid solubility, and a high degree of ionization will impede but not totally prevent the transfer of a drug across the placenta. Muscle relaxants such as curare and succinylcholine which are highly ionized do cross the placenta but only to a limited extent.[24, 25]

Despite the usefulness of Fick's law of diffusion in describing the transfer of anesthetic drug across the placenta[6] the law assumes that membrane characteristics remain constant. Local or general anesthetics interact with and physically change lipid membrane properties such as fluidity and structure[26] and, therefore, may change diffusion constants. Nevertheless, from a clinical standpoint, Fick's law is important in that it emphasizes the role played by Cm, i.e. the maternal concentration of drug. This is the quantity in Fick's equation that anesthesiologists can control so readily.

Fetal Factors

Fetal uptake, distribution, metabolism and elimination determine drug disposition and physiologic effects once a drug has diffused across the placental exchange site.

FETAL UPTAKE OF DRUGS

Fetal uptake is determined by solubility of the drug in fetal blood (which includes drug dissolved in plasma water as well as drug bound to red cell and plasma protein components); the quantity and distribution of fetal blood flow to the intervillous space; and the concentration of drug in fetal blood returning to the placenta (Figure 5.2). In addition, the pH gradient existing between maternal and fetal blood influences the concentration of drug at equilibrium. For example, local anesthetics are weak bases, with pKa's ranging from 7.6 for mepivacaine to 8.9 for procaine. At a higher hydrogen ion concentration (or lower pH) more local anesthetic exists in the ionized state. At pH 7.40 lidocaine is 24 per cent non-ionized, whereas at pH 7.0, 11 per cent exists in the non-ionized form. Thus a 0.40 pH gradient would cause a 54 per cent increase in the amount of ionized drug. Such a pH gradient may exist between a mother and an asphyxiated fetus. Because the ionized form of the drug does not pass through lipid membranes as readily as the lipid-soluble, non-ionized form, a weakly basic drug may accumulate in the more acid fetal blood. Recent clinical and laboratory evidence suggests that this phenomenon of "ion-trapping" may indeed occur. Brown et al.[27] found high umbilical vein (UV) to maternal vein (MV) concentration ratios of lidocaine and mepivacaine in neonates with umbilical artery pH values of 7.03 to 7.23. Biehl et al.[28] induced acidosis in fetal lambs during constant-rate lidocaine infusion into the mother. Higher fetal blood lidocaine concentrations were seen during fetal acidosis (pH 6.90 to 7.18) than when fetal pH was normal (7.30 to 7.35). Correction of fetal acidosis with bicarbonate (fetal pH 7.22 to 7.40) resulted in a decrease in fetal blood lidocaine concentration (Figure 5.6). Although "ion trapping" may account for the higher fetal blood levels of local anes-

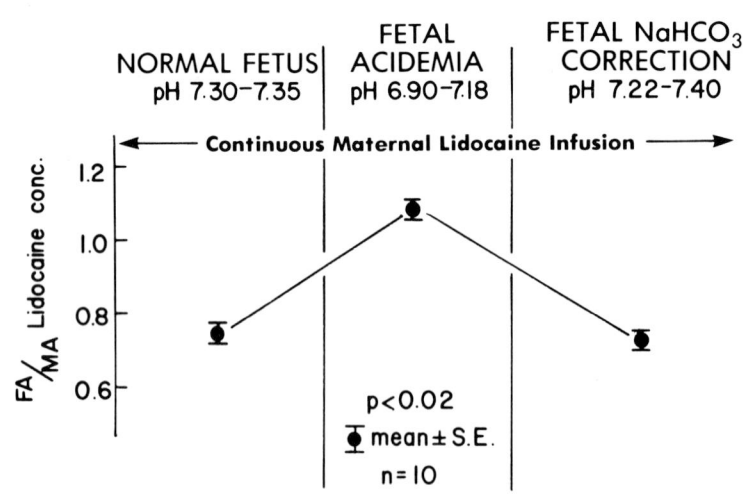

Figure 5.6. Fetal to maternal arterial (*FA/MA*) lidocaine ratios were significantly higher during fetal acidemia than during control or during pH correction with bicarbonate. (Reprinted by permission from Biehl D, Shnider SM, Levinson G, et al.: Placental transfer of lidocaine: Effects of fetal acidosis. Anesthesiology 48: 409, 1978.)

thetics and narcotics, reduced fetal clearance of these drugs due to alterations in fetal cardiac output, umbilical or hepatic blood flow or changes in the blood to tissue distribution of these drugs during metabolic acidosis might also explain the observed findings. Tissue levels of lidocaine in the non-pregnant adult rabbit during metabolic or respiratory acidosis, for example, are higher than those in blood.[29]

Fetal umbilical blood flow to the placental exchange site is obviously essential for fetal drug uptake (Figure 5.7). Fetal placental flow in the lamb is 200 to 250 ml/min/kg body weight, representing approximately 50 per cent (Figure 5.8) of the combined ventricular output.[12, 30] The fraction of combined ventricular output perfusing the placenta increases with fetal asphyxia[31] and may decrease with cord compression. The influence of changes in the quantity of fetal umbilical blood flow on fetal drug absorption is unknown. Further complicating the understanding of hemodynamic factors in fetal drug uptake is the non-homogeneity of maternal and fetal blood flow in the placenta.[32, 33] Inasmuch as most anesthetic drugs (similar to O_2 placental transfer) cross the placenta by a process of flow-dependent passive diffusion, changes in the maternal to fetal circulation ratios in various parts of the placenta undoubtedly modulate drug transfer. Little information is available in this area.

FETAL DISTRIBUTION OF DRUGS

The fetal circulation is unique in several ways and greatly modifies drug distribution (Figure 5.9). Umbilical venous blood returning from the placenta either perfuses the liver or flows through the ductus venosus.[34] Fetal hepatic perfusion may protect against attainment of high drug levels on the arterial side of the fetal circulation.[35, 36] Dilution of umbilical venous blood in the fetal right atrium and shunting of blood

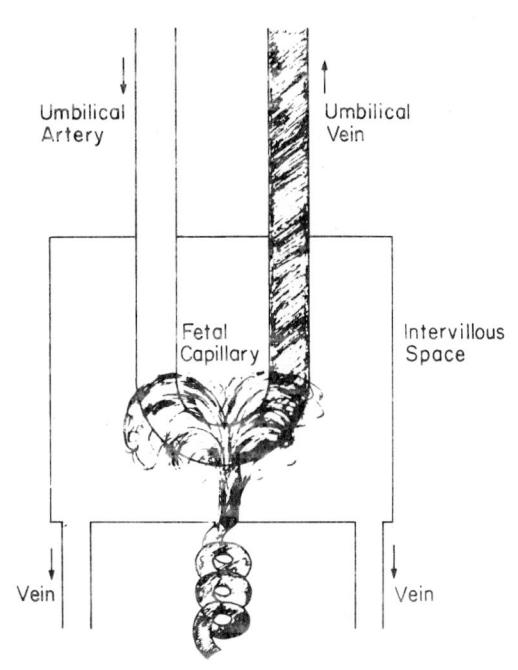

Figure 5.7. Circulatory pathways at the intervillous space. The fetal umbilical artery carries blood to the intervillous space, where exchange of oxygen, carbon dioxide and drug occurs. The maternal spinal artery enters at the base, and fountain-like spurts of blood bathe the branching villi which contain fetal capillaries. Blood returns to the fetus via the umbilical vein, while uterine veins drain maternal blood from the intervillous space. Hemodynamic alterations may occur at several sites: umbilical artery or vein (cord compression); intervillous space (fetal capillary compression with increased intrauterine pressure); uterine vein (vena caval obstruction with a parturient in the supine position); or uterine artery (spinal hypotension or α-adrenergic stimulation). How hemodynamic changes influence placental transfer is poorly understood.

across the foramen ovale and ductus arteriosus also modify fetal drug distribution.

The concentration of drug returning to the placenta in umbilical arterial blood (Cf) is determined by the quantity of drug entering the fetal circulation (the input), fetal tissue uptake, fetal pH, protein binding mepivacaine during caudal anesthesia, postmortem tissue drug concentrations in liver, brain and kidney[37] were many times greater than blood concentrations.

Fetal red blood cell and serum proteins bind local anesthetics to a lesser degree than do maternal red cells and proteins.[38] This may be clinically significant because at a given total drug concentration, more drug would be in the unbound free form, the fraction presumably responsible for physiologic effects[17] (Figure 5.10).

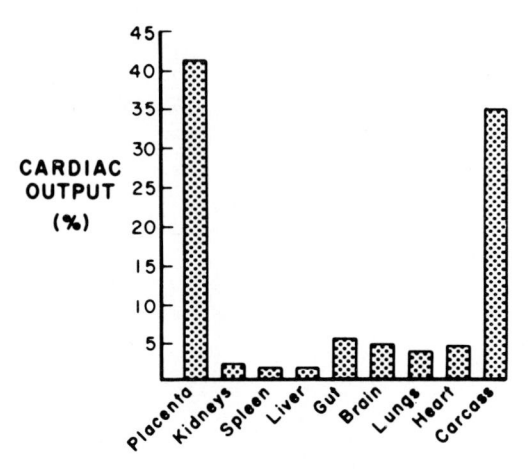

Figure 5.8. Per cent distribution of combined ventricular output in fetal lamb near term (measured with radioactive microspheres). (Reprinted by permission from Pang LM, Mellins RB: Neonatal cardiorespiratory physiology. Anesthesiology 43: 171, 1975.)

FETAL METABOLISM AND EXCRETION OF DRUGS

Fetal hepatic enzyme activity is generally less than in adults. Oxidative and conjugative detoxification pathways, both of which are involved in the metabolism of

Table 5.2
Factors Which Determine the Concentration of Free Drug in Fetal Umbilical Arterial Blood (Cf)

Umbilical venous blood concentration (input)
Fetal pH
Fetal protein binding
Fetal tissue uptake
Non-placental routes of fetal drug elimination
    Fetal hepatic metabolism
    Fetal renal excretion

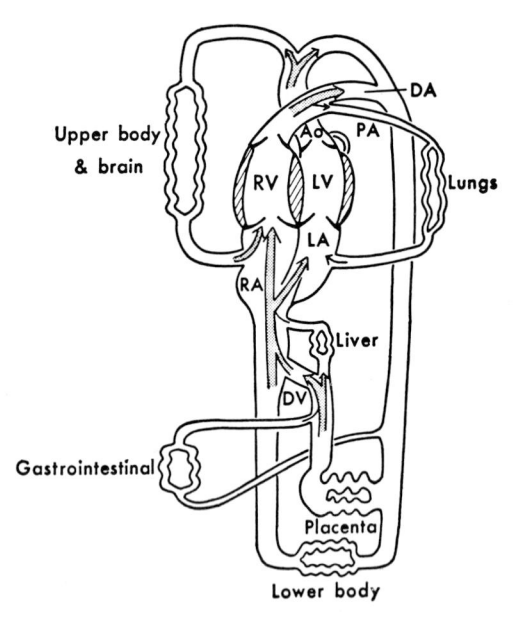

Figure 5.9. The fetal circulation. (Reprinted by permission from Rudolph AM: *Congenital Disease of the Heart*. Year Book Medical Publishers, Chicago, 1974.)

and, possibly, non-placental routes of fetal drug elimination (Table 5.2). Fetal tissue affinity for local anesthetics is high.[35] After inadvertent direct fetal administration of

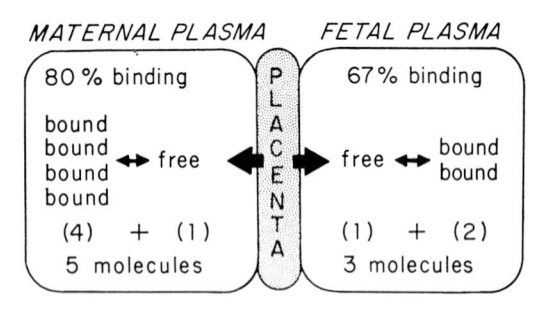

Figure 5.10. Differential protein binding of drug by maternal and fetal blood would account for differences in *total* drug concentrations on both sides of the placenta when free drug concentrations were, in fact, equal. (Reprinted by permission from DeJong RH: *Local Anesthetics*. Charles C Thomas, Springfield, Ill., 1976, p 204.)

Table 5.3
Percentage of Neonates with High Scores Following Either No Maternal Extradural Anesthesia or Maternal Extradural Anesthesia with Chloroprocaine, Bupivacaine, Lidocaine or Mepivacaine.

	Nonextradural (n = 13)	Chloroprocaine (n = 69)	Bupivacaine (n = 20)	Lidocaine or Mepivacaine (n = 28)
Age on examination	8 hr	4–24 hr	2–4 hr	8 hr
Tone	100	97	95	57*
Rooting	85	77	85	46†
Moro response	100	97	100	50*
Habituation: pinprick	100	97	100	82†

* $p < .01$.
† $p < .05$.
(Reprinted by permission from Brown WU Jr: Guest discussion. In Hodgkinson R, Marx GF, Kim SS, et al.: Neonatal neurobehavioral tests following vaginal delivery under ketamine, thiopental, and extradural anesthesia. Anesth Analg (56: 548, 1977.)

many drugs, are deficient in the fetal or neonatal animal.[39] In humans, although fetal metabolism of amide local anesthetics has not been studied, indirect evidence suggests that the human fetus can metabolize these drugs. Although hepatic cytochrome P-450 activity is absent in fetuses of several animal species either early or late in gestation, human fetal liver microsomes have significant cytochrome P-450 levels and NADPH cytochrome C reductase as early as the fourteenth week of gestation.[3, 40, 41] This suggests that even the premature human fetus can metabolize numerous drugs, including most local anesthetics. However, for some local anesthetics, such as mepivacaine, human **neonatal** metabolism appears very limited or non-existent and the drug is excreted via the kidney unchanged.[42]

ANESTHETIC EFFECTS ON THE NEONATE

Traditionally, neonatal drug effects have been assessed by Apgar scores, time-to-sustained respiration and umbilical cord blood gases. Recently a neonatal neurobehavioral examination[43-45] has been developed and used to evaluate the newborn after maternal administration of a variety of drugs. Subtle, although transient, neurobehavioral changes in infants born after maternal epidural anesthesia with lidocaine or mepivacaine have been demonstrated. Similar neurobehavioral changes do not occur after maternal epidural administration of bupivacaine,[45] 2-chloroprocaine[46] or etidocaine[47] (Table 5.3). The neonatal effects of drugs will be discussed in detail in later chapters.

References

1. Finnegan L: Clinical effects of pharmacologic agents on pregnancy, the fetus, and the neonate. Ann NY Acad Sci 281:74, 1976.
2. Mirkin BL: Research goals in developmental pharmacology. In *Perinatal Pharmacology: Problems and Priorities*, J Dancis and JC Hewang, eds. Raven Press, New York, 1974, p 221.
3. Yaffe SJ, Juchau MP: Perinatal pharmacology. Annu Rev Pharmacol 14:219, 1974.
4. Yaffe SJ, Stern L: Clinical implications of perinatal pharmacology. In *Perinatal Pharmacology and Therapeutics*, BL Mirkin, ed. Academic Press, New York, 1976, p 355.
5. Herbst AL, Ulfelder H, Paskanzer DC: Adenocarcinoma of the vagina. Association of maternal stilbesterol therapy with tumor appearance in young women. N Engl J Med 284:878, 1971.
6. Mirkin BL, Singh S: Placental transfer of pharmacologically active molecules. In *Perinatal Pharmacology and Therapeutics*, BL Mirkin, ed. Academic Press, New York, 1976, p 1.
7. Mirkin BL: Drug distribution in pregnancy. In *Fetal Pharmacology*, L Boréus, ed. Raven Press, New York, 1973, p 1.
8. Mirkin BL: Maternal and fetal distribution of drugs in pregnancy. Clin Pharmacol Ther 14:643, 1973.

9. Levinson G, Shnider SM: Placental transfer of local anesthetics: Clinical implications. In *Parturition and Perinatology*, GF Marx, ed. F. A. Davis, Philadelphia, 1973, p 173.
10. Mirkin BL: Perinatal pharmacology: Placental transfer, fetal localization, and neonatal disposition of drugs. Anesthesiology 43:156, 1975.
11. Assali NS, Douglass RA, Baird WM, et al.: Measurement of uterine metabolism. IV. Results in normal pregnancy. Am J Obstet Gynecol 66:248, 1953.
12. Comline RS, Silver M: Placental transfer of blood gases. Br Med Bull 31:25, 1975.
13. Makowski EL, Meschia G, Droegemueller W, et al.: Distribution of uterine blood flow in the pregnant sheep. Am J Obstet Gynecol 101:409, 1968.
14. Covino BG, Vassallo HG: *Local Anesthetics: Mechanisms of Action and Clinical Use*. Grune & Stratton, New York, 1976, p 100.
15. Lund PC, Bush DF, Covino BG: Determinants of etidocaine concentration in the blood. Anesthesiology 42:497, 1975.
16. Shnider SM, Way EL: The kinetics of transfer of lidocaine (Xylocaine®) across the human placenta. Anesthesiology 29:944, 1968.
17. DeJong RH: *Local Anesthetics*. Charles C Thomas, Springfield, Ill., 1977, p 197.
18. Tucker GT, Mather LE: Pharmacokinetics of local anesthetic agents. Br J Anaesth 47:213, 1975.
19. Magno R, Berlin A, Karrlson K, et al.: Anesthesia for cesarean section. IV. Placental transfer and neonatal elimination of bupivacaine following epidural analgesia for elective cesarean section. Acta Anaesth Scand 20:141, 1976.
20. Tucker GT: Plasma binding and disposition of local anesthetics. Int Anesthesiol Clin 13:33, 1975.
21. Poppers PJ: Evaluation of local anaesthetic agents for regional anaesthesia in obstetrics. Br J Anaesth 47:322, 1975.
22. Morishima HO, Finster M, Pedersen H, et al.: Placental transfer and tissue distribution of etidocaine and lidocaine in guinea pigs. In *Abstracts of Scientific Papers*, Annual Meeting, American Society of Anesthesiologists, Chicago, 1975, p 83.
23. Gillette JR, Stripp B: Pre- and postnatal enzyme capacity for drug metabolite production. Fed Proc 34:172, 1975.
24. Drábková J, Crul JF, van der Kleihn E: Placental transfer of ^{14}C labelled succinylcholine in near-term Macaca mulatta monkeys. Br J Anaesth 45:1087, 1973.
25. Kivalo I, Saarikoski S: Placental transfer of ^{14}C-dimethyl tubocurarine during caesarean section. Br J Anaesth 48:239, 1976.
26. Strichartz G: Molecular mechanisms of nerve block by local anesthetics. Anesthesiology 45:421, 1976.
27. Brown WU Jr, Bell GC, Alper MH: Acidosis, local anesthetics and the newborn. Obstet Gynecol 48:27, 1976.
28. Biehl D, Shnider SM, Levinson G, et al.: Placental transfer of lidocaine: Effects of fetal acidosis. Anesthesiology 48:409, 1978.
29. Sjöstrand U, Widman B: Distribution of bupivacaine in the rabbit under normal and acidotic conditions. Acta Anaesth Scand (Suppl) 50:5, 1973.
30. Rudolph AM, Heymann MA: The circulation of the fetus in utero. Circ Res 21:163, 1967.
31. Rudolph AM: *Congenital Disease of the Heart*. Year Book Medical Publishers, Chicago, 1974, p 1.
32. Power GG, Hill EP, Longo LD: Analysis of uneven distribution of diffusing capacity and blood flow in the placenta. Am J Physiol 222:740, 1972.
33. Power GG, Longo LD, Wagner NN, et al.: Uneven distribution of maternal and fetal placental blood flow, as demonstrated using macroaggregates, and its response to hypoxia. J Clin Invest 46:2053, 1967.
34. Pang LM, Mellins RB: Neonatal cardiorespiratory physiology. Anesthesiology 43:171, 1975.
35. Finster M, Morishima HO, Boyes RN, et al.: The placental transfer of lidocaine and its uptake by fetal tissues. Anesthesiology 36:159, 1972.
36. Finster M, Morishima HO, Mark LC, et al.: Tissue thiopental concentrations in the fetus and newborn. Anesthesiology 36:155, 1972.
37. Sinclair JC, Fox HA, Lentz UF, et al.: Intoxication of the fetus by a local anesthetic, a newly recognized complication of maternal caudal anesthesia. N Engl J Med 273:1173, 1965.
38. Mather LE, Long G, Thomas J: The binding of bupivacaine to maternal and foetal plasma proteins. J Pharm Pharmacol 23:359, 1971.
39. Dawkins MJ: Biochemical aspects of developing function in newborn mammalian liver. Br Med Bull 22:27, 1966.
40. Waddell WJ, Marlowe GC: Disposition of drugs in the fetus. In *Perinatal Pharmacology and Therapeutics*, BL Mirkin, ed. Academic Press, New York, 1976, p 119.
41. Yaffe SJ: Developmental factors influencing interactions of drugs. Ann NY Acad Sci 281:90, 1976.
42. Brown WU Jr, Bell GC, Lurie AO, et al.: Newborn blood levels of lidocaine and mepivacaine in the first postnatal day following maternal epidural anesthesia. Anesthesiology 42:698, 1975.
43. Scanlon JW, Alper MH: Perinatal pharmacology and evaluation of the newborn. Int Anesthesiol Clin 11:163, 1973.
44. Scanlon JW, Brown WU Jr, Weiss JB, et al.: Neurobehavioral responses of newborn infants after maternal epidural anesthesia. Anesthesiology 40:121, 1974.
45. Scanlon JW, Ostheimer GW, Lurie AO, et al.: Neurobehavioral responses and drug concentrations in newborns after maternal epidural anesthesia with bupivacaine. Anesthesiology 45:400, 1976.
46. Hodgkinson R, Marx GF, Kim SS, et al.: Neonatal neurobehavioral tests following vaginal delivery under ketamine, thiopental, and extradural anesthesia. Anesth Analg 56:548, 1977.
47. Lund PC, Cwik JC, Gannon RT, et al.: Etidocaine for caesarean section—effects on mother and baby. Br J Anaesth 49:457, 1977.

SECTION TWO

ANESTHESIA FOR VAGINAL DELIVERY

CHAPTER 6

Psychological Anesthesia for Obstetrics

Jay S. DeVore, M.D.

The experience of childbirth ranges from agony to ecstasy. For many women fear and anxiety contribute to the pain generated by uterine contractions, cervical dilation and perineal distension. Therefore, especially in recent years, there has been increasing emphasis placed on education and preparation for childbirth and on psychological methods of anesthesia. There is a growing belief that preparation for childbirth can diminish the amount of anesthetic and analgesic drugs used during labor and delivery. Furthermore, in the prepared mother, childbirth is more likely to be an enjoyable experience which will influence maternal feelings towards her child for years to come. Preparation of the father, so that both parents may participate in the birth of the child, has also become popular.

A number of different methods of psychological anesthesia have been used with varying degrees of success. These include (1) hypnosis; (2) "natural childbirth," as described by Dick-Read in his book, *Childbirth without Fear*[1]; (3) "psychoprophylaxis," as described by Lamaze in his book *Painless Childbirth*[2]; (4) acupuncture; (5) the LeBoyer technique as described in his book *Birth without Violence*.[3] These techniques have been used with a variety of combinations and modifications.

HYPNOSIS

Hypnosis has been used as a method of pain relief in childbirth for many years.[4] The hypnoidal trance achieves maternal analgesia with no obstruction of airway reflexes or hypotension and no drug depression of the neonate.[5] Furthermore, several investigators have claimed that hypnosis shortens labor[6] and that the acid-base status of the neonate is better at birth and in the hour following than if general anesthesia is used[5] (Figure 6.1).

Patients who may be candidates for hypnosis, namely those with extreme anxiety or in whom there might be contraindications to more conventional anesthetic techniques, can be evaluated for hypnotic suggestibility by any of several techniques. The eye roll test of Speigel[7] is simple and reliable. Those with high susceptibility can be conditioned for full hypnoanalgesia but those with low susceptibility should be cautioned that supplemental chemical anesthesia may be necessary.

Preparation of the patient for hypnosis for childbirth consists of a series of conditioning sessions approximately 30 minutes in length. With each session greater degrees of trance are induced until a level of analgesia, generally of the hand, is achieved. The patient is then conditioned to transfer the analgesia from the hand to the abdomen and perineum to provide pain relief for labor and delivery. The well conditioned patient will be able to perform these maneuvers without the hypnotist actually being present at the time of delivery.

Hypnoanalgesia for childbirth is not widely used currently. Aside from the

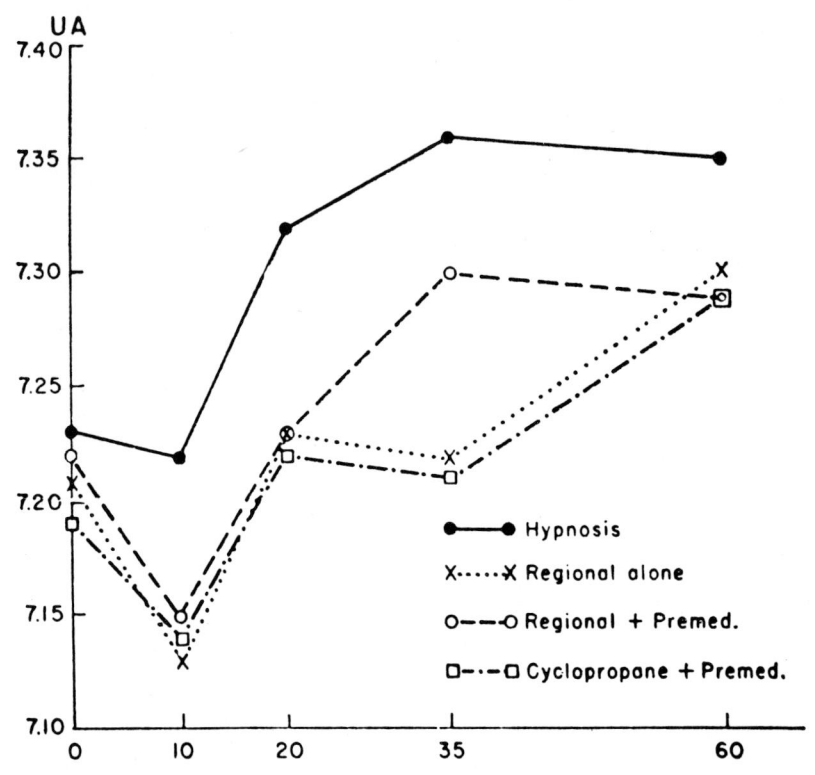

Figure 6.1. Mean serial arterial blood pH values in first hour after birth. Umbilical artery (*UA*) blood averages are plotted at zero time. Time in minutes is shown on *horizontal axis*; pH is shown on *vertical axis*. (Reprinted by permission from Moya F, James LS: Medical hypnosis for obstetrics. JAMA 174:2026, 1960.)

time-consuming aspects of hypnosis, occasional undesirable effects have been noted. Rosen[8] described the danger of hypnosis practiced by improperly trained physicians. Wahl[9] reported complications of hypnosis in obstetrics which ranged from states of acute anxiety to frank psychosis. He suggested as strong contraindications to the use of hypnosis for childbirth: history of psychosis or psychoneurotic hysterical conversion reactions; ambivalence regarding birth or motherhood; nightmares in the last trimester.

NATURAL CHILDBIRTH

Other methods of psychological analgesia have been more widely used than hypnosis. The "natural childbirth" method of Dick-Read,[1] popular in the 1940's, was rather authoritarian and relied on psychological principles that are not totally compatible with today's thinking. The basis of his approach was that anxiety, fear and pain were interlinked and that a simple and fearless approach to labor could render it painless. He believed that during complicated labor uterine contractions should be painless because "there is no physiologic function in the body which gives rise to pain in the normal course of health."[1]

PSYCHOPROPHYLAXIS

The psychoprophylactic method of Lamaze[2] is currently the most popular technique. This technique relies on positive conditioning and the education of the patient regarding the process of childbirth. The basis for psychoprophylaxis is the belief that the pain of labor and delivery can be suppressed by reorganization of cerebral cortical activity. Conditioned pain reflexes associated with uterine contractions and perineal distention can be replaced by newly created "positive" conditioned reflexes. For example the patient is taught to respond when a contraction begins by immediately taking a deep "cleansing breath," gently exhaling and then breathing in a specific shallow pattern until the contraction ends. She also focuses her eyes on a specific object or location away from herself, concentrates on release of muscle tension, maintaining the proper breathing rhythm and the reassuring words of her coach (usually her husband). The increased concentration required by these activities distract from or inhibit the painful sensations associated with the uterine contraction. Preparation usually begins 6 weeks prior to delivery. Instruction includes normal anatomy and physiology of pregnancy, labor and delivery, which in itself reduces the fear and anxiety which so often arises from the unknown.

Although it may appear that there is a certain similarity between psychoprophylaxis and hypnosis, proponents of psychoprophylaxis believe that hypnosis results in a loss of free will which their method does not. Samko and Schoenfeld[10] investigated the relationship between the successful use of the Lamaze technique and hypnotic susceptibility and reported no correlation.

Psychoprophylaxis reduces the amount of chemical anesthesia required by the mother.[11] However, widespread experience indicates that between one-third and two-thirds of mothers receiving Lamaze preparation will request additional pharmacologic analgesia or regional blocks.[12]

Patients with Lamaze training must be made aware that their preparation is no guarantee of a painless labor. They should be informed about anesthetic aids and must not be judged as failures if anesthesia is requested or required. Indeed, excessive maternal pain or severe anxiety over failure might result in more detriment to the fetus than the judicious use of pharmacologic analgesia.[13] There is increasing evidence that analgesic and anesthetic drugs administered to the mother may cross the placenta and sedate the fetus. Some have therefore advocated not using anesthesia for childbirth. Myers[13] and Morishima et al.[14] have shown, however, that psychological stress to the primate mother during labor can cause hypoxia and acidosis in the fetus, probably due to decreased uterine blood flow (Figure 6.2). Shnider et al.[15] have demonstrated in the pregnant ewe that maternal stress results in increased plasma norepinephrine levels and reduced uterine blood flow (Figure 6.3). In addition, high levels of maternal catecholamines can also cause inefficient contractions of the uterus. Therefore, avoidance of chemical analgesia must not be taken to an extreme that results in harm to the fetus or rejection of the newborn due to the unpleasantness of labor and delivery.

Regional anesthesia would seem to be a reasonable compromise, allowing maternal awareness and paternal presence but minimizing the stress associated with labor. However, there have been complaints by some patients that the removal of pain deprives them of a major portion of the experience of childbirth. Billewicz-Driemel and Milne[16] studied whether or not this feeling of deprivation is real and whether there are any consequences of it. They found that a small percentage of patients receiving epidural analgesia felt deprived, but there did not seem to be any long-term psychological effects of this phenomenon.

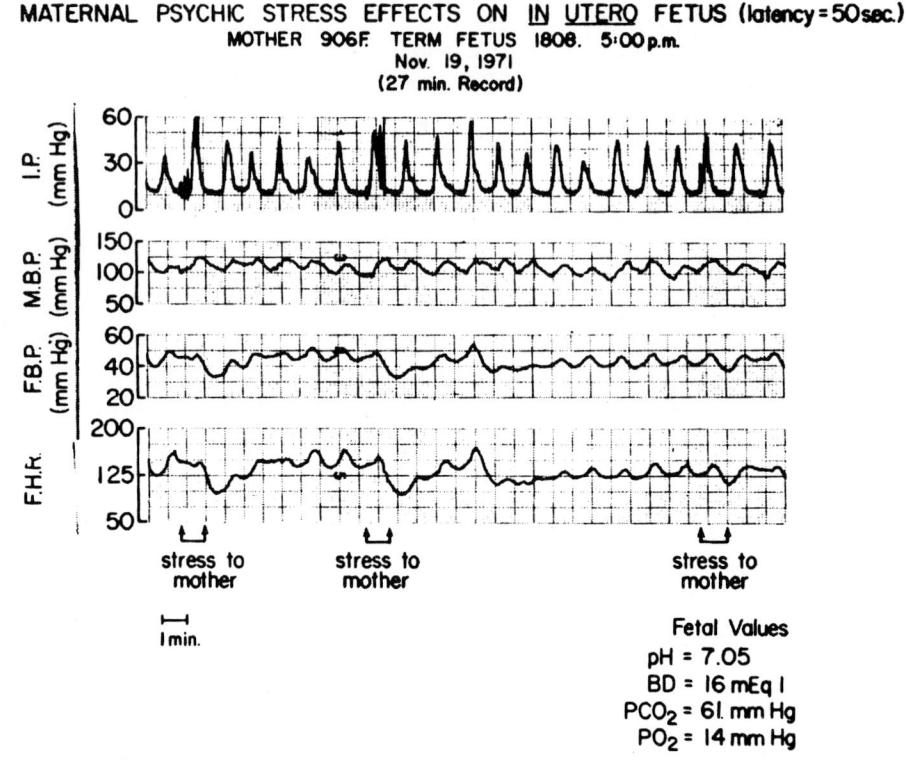

MATERNAL PSYCHIC STRESS EFFECTS ON IN UTERO FETUS (latency = 50 sec.)
MOTHER 906F. TERM FETUS 1808. 5:00 p.m.
Nov. 19, 1971
(27 min. Record)

Fetal Values
pH = 7.05
BD = 16 mEq l
PCO_2 = 61 mm Hg
PO_2 = 14 mm Hg

Figure 6.2. The effects of three 1-minute episodes of "contrived" psychological stress stimulation of a pregnant monkey timed with a stopwatch. In two instances, the fetus responded with clear-cut episodes of bradycardia. (Reprinted by permission from Myers RE: Maternal psychological stress and fetal asphyxia: A study in the monkey. Am J Obstet Gynecol 122:47, 1975.)

The question of whether or not Lamaze preparation results in better babies was addressed by Scott and Rose.[11] They compared prepared and unprepared mothers and found that, although the prepared mothers did indeed require less analgesia (Table 6.1), the neonatal outcome was indistinguishable. There is no question, however, that preparation for the event of childbirth is of benefit to almost all women and, regardless of the type of anesthesia used, can make the experience more pleasant.[17]

ACUPUNCTURE

Acupuncture has been practiced in China for more than a thousand years, for both its therapeutic and its analgesic properties.[18] Recent reports have stimulated interest in the value of acupuncture as an alternative to conventional anesthesia.[19,20] It is only natural that acupuncture would receive attention as a possible obstetric anesthetic, inasmuch as it would seem to be completely safe for mother and newborn. Because oriental women traditionally have delivered their children without anesthesia, there are no traditional acupuncture points for vaginal delivery. In China, acupuncture anesthesia for surgery is reported to be successful in about 70 per cent of patients. However, this success depends on careful patient selection, together with sociological indoctrination and motivation of the patient.[20] Patients lack-

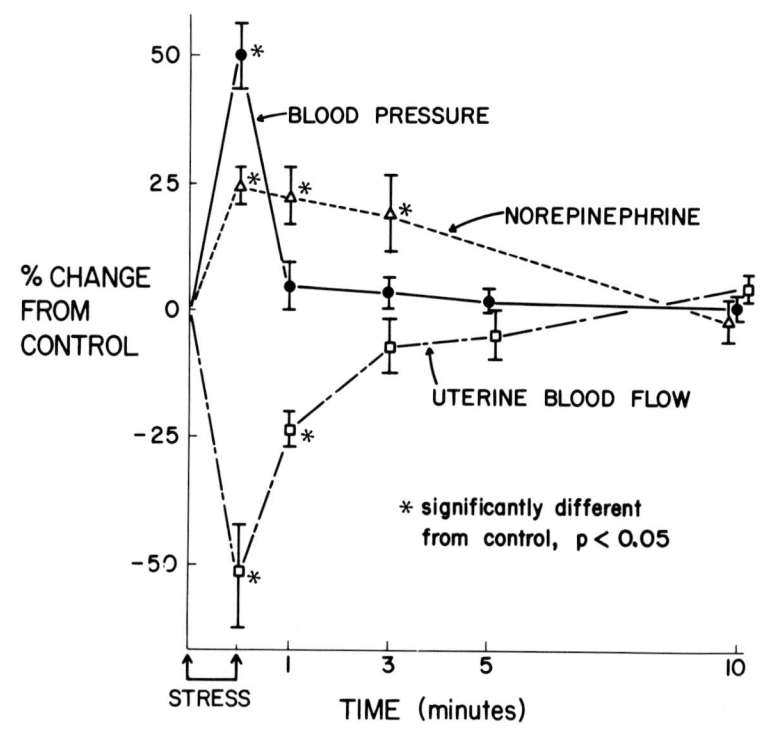

Figure 6.3. Effect of electrically induced stress (30 to 60 seconds) on maternal arterial blood pressure, plasma norepinephrine levels and uterine blood flow. All values subsequent to control are given as mean percentage change with standard error. (Reprinted by permission from Shnider SM, Wright RG, Levinson G, et al.: Uterine blood flow and plasma norepinephrine changes during maternal stress in the pregnant ewe. Anesthesiology. 50:526, 1979.)

ing this cultural background and pre-anesthetic management have not shown encouraging results. These factors suggest that hypnosis may be an important element in successful acupuncture, although other studies have suggested that successful response to acupuncture does not correlate with hypnotic susceptibility.

Several American investigators have attempted to provide analgesia for labor and delivery, choosing acupuncture points used for vaginal hysterectomy and dysmenorrhea[21,22] (Figure 6.4). Wallis et al.[21] studied manual and electrical acupuncture in 21 motivated volunteers. Nineteen of 21 patients had inadequate analgesia (Figure 6.5). Only two patients, both of whom received manual acupuncture, reported significant relief of pain. Both had practiced a natural childbirth technique. None of the 21 subjects was judged by the investigators to have adequate analgesia. Alternative methods of analgesia were requested by 16 patients. Five patients did not request further analgesia; of these, three practiced natural childbirth methods.

LeBOYER TECHNIQUE

The French obstetrician, Frederick LeBoyer, has received much attention for his discussion of the concept of "childbirth without violence."[3] He believes that the noise, bright lights and other stimulation associated with the traditional delivery cause undue psychologic trauma to the

Table 6.1
Pharmacologic Methods of Pain Relief Used during Labor and Delivery*

Analgesia and Anesthesia	Lamaze Group	Control Group	P Value
	no. of mothers		
None during first stage of labor	36	9	< 0.001
Sedatives or tranquilizers	28	39	NS†
Narcotics	84	109	< 0.001
Paracervical	13	15	NS
Epidural or caudal	18	52	< 0.001
Saddle	6	8	NS
General anesthesia	4	5	NS
Pudendal	83	59	< 0.001
Local infiltration only	13	5	NS

* Reprinted by permission from Scott JR, Rose NB: Effect of psychoprophylaxis (Lamage preparation) on labor and delivery in primiparas. N Engl J Med 294:1205, 1976.

† NS, not significant.

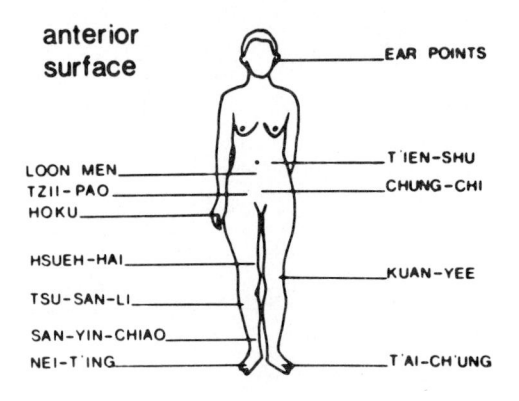

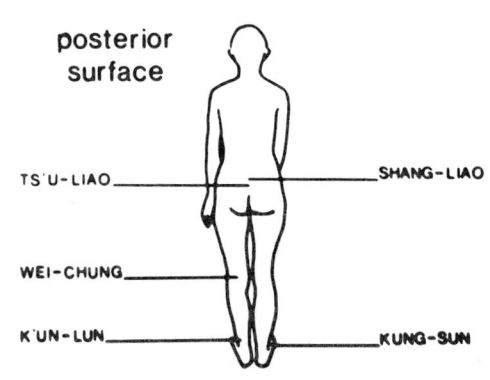

Figure 6.4. Sites of acupuncture points chosen by the acupuncturist to provide analgesia during labor. (Reprinted by permission from Wallis L, Shnider SM, Palahniuk RJ, et al.: An evaluation of acupuncture analgesia in obstetrics. Anesthesiology 41: 596, 1974.)

newborn. His solution is to perform deliveries in near silence and semi-darkness and to avoid stimulation of the newborn to prevent crying. Although there is no doubt that there is unnecessary noise in most delivery rooms, the author believes good lighting is essential to evaluate the condition of the newborn and to care for the mother. LeBoyer's method of placing the baby on the mother's abdomen with the umbilical cord still intact and pulsating can result in a loss of blood from the newborn to the placenta which can be deleterious. Furthermore, the author believes there is a rather subtle suggestion in his technique that newborns who cannot survive without active resuscitation are already permanently damaged and intervention should be avoided. This, of course, is not true (see Chapter 26).

FAMILY-CENTERED MATERNITY CARE

Currently, one of the most widely discussed areas in the psychology of childbirth is the concept of family-centered maternity care. The belief is that the interaction between mother, father and child in the first few minutes of life can greatly influence the entire relationship of the child with its environment. Proponents of this philosophy believe that the traditional hospital maternity care is doctor-centered

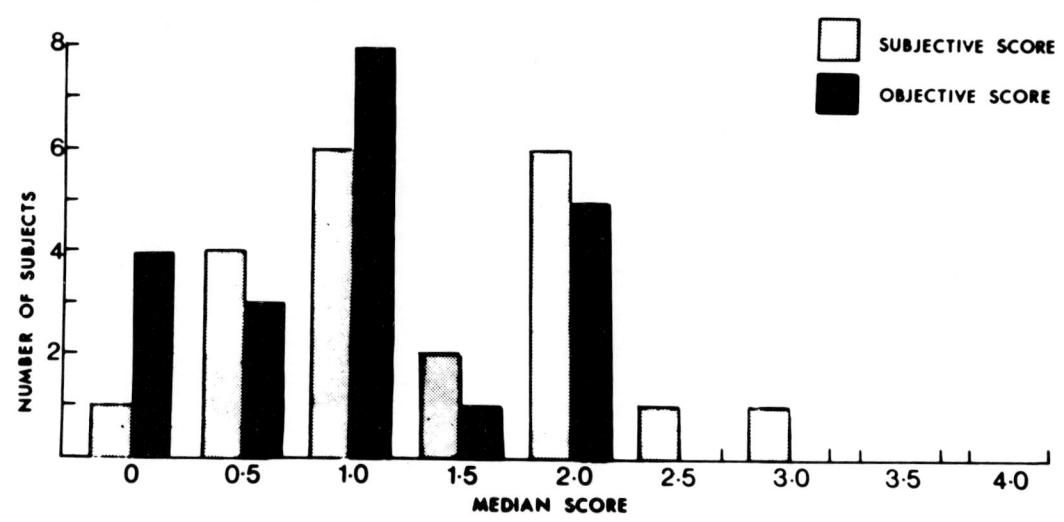

Figure 6.5. Histogram representing median analgesia scores during acupuncture treatment for all 21 subjects in the study. Subjective and observer scores are shown for each patient. Scores ≤ 2 were considered to indicate inadequate analgesia. (Reprinted by permission from Wallis L, Shnider SM, Palahniuk RJ, et al: An evaluation of acupuncture analgesia in obstetrics. Anesthesiology 41:596, 1974.)

and sacrifices the individuality of the patient and the psychologic well-being of the newborn for the convenience of the hospital staff. This has led to the current rebirth of interest in home deliveries. Advocates of home deliveries point out that the vast majority of deliveries are perfectly normal and do not require the intervention of a physician. This unfortunate idea ignores the fact that it is impossible to predict accurately which patients will develop problems during labor and that when a problem does occur, immediate intervention is often necessary to preserve the life of both the mother and the baby. Recent data from 11 state health departments showed that out-of-hospital births posed two to five times greater risk to a baby's life than hospital births.[23] For example, in 1975 California had a perinatal mortality rate of 20 per 1,000 births in the hospital in contrast to 42.3 per 1,000 births for home deliveries. In response to some of the objections to traditional hospital maternity care, the concept of the "birthing room" has been devised. This is a room in which the mother both labors and delivers her baby. The room is in a hospital maternity suite, but an attempt is made to provide a rather home-like atmosphere. Patients are encouraged to bring their own personal effects. The presence of the father is encouraged. Much latitude is allowed in the management of labor. However, all emergency facilities are immediately at hand. Thus, what is provided is, in effect, a home delivery in the hospital.

PRENATAL ANESTHESIA VISITS

In an effort to allay the anxieties of obstetric patients, some anesthesiologists set up prenatal anesthesia clinics. In these situations the obstetric patient is given the opportunity to make an individual appointment with an anesthesiologist prior to the onset of her labor. In the relaxed atmosphere of an office, a medical history is taken, the choices of anesthesia are discussed and the patient's questions are answered. If individual interviews are impractical, then a session during which an anesthesiologist will meet with a group of expectant parents to discuss anesthetic alternatives and answer questions should be arranged. A prenatal anesthetic visit can avoid much of the anxiety which so often occurs on the labor floor when an anesthesiologist is called to see a patient, writhing in pain, about whom he knows nothing. Additionally, many of the patient's misconceptions regarding obstetric anesthesia can be corrected, and frequently imagined conflicts between the so-called natural childbirth methods and anesthesia can be resolved. Many obstetric anesthesia units distribute a brochure to prospective parents describing pain relief in childbirth. An example of such a brochure is reprinted below.

APPENDIX

Pain Relief in Childbirth

University of California, San Francisco

The Department of Anesthesia at the University of California, San Francisco, provides a 24-hour service assuring that there will be an anesthesiologist (a physician specially trained in anesthesia) to administer your anesthetic. In choosing an anesthetic or the method of anesthesia, the anesthesiologist has the same objective as your obstetrician; that is, a healthy, happy mother and baby.

There are certain circumstances which will have an important bearing on the choice of your anesthetic. There is no routine method of anesthesia for childbirth. The type of anesthetic will be determined at the time of delivery by your condition and that of your baby. This choice is usually made after you have been admitted to Obstetrics.

At that time, after your initial examination by an obstetrician, an anesthesiologist will visit you to ask a few questions. These questions usually include: What is your expected delivery date? Do you have a history of allergies? When was your last meal? Have you ever had surgery or a medical illness?

He will also discuss the various ways you can overcome the discomfort of contractions. Many choices and possibilities are now available, and this is fortunate, since patients differ in their response to labor pains and to medication. The need for pain relief and the proper selection of sedation must be determined for each individual patient. This pamphlet will help you to understand better some of the ways used to relieve and prevent undue discomfort during childbirth.

YOU CAN HELP

As soon as you know your labor has started, *refrain from taking any liquids or solid foods*. If you are in doubt whether or not labor has started, take only such clear liquids as tea or ginger ale, those that you can see through.

It is most important that you realize your obstetrician and anesthesiologist are primarily interested in the welfare of you and your baby. Your wishes and choices of pain relief and anesthetic will be considered. Place your confidence in the judgment of the obstetrician and anesthesiologist attending you. If situations arise during labor and delivery that indicate the use of a particular method of pain relief or anesthesia, let your physicians advise you,

PSYCHOLOGICAL ANESTHESIA FOR OBSTETRICS

for they know what is best and necessary for you in your particular situation.

MEDICATION DURING LABOR

If you need medication, it will be given. The kind of medication and the time to take it will be determined by your obstetrician, according to your reactions and the condition of your baby. Medication will help you relax and rest between contractions and may, if you wish, help you to sleep. On occasion, a "regional" method of anesthesia, called caudal or epidural, may be used. This method freezes or numbs the areas where discomfort is felt or expected. In addition, Cyprane inhalers may be used. These devices contain Penthrane, a sweet and pleasant smelling vapor. You can relieve your discomfort by holding this inhaler and administering the vapor yourself during contractions.

ANESTHESIA FOR DELIVERY

The choice of an anesthetic for delivery depends on many factors, and often the final decision cannot be made until you are in labor, or it must be changed at the actual time of delivery. The methods of anesthesia fall into two principal groups, those that relieve pain by putting you to sleep (general anesthesia), and those that produce a loss of pain or numbness locally or in one region of the body (regional anesthesia). It should be remembered that all anesthetics that make you sleepy have, to some extent, the same effect on your baby.

General Anesthesia

The general anesthetic method includes the injection of an anesthetic into a vein in the arm followed by the inhalation of a gas or vapor from the mask of an anesthetic machine. The most frequent and serious problem with this method of anesthesia occurs when patients vomit and inhale their stomach contents into their lungs. This is the reason your obstetrician and anesthesiologist are interested in the time of your last meal. Since most digestion stops when labor starts, a 6-hour lapse of time is desirable, if a general anesthetic is to be given for a normal delivery. Unexpected problems may make special precautions necessary for the use of a general anesthetic under less ideal conditions.

Regional Anesthesia

Regional anesthetic methods cause numbness in an area where pain occurs. Usually these methods do not make you sleepy and have no effect on the baby. You may then have the pleasant experience of watching the birth of your baby while being virtually free from pain. Regional anesthetics may be administered in several ways. You obstetrician will select the most suitable method for you.

Local Infiltration. The simplest form of regional anesthesia is local infiltration or one of the block methods. These are easy to administer and remove a great deal of the pain. These methods are used just before delivery.

Epidural or caudal. Epidural or caudal methods of anesthesia freeze a larger area and are usually administered when labor is well advanced and can be continued for the actual delivery.

Spinal. Many mothers, obstetricians, and anesthesiologists prefer spinal anesthesia (saddle block). It gives rapid and complete pain relief and does not disturb mother or baby. This method is administered just before the baby is delivered.

NATURAL CHILDBIRTH

If you prefer a form of natural childbirth or wish to participate in childbirth education classes, it is suggested that you discuss this with your obstetrician as early in pregnancy as possible. He will explain its advantages and limitations. Preparation for childbirth frequently enables you to reduce either the need for pain medication or its frequency. Nevertheless, medication is available during childbirth if you need it. In short, childbirth education classes provide you with a greater knowledge of the processes of labor and delivery.

IN SUMMARY

The entire team—you (the patient), the obstetrician, and the anesthesiologist—have in mind but one principal objective: a healthy, happy mother and baby.

References

1. Dick-Read G: *Childbirth without Fear,* ed 2. Harper & Row, New York, 1959.
2. Lamaze F: *Painless Childbirth: Psychoprophylactic Method.* Burke, London, 1958.
3. LeBoyer F: *Birth without Violence.* Wildwood House, London, 1975.
4. August RV: *Hypnosis in Obstetrics.* McGraw-Hill, New York, 1961.
5. Moya F, James LS: Medical hypnosis for obstetrics. JAMA 174:2026, 1960.
6. Flowers CE, Littlejohn TW, Wells HB: Pharmacologic and hypnoid analgesia. Obstet Gynecol 16:210, 1960.
7. Spiegel H: An eye-roll test for hypnotizability. Am J Clin Hypn 15:25, 1972.
8. Rosen H: Hypnosis—applications and misapplications. JAMA 172:683, 1960.
9. Wahl CW: Contraindications and limitations of hypnosis in obstetric analgesia. Am J Obstet Gynecol 84:1869, 1962.
10. Samko MR, Schoenfeld LS: Hypnotic susceptibility and the Lamaze childbirth experience. Am J Obstet Gynecol 121:631, 1975.
11. Scott JR, Rose NB: Effect of psychoprophylaxis (Lamaze preparation) on labor and delivery in primiparas. N Engl J Med 294:1205, 1976.
12. Shnider SM: Personal Communication.
13. Myers RE: Maternal psychological stress and fetal asphyxia: A study in the monkey. Am J Obstet Gynecol 122:47, 1975.
14. Morishima HO, Pedersen H, Finster M: The influence of maternal psychological stress on the fetus. Am J Obstet Gynecol 131:286, 1978.
15. Shnider SM, Wright RG, Levinson G, et al.: Uterine blood flow and plasma norepinephrine changes during maternal stress in the pregnant ewe. Anesthesiology 50:524, 1979.
16. Billewicz-Driemel AM, Milne MD: Long term assessment of extradural analgesia for the relief of pain in labour. II. Sense of deprivation after extradural analgesia in labour: Relevant or not? Br J Anaesth 48:139, 1976.
17. Doering SG, Entwisle DR: Preparation during pregnancy and ability to cope with labor and delivery. Am J Orthopsychiatry 45:825, 1975.
18. Veith I: Acupuncture in traditional Chinese medicine—an historical review. Calif Med 118:70, 1973.
19. Reston J: Now, about my operation in Peking. In *The New York Times Report from Red China.* F Ching, ed. Quadrangle Books, New York, 1971, p. 304.
20. Dimond EG: Acupuncture anesthesia: Western medicine and Chinese traditional medicine. JAMA 218:1558, 1971.
21. Wallis L, Shnider SM, Palahniuk RJ, et al.: An evaluation of acupuncture analgesia in obstetrics. Anesthesiology 41:596, 1974.
22. Abouleish E, Depp R: Acupuncture in obstetrics. Anesth Analg 54:82, 1975.
23. American College of Obstetricians and Gynecologists: *ACOG Newsletter,* vol 22, number 2, February 1978.

CHAPTER 7

Systemic Medication for Labor and Delivery

Gershon Levinson, M.D.
Sol M. Shnider, M.D.

Despite the increasing use of regional analgesia during labor, systemic medications are still widely used to relieve pain and anxiety. There is no ideal, universally applicable analgesic agent for use during childbirth. All systemic medications used for pain relief in labor cross the placenta and may have a depressant effect on the fetus. The amount of depression will depend on the dose of the drug, the route and time of administration before delivery and the presence of obstetric complications.

The systemic drugs administered during labor may be classified into five broad groups:

1. Sedative-tranquilizers are generally used during the first stage of labor, either alone or in combination with a narcotic.

2. Narcotics are used to relieve pain during the first and second stages of labor.

3. Dissociative or amnesic drugs, such as ketamine or scopolamine, are used infrequently. Ketamine in low subanesthetic doses may be used as an analgesic during the second stage of labor or as an adjunct to regional anesthesia for cesarean section. Scopolamine has been used as an amnesic drug.

4. Neuroleptanalgesia with a drug preparation such as Innovar is not commonly used prior to birth.

5. Antagonists are drugs used to reverse possible adverse effects of the above medications.

SEDATIVE-TRANQUILIZERS

The amount of anxiety and fear a woman experiences during labor and delivery can be minimized by proper psychological preparation and the continuous presence of supportive attendants and a sympathetic husband. In practice, however, many women still require some pharmacologic intervention to reduce their anxiety. Furthermore, these drugs promote sleep, and this hypnotic effect may be especially beneficial in early labor. In addition, all the phenothiazines, as well as drugs such as hydroxyzine and droperidol are potent antiemetics and will reduce the nausea and vomiting commonly seen during labor.

Barbiturates

The use of short- or medium-acting barbiturates such as secobarbital (Seconal), pentobarbital (Nembutal) or amobarbital (Amytal) is no longer popular. These sedative-hypnotic drugs possess no analgesic action and, indeed, may produce an antianalgesic effect.[1,2] In the presence of severe pain, administration of these drugs may result in an excited, disoriented and unmanageable parturient.

With low doses (secobarbital 50 to 200 mg intramuscularly) there is no significant maternal respiratory depression.[3] In larger doses or with the addition of narcotics to smaller doses, barbiturates are associated with respiratory depression and obtundation of protective airway reflexes.

The principal objection to the use of barbiturates in obstetrics is their prolonged depressant effects on the neonate. All the barbiturates rapidly cross the placenta, and equilibrium between mother and fetus is achieved in minutes (Figure 7.1).[4,5] Shnider and Moya[6] showed that the addition of secobarbital (100 mg intramuscularly or 200 mg p.o.) to meperidine (50 to 100 mg intramuscularly) increased the incidence of depressed newborns. High doses of barbiturates alone (600 to 1,000 mg) have been reported to produce neonatal somnolence, flaccidity, hypoventilation, and failure to feed for up to 2 days.[7] Even with smaller doses, resulting in no apparent clinical depression as ascertained by the Apgar score, the newborn's attention span may be decreased for 2 to 4 days.[8]

Currently, the primary indication for the use of barbiturates is as a sedative-hypnotic during the early latent phase of labor when delivery is not anticipated for 12 to 24 hours.

Phenothiazine Derivatives and Hydroxyzine

Promethazine (Phenergan) and propiomazine (Largon) are phenothiazine de-

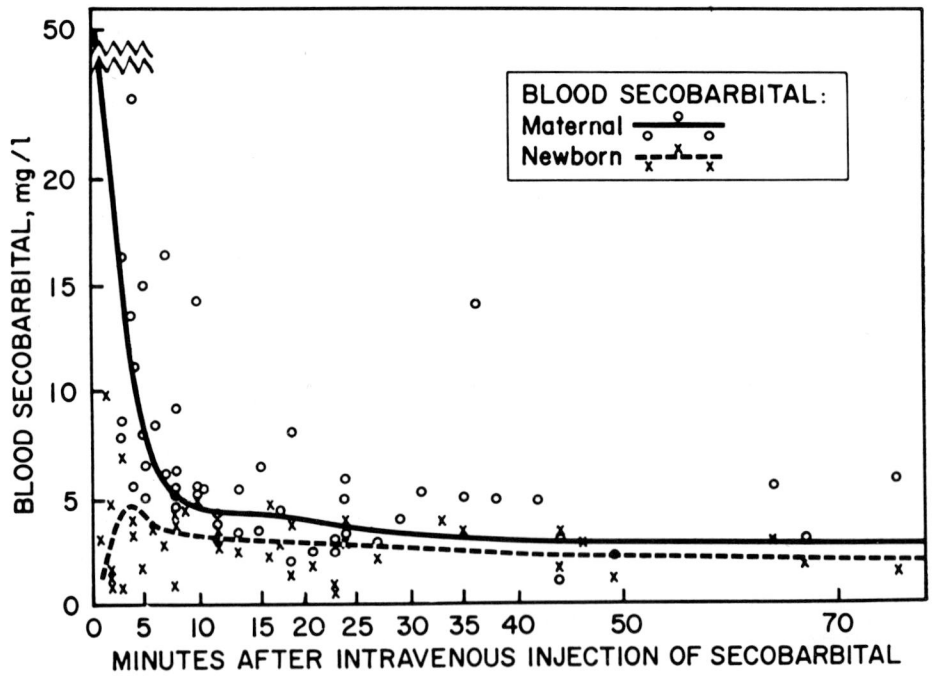

Figure 7.1. Scattergram of blood levels of secobarbital in maternal venous and umbilical cord blood after a single intravenous injection of 250 mg of sodium secobarbital from 1 to 75 minutes before delivery. Secobarbital crosses the placenta rapidly and the neonatal blood level at delivery is approximately 70 per cent of that in the mother. (Reprinted by permission from Root B, Eichner E, Sunshine I: Blood secobarbital levels and their clinical correlation in mothers and newborn infants. Am J Obstet Gynecol 81:948, 1961.)

rivatives which may be useful during labor to relieve anxiety. Chlorpromazine (Thorazine), promazine (Sparine) and prochlorperazine (Compazine)—also phenothiazine derivatives—are not as popular because they possess greater α-adrenergic blocking properties, resulting in hypotension. Hydroxyzine (Vistaril), although chemically unrelated to the phenothiazines, has similar ataractic properties.

Promethazine, propiomazine and hydroxyzine seem to be equally effective in relieving anxiety, reducing narcotic requirements and controlling emesis. Differences between these drugs are relatively minor. Propiomazine has a shorter onset time and duration than promethazine.[9] Promethazine is a respiratory stimulant, whereas propiomazine is a mild respiratory depressant. Hydroxyzine has a slight disadvantage in that it cannot be used intravenously.

Despite the rapid placental transfer and decrease in beat-to-beat variability of the fetal heart rate, these drugs in the recommended doses do not seem to cause neonatal depression. For example, Powe et al.[9] compared three intramuscular analgesic regimens: meperidine 50 mg; meperidine 50 mg plus promethazine 50 mg; and meperidine 50 mg; and meperidine 50 mg plus propiomazine 20 mg. Although increasing the sedation in the mother, the incidence of depressed newborns was not increased by the addition of either tranquilizer to the narcotic. Similarly, hydroxyzine 50 to 100 mg combined with a narcotic or by itself produced increased tranquility without increased neonatal depression.[10-12]

Diazepam

Diazepam (Valium) is used as a sedative, a narcotic adjuvant, an anticonvulsant in treating toxemia and as a pre-medicant for cesarean section. It is a benzodiazepine derivative structurally and pharmacologically related to chlordiazepoxide (Librium). Like the other tranquilizers, diazepam can reduce maternal anxiety and narcotic requirements without prolonging labor or increasing the incidence of neonatal respiratory depression.

Despite the fact that diazepam is the most popular and widely prescribed tranquilizer in the world, its use in obstetrics is controversial. The drug rapidly crosses the placenta, and maternal and fetal blood levels are approximately equal within minutes of an intravenous dose.[13] Some have reported that at birth fetal blood levels may actually exceed maternal levels (Figure 7.2).[14-16] Furthermore, although the neonate is capable of metabolizing small doses of diazepam, when the total maternal dosage during labor exceeds 30 mg, the drug and its active metabolite persist in pharmacologically active concentrations for at least a week in the neonate.[14] The principal adverse effects of large doses of diazepam are hypotonia, lethargy, decreased feeding and hypothermia.[14, 17-19]

In small doses, the authors and other investigators[15, 20] have found minimal fetal and neonatal effects. Although beat-to-beat variability of the fetal heart rate is markedly decreased even with small intravenous doses (5 to 10 mg),[20] there are no adverse effects on fetal or neonatal acid-base or clinical status.[15, 21] The authors have recently studied the effects of small doses (2.5 to 10 mg) of intravenous diazepam as an antianxiety medication in patients undergoing cesarean section under regional anesthesia.[22] They found that these small doses did not sedate the newborn—as evidenced by total Apgar scores—and did not alter umbilical vein or artery oxygen or acid-base status but did decrease newborn muscle tone. The Scanlon neurobehavioral examination also showed decreased tone at 4 hours but not at 24 hours of age.

A theoretical objection to the use of diazepam in obstetrics has been raised by the work of Schiff et al.[23] These investigators found that the sodium benzoate,

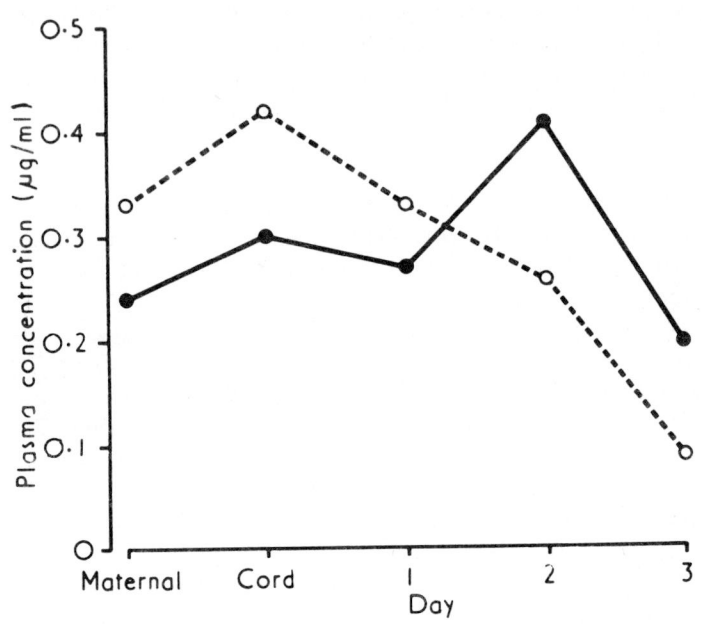

Figure 7.2. Mean plasma concentrations of diazepam and desmethyldiazepam showing crossover in degradation curves. O-O, diazepam; ●-●, desmethyldiazepam. (Reprinted by permission from Cree IE, Meyer J, Hailey DM: Diazepam in labour: Its metabolism and effect on the clinical condition and thermogenesis of the newborn. Br Med J 4:251, 1973.)

which is used as a buffer in the injectable form of the drug, is a potent bilirubin-albumin uncoupler. The displacement of lipid-soluble bilirubin from its albumin-binding sites would increase the susceptibility of the infant to kernicterus. These workers, therefore, advised caution in using the drug as a relaxant for infants receiving mechanical intermittent positive-pressure respiration or for the control of convulsions in the neonate when serum bilirubin levels are increased. In parturients, only small doses of diazepam are required and would seem very unlikely to cause subsequent problems with bilirubin binding in the neonate.[24] Furthermore, the maternal liver should rapidly metabolize the sodium benzoate.

The authors believe that small intravenous doses of diazepam (2.5-mg doses up to a total of 10 mg) can help allay extreme apprehension and anxiety without producing significant adverse fetal or neonatal effects. When larger doses are used, as for example in the therapy of preeclampsia-eclampsia, particular care should be taken to maintain a warm environment for the newborn, and these infants should be observed carefully for at least 36 hours after delivery.

NARCOTICS

Narcotics are the most effective systemic medication for the relief of pain. Although a wide variety of narcotics are available only a few are used currently in obstetrics. These include morphine, meperidine (Demerol), alphaprodine (Nisentil), pentazocine (Talwin) and fentanyl (Sublimaze). Oxymorphone (Numorphan) and anileridine (Leritine) are not widely used in obstetrics because they have no advantages over meperidine and seem to be more depressant to the neonate than other narcotics.[25, 26]

SYSTEMIC MEDICATION FOR LABOR AND DELIVERY

No narcotic currently available can produce effective analgesia without some respiratory depression. **Complete analgesia** for labor and delivery cannot be achieved in most parturients without also producing severe hypoventilation, obtundation of reflexes and postural hypotension. Therefore, narcotics are used to reduce pain rather than completely eliminate it. Because all narcotics in appropriate doses produce comparable pain relief, the choice of drug depends on potential maternal and neonatal side effects and the desired onset and duration of action.

Respiratory depression is the most significant side effect of narcotic administration. In equianalgesic doses most narcotics probably produce a comparable shift of the carbon dioxide response curve to the right. Some narcotics such as fentanyl[27] and alphaprodine[28] may produce an extremely rapid, transient shift in the response curve. The peak respiratory depression of these narcotics may be of much greater magnitude than equianalgesic doses of other narcotics (Figure 7.3). Usually, serious problems do not occur with small doses of fentanyl and alphaprodine because of the short duration of the respiratory depression, but apnea may occasionally occur even with therapeutic doses (Figure 7.4).

Another potentially serious side effect of all narcotics is orthostatic hypotension resulting from peripheral vasodilation.[29] When the usual analgesic doses of narcotics are administered to parturients in the horizontal position, maternal blood pressure, heart rate and rhythm are unaffected. If these patients, however, are allowed to ambulate or sit up or are moved too vigorously, severe hypotension with maternal and fetal distress may develop. Frequent monitoring of blood pressure is mandatory.

Narcotics produce nausea and vomiting probably by direct stimulation of the chemoreceptor trigger zone in the medulla.

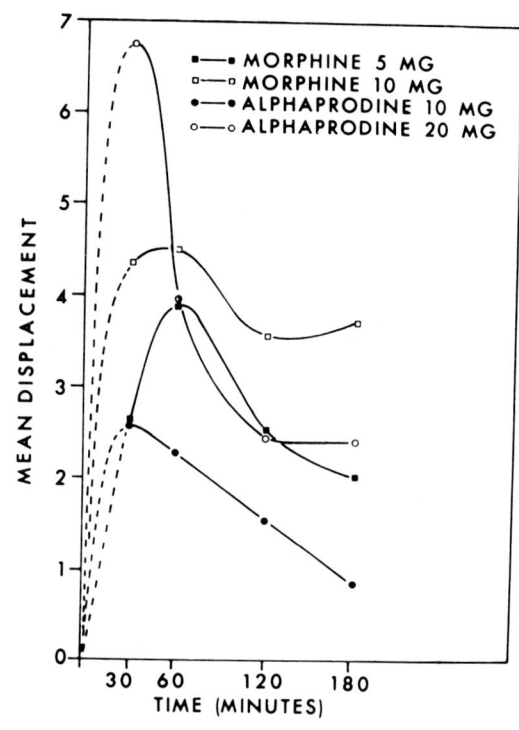

Figure 7.3. Mean displacement of respiratory response to carbon dioxide plotted as time-effect curves. Each medication was administered intramuscularly to six subjects. The initial peak effect of alphaprodine may have been missed for both doses. (Reprinted by permission from Forrest WH, Bellville JW: Respiratory effects of alphaprodine in man. Obstet Gynecol 31:61, 1968.)

The emetic effects are dose-related, and equianalgesic doses of the commonly used narcotics usually produce equal amounts of nausea and vomiting. Some patients, however, seem to be more sensitive to nausea with some narcotics than with others.

Although narcotics usually stimulate smooth muscle, gastric motility is decreased. During active labor, meperidine 100 mg and scopolamine 0.4 mg have been reported to produce retention of 20 to 43 per cent of a test meal at 3 hours and 12 to 37 per cent at 5 hours.[30]

During the latent or early stages of labor

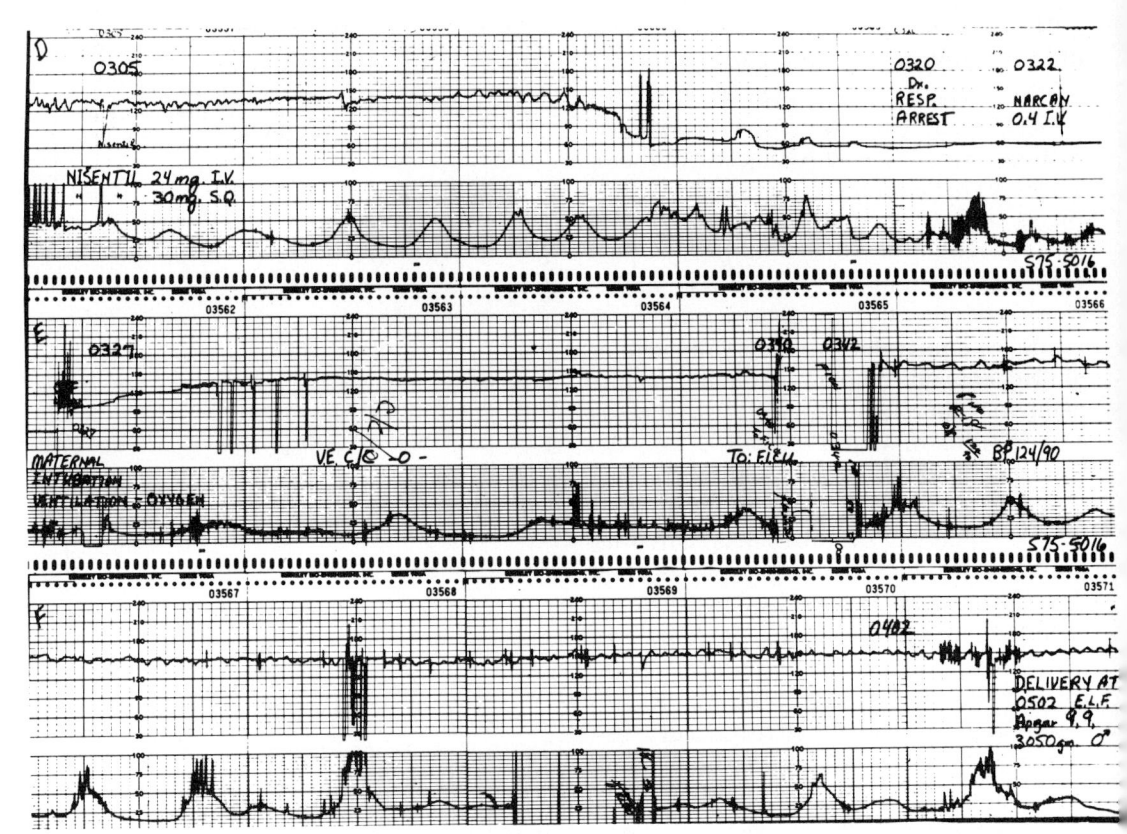

Figure 7.4. Continuous fetal heart rate monitor strip from a patient who received Nisentil intravenously and subcutaneously. Ten minutes after medication a sustained fetal bradycardia developed and a maternal respiratory arrest was noted shortly thereafter. The mother was treated with Narcan, endotracheal intubation and controlled ventilation with 100 per cent oxygen. Fetal heart rate rapidly improved, and a vigorous neonate was delivered 2 hours later. (Labor record kindly provided by R. H. Paul, M.D., University of Southern California, Los Angeles.)

narcotics, like all analgesic agents, may decrease uterine activity, slow cervical dilation and retard the progress of labor.[31] Once labor is well established narcotics have been reported to shorten labor and correct incoordinate uterine contractions.[32, 33] The mechanism of these effects seems to be related to relief of anxiety and pain rather than direct action on uterine muscle. Low spinal anesthesia also exerts these actions.

All narcotics are rapidly transferred across the placenta[34-36] and are capable of producing neonatal respiratory depression and changes in neurobehavioral status.

With most narcotics the maximum neonatal depression of Apgar scores occurs in newborns delivered 2 to 3 hours after maternal intramuscular administration.[6, 37, 38]

Meperidine (Demerol)

Meperidine is the most popular narcotic currently used in obstetrics. The usual dosage is 50 to 100 mg intramuscularly or 25 to 50 mg intravenously. The peak analgesic effect occurs 40 to 50 minutes after intramuscular and 5 to 10 minutes after intravenous administration. The duration of action is 3 to 4 hours.

SYSTEMIC MEDICATION FOR LABOR AND DELIVERY

The placental transfer and the fetal and neonatal effects of this drug have been studied extensively. Meperidine reaches the fetal circulation within 90 seconds of intravenous administration to the mother, and the fetal and maternal concentrations achieve equilibrium within 6 minutes (Figure 7.5).[39] In most studies, at delivery maternal and umbilical cord blood levels are similar.[40,41]

The effects of meperidine on the fetus include altered electroencephalogram,[42] decreased or arrested respiratory movements[43] and decreased beat-to-beat variability.[44] The effect of meperidine on fetal blood pressure, heart rate, arterial oxygen and acid-base status has been studied in pregnant ewes. Intravenous injections of small doses to the mother did not affect these variables.[45]

Maternally administered meperidine may produce neonatal depression as evidenced by prolonged time-to-sustained respirations (TSR), decreased Apgar scores,[6] lower oxygen saturation,[46] decreased minute volume,[38] respiratory acidosis[47] and abnormal neurobehavioral examinations.[48,49] These effects are related to the dose and to the time interval between maternal administration and delivery of the infant. Shnider and Moya[6] studied a group of parturients with no medical or obstetric complications. If meperidine was given within 1 hour of birth, there was no statistically significant difference in the incidence of depressed babies compared

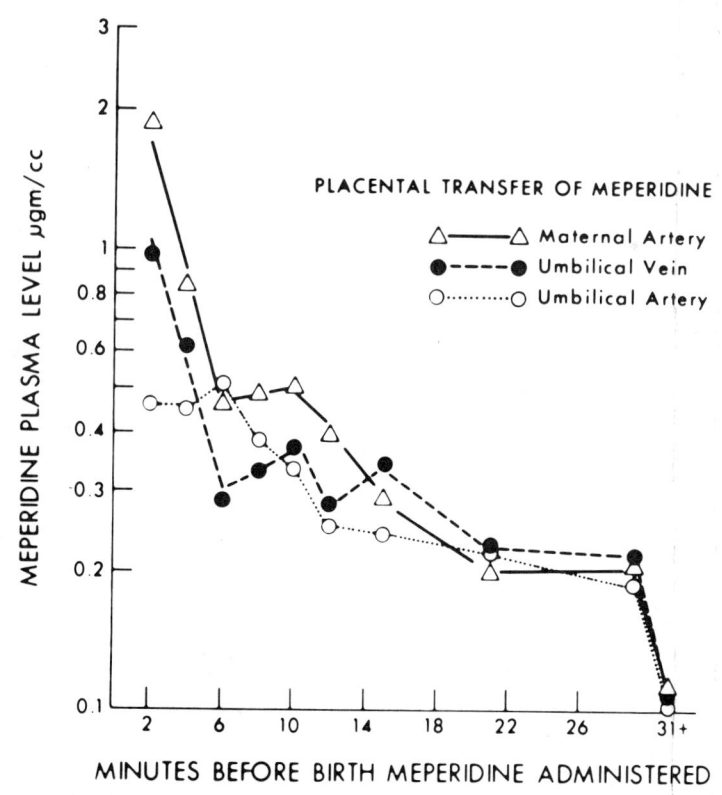

Figure 7.5. Plasma levels of meperidine at delivery after maternal intravenous administration of 50 mg at various intervals from 30 seconds to 4 hours before delivery. (Drawn from data in Shnider SM, Way EL, Lord MJ: Rate of appearance and disappearance of meperidine in fetal blood after administration of narcotic to the mother. Anesthesiology 27:227, 1966.)

to a control, unmedicated group (Figure 7.6). This was found even when the mother received up to 100 mg of drug. However, there was a significant increase in the percentage of depressed babies born during the second hour after drug administration. This was true even if mothers had received only 50 mg of meperidine. Increased doses tended to prolong the period in which significant neonatal depression was observed. The addition of a barbiturate not only prolonged the period but also increased the percentage of neonatal depression (Figure 7.7).

The reason for the delay in the appearance of neonatal depression is unclear. One possibility is delayed uptake of drug after intramuscular administration. Another may be the presence of a pharmacologically active metabolite rather than the parent compound. Using a non-specific colorimetric assay, Morrison et al.[50, 51] reported that after intravenous administration of meperidine to pregnant women, there were three distinct types of metabolic patterns. Neonatal depression was associated with two of these patterns in which high and prolonged blood levels of unidentified metabolites were found. Of the known metabolites of meperidine only normeperidine is known to be a central nervous system depressant. Kuhnert et al.[52] reported that normeperidine levels in umbilical cord blood were highest 4 hours or more after administration of a single intravenous dose of meperidine to the mother. However, Freeman et al.[53] have shown that normeperidine levels in umbilical cord blood are low and are unrelated to the time from maternal administration of meperidine to the delivery of the baby. Thus, the reason for the apparent safe period after intramuscular meperidine is as yet unexplained.

Neonatal depression after meperidine may be prolonged. Oxygen saturation is

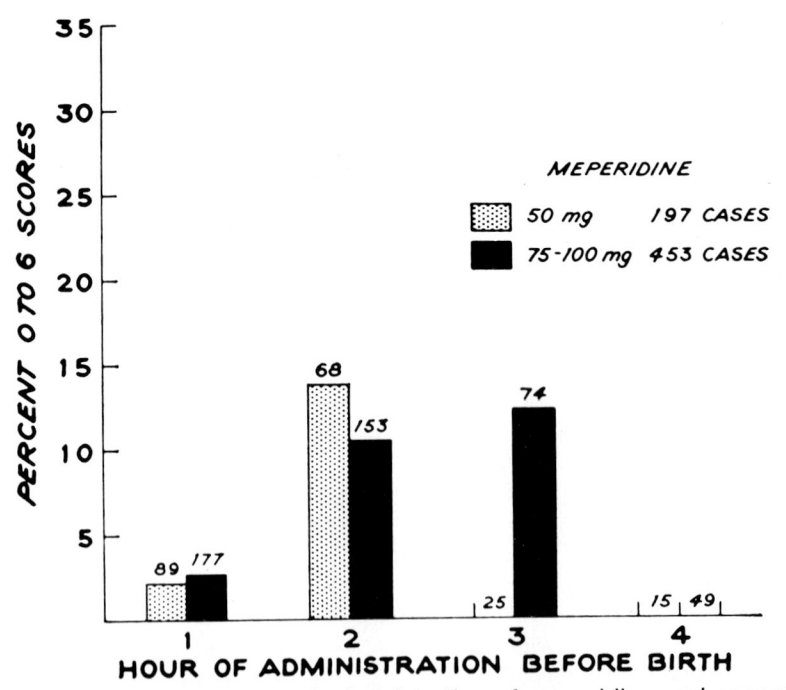

Figure 7.6. Correlation of the time of administration of meperidine and neonatal depression according to Apgar scores. (Reprinted with permission from Shnider SM, Moya F: Effects of meperidine on the newborn infant. Am J Obstet Gynecol 89:1009, 1964.)

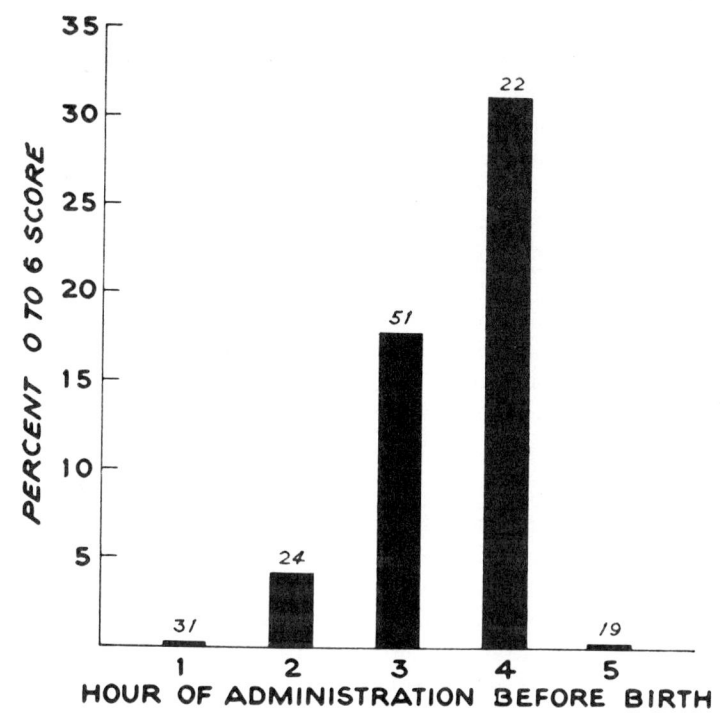

Figure 7.7. Correlation of the time of administration of meperidine-secobarbital and neonatal depression according to Apgar scores. (Reprinted with permission from Shnider SM, Moya F: Effects of meperidine on the newborn infant. Am J Obstet Gynecol 89: 1009, 1964.)

significantly depressed for at least 30 minutes after birth in full-term babies of mothers who receive 100 mg of meperidine 2 to 4 hours before birth.[46] Neonatal hypercapnia may persist for up to 5 hours.[47] Depression of habituation to an auditory stimulus as well as other subtle neurobehavioral changes are directly proportional to the dose of meperidine (50 to 150 mg) given to the mother and have been found to be present 20 to 60 hours after birth.[48,49] Recent studies indicate that the neonate requires 3 to 6 days to eliminate the drug completely.[54] The elimination half-life of meperidine is about 23 hours in the newborn,[55] compared with 3 to 5 hours in normal adults.

Alphaprodine (Nisentil)

Alphaprodine has achieved great popularity in many obstetric units because of its rapid onset and short duration. The peak analgesic effect occurs 5 to 10 minutes after subcutaneous and 1 to 2 minutes after intravenous administration. The duration of action is 1 to 2 hours. Recommended use is "initially 40 to 60 mg subcutaneously after cervical dilatation has begun, repeated as required at two-hour intervals."[56] The authors believe this dosage is excessive and potentially dangerous. Although 40 to 60 mg of alphaprodine do produce the same analgesic effects as 10 mg of morphine or 80 to 100 mg of meperidine, the respiratory depression produced is much greater. At their respective peaks of respiratory depressant activity, alphaprodine 19 mg produces the same respiratory depression as morphine 10 mg.[28] When these effects are mathematically extrapolated over a 3-hour period, alphaprodine 28 mg produces equivalent respiratory depression to morphine 10 mg. Therefore, the authors believe that alphaprodine should be administered in doses no greater than 20 to 30 mg subcutaneously or 10 to 20 mg intravenously and repeated if necessary.

The fetal and neonatal effects of alphaprodine have not been studied extensively but would seem to be similar to other narcotics.[57,58] The time of maximum neonatal depression after maternal administration of alphaprodine has not been determined.

Morphine

Morphine is no longer popular in obstetrics. When used it is usually administered in doses of 5 to 10 mg intramuscularly or 2 to 3 mg intravenously. The peak analgesic effect is 1 to 2 hours after intramuscular administration and 20 minutes after intravenous administration. The duration of action is 4 to 6 hours. In equianalgesic doses morphine produces more respiratory depression of the newborn than does meperidine (Figure 7.8).[59]

Because of the delayed onset and prolonged duration of action in the mother, coupled with the greater sensitivity of the newborn's respiratory center to morphine, meperidine has replaced morphine as an obstetric analgesic.

Pentazocine (Talwin)

Pentazocine is a synthetic analgesic with both agonistic action and weak opioid antagonistic activity. It may precipitate withdrawal symptoms if administered to narcotic addicts. Pentazocine is usually administered in doses of 20 to 30 mg intramuscularly or 10 to 20 mg intravenously. Analgesia occurs within 10 to 20 minutes after intramuscular administration or 2 to 3 minutes after intravenous administration. The duration of action is 3 to 4 hours.

The side effects of pentazocine, includ-

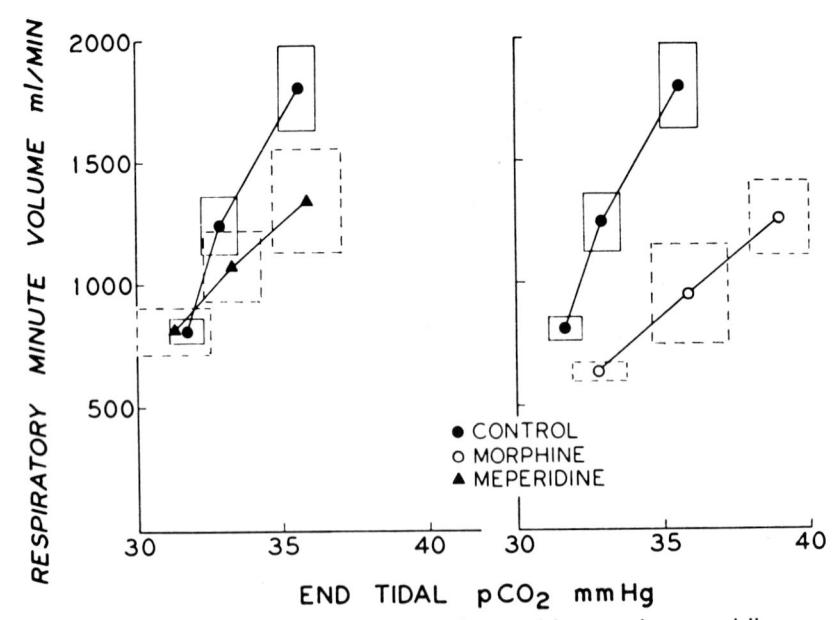

Figure 7.8. Effect of equianalgesic doses of morphine and meperidine on the CO_2 response curve in the newborn. The standard error of the means is indicated by the *rectangles* about each *point*. (Reprinted with permission from Way WL, Costley EC, Way EL: Respiratory sensitivity of the newborn infant to meperidine and morphine. Clin Pharmacol Ther 6:454, 1965.)

ing respiratory depression and delayed gastric emptying, are similar to other narcotics. Possible advantages include less postural hypotension, nausea and vomiting.[36, 60] With doses above 60 mg, psychotomimetic effects—such as nightmares, hallucinations and bizarre thoughts—have been reported.[61]

Pentazocine rapidly crosses the placenta. Within 10 minutes of intravenous administration fetal blood levels are approximately two-thirds of maternal levels. Compared to meperidine there do not seem to be any significant differences in neonatal depression with equianalgesic doses of pentazocine.[36, 60, 62]

Fentanyl (Sublimaze)

Fentanyl is a rapid-acting narcotic analgesic with properties similar to those of morphine. Fentanyl 100 µg is equianalgesic to morphine 10 mg. The usual doses are 50 to 100 µg intramuscularly and 25 to 50 µg intravenously. Intravenously administered fentanyl produces analgesia almost immediately; the peak effect follows within 3 to 5 minutes, and the duration of action is 30 to 60 minutes. After intramuscular administration analgesia begins in 7 to 8 minutes, peaks at about 30 minutes and lasts 1 to 2 hours.

Clinically, the drug is usually administered in combination with droperidol. By itself, fentanyl has not been used extensively in obstetrics. There is no reason to believe that it does not rapidly cross the placenta and produce fetal and neonatal effects comparable to equianalgesic doses of other narcotics.

DISSOCIATIVE OR AMNESIC DRUGS

Ketamine (Ketalar, Ketaject)

Intramuscular or intravenous administration of ketamine produces a state referred to as "dissociative anesthesia," which is characterized by intense analgesia with only superficial sleep. In obstetrics the drug may be used in lieu of thiopental as an induction agent for general anesthesia (1 mg/kg) or in very small doses (0.25 mg/kg) in lieu of inhalation analgesia as a systemic analgesic in the awake parturient.

In both dose ranges the drug produces minimal respiratory depression and usually increases arterial blood pressure 10 to 25 per cent. Undesirable hypertension may occur, and the drug should not be given to patients with high blood pressure. In the bleeding hypotensive patient, the cardiovascular stimulation is desirable, and ketamine may be the preferred induction agent for general anesthesia. Protective pharyngeal and laryngeal reflexes are maintained with low-dose ketamine, but with larger doses laryngeal incompetence and aspiration have been reported.[63-65] Emergence delirium and hallucinations are common with high doses in unpremedicated patients.[66] With low doses most patients experience a dream-like state which is rarely unpleasant.

Because ketamine has vasopressor effects and many vasoactive compounds decrease uterine blood flow, several investigators have examined the effects of ketamine on uterine perfusion. In both pregnant ewes and monkeys the increase in maternal blood pressure was not associated with a reduction in uterine blood flow.[67, 68] Ketamine produces a dose-related oxytocic effect on uterine tone. With low doses (0.25 to 1.0 mg/kg) these effects are clinically insignificant (Figure 7.9). With doses of 2 mg/kg, uterine tone increases almost 40 per cent.[69] Ketamine crosses the placenta rapidly but does not produce neonatal depression unless used in doses above 1 mg/kg (Figure 7.10).[70, 71] At higher doses low Apgar scores and neonatal muscular hypertonicity have been reported. In several instances, even with endotracheal intubation, ventilation

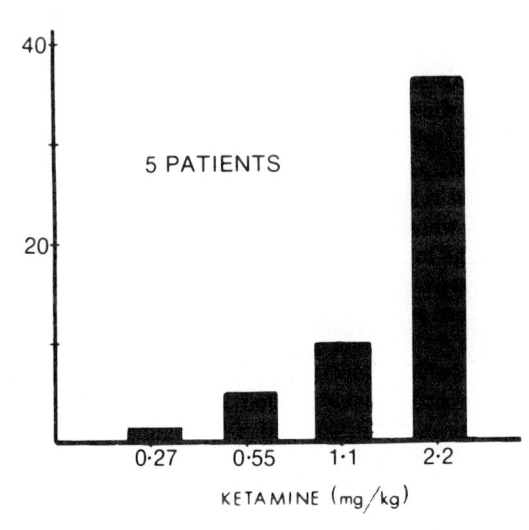

Figure 7.9. Mean increases in uterine tone produced by cumulative doses of ketamine. (Reprinted with permission from Galloon S: Ketamine for obstetric delivery. Anesthesiology 44:523, 1976.)

of the infant has been difficult because of excessive muscle tone.

Low-dose Ketamine (Table 7.1)

Ketamine in intermittent intravenous doses of 10 to 15 mg can be titrated to produce intense maternal analgesia without loss of consciousness.[72] Onset of action is less than 30 seconds, and recovery is rapid (4 minutes) as evidenced by orientation to time, place and person. Undesirable hallucinations are minimal, especially if the anesthesiologist provides pleasant verbal reassurance and encouragement.

Low-dose ketamine is particularly useful for parturients in whom imminent vaginal delivery of the fetus is expected or for parturients with spotty regional analgesia for either vaginal delivery or cesarean section. After the initial dose, the patient should remain awake and responsive and the dose may be repeated at intervals of 2 to 5 minutes. The total dose should not exceed 100 mg over a 30-minute period. Amnesia for delivery is common and may be undesirable.

High-dose Ketamine

When ketamine is used in a single intravenous dose of 1 mg/kg for induction of general anesthesia for cesarean section, neonatal neurobehavioral tests are higher than after thiopental 4 mg/kg.[73] The Apgar scores and fetal acid-base status at birth are similar after ketamine or thiopental anesthesia.[74, 75] However, it is unlikely that ketamine will replace thiopental as the routine induction agent of choice because of ketamine's psychotomimetic properties. On the other hand, ketamine offers distinct advantages over thiopental in the severely hypotensive, hypovolemic parturient or the patient with severe asthma.[76] Ketamine should not be administered to the obstetric patient in doses greater than 1 mg/kg, because an unacceptably high incidence of neonatal depression and uterine hypertonus is found.

Scopolamine (Hyoscine)

Scopolamine, like atropine, is a belladonna derivative with vagolytic action. The drug, producing inhibition of acetylcholine at muscarinic and nicotinic receptor sites, results in decreased salivary secretions and gastric motility.[77] Placental transfer is rapid; after intravenous administration (0.3 to 0.6 mg) fetal tachycardia and loss of beat-to-beat variability are produced within 10 to 25 minutes and last 60 to 90 minutes.[78, 79] Unlike atropine, scopolamine crosses the blood-brain barrier and produces profound amnesia and mild sedation, presumably by its anticholinergic actions in the central nervous system.[80] Amnesia does not occur until at least 20 minutes after intravenous administration. Scopolamine does not possess analgesic properties and, like most sedatives, will result in severe agitation, marked excitement and loss of inhibitions in the presence of severe pain. Hallucinations and

SYSTEMIC MEDICATION FOR LABOR AND DELIVERY

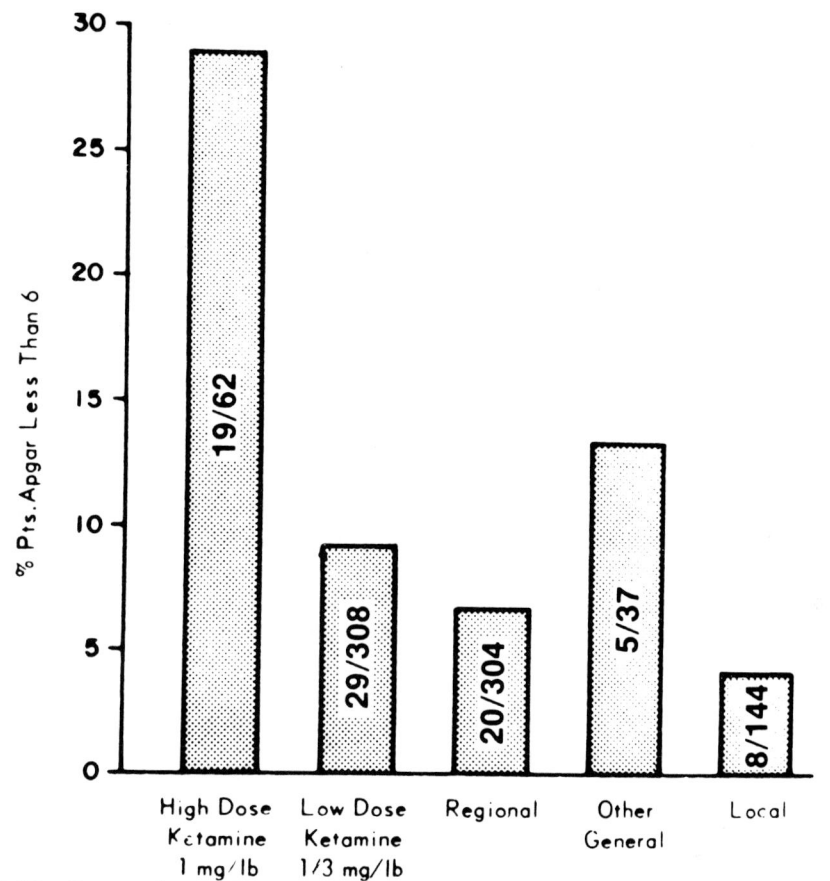

Figure 7.10. Comparison of high-dose and low-dose ketamine anesthesia with regional, local and other general anesthetics. (Reprinted with permission from Janeczko GF, El-Etr AA, Younes S: Low-dose ketamine anesthesia for obstetrical delivery. Anesth Analg 53:829, 1974.)

Table 7.1
Low-dose Ketamine Analgesia: A Suggested Technique

1. Administer 15 to 30 ml of antacid.
2. Check blood pressure.
3. Administer an initial dose of ketamine 10 to 15 mg, but not to exceed 0.25 mg/kg.
4. Maintain continuous verbal contact with patient to provide reassurance and monitor her sensorium.
5. If necessary, give additional 10- to 15-mg doses of ketamine every 2 to 5 minutes, up to a maximum total dose of 100 mg.

delirium are common if a parturient in active labor is given scopolamine without adequate narcotics. "Twilight sleep," once a popular analgesic-amnesic technique, consisted of the administration of a single dose of morphine and scopolamine during labor followed by later injections of scopolamine only. Maternal amnesia for labor and delivery was intense, neonatal narcotic depression was common and the parturient was difficult to manage. Scopolamine per se has no adverse effects on the progress of labor or significant respiratory depressant effects on the neonate.[7]

The authors believe that scopolamine has little place as a sedative during labor, because maternal amnesia is no longer desired by most parturients. No good data exist to prove that scopolamine, when used as a pre-medicant prior to general anesthesia for cesarean section, decreases the incidence of maternal awareness for the operation.

NEUROLEPTANALGESIA

The state of psychic indifference to environmental stimuli produced by the combination of a major tranquilizer with a potent narcotic is known as neuroleptanalgesia. The most popular mixture of this type, Innovar, consists of droperidol (Inapsine) 2.5 mg/ml and fentanyl 0.05 mg/ml. Droperidol is a potent, long-acting tranquilizer with little or no direct effect on respiration, heart rate, myocardial contractile force or cardiac output. It is an adrenergic blocking agent and can cause peripheral vasodilation and hypotension, particularly in hypovolemic patients. Droperidol, like other butyrophenones, may occasionally produce undesirable restlessness and extrapyramidal dyskinesia. Although most of the sedative-tranquilizer drugs possess antiemetic actions, droperidol seems to be vastly superior in this regard. Nausea and vomiting are not uncommon in parturients, especially in those receiving narcotics, and the antiemetic activity of droperidol is one of its most attractive properties. Fentanyl, the narcotic portion of Innovar, has been discussed previously.

Neuroleptanalgesia for childbirth is not a popular technique because of the potential for profound depressant effects on the newborn. The few studies available have indicated that Innovar probably does not cause more neonatal depression than other narcotic-tranquilizer combinations. For example, Ovadia and Halbrecht[81] administered Innovar for normal vaginal deliveries to 100 women. They gave 3 to 5 ml intramuscularly when the cervix was 4-cm dilated, followed by smaller doses at 30-minute intervals if necessary. No medication was given after the cervix was fully dilated. They found that most of the women had considerably less discomfort, were able to sleep quietly between contractions and were generally more cooperative than patients receiving a Demerol-Phenergan combination. Innovar decreased the duration and frequency of contractions, and almost all their patients received oxytocin or vacuum extraction. All the neonates had Apgar scores greater than 7, and none required any form of resuscitation. The lack of fetal depression was attributed to the short duration of action of fentanyl.

Although a few investigators have used Innovar for cesarean section without adverse maternal or fetal effects, most commonly the droperidol component has been administered during induction and the fentanyl withheld until after the umbilical cord is clamped[82] to avoid neonatal respiratory depression.

ANTAGONISTS

Physostigmine (Antilirium)

Physostigmine is an anticholinesterase agent which, unlike its analogue neostigmine, rapidly crosses the blood-brain barrier and increases central nervous system acetylcholine. It is extremely effective in reversing the delirium and sedation produced by scopolamine and other sedative drugs with anticholinergic activity.[83, 84] Some preliminary reports indicate that it may be effective in reversing the sedative effects of diazepam,[85] Innovar[86] and ketamine.[87] The usual dose is 0.5 to 2.0 mg intravenously given in 0.5-mg increments. Total doses of 3 to 4 mg are occasionally necessary. The duration of action is 1 to 2 hours. Although bradycardia after physostigmine administration is uncommon, atropine should be readily available.

The drug has been used in obstetrics and found to be a safe and rapidly effective agent for reversing the delirium and somnolence produced by scopolamine. When used prior to delivery it is not associated with fetal bradycardia. The drug will reverse the decreased beat-to-beat variability produced by atropine and scopolamine.[79] The clinical condition of newborns from mothers who have received physostigmine does not seem to be adversely affected.[83, 84]

Naloxone (Narcan)

Naloxone is currently the preferred narcotic antagonist. Unlike nalorphine (Nalline) and levallorphan (Lorfan) it has no agonist activity and thus produces no cardiorespiratory or central nervous system depression. Narcotic antagonists have been administered in three ways: (1) to the mother with each dose of narcotic, (2) to the mother 10 to 15 minutes before delivery and (3) to the neonate immediately after delivery.

The rationale for administering a narcotic and a narcotic antagonist simultaneously is to provide maximum analgesia with minimal respiratory depression. Numerous studies have proved[88] that the antagonists will reverse the analgesia as well as the respiratory depression and, therefore, offer no advantage.

The rationale for administering naloxone just before delivery is to allow placental transfer and intrauterine reversal of narcotic depression in the fetus and neonate.[89] Many consider this approach inadvisable, because removal of maternal analgesia immediately before delivery is unfair to the mother, may result in an uncontrollable and difficult delivery and is usually unnecessary insofar as the neonate is concerned.

The rationale for administering naloxone routinely to all neonates whose mothers have received narcotics within 4 hours of delivery is that even apparently vigorous babies will have some central nervous system depression and alteration of neurobehavioral status.[49, 90] The objection to this approach is based on the lack of documentation of long-term safety of naloxone. The short-term safety of naloxone is well documented. Even when administered in excessive doses no adverse effects are found.

However, it has become apparent that opiate receptors and endogenous opioid substances (enkephalins and endorphans) may have a normal physiologic function.[91, 92] These compounds may be important neurotransmitters and be involved in hypothalamic-pituitary function and the integration of sensory stimuli. Naloxone acts by displacing narcotics from the receptor sites in the central nervous system and blocks the physiologic effects of enkephalins and endorphans; theoretically, it may adversely influence the neonate's response to stress. Until further studies are performed the routine administration of naloxone to all neonates is not recommended.

It should be emphasized that adverse neonatal effects of naloxone have never been demonstrated and the drug should not be withheld when indicated. Parturients who receive an absolute or relative overdose of narcotics, as evidenced by obtundation or hypoventilation, should receive naloxone. Depressed infants who have a high probability of being narcotized and do not respond to routine resuscitation with oxygenation, ventilation and tactile stimulation should also receive naloxone.

In adults the usual initial dose is 0.4 mg intravenously. The neonatal dose is 0.01 mg/kg either intravenously or, if perfusion is good, intramuscularly. Effects are seen within minutes and last 1 to 2 hours. Because of the relatively short duration of action of naloxone, the narcotically overdosed mother or neonate must be observed carefully and repeat doses of the antagonist administered if necessary. Naloxone should not be used in narcotic addicts or their neonates because acute withdrawal symptoms may be precipitated.

References

1. Clutton-Brock JC: Some pain threshold studies with particular reference to thiopentone. Anaesthesia 15:71, 1960.
2. Dundee JW: Alterations in response to somatic pain associated with anaesthesia. II. The effect of thiopentone and pentobarbitone. Br J Anaesth 32:407, 1960.
3. Keats AS, Kurosu Y: Increased ventilation after pentobarbital in man. Surv Anesthesiol 1:473, 1957.
4. Root B, Eichner E, Sunshine I: Blood secobarbital levels and their clinical correlation in mothers and newborn infants. Am J Obstet Gynecol 81:948, 1961.
5. Kosaka Y, Takahashi T, Mark LC: Intravenous thiobarbiturate anesthesia for cesarean section. Anesthesiology 31:489, 1969.
6. Shnider SM, Moya F: Effects of meperidine on the newborn infant. Am J Obstet Gynecol 89:1009, 1964.
7. Snyder FF: *Obstetric Analgesia and Anesthesia.* W. B. Saunders, Philadelphia, 1949.
8. Irving FC: Advantages and disadvantages of barbiturates in obstetrics. R I Med J 28:493, 1945.
9. Powe CE, Kiem IM, Fromhagen C, et al.: Propiomazine hydrochloride in obstetrical analgesia. JAMA 181:290, 1962.
10. Benson C, Benson RC: Hydroxyzine-meperidine analgesia and neonatal response. Am J Obstet Gynecol 84:37, 1962.
11. Brelje MC, Garcia-Bunuel R: Meperidine-hydroxyzine in obstetric analgesia. Obstet Gynecol 27:350, 1966.
12. Zsigmond EK, Patterson RL: Double blind evaluation of hydroxyzine hydrochloride in obstetric anesthesia. Anesth Analg 46:275, 1967.
13. Cavanagh D, Condo CS: Diazepam: A pilot study of drug concentrations in maternal blood, amniotic fluid and cord blood. Curr Ther Res 6:122, 1964.
14. Cree IE, Meyer J, Hailey DM: Diazepam in labour: Its metabolism and effect on the clinical condition and thermogenesis of the newborn. Br Med J 4:251, 1973.
15. Scher J, Hailey DM, Beard RW: The effects of diazepam on the fetus. J Obstet Gynaecol Br Commonw 79:635, 1972.
16. DeSilva JAF, D'Aconte L, Kaplan J: The determination of blood levels and the placental transfer of diazepam in humans. Curr Ther Res 6:115, 1964.
17. Flowers CE, Rudolph AJ, Desmond MM: Diazepam (Valium) as an adjunct in obstetric analgesia. Obstet Gynecol 34:68, 1969.
18. Shannon RW, Fraser GP, Aitken RG, et al.: Diazepam in preeclamptic toxaemia with special reference to its effect on the newborn infant. Br J Clin Pract 26:271, 1972.
19. Owen JR, Irani SF, Blair AW: Effect of diazepam administered to mothers during labour on temperature regulation of neonate. Arch Dis Child 47:107, 1972.
20. Hon E: *An Atlas of Fetal Heart Rate Patterns.* Harty Press, New Haven, Conn., p 231.
21. Yeh SY, Paul RH, Cordero L, et al.: A study of diazepam during labor. Obstet Gynecol 43:363, 1974.
22. Rolbin SH, Wright RG, Shnider SM, et al.: Diazepam during cesarean section: Effects on neonatal Apgar scores, acid-base status, neurobehavioral assessment and maternal and fetal plasma norepinephrine levels. *Abstracts of Scientific Papers,* Annual Meeting, American Society of Anesthesiologists, New Orleans, 1977, p. 449.
23. Schiff D, Chan G, Stern L: Fixed drug combinations and the displacement of bilirubin from albumin. Pediatrics 48:139, 1971.
24. Nathenson G, Cohen MI, McNamara H: The effect of Na benzoate on serum bilirubin of the Gunn rat. J Pediatr 86:799, 1975.
25. Sentor MH, Solomon E, Kohl SG: An evaluation of oxymorphone in labor. Am J Obstet Gynecol 84:956, 1962.
26. Flowers CE: *Obstetrical Analgesia and Anesthesia.* Harper & Row, New York, 1967, p 76.
27. Downes JJ, Kemp RA, Lambersen CJ: The magnitude and duration of respiratory depression due to fentanyl and meperidine in man. J Pharmacol Exp Therap 158:416, 1967.
28. Forrest WH, Bellville JW: Respiratory effects of alphaprodine in man. Obstet Gynecol 31:61, 1968.
29. Eckenhoff JE, Oech SR: The effects of narcotics and antagonists upon respiration and circulation in man. Clin Pharmacol Ther 1:483, 1960.
30. La Salvia LA, Steffen EA: Delayed gastric emptying time in labor. Am J Obstet Gynecol 59:1075, 1950.
31. Friedman EA: The functional divisions of labor. Am J Obstet Gynecol 109:274, 1971.
32. DeVoe SJ, DeVoe K Jr, Rigsby WC, et al.: Effect of meperidine on uterine contractility. Am J Obstet Gynecol 105:1004, 1969.
33. Filler WW Jr, Hall WC, Filler NW: Analgesia in obstetrics. Am J Obstet Gynecol 96:832, 1967.
34. Apgar V, Burns JJ, Brodie BB, et al.: Transmission of meperidine across human placenta. Am J Obstet Gynecol 64:1368, 1952.
35. Moya F, Thorndike V: Passage of drugs across the placenta. Am J Obstet Gynecol 84:1778, 1962.
36. Moore J, Carson RM, Hunter RJ: A comparison of the effects of pentazocine and pethidine administered during labour. J Obstet Gynaecol Br Commonw 77:830, 1970.
37. Shute E, Davis M: The effect on the infant of morphine administered in labor. Surg Gynecol Obstet 57:727, 1933.
38. Roberts H, Kane KM, Percival N, et al.: Effects of some analgesic drugs used in childbirth. Lancet 1:128, 1957.
39. Shnider SM, Way EL, Lord MJ: Rate of appearance and disappearance of meperidine in fetal blood after administration of narcotic to the mother. Anesthesiology 27:227, 1966.
40. Beckett AH, Taylor JF: Blood concentrations of pethidine and pentazocine in mother and infant at time of birth. J Pharm Pharmacol (Suppl)19:50S, 1967.

41. Moore J, McNabb TG, Glynn JP: The placental transfer of pentazocine and pethidine. Brit J Anaesth (Suppl)45:798, 1973.
42. Rosen MG, Scibetta JJ, Hochberg CJ: Human fetal electroencephalogram. III. Pattern changes in presence of fetal heart rate alterations and after use of maternal medications. Obstet Gynecol 36:132, 1970.
43. Boddy K, Dawes GS: Fetal breathing. Br Med Bull 31:3, 1975.
44. Yeh SY, Forsythe A, Hon EH: Quantification of fetal heart beat-to-beat interval differences. Obstet Gynecol 41:355, 1973.
45. Jenkins VR II, Dilts PV Jr: Some effects of meperidine hydrochloride on maternal and fetal sheep. Am J Obstet Gynecol 109:1005, 1971.
46. Taylor ES, vonFumetti HH, Essig LL, et al.: The effects of Demerol and trichloroethylene on arterial oxygen saturation in the newborn. Am J Obstet Gynecol 69:348, 1955.
47. Koch G, Wandel H: Effect of pethidine on the postnatal adjustment of respiration and acid-base balance. Acta Obstet Gynecol Scand 47:27, 1968.
48. Brackbill Y, Kane J, Manniello RL: Obstetric meperidine usage and assessment of neonatal status. Anesthesiology 40:116, 1974.
49. Hodgkinson R, Bhatt M, Kim SS, et al.: Double blind comparison of the neurobehavior of 920 neonates following the administration of different doses of meperidine to the mother. In *Abstracts of Scientific Papers*, Annual Meeting, American Society of Anesthesiologists, San Francisco, 1976, p 255.
50. Morrison JC, Wiser WL, Rosser SI, et al.: Metabolites of meperidine related to fetal depression. Am J Obstet Gynecol 115:1132, 1973.
51. Morrison JC, Whybrew WD, Rosser SI, et al.: Metabolites of meperidine in the fetal and maternal serum. Am J Obstet Gynecol 126:997, 1976.
52. Kuhnert BR, Kuhnert PM, Rosen MG: Meperidine and normeperidine levels in the mother, fetus and neonate following meperidine administration during labor. In *Abstracts of Papers Presented*, Annual Meeting, Society for Obstetric Anesthesia and Perinatology, Memphis, 1978, p 58.
53. Freeman DS, Gjika HB, Van Vunakis H: Radioimmunoassay for normeperidine: Studies on the N-dealkylation of meperidine and anileridine. J Pharmacol Exp Therap 203:203, 1977.
54. Cooper LV, Stephen GW, Aggett PJA: Elimination of pethidine and bupivacaine in the newborn. Arch Dis Child 52:638, 1977.
55. Caldwell J, Wakile LA, Notarianni LJ, et al.: Maternal and neonatal disposition of pethidine in childbirth: A study using quantitative gas chromatography-mass spectrometry. Life Sci 22:589, 1978.
56. *Physicians' Desk Reference*, ed 32 Medical Economics, Oradell, N J, 1978, p 1407.
57. Gillam JS, Hunter GW, Darner CB, et al.: Meperidine hydrochloride and alphaprodine as obstetric analgesic agents. Am J Obstet Gynecol 75:1105, 1958.
58. Powell PO Jr, Savage JE: Nisentil in obstetrics. Obstet Gynecol 2:658, 1953.
59. Way WL, Costley EC, Way EL: Respiratory sensitivity of the newborn infant to meperidine and morphine. Clin Pharmacol Ther 6:454, 1965.
60. Mowat J, Garrey MM: Comparison of pentazocine and pethidine in labour. Br Med J 2:757, 1970.
61. Paddock R, Beer EG, Bellville JW, et al.: Analgesic and side effects of pentazocine and morphine in a large population of postoperative patients. Clin Pharmacol Ther 10:355, 1969.
62. Duncan SLB, Ginsburg J, Morris NF: Comparison of pentazocine and pethidine in normal labor. Am J Obstet Gynecol 105:197, 1969.
63. Penrose BH: Aspiration pneumonitis following ketamine induction. Anesth Analg 51:41, 1972.
64. Meer FM, Downing JW, Coleman AJ: An intravenous method of anesthesia for caesarean section. II. Ketamine. Br J Anaesth 45:191, 1973.
65. Taylor PA, Towey RM: Depression of laryngeal reflexes during ketamine anesthesia. Br Med J 2:688, 1971.
66. Bovill JG, Dundee JW, Coppell DL, et al.: Current status of ketamine anaesthesia. Lancet 1:1285, 1971.
67. Levinson G, Shnider SM, Gildea J, et al.: Maternal and foetal cardiovascular and acid base changes during ketamine anaesthesia. Br J Anaesth 45:1111, 1973.
68. Eng M, Berges PU, Bonica JJ: The effects of ketamine on uterine blood flow in the monkey. In *Abstracts of Scientific Papers*, Annual Meeting, Society for Gynecological Investigation, Atlanta, 1973, abstract 75, p 48.
69. Galloon S: Ketamine for obstetric delivery. Anesthesiology 44:522, 1976.
70. Little B, Chang T, Chucot L, et al.: Study of ketamine as an obstetric agent. Am J Obstet Gynecol 113:247, 1972.
71. Janeczko GF, El-Etr AA, Younes S: Low-dose ketamine anesthesia for obstetrical delivery. Anesth Analg 53:829, 1974.
72. Akamatsu TJ, Bonica JJ, Rehmet R, et al.: Experiences with the use of ketamine for parturition. I. Primary anesthetic for vaginal delivery. Anesth Analg 53:284, 1974.
73. Hodgkinson R, Marx GF, Kim SS, et al.: Neonatal neurobehavioral tests following vaginal delivery under ketamine, thiopental and extradural anesthesia. Anesth Analg 56:548, 1977.
74. Pelz B, Sinclair DM: Induction agents for caesarean section: A comparison of thiopentone and ketamine. Anaesthesia 28:37, 1973.
75. Downing JW, Mahomedy MC, Jeal DE, et al.: Anaesthesia for caesarean section with ketamine. Anaesthesia 31:883, 1976.
76. Corssen G, Gutierrez J, Reves JG, et al.: Ketamine in the anesthetic management of asthmatic patients. Anesth Analg 51:588, 1972.
77. Eger EI II: Atropine, scopolamine and related compounds. Anesthesiology 23:365, 1962.
78. Hellman LM, Morton GW, Wallach EE: An analysis of the atropine test for placental transfer in 28 normal gravidas. Am J Obstet Gynecol 87:650, 1963.
79. Boehm FH, Smith BE, Egilmez A: Physostigmine's effect on diminished fetal heart rate vari-

ability caused by scopolamine. In *Abstracts of Scientific Papers*, Annual Meeting, Society for Obstetric Anesthesia and Perinatology, Philadelphia, 1975, p.18.
80. Safer DJ, Allen RP: The central effects of scopolamine in man. Biol Psychiatry 3:347, 1971.
81. Ovadia L, Halbrecht I: Neuroleptanalgesia: A new method of anesthesia for normal childbirth. Harefuah 72:143, 1967.
82. McGowan SW: Droperidol in obstetric practice. In *The Application of Neuroleptanalgesia in Anesthetic and Other Practice*, NW Shepard, ed. Pergamon Press, New York, 1965, p. 69.
83. Smiler BG, Bartholomew EG, Sivak BV, et al.: Physostigmine reversal of scopolamine delirium in obstetric patients. Am J Obstet Gynecol 116:326, 1973.
84. Smith DB, Clark RB, Stephens SR: Physostigmine reversal of sedation in parturients. Anesth Analg 55:478, 1976.
85. Larson GF, Hurlbert BJ, Wingard DW: Physostigmine reversal of diazepam-induced depression. Anesth Analg 56:348, 1977.
86. Bidwai AV, Cornelius CR, Stanley TH: Reversal of Innovar-induced post-anesthetic somnolence and disorientation with physostigmine. Anesthesiology 44:249, 1976.
87. Balmer HGR, Wyte SR: Antagonism of ketamine by physostigmine. Br J Anaesth 49:510, 1977.
88. Teleford J, Keats AS: Narcotic-narcotic antagonist mixtures. Anesthesiology 22:465, 1961.
89. Clark RB: Transplacental reversal of meperidine depression in the fetus by naloxone. J Arkansas Med Soc 68:128, 1971.
90. Gerhardt T, Bancalari E, Cohen H, et al.: Use of naloxone. J Pediatr 90:1009, 1977.
91. Snyder SH: Opiate receptors in the brain. N Engl J Med 296:266, 1977.
92. Kosterlitz HW, Hughes J: Possible physiological significance of enkephalin, an endogenous ligand of opiate receptors. Adv Pain Res Therap 1:641, 1976.

CHAPTER 8

Regional Anesthesia for Labor and Delivery

Sol M. Shnider, M.D.
Gershon Levinson, M.D.
David H. Ralston, M.D.

Regional anesthesia for labor and vaginal delivery has gained widespread use because of its effectiveness and, when properly conducted, its safety. Regional blocks provide analgesia while allowing the parturient to be awake and able to participate in labor and delivery. In contrast to parenteral or general inhalation anesthesia techniques, regional anesthesia decreases the likelihood of fetal drug depression and maternal aspiration pneumonitis. The most common forms of regional anesthesia are spinal, lumbar epidural, caudal, paracervical, pudendal and local perineal infiltration. Each technique has a specific application and can be used to block some or all of the nerves carrying the pain impulses.

PAIN PATHWAYS

The pain of labor arises primarily from nociceptors in uterine and perineal structures. Nerve fibers transmitting pain sensation during the first stage of labor travel with sympathetic fibers and enter the neuraxis at the tenth, eleventh and twelfth thoracic and first lumbar spinal segments (Figure 8.1). These fibers synapse in, and make connections with, other ascending and descending fibers in the dorsal horn, particularly in lamina V (Figures 8.2 and 8.3). In late first-stage and second-stage labor, pain impulses increasingly originate from pain-sensitive areas in the perineum and travel via the pudendal nerve to enter the neuraxis at the second, third and fourth sacral segments. The afferent sensory component of pain can be largely relieved by blockade of the neural pathways at several anatomic sites. A list of regional obstetric anesthetic techniques and examples of each are given in Table 8.1 and Figure 8.4.

MANAGEMENT OF COMPLICATIONS

Before performing any regional block in obstetrics, the physician must be prepared for the management of possible complications. The most serious life-threatening complications—severe hypotension, local anesthetic convulsions, total spinal anesthesia with respiratory arrest and vasopressor-induced hypertension—are discussed below. Neurologic complications of regional anesthesia are discussed in chapter 20.

Any room in which anesthesia is per-

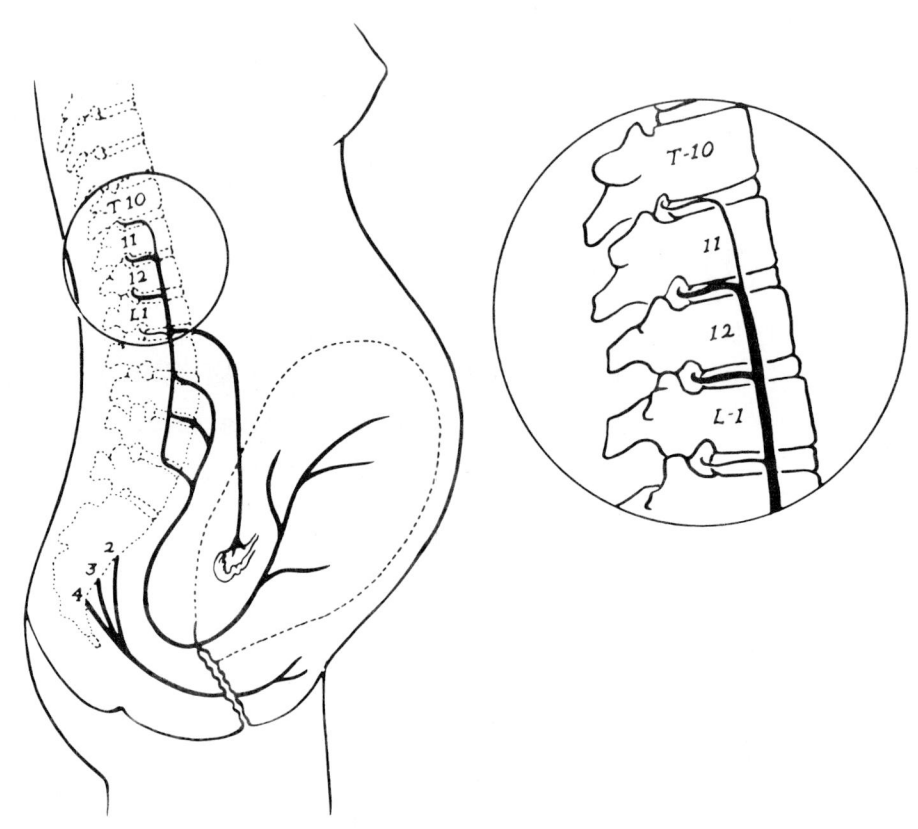

Figure 8.1. Parturition pain pathways. Afferent pain impulses from the cervix and uterus are carried by nerves which accompany sympathetic fibers and enter the neuraxis at T10, T11, T12 and L1 spinal level. Pain pathways from the perineum travel to S2, S3 and S4 via the pudendal nerve. (Reprinted by permission from Bonica JJ: The nature of pain of parturition. Clin Obstet Gynaecol 2:511, 1975.)

formed should have the following items immediately available before starting the block: apparatus for monitoring blood pressure, oxygen with positive pressure breathing apparatus and mask, suction with a wide-bore suction catheter, oral and nasal airways, a laryngoscope and endotracheal tubes, thiopental or diazepam to stop a convulsion and ephedrine to treat hypotension. Prior to placing any block an intravenous route should be established. The bed should be capable of being placed in the Trendelenburg (head-down) position rapidly. The suggested contents of a mobile resuscitation cart are listed in Table 8.2. The cart should be checked prior to starting a block.

Hypotension

Hypotension remains the most common side effect of major conduction anesthesia for vaginal delivery[1]; it is discussed fully in chapter 18. The incidence and severity of hypotension depend on the height of the block, maternal position, the addition of epinephrine to the local anesthetic, the physical status of the parturient and the prophylactic means taken to avoid hypotension. Measures to reduce the incidence of hypotension include administration of fluids prior to the block, left uterine displacement and prophylactic administration of ephedrine.[2-4] If hypotension occurs, more left uterine displacement should be applied, the patient placed in the Trendelenburg position, and intravenous fluids administered rapidly. If blood pressure is not restored within 30 to 60 seconds, ephedrine 10 to 15 mg should be given intravenously and oxygen administered by face mask. Transient maternal hypotension, if recognized and treated promptly, does not lead to maternal or neonatal morbidity.[1]

Local Anesthetic Convulsions

Central nervous system toxicity occurs when a critical arterial blood (and brain tissue) concentration of local anesthetic is exceeded. High blood levels result from inadvertent intravascular injection, accumulation of local anesthetic during repeated injections over a prolonged period of time and rapid systemic absorption of local anesthetic from a highly vascular area. The rate of administration, the total dose of drug and the physical status of the patient affect tolerance to local anesthetics.[5] Inadvertent intravascular injection may occur with **any** regional anesthetic technique, including paracervical and pudendal blocks.[6] Therefore, when a needle or catheter is placed, aspiration should be performed before drug injection to determine whether a blood vessel has been entered. The elimination half-life of amide local anesthetics is 2 to 3 hours. Therefore, systemic accumulation of amide local anesthetics to near toxic levels may occur with large doses repeated at frequent intervals. During properly conducted regional anesthesia, toxic concentrations of local anesthetics resulting from absorption are rarely seen.[5,7] The potential risk of systemic accumulation can be min-

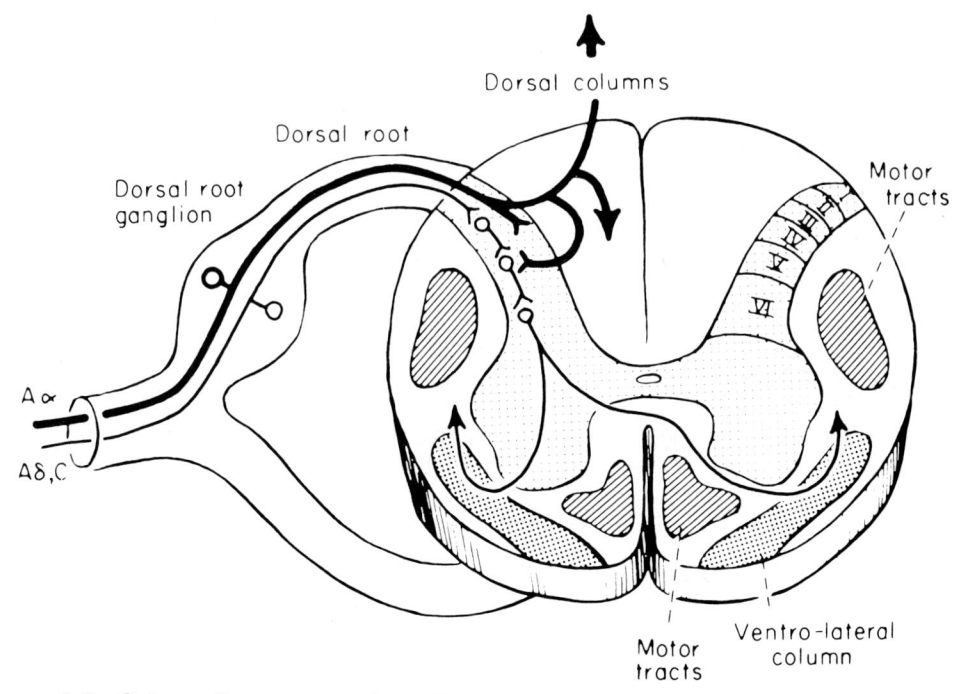

Figure 8.2. Schematic cross-section of the spinal cord. Aδ and C fibers make multiple synaptic connections in the dorsal horn. Cell bodies in lamina V send axons to the ipsilateral and contralateral ventral column to make up the spinothalamic system. (Reprinted by permission from Bonica JJ: The nature of pain of parturition. Clin Obstet Gynaecol 2:500, 1975.)

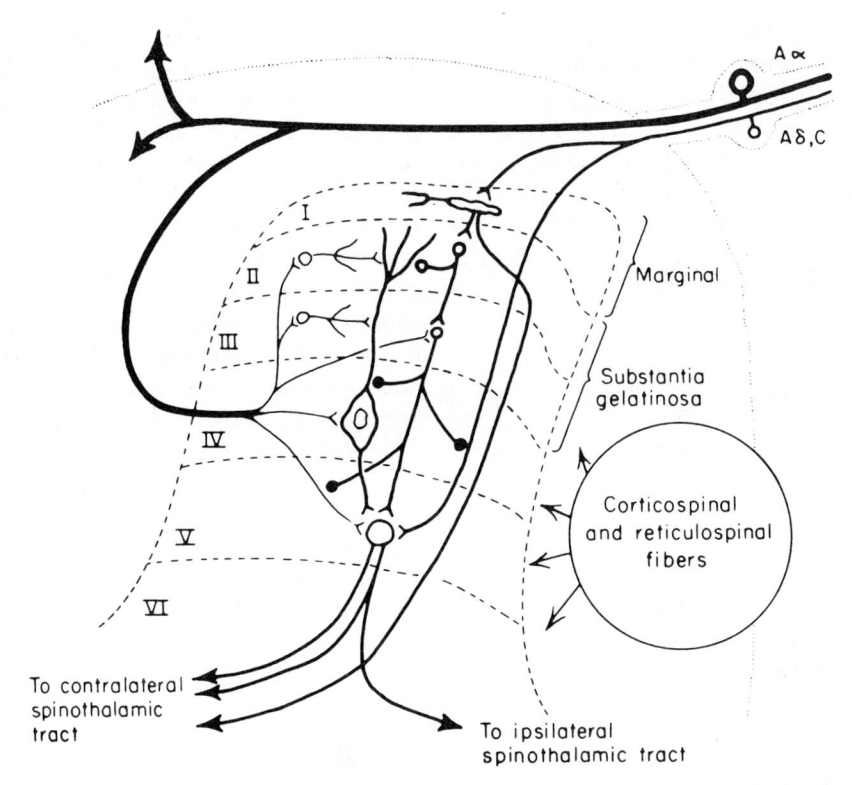

Figure 8.3. A simplified model of the synaptic connections within the six laminae of the dorsal horn. Pain impulses during parturition are transmitted via Aδ and C fibers to the dorsal horn, where multiple synaptic connections are made. Descending corticospinal and reticulospinal fibers carry impulses which may modulate pain information at the dorsal horn, a possible neurophysiologic mechanism for cortical modification of afferent pain stimuli. (Reprinted by permission from Bonica JJ: The nature of pain of parturition. Clin Obstet Gynaecol 2:501, 1975.)

imized by using the smallest quantity of drug necessary to achieve the desired anesthesia and by using agents which are rapidly metabolized and intrinsically less toxic, such as chloroprocaine.[8] The use of epidural catheters in both sacral and lumbar areas (double-catheter technique) may also minimize total local anesthetic drug requirement, although no data are currently available to support this claim.

The reported incidence of convulsions during obstetric regional anesthesia is low, varying from 0.03 to 0.5 per cent (Table 8.3). Of note is the lack of resultant maternal morbidity or mortality, suggesting that local anesthetic-induced toxic reactions, if properly treated, should not cause permanent sequelae. A summary of the symptoms and signs of local anesthetic toxic reactions is shown in Table 8.4. Treatment involves:

1. Early recognition of the reaction. By constant observation of the patient and her vital signs and by talking to her, it is possible to become aware of the impending toxic reaction and to take steps to prevent it from becoming serious.

2. Prevention of progression of the reaction. Small doses of barbiturates given intravenously may prevent convulsions.

The depressant effect of the barbiturate may intensify the depression which results from the local anesthetic, but small doses of thiopental (Pentothal), 50 to 75 mg, or diazepam (Valium), 5 mg, repeated as needed are probably safe. At the same time, oxygen should be given by mask so that the patient is well oxygenated should a convulsion occur.

3. Maintenance of oxygenation despite convulsions and/or vomiting. Convulsions are not lethal, but the anoxia that they produce is. If, after clearing the airway of foreign material, it becomes impossible to oxygenate the convulsing patient with positive pressure breathing apparatus, it may be necessary to paralyze her with 60 to 80 mg of succinylcholine and intubate her trachea with a cuffed endotracheal tube.

4. Support of the circulation. Elevation of the legs and rapid administration of intravenous fluids and vasopressors may be needed to support the depressed circulation.

5. Treatment of cardiac arrest. Cardiac arrest should be treated in the usual way, with external cardiac massage, defibrillation if necessary, sodium bicarbonate and appropriate cardiotonic drugs, such as dopamine, epinephrine and isoproterenol. Left uterine displacement should be maintained if possible.

6. Consideration of the fetus. As soon as possible, the condition of the fetus should be assessed to enable the obstetrician to decide the subsequent course of delivery. Prompt maternal resuscitation usually will restore uterine blood flow and fetal oxygenation and will allow fetal excretion of local anesthetic to the mother via the placenta.[19]

Total Spinal

Total spinal anesthesia may occur from an excessive spread of local anesthetic administered intrathecally, extradurally or perhaps even subdurally. Dural perfora-

Table 8.1
Regional Anesthetic Techniques in Obstetrics

Technique	Example	Area of Anesthesia
Infiltration	Local for episiotomy	Perineal skin and subcutaneous tissue
	Local for cesarean section	Skin, subcutaneous tissue fascia, peritoneum
Peripheral neural blockade		
Single nerve	Pudendal	S2–S4
Plexus	Lumbar Sympathetic	T10–L1
	Paracervical	T10–L1
Central neural blockade		
Epidural	Lumbar	
	Standard	T10–S5
	Segmental	T10–L1
	Caudal	
	Standard	T10–S5
	High catheter	T10–S5
	Low catheter	S2–S5
	Combined	
	Segmental	T10–L1
	+	+
	Low caudal	S2–S5
Subarachnoid	Standard	T10–S5
	Low (saddle)	S1–S5

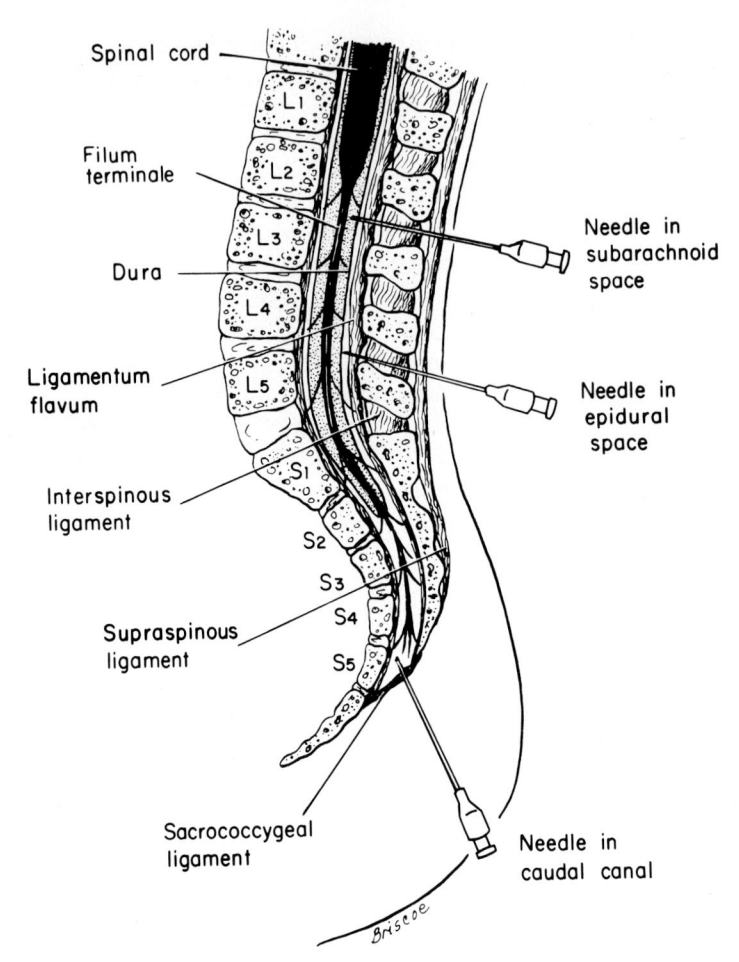

Figure 8.4. Schematic diagram of lumbo-sacral anatomy showing needle placement for subarachnoid, lumbar epidural and caudal blocks.

tion by an epidural catheter may occur when the catheter is initially inserted or during the course of a previously uneventful continuous epidural anesthetic.[20] Although infrequent, the possibility of total spinal anesthesia necessitates the immediate presence of personnel who can promptly diagnose and treat this complication.

Treatment consists of establishing an airway and ventilating with oxygen. Endotracheal intubation should be performed as soon as possible to protect the airway from aspiration. The Trendelenburg position and left uterine displacement should be used to increase venous return to the heart. Fluids and ephedrine should be administered as necessary to maintain blood pressure.

Vasopressor-induced Hypertension

Inadvertent intravascular injection of as little as 5 to 10 µg of epinephrine may cause maternal hypertension from α-adrenergic stimulation. This reaction is brief because of the short half-life of epinephrine. The interaction of vasoactive drugs and ergot derivatives may also lead to severe maternal hypertension and possible cerebrovascular accidents.[21] Particularly dangerous is the combination of a purely α-adrenergic agent, such as methoxamine, and the ergot derivatives ergonovine and methylergonovine. Ephedrine, when used alone, may also be associated with postpartum hypertension.[21] Prophylactic vasopressors or anesthetic solutions containing epinephrine should be avoided in parturients with pre-existing hypertension. If acute postpartum hypertension occurs, treatment includes: (1) chlorpromazine (Thorazine) 2.5 mg intravenously given at 15-second intervals to a maximum dose of 15 mg or (2) trimethaphan (Arfonad) drip (500 mg in 500 ml), (3) phentolamine (Regetine) 5 mg intravenously or nitroprusside (Nipride) drip (50 mg in 500 ml).

TECHNIQUES OF REGIONAL ANESTHESIA

Lumbar Epidural Anesthesia (Table 8.5 and Figures 8.5 to 8.7)

Once labor is well established—i.e. cervical dilation is usually 6 to 8 cm in a nullipara or 4 to 6 cm in a multipara, with strong (50 to 70 mm Hg) contractions lasting 1 minute and occurring 3 minutes apart—a continuous lumbar epidural

Table 8.2
Resuscitation Cart

Positive pressure breathing apparatus
Oxygen supply
Laryngoscope: adult and infant blades
Endotracheal tubes: adult—6.5, 7.0, 7.5, 8.0
  infant—2.5, 3.0, 3.5
Stylets: adult and infant
Oral airways: adult and infant
Nasal airways
Suction catheters: adult and infant
Board for closed-chest massage
Drugs: ephedrine   atropine, dopamine,
  $CaCl_2$ thiopental, or diazepam
  $NaHCO_3$ hydralazine, phentolamine,
  epinephrine   succinylcholine,* curare
  naloxone   heparin, trimethaphan,*
                  thorazine
Naso-gastric tubes
I.V. supplies, plasma expanders and electrolyte solution, syringes, needles, plastic indwelling catheters
Each labor room should contain an oxygen supply, suction and bed capable of rapid Trendelenburg position. An ECG monitor and defibrillator should be readily available.

* Often kept in the refrigerator.

Table 8.4
Signs and Symptoms of Local Anesthetic-induced Systemic Toxicity

Central nervous system
  Cerebral cortex
    Stimulation—restlessness, nervousness, incoherent speech, metalic taste, dizziness, blurred vision, tremors and convulsions
    Depression—unconsciousness
  Medulla
    Stimulation—increased blood pressure, heart and respiratory rate, nausea and vomiting
    Depression—hypotension, apnea and asystole
Cardiovascular
  Heart—bradycardia, ventricular tachycardia and fibrillation, decreased contractility
  Blood vessels—vasodilation and hypotension
Uterus
  Uterine vasoconstriction and uterine hypertonus resulting in fetal distress

Table 8.3
Incidence of Major Complications during Regional Anesthesia in Obstetrics

Regional Technique	Number of Parturients	Toxic Reactions	Resultant Morbidity	Total Spinal	Permanent Paralysis	References
Lumbar epidural	13,817	0.03–0.5	0	0–0.03	0	9–11
Caudal epidural	18,642	0.05–0.3	0	0.06	0	12–15
Subarachnoid	29,102	—	—	0.1	0.01–0.05	16–18

Table 8.5
Lumbar Epidural and Caudal Anesthesia for Labor and Vaginal Delivery: Suggested Techniques

Labor should be well established: Cervical dilation 6 to 8 cm in nulliparas, 4 to 6 cm in multiparas; earlier if oxytocin induction or augmentation are used.
1. Check resuscitation equipment and oxygen delivery system.
2. Start I.V. with 16- or 18-gauge plastic indwelling catheter.
3. Apply blood pressure cuff and check control pressure.
4. Administer 500 ml of balanced salt solution before starting block in all patients except in those with preeclampsia. In preeclamptics administer 250 ml of plasmanate and 250 ml of balanced salt solution.

Lumbar Epidural	*Caudal*
5. Position patient: Lateral decubitus is most commonly used, but sitting position may be useful in very obese patients. Have nurse available to reassure patient, to help with positioning and to prevent movement during placement of the block.	5. Position patient: Lateral decubitus is most commonly used, but prone position with bolster under hips is also popular. Have nurse available to reassure patient, to help with positioning and to prevent movement during placement of the block.
6. Prep and drape the lumbar area.	6. Prep and drape the caudal area.
7. Palpate lumbar spinous processes and choose widest interspace below L2.	7. Using the coccyx as a landmark for the midline, palpate the sacral hiatus and the sacrococcygeal ligament.
8. A large-gauge Tuohy or Crawford needle (16- to 18-gauge) is placed in the epidural space in the usual manner.	8. Place a 16- to 18-gauge Tuohy or Crawford needle in the caudal canal in the usual manner.
a. Midline approach is most popular but lateral or paramedian approach is used by some.	a. After positioning the needle, remove drapes and perform rectal examination to exclude the possibility of inadvertent puncture of the rectum, cervix and fetal presenting part and subsequent anesthetic intoxication of the fetus.
b. Loss of resistance technique with air or saline-filled syringe most commonly used. Negative pressure method, e.g. hanging drop, is also used, but the incidence of dural puncture may be higher.	b. Change gloves, replace drape and pass catheter through needle.
9. Aspirate for blood or CSF.	9. Aspirate for blood or CSF.
10. Administer first local anesthetic dose through needle. Authors recommend chloroprocaine 2 per cent or bupivacaine 0.25 or 0.5 per cent.	10. Administer local anesthetic. Authors recommend chloroprocaine 2 per cent or bupivacaine 0.25 per cent.

11. Inject a 2-ml test dose and wait at least 3 minutes to determine whether a spinal block occurs. If not, inject 5 ml of local anesthetic, wait 30 to 60 seconds to determine whether an intravascular injection occurs (tinnitus, apprehension, tingling) then inject the remainder of the anesthetizing dose.

| 12. For segmental epidurals the above is the usual initial dose. Insert catheter and remove needle. Catheter should be no more than 1 to 2 cm into the epidural space to prevent one-sided or single dermatome blocks. Aspirate catheter for blood or CSF. If negative, inject test dose of local anesthetic. | 12. For a T10 level a total volume of 15 to 20 ml of local anesthetic is usually necessary. |

REGIONAL ANESTHESIA FOR LABOR AND DELIVERY

Table 8.5—*continued*

13. Maintain patient in lateral position throughout labor to prevent aortocaval compression. If one-sided block occurs, place the patient on the unanesthetized side and give more local anesthetic. If the supine position is mandatory for fetal scalp sampling or vaginal examination, duration of the procedure should be as short as possible.
14. Monitor blood pressure every 1 to 2 minutes for the first 10 minutes after injection of local anesthetic, then every 5 to 10 minutes until the block wears off.
15. During the first 20 minutes after the initial dose and after any top-up dose the patient must be observed continuously and not left unattended.
16. If hypotension occurs (fall in systolic blood pressure of 20 to 30 per cent or to below 100 mm Hg) assure left uterine displacement. Infuse intravenous fluids rapidly, place patient in 10° to 20° Trendelenburg position and administer oxygen by well fitting face mask. If blood pressure is not restored within 1 to 2 minutes then administer ephedrine 2.5 to 10 mg I.V. Repeat if necessary.
17. When possible continuously monitor fetal heart rate and uterine contractions by electronic means before and after instituting an epidural block.
18. Check labor progress by vaginal examination at frequent intervals.
19. Aspirate catheter for blood for CSF and administer test dose before each top-up dose.

20. With lumbar epidural anesthesia maintain segmental block during labor with repeated injections until perineal anesthesia is required. Then place patient in semirecumbent or sitting position and administer 10 to 20 ml of local anesthetic. Authors recommend chloroprocaine 3 per cent.	20. With caudal anesthesia use 3 per cent chloroprocaine for delivery.

21. After delivery and episiotomy repair remove catheter and check for hypotension when the patient's legs are taken out of stirrups.

---

block may be administered. The authors have found that chloroprocaine 2.0 per cent or bupivacaine 0.25 to 0.5 per cent produces excellent sensory analgesia with minimal motor blockade. The choice and selection of local anesthetics is fully discussed by Bromage in chapter 9.

After placement of a plastic catheter in the epidural space its position must be verified by injecting a test dose. It is important to realize that the small test dose used to ascertain a spinal block is usually too small to recognize an intravascular injection. Therefore, the authors recommend two test doses as described in Table 8.5. Analgesia is established by injecting a total of 4 to 10 ml of the local anesthetic. The mother is maintained on her side to prevent supine hypotension. If unilateral analgesia occurs, the patient is turned to the opposite side and more local anesthetic (5 to 10 ml) is injected. Segmental anesthesia is provided during labor with repeated injections until perineal anesthesia is required. With perineal distension by the fetal presenting part, the patient is placed in the sitting position, and 10 to 20 ml of drug are administered. Here the authors favor chloroprocaine 3.0 per cent to produce rapid onset of profound analgesia and muscle relaxation.

Caudal Anesthesia (Table 8.5)

A caudal block is also administered after labor is well established. Caudal blocks are

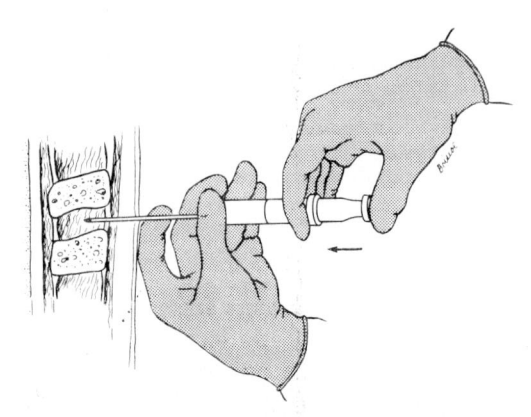

Figure 8.5. Loss-of-resistance technique for identifying epidural space. Needle is placed in interspinous ligament, and resistance to pressure on plunger of syringe is determined. Needle is stabilized with left hand while thumb of right hand applies intermittent pressure to plunger.

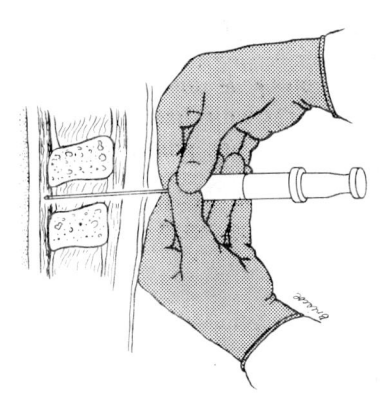

Figure 8.6. Needle is slowly advanced with both hands to prevent too rapid progression and inadvertent dural puncture. Following each incremental advance, intermittent pressure is applied to plunger.

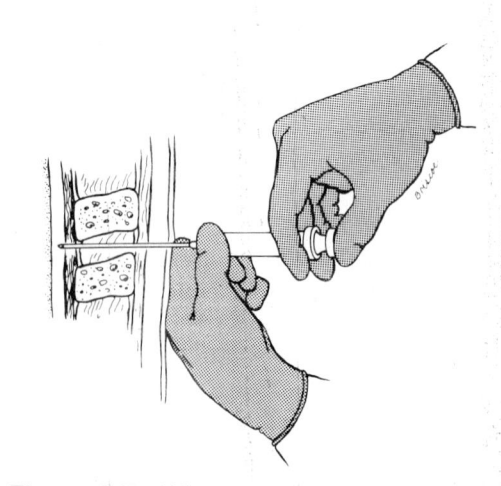

Figure 8.7. When needle passes through ligamentum flavum and enters the epidural space, there will be a sudden loss of resistance.

part and subsequent anesthetic intoxication of the fetus (Figures 8.10 to 8.12).[22] After replacing drapes and gloves the caudal catheter is introduced through the needle. After aspiration a test dose of local anesthetic is given through the needle and/or catheter, because it is possible to puncture the dural sac which ends at the second sacral vertebra or a dural sleeve of a sacral nerve root and produce spinal anesthesia. The volume necessary to provide a T10 block varies between 15 and 20 ml with subsequent doses of 15 ml to maintain analgesia. Placing the patient in a head-down position may be necessary to achieve a T10 block with smaller volumes of drug.

Lumbar epidural may be preferable to caudal anesthesia for the following reasons: (1) segmental T10 to T12 levels can be achieved in early labor when sacral anesthesia is not required; (2) less drug is needed during labor; (3) pelvic muscles retain their tone, and rotation of the fetal head is more easily accomplished; and (4) even though there is an increased risk of dural puncture, often a lumbar epidural is technically easier for the anesthesiologist to administer and less painful for the pa-

performed in patients positioned either on their side (Figure 8.8) or prone with a bolster placed under the thighs. Using the coccyx as a landmark for the midline, the sacral cornu and sacrococcygeal ligament are palpated (Figure 8.9). Once the needle is placed in the canal, the drapes are removed and a rectal examination is performed to exclude the possibility of inadvertent puncture of the fetal presenting

REGIONAL ANESTHESIA FOR LABOR AND DELIVERY

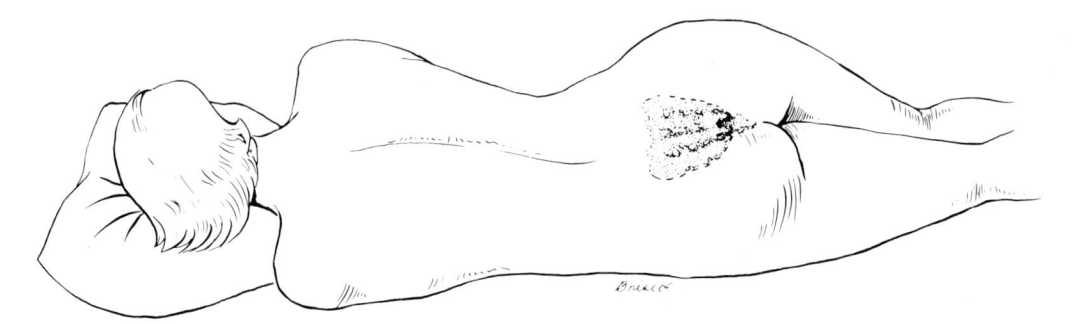

Figure 8.8. Lateral position for caudal block. Note forward tilt of upper hip. For the right-handed physician the patient should lie on her left side.

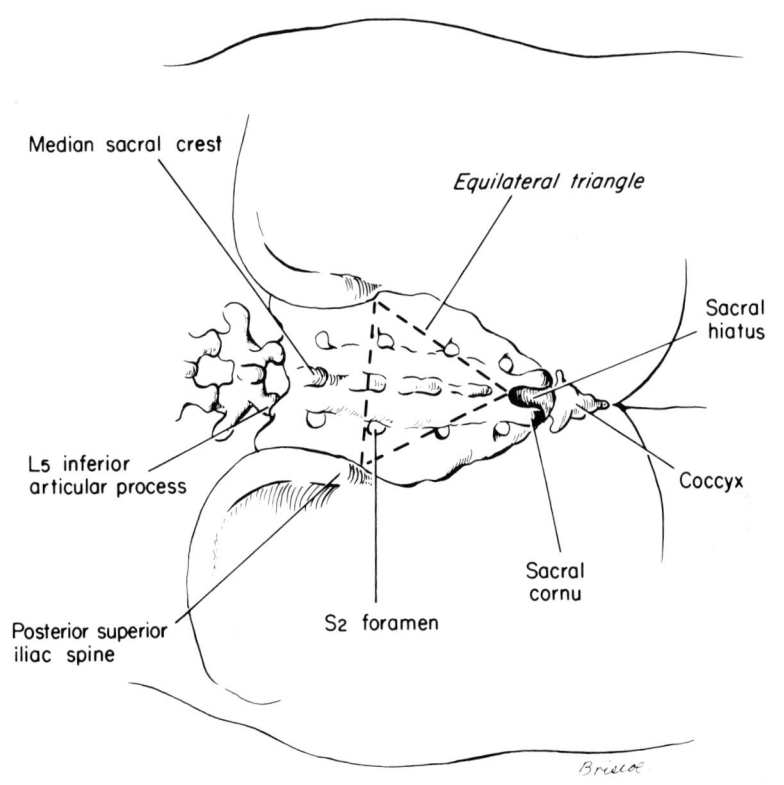

Figure 8.9. Schematic diagram of sacrum showing bony landmarks for identifying sacral cornua and sacral hiatus. Sacral hiatus is usually located 2½ inches above tip of coccyx or at the apex of an equilateral triangle formed by posterior superior iliac spines and sacrococcygeal ligament.

tient during the placement of the needle than a caudal anesthetic. Caudal anesthesia administered just before delivery has advantages over lumbar epidural anesthesia in that the onset of perineal anesthesia and muscle relaxation is more rapid.

Double-catheter Technique

This technique consists of inserting two catheters, a lumbar epidural catheter for pain relief during stage one labor and a caudal catheter for delivery. Usually the

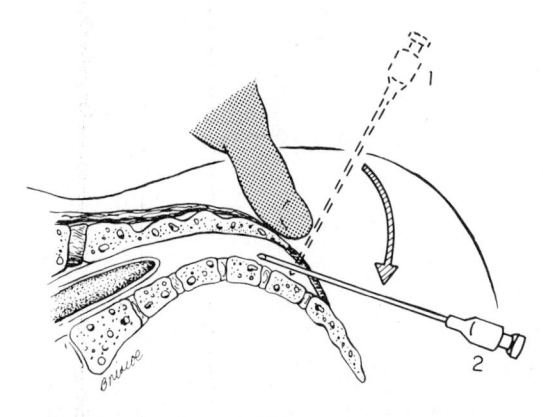

Figure 8.10. Technique of caudal anesthesia. Thumb is placed between sacral cornua at apex of sacral hiatus. Needle is inserted through sacrococcygeal ligament at an angle of approximately 45° (needle position 1). Once ligament is penetrated, needle is repositioned as shown and advanced 1 to 2 cm into caudal canal (needle position 2).

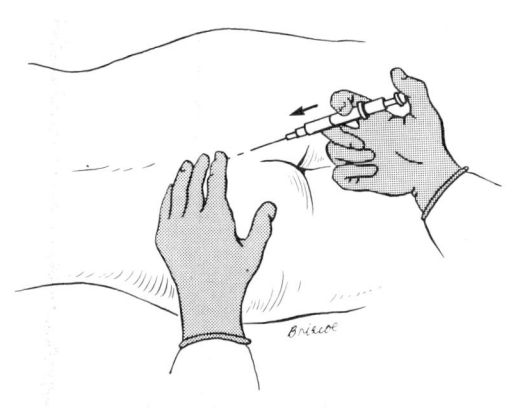

Figure 8.11. Position of needle in caudal canal verified by rapidly injecting a 2- to 3-ml bolus of saline and not palpating an impulse under the finger tips.

caudal catheter is inserted immediately after the epidural catheter, because this is more convenient for both the physician and the patient. Also, labor pains can be diminished during performance of the caudal block.

The double-catheter technique has several advantages. It allows the use of a smaller total dose of local anesthetic. It also permits one to achieve a segmental block (T10 to L1) early in labor, and then, at the time of delivery, by not injecting the lumbar epidural catheter but instead activating the caudal catheter, allows the mother to feel contractions, have maximum ability to push and still have profound perineal anesthesia. These conditions are ideal for breech delivery (chapter 12).

The technique is not currently popular because of the added hazards and discomfort of two needle and catheter insertions. In addition, either lumbar epidural or caudal alone may be used satisfactorily to achieve analgesia for a normal labor and delivery.

Spinal Anesthesia (Table 8.6)

Spinal, often called saddle block, anesthesia is administered immediately before delivery. A small dose of hyperbaric local anesthetic, e.g. tetracaine 3 mg or lidocaine 15 to 20 mg, injected into the subarachnoid space with the patient in the sitting position is needed to accomplish sacral anesthesia. More commonly, however, a T10 to S5 dermatome anesthetic distribution is

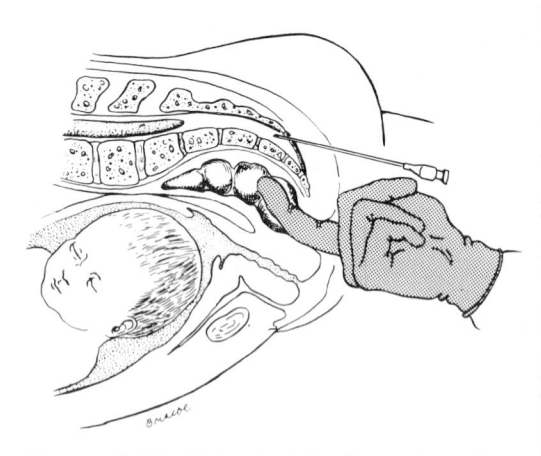

Figure 8.12. Prior to injection of medication or placement of catheter, a rectal examination is performed to rule out inadvertent misplacement of needle with rectal or fetal puncture.

Table 8.6
Spinal Anesthesia for Vaginal Delivery: A Suggested Technique

Perform spinal anesthesia in delivery room.
Check resuscitation equipment and anesthesia machine prior to block.
Start I.V. with plastic indwelling catheter and infuse 500 to 1,000 ml of solution rapidly.
Apply blood pressure cuff and check control pressure.
Position patient; the sitting position is most common. Lateral decubitus with reverse Trendelenburg may be used, especially in the multigravida in whom fetal descent may be very rapid.
Prep and drape lumbar area.
Palpate lumbar spinous processes and choose widest interspace below L2.
Use a 25-gauge spinal needle if possible and place in subarachnoid space in the usual manner.
Inject tetracaine 4 mg or lidocaine 30 mg immediately after a uterine contraction when the patient is relaxed and not straining.
Maintain patient in sitting or reverse Trendelenburg position for 30 seconds and then place supine with legs in stirrups.
Monitor blood pressure every 1 to 2 minutes for the first 10 minutes after injection of local anesthetic, then every 5 to 10 minutes.
If hypotension occurs (fall in systolic blood pressure of 20 to 30 per cent or to below 100 mm Hg) assure left uterine displacement. Infuse intravenous fluids rapidly, place patient in 10° to 20° Trendelenburg position and administer oxygen by well fitting face mask. If blood pressure is not restored within 1 to 2 minutes then administer ephedrine 2.5 to 10 mg I.V. Repeat if necessary.
Following delivery and episiotomy repair, check for hypotension when the patient's legs are taken out of stirrups.

---

desired and can be accomplished with slightly larger doses of tetracaine (4 to 5 mg) or lidocaine (30 to 40 mg). Small-bore needles, such as 25 or 26 gauge, will decrease the incidence of post-dural puncture headache.[23] Care must be taken not to administer the drug just before or during a uterine contraction lest the accompanying Valsalva maneuver result in an excessively high anesthetic level.

Contraindications to Epidural, Caudal and Spinal Anesthesia

There are relatively few absolute contraindications to major conduction anesthesia. These include: (1) patient refusal, (2) infection at site of needle injection, (3) hypovolemic shock and (4) coagulopathies. There are no studies on the use of epidural anesthesia in patients receiving mini-dose heparin and having a normal partial thromboplastin time.

Pre-existing neurologic disease of the spinal cord or peripheral nerves is a relative contraindication, but at times regional anesthesia may be in the best interest of the mother and neonate. Each case should be evaluated individually.

Paracervical Block Anesthesia

Paracervical block is a relatively simple method used by obstetricians to provide analgesia during labor. Local anesthesia is injected submucosally into the fornix of the vagina lateral to the cervix. Frankenhauser's ganglion, containing all the visceral sensory nerve fibers from the uterus, cervix and upper vagina, is anesthetized. The somatic sensory fibers from the perineum are not blocked; thus, the technique is only effective during the first stage of labor. The major disadvantage of paracervical block anesthesia is the relatively high frequency of fetal bradycardia following the block. This bradycardia is associated with fetal acidosis and an increased likelihood of neonatal depression. Bradycardia usually develops within 2 to 10 minutes and lasts from 3 to 30 minutes. The etiology of bradycardia is still unclear, but evidence suggests that it is related to a combination of decreased uterine blood flow from uterine vasoconstriction from the local anesthetic applied in close proximity to the artery (Figure 8.13) and from high fetal blood levels of local anesthetics.[24] Fetal drug levels in infants with bradycardia are occasionally higher than simultaneously drawn maternal levels, suggesting that local anesthetics may reach the fetus by a more direct route than maternal systemic absorption. Some investigators have postulated that high concentrations of local anesthetics reach the fetus by diffusion across the uterine arteries.

Although the precise cause of fetal bradycardia may be controversial, the significance is not. Paracervical block bradycardia indicates fetal distress. Increased neonatal morbidity and, indeed, mortality occur when bradycardia follows paracervical block. Currently, American and European medical journals contain reports of more than 50 perinatal deaths associated with paracervical block. Because of the potential fetal and neonatal hazards, the authors believe that this technique should not be used in cases of utero-placental insufficiency or where there is pre-existing fetal distress. There may be exceptions if other anesthetic techniques are contraindicated or pose a greater hazard to the mother or fetus.

When the technique is used the drug dosage must be kept to a minimum. Safe use of this technique requires that injections be superficial—that is, just below the mucosa—aspiration be done before injection and the fetal heart rate monitored closely after the injection. The block is performed with the patient in the lithotomy position. A needle is placed through the vaginal mucosa just lateral to the cervix at the three o'clock position. After aspiration for blood, 5 to 10 ml of a low-concentration local anesthetic are injected. The fetal heart rate is monitored continuously during the next 5 minutes. If there is no bradycardia, the block is repeated on the other side just lateral to the cervix at the nine o'clock position with the same volume of drug. The fetal heart rate and maternal blood pressure and pulse are monitored closely during the next 10 minutes. The duration of pain relief will vary from 40 minutes with 1.5 per cent chloroprocaine to 90 minutes with 1 per cent mepivacaine. The block may be repeated at intervals depending on the duration of action of the local anesthetic. If the cervix has reached 8 cm of dilation the block should be used with caution lest an injection into the fetal scalp occur.

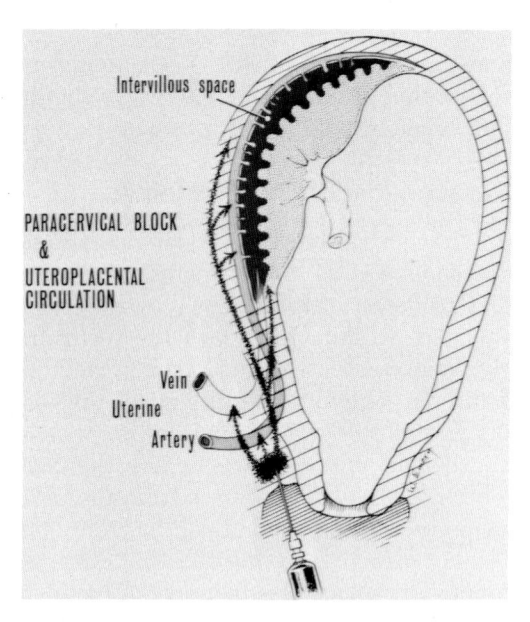

Figure 8.13. Diagram of paracervical area in relation to utero-placental circulation. (Reprinted by permission from Asling JH, Shnider SM, Margolis AJ, et al.: Paracervical block anesthesia in obstetrics. II. Etiology of fetal bradycardia following paracervical block anesthesia. Am J Obstet Gynecol 107:626, 1970.)

Lumbar Sympathetic Block

Bilateral lumbar sympathetic block interrupts the pain impulses from the uterus, cervix and upper third of the vagina and may be used to provide analgesia during the first stage of labor. For relief of perineal pain during the second stage, pudendal nerve blocks or a subarachnoid block must be added.

The lumbar sympathetic block is usually performed at the level of the second lumbar vertebra. Using a 22-gauge, 10-cm needle, the transverse process is located; the needle is then redirected and advanced an additional 5 cm so that the tip is at the anterolateral surface of the vertebral column just anterior to the medial attachment of the psoas muscle.[25] The needle is aspirated in two planes to detect blood or cerebrospinal fluid, and then 10 ml of local anesthetic are injected. This volume will allow the anesthetic to spread along the length of the sympathetic chain. The procedure must be performed on both sides. Bupivacaine 0.5 per cent will provide 2 to 3 hours of anesthesia.

Following the block the patient must be monitored as closely as with a lumbar epidural or caudal anesthetic. Maternal hypotension may occur and is especially common with larger volumes of local anesthetic which spread to and anesthetize the celiac plexus and splanchnic nerves. Systemic toxic reactions from inadvertent intravascular injection or accidental spinal or epidural injections may also occur. Consequently, prior to performing the block, preparations for these complications must be made. There is some evidence that lumbar sympathetic block accelerates the first stage of labor,[26] and it should be used cautiously in the presence of rapidly progressive labor lest tumultuous contractions result.[27]

Compared to continuous lumbar epidural analgesia, lumbar sympathetic block is a technically more difficult block to perform, involves more painful needle placement and does not provide second-stage analgesia. Consequently, it is seldom performed in obstetrics.

Pudendal Block and Local Perineal Infiltration Anesthesia

These blocks are usually administered by the obstetrician just before delivery. Pudendal block is most commonly performed transvaginally. With the patient in the lithotomy position the physician palpates the ischial spine, places a needle guide (Iowa trumpet) under the spine and introduces a 20-gauge needle through the guide until the point rests on the vaginal mucosa. The needle is advanced approximately ½ inch, piercing the sacrospinous ligament; after aspirating for blood, 10 ml of local anesthetic, lidocaine or mepivacaine 1 per cent or chloroprocaine 2 per cent, are injected. The technique is then repeated on the opposite side.

References

1. Shnider SM: Experience with regional anesthesia for vaginal delivery. In The Anesthesiologist, Mother and Newborn, SM Shnider and F Moya, eds. Williams & Wilkins, Baltimore, 1974, p 38.
2. Clark RB: Prevention of spinal hypotension associated with cesarean section. Anesthesiology 45:670, 1976.
3. Gutsche BB: Prophylactic ephedrine preceding spinal analgesia for cesarean section. Anesthesiology 45:462, 1976.
4. Wollman SB, Marx GF: Acute hydration for prevention of hypotension of spinal anesthesia in parturients. Anesthesiology 29:374, 1968.
5. Moore DC, Bridenbaugh LD, Thompson GE, et al.: Factors determining dosages of amide-type local anesthetic drugs. Anesthesiology 47:263, 1977.
6. Grimes DA, Cates W Jr: Deaths from paracervical anesthesia used for first-trimester abortion. N Engl J Med 295:1397, 1976.
7. Poppers PJ: Evaluation of local anaesthetic agents for regional anaesthesia in obstetrics. Br J Anaesth 47:322, 1975.
8. Zsigmond EK: Obstetric use of 2-chloroprocaine. N Engl J Med 289:868, 1973.
9. Adamson DH: Continuous epidural anesthesia in the community hospital. Can Anaesth Soc J 20: 687, 1973.
10. Crawford JS: The second thousand epidural blocks in an obstetric hospital practice. Br J Anaesth 44:1277, 1972.
11. Kandel PF, Spoerel WE, Kinch RAH: Continuous epidural analgesia for labour and delivery. Review of 1000 cases. Can Med Assoc J 95:947, 1966.
12. Bush RC: Caudal analgesia for vaginal delivery.

II. Anesthesiology 20:186, 1959.
13. Dogu TS: Continuous caudal analgesia and anesthesia for labor and vaginal delivery. Obstet Gynecol 33:92, 1969.
14. Epstein HM, Sherline DM: Single-injection caudal anesthesia in obstetrics. Obstet Gynecol 33: 496, 1969.
15. Gunther RE, Bellville JW: Obstetrical caudal anesthesia. II. A randomized study comparing 1 per cent mepivacaine with 1 per cent mepivacaine plus epinephrine. Anesthesiology 37:288, 1972.
16. Burge ES, Baldwin CE Jr: The use of spinal anesthesia in obstetrics at the Evanston Hospital. Am J Obstet Gynecol 71:973, 1956.
17. Ebner H: An evaluation of spinal anesthesia in obstetrics. Anesth Analg 38:378, 1959.
18. Phillips OC, Nelson AT, Lyons WB, et al.: Spinal anesthesia for vaginal delivery. Obstet Gynecol 13:437, 1959.
19. Morishima HO, Adamsons K: Placental clearance of mepivacaine following administration to the guinea pig fetus. Anesthesiology 28:343, 1967.
20. Philip JH, Brown WU Jr: Total spinal anesthesia late in the course of obstetric bupivacaine epidural block. Anesthesiology 44:340, 1976.
21. Cassady GN, Moore CD, Bridenbaugh LD: Postpartum hypertension after use of vasoconstrictor and oxytocic drugs. JAMA 172:1011, 1960.
22. Sinclair JC, Fox HA, Lentz JF, et al.: Intoxication of fetus by a local anesthetic, a newly recognized complication of maternal caudal anesthesia. N Engl J Med 273:1173, 1965.
23. Greene BA: A 26-gauge lumbar puncture needle. Its value in the prophylaxis of headache following spinal analgesia for vaginal delivery. Anesthesiology 11:464, 1950.
24. Ralston DH, Shnider SM: The fetal and neonatal effects of regional anesthesia in obstetrics. Anesthesiology 48:34, 1978.
25. Bonica JJ: *Principles and Practice of Obstetric Analgesia and Anesthesia*, vol 1. F. A. Davis, Philadelphia, p 253.
26. Hunter CA: Uterine motility studies during labor. Observations on bilateral sympathetic nerve block in the normal and abnormal first stage of labor. Am J Obstet Gynecol 85:681, 1963.
27. James FM III: Clinical obstetrical anesthesia: Labor and delivery. In *Annual Refresher Course Lectures*, lesson 126A. American Society of Anesthesiologists, Chicago, 1978.

CHAPTER 9

Choice of Local Anesthetics in Obstetrics

Philip R. Bromage, M.B., B.S. (Lond.), F.F.A.R.C.S., F.R.C.P.(C)

A large number of local anesthetics are available for relief of pain in labor. Selection is bewildering, and the anesthesiologist is left wondering whether the choice really matters provided the selected drug works effectively and does no apparent harm. This chapter will attempt to set out guidelines to indicate the major advantages and disadvantages of the agents that are currently available and to suggest which drugs and concentrations are likely to be better than others under different circumstances.

DESIDERATA

As with any choice, the question must be asked: What do we really want? All too often this essential preliminary to the act of selection has not been thought through, but in the context of obstetric anesthesia most of the information that is needed to make a rational selection has been amassed by laborious investigation over the past 40 years. Five basic requirements must be met, as set out in Table 9.1.

The drug must do the clinical job intended. It must provide effective analgesia, and, obviously, it must be safe to the mother. The fetus must not be jeopardized. In terms of the three p's outlined in Table 9.1, this means that the expulsive forces of labor must be unaffected. In addition, tone should be preserved in the muscles of the birth canal so that rotation of the fetal head occurs in a normal fashion as the presenting part descends. Finally, and very important, the fetus, or the **passenger**, must not be intoxicated by placental transfer of potentially depressing drugs. This implies that dosages should be kept to a minimum consistent with efficacy, and that every means should be sought to minimize placental transfer.

The emphasis on these five requirements will shift depending on whether delivery is by the vaginal route, when it is important to preserve normal tone in the **powers** and the **passages**, or by cesarean section, when it is not. Also, vaginal delivery requires less intense analgesia than abdominal section; therefore, as a general rule, one may expect that more dilute solutions of local anesthetics will be adequate for labor and vaginal delivery.

LOCAL ANESTHETIC AGENTS: GENERAL CONSIDERATIONS

Having decided what we want, let us look at what is available, with particular emphasis on the qualities that will spare the fetus unnecessary depression.

Ester-linked Agents

Local anesthetics are divided into two main pharmacologic genera depending on

Table 9.1
Requirements of a Local Anesthetic Agent for Obstetrics

Effective and controllable analgesia
Maternal safety
No weakening of maternal **powers**
No alteration of maternal **passages**
No depression of the **passenger**

Table 9.2
Half-life of Chloroprocaine (in Seconds)*

	mean ± SD
Mothers (n = 7)	20.9 ± 5.8
Umbilical cords (n = 7)	42.6 ± 11.2
Male controls (n = 6)	20.6 ± 4.1
Female controls (n = 5)	25.2 ± 3.7
Homozygous atypical cholinesterase carriers (n = 10)	106.0 ± 45.0

* Reprinted by permission from O'Brien JE, Abbey V, Hinsvark O, et al.: Metabolism and measurement of 2-chloroprocaine, an ester-type anesthetic. J Pharm Sci. 68:75, 1979.

their molecular structure: those with ester-type linkage in the molecule and those with an amide linkage (Figure 9.1). The esters, such as procaine, chloroprocaine and tetracaine, are broken down in the blood stream by plasma pseudocholinesterase at different speeds, with chloroprocaine having the fastest rate of hydrolysis. Paraaminobenzoic acid, the end product of ester cleavage, passes across the placenta very freely, but it does not appear to cause appreciable fetal depresssion.[1] Some esters, such as piperocaine (Metycaine) are broken down more readily by the liver than by plasma pseudocholinesterase.[2]

CHLOROPROCAINE (NESACAINE)

Current evidence indicates that chloroprocaine is one of the safest agents for use in obstetrics. Its speed of breakdown is very fast in the presence of normal pseudocholinesterase. The in vitro plasma half-life is 21 seconds for maternal blood and 43 seconds for umbilical cord blood (Table 9.2). Thus, it is unlikely to reach the fetus in appreciable amounts. If any of the drug reached the fetus, it would probably be rapidly hydrolyzed. Chloroprocaine has most of the attributes of a successful local anesthetic for obstetrics. It has a fast onset, good quality of sensory blockade and great safety due to its rapid rate of hydrolysis. However, it has a very short duration of action, lasting often only 35 to 50 minutes in plain solution and 50 to 65 minutes when epinephrine is added. Therefore, frequent repeated injections are needed when prolonged analgesia is required. A concentration of 1.5 to 2.0 per cent is adequate for relief of first stage labor pain, but a 3 per cent concentration is required for perineal analgesia and relaxation or for cesarean section.

PIPEROCAINE (METYCAINE)

Piperocaine enjoyed a period of popularity in the 1940's and 1950's, but its slow hydrolysis rate gives it no advantage in terms of fetal toxicity, and it was discarded in favor of the more effective amide agents, such as lidocaine.

TETRACAINE (PONTOCAINE)

Tetracaine has a long duration of action and might seem to be a desirable ester-linked agent for use in labor. Although tetracaine remains one of the most effective and popular drugs for subarachnoid block, it is a poor choice in epidural analgesia. For reasons that are not altogether clear, epidural tetracaine produces a relatively profound motor block but somewhat skimpy analgesia.[3] This pattern of dissociated blockade is particularly undesirable in obstetrics, where sensory analgesia is needed but where motor block interferes with the active management of parturition.

Dibucaine (Nupercaine)

Dibucaine is a very potent and long-lasting quinoline derivative formerly used extensively for infiltration and epidural

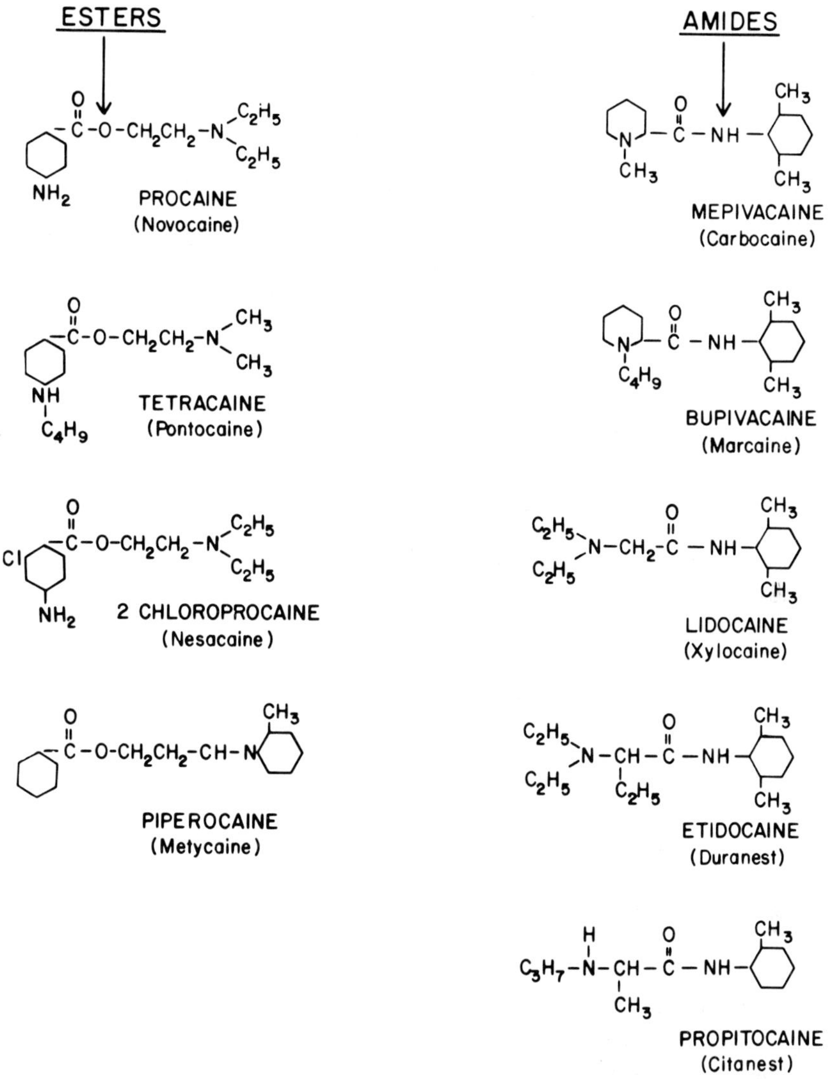

CHOICE OF LOCAL ANESTHETICS IN OBSTETRICS   111

Figure 9.1. Representative local anesthetic structures.

blockade. Dibucaine is not a very successful local anesthetic, except in the subarachnoid space. Spinal anesthesia with hyperbaric dibucaine (5 mg/ml in 6 per cent glucose) is reliable, effective and long-lasting, and it is an excellent choice for saddle block anesthesia in obstetrics. At the present time injectable dibucaine is not readily available in the United States.

Amide-linked Agents

The amide-linked agents include the most powerful and effective local anesthetics available today. Unfortunately these drugs are all broken down in the liver, and their half-lives are long. They have relatively low molecular weights (under 325) and high lipid solubilities, and they all pass the placenta to greater or lesser degrees. The ease of placental transfer is also determined by their degree of ionization at physiologic pH. Transfer is favored by a high proportion of un-ionized drug, and this in turn is favored by a low dissociation constant, or pKa. For example, the four agents—lidocaine, etidocaine, mepivacaine and bupivacaine—can be ranked in order of pKa and diffusibility thus:

Mepivacaine (pKa, 7.65) > Etidocaine (pKa, 7.76) > Lidocaine (pKa, 7.85) > Bupivacaine (pKa, 8.05)

From this scale it can be seen that mepivacaine is likely to show the greatest degree of placental transfer and bupivacaine the least, an expectation that is borne out in practice.

Protein binding also influences toxicity and placental transfer to a marked degree.[4,5] Because local anesthetics are only pharmacologically active in the unbound form, agents with strong protein binding are generally less toxic than those with weak binding characteristics. Again, bupivacaine stands out as a very favorable agent in this regard, because it is bound about twice as extensively as lidocaine. Very little active drug is left free to diffuse across the placenta.

Five of the more important amide drugs are briefly reviewed.

MEPIVACAINE (CARBOCAINE)

Mepivacaine is an effective agent with a slightly longer action than lidocaine. Unfortunately, its propensity to reach the fetus is significantly greater than other amides.[6,7] This combined with its long half-life in the neonate (9 hours versus lidocaine at less than 3 hours[8]) has led to its decline in obstetric practice.

PRILOCAINE (CITANEST)

Prilocaine was launched with high hopes that its rapid breakdown and low acute toxicity would make it a useful drug for obstetrics. Regrettably the phenolic breakdown product of prilocaine, α-orthotoluidine, causes methemoglobinemia in doses above 600 mg.[9,10] Because the fetus is vulnerable to any reduction of oxygen supply, it is generally agreed that the risk of methemoglobinemia is a contraindication to the use of prilocaine for relief of pain in labor.[11]

LIDOCAINE (XYLOCAINE)

For many years lidocaine hydrochloride was the standard agent for epidural analgesia in labor. Lidocaine provides dependable analgesia with a duration of action of about 60 minutes without epinephrine and 75 minutes when epinephrine 1/200,000 is added. Although placental transfer is appreciable, Apgar scores are usually high.[12,13] However, neurobehavioral studies in the newborn indicate transient changes not found with bupivacaine or 2-chloroprocaine[14] (Table 5.3). Primarily for this reason, the drug is losing some popularity in obstetrics.

The carbonated solution of lidocaine is dramatically effective, and the equivalent concentration to 2 per cent lidocaine HCl is unsurpassed for its speed and quality of analgesia.[15-17] The superb quality of analgesia makes it an ideal agent, the author believes, for cesarean section under epidural blockade. Carbonated lidocaine has been in use for some years in Canada, but, in spite of its obvious advantages, it is not yet available in the United States.

ETIDOCAINE (DURANEST)

Etidocaine, a long-acting congener of lidocaine, has recently been launched on the market in a flurry of controversy. The drug is interesting in that it seems to cause a striking degree of motor block in epidural analgesia, whereas its quality of sensory blockade is less impressive. Some investigators have had a precisely contrary impression. Poppers et al.[18] have claimed that great freedom from motor blockade is found with the 0.25 and 0.5 per cent concentrations. However, the general concensus of opinion is that etidocaine produces an inordinate amount of motor weakness compared with other agents.[19-22] This propensity to cause motor blockade makes etidocaine a poor choice for the management of pain in active labor. On the positive side, etidocaine is heavily protein-bound and very little of the agent passes the placenta[23]; neonatal neurobehavioral scores are unaffected. Accordingly, it is suitable for cesarean section, where birth is passive and where muscle activity is not required.

BUPIVACAINE (MARCAINE)

Bupivacaine is a congener of mepivacaine, with three methyl groups added to the piperidine ring of the mepivacaine molecule. This important agent was introduced into clinical practice by Telivuo[24] in 1963.

Bupivacaine has three advantages in obstetric practice: (1) the drug is heavily protein-bound; (2) the quality of analgesia is high in relation to the degree of motor block; (3) the duration is long, especially when epinephrine is added. The drug provides effective relief of first-stage labor pain in dilutions down to 0.125 per cent.[25] Bupivacaine is currently established as the safest and most effective amide-linked local anesthetic for obstetric anesthesia. The choice of concentration will be discussed later in this chapter.

Epinephrine as a Vasoconstrictive Adjuvant

The place of epinephrine in obstetrical regional anesthesia is controversial, and opinions for and against the use of epinephrine as a vasoconstrictor are sharply divided. On the one hand, absorbed epinephrine tends to reduce uterine blood flow, inhibit uterine contractility and slow labor; on the other hand, epinephrine 1/300,000 to 1/200,000 improves the quality of analgesic and motor blockade (Figure 9.2) and reduces vascular uptake. The effects of epinephrine added to local anesthetic solution are discussed in detail in chapters 3, 4 and 5.

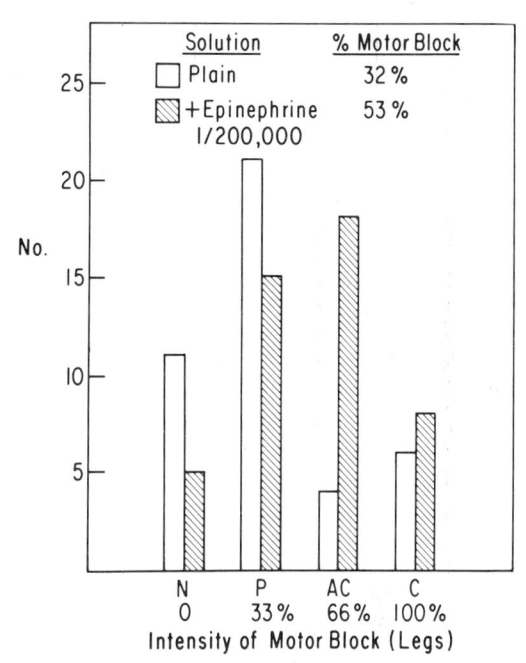

Figure 9.2. Epidural bupivacaine 0.75 per cent; quality of motor blockade with and without epinephrine 1/200,000. Nil (*N*), full movement of legs and feet, 0 per cent. Partial (*P*), able to move feet freely, just able to move knees, 33 per cent. Almost complete (*AC*), unable to move knees, able to move feet, 66 per cent. Complete (*C*), unable to move knees or feet, 100 per cent. Plain 0.75 per cent bupivacaine: 32 per cent motor block. 0.75 per cent bupivacaine plus epinephrine: 53 per cent motor block.

SELECTION OF AGENTS AND CONCENTRATIONS FOR SPECIAL TASKS

Cesarean Section

Analgesic requirements for cesarean section are very different from those for vaginal delivery. First, motor power is not required for expulsion of the fetus. Second, analgesia must be profound in order to provide good interruption of operative stimuli. Third, segmental analgesia must extend up to the fourth to sixth thoracic segment in order to secure analgesia of the entire abdominal cavity. Some authorities recommend that analgesia to the eighth thoracic segment is sufficient,[26] but in the author's experience, patients complain and become restless unless blockade reaches at least the costal margin. These clinical goals must be achieved by techniques and agents that provide profound and extensive segmental blockade without causing fetal depression. Subarachnoid and lumbar epidural blockade are the only two feasible techniques for the task. Caudal anesthesia requires excessively large amounts of local anesthetic, and it is not recommended for cesarean section.

SUBARACHNOID BLOCKADE

Subarachnoid block is favored by many as the technique of choice for cesarean section. It has great esthetic appeal, in that intense and extensive analgesia is obtained from a tiny dose of local anesthetic, and blood concentrations of local anesthetic never reach a level that can possibly have any depressant effect on the fetus. Weighed against this advantage, however, is the difficulty of controlling segmental spread of analgesia and preventing maternal hypotension. It is difficult to predict the upper level of anesthesia with any degree of precision, and commonly employed dose schedules may result in anesthesia that extends anywhere between T_{10} and T_2 and sometimes even higher. The great rapidity of sympathetic blockade is prone to causing precipitous changes of cardiovascular dynamics. As a result the incidence of arterial hypotension is high, even when prophylactic measures of pre-hydration and left uterine displacement are taken, and corrective vasopressor treatment is often needed.[19, 27]

Subarachnoid and epidural blockade spread further in obstetric patients than in the normal population, and most recommended dose schedules for subarachnoid anesthesia in cesarean section are on the low side for safety's sake. The reader should be aware that in following the dose schedules in this chapter, a fair proportion of inadequate blocks will be encountered, where the upper level of spinal analgesia fails to reach as high as T_6. Table 9.3 outlines the generally accepted dose requirements for cesarean section under subarachnoid block.

EPIDURAL ANALGESIA

Unlike subarachnoid block, epidural analgesia requires dosages large enough to cause appreciable transfer of local anesthetic across the placenta, with the resulting possibility of fetal depression. Blockade, however, comes on more slowly, and the maternal cardiovascular system is more readily controlled than in the precipitous onset of subarachnoid block. Moreover, when a continuous catheter technique is used, dosage can be titrated to achieve a more precise segmental level, and an inadequate initial level can be raised by injecting a small supplementary dose.

At the present time, choice of agent for epidural analgesia is narrowed to three or possibly four drugs that stand out as superior for the special requirements of pain relief for cesarean section. These are chloroprocaine, bupivacaine, etidocaine and carbonated lidocaine.

Chloroprocaine. Chloroprocaine 3 per cent provides satisfactory analgesia for cesarean section. Epinephrine 1/200,000 can be added to prolong the duration of anes-

Table 9.3.
Subarachnoid Block for Cesarean Section: Dose Requirements

Drug	Dose	Predicted Spread*	Duration†
	mg		hrs
Dibucaine	6–7	T_7	3–3½
Tetracaine	8	(T_{10}–T_1)	2½–3
Lidocaine	50–75		1½–2

* Average and range.
† With epinephrine 0.2 ml 1:1,000.

thesia. Volumes between 15 ml and 22 ml are needed to carry analgesia up to T6. Blockade is powerful but somewhat short-acting, with a duration of about 1 hour before the upper level of analgesia falls appreciably. A top-up dose is necessary 35 to 45 minutes after the first dose. Because chloroprocaine is rapidly broken down in the plasma, little or no placental transfer takes place, and fetal uptake is negligible.

Bupivacaine. Because low concentrations of bupivacaine (of the order of 0.25 per cent) do not give adequate surgical anesthesia, it is necessary to use 0.5 per cent solution in volumes of 17 to 18 ml (i.e. 85 to 90 mg of bupivacaine) in order to obtain satisfactory operating conditions. Bupivacaine 0.75 per cent concentration has become increasingly popular because of its fast onset and great reliability. McGuinness et al.[28] used 0.75 per cent bupivacaine without epinephrine in volumes of 22 ml (i.e. 165 mg) for elective cesarean section. At delivery maternal blood levels averaged 720 ng/ml and umbilical venous levels 210 ng/ml, levels comparable to those reported by Magno et al.[29] (Figure 9.3). These blood levels were not associated with maternal or neonatal toxicity. The neonates were compared to a control group delivered under spinal anesthesia with tetracaine 10 mg. In both groups the babies were vigorous at birth with normal acid-base status. There were no differences within the two groups in respect to their neurobehavioral status measured by the Scanlon examination at 4 and 24 hours of age. These investigators concluded that bupivacaine 0.75 per cent offers advantages over the other local anesthetics for cesarean section.

The addition of epinephrine to 0.75 per

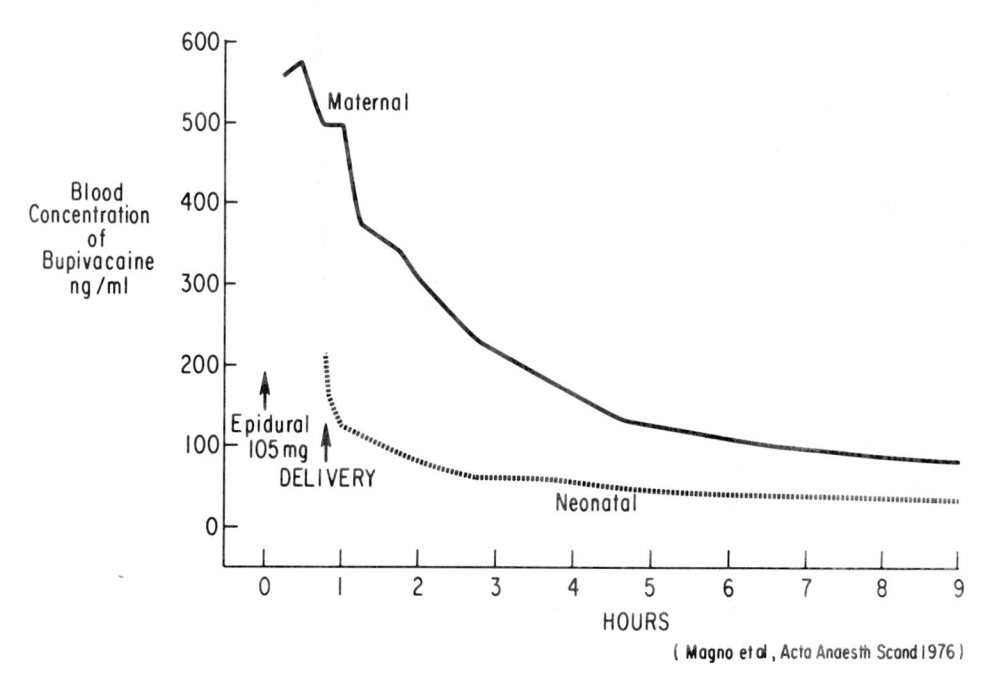

Figure 9.3. Cesarean section with 0.75 per cent plain bupivacaine. Average maternal dose is 105 mg. Serial plasma concentrations in mothers and infants. (Reprinted by permission from Magno R, Berlin A, Karlsson K, et al.: Anesthesia for cesarean section. IV. Placental transfer and neonatal elimination of bupivacaine following epidural analgesia for elective cesarean section. Acta Anaesth Scand 20:141, 1976.)

cent bupivacaine is not recommended. It causes marked motor paralysis of the legs for about 3 hours. This prolonged immobility is undesirable because it encourages venous stasis and clot formation in the deep veins of the calf, and it may contribute to the occurrence of thromboembolism.

Etidocaine. Etidocaine is a long-acting drug with a high degree of protein binding, and it appears to undergo relatively slight placental transfer.[23] Motor blockade is intense when the 1 per cent solution is used with 1/200,000 epinephrine, and it provides good conditions for abdominal surgery.[20] However, as with 0.75 per cent bupivacaine, prolonged post-operative immobility is an undesirable feature, and the agent has not had very widespread appeal.

Carbonated lidocaine. Carbonated lidocaine is outstanding for speed of onset and reliability in cesarean section, but inasmuch as it is still unavailable in the United States after more than 12 years of experience in Canada, it will not be discussed further. Readers are referred to published clinical studies for details of dosage, performance and placental transfer.[16, 17]

Vaginal Delivery

As set out at the beginning of this chapter, the analgesic requirements for vaginal delivery are quite clear-cut. Analgesia must be effective, controllable, and safe, and there should be no depression of the three p's, that is, the powers of labor, the tone of the birth passages or the baby, the passenger traveling through those passages. Effective analgesia must not be bought at the expense of excessive dosage and consequent fetal depression. The art of choice lies in delicate compromise and in choosing the least dose that will do the job. This implies rather close supervision of the patient to ensure that the delicate balance between effective analgesia and fetal depression does not tip one way or the other. The agents currently available are good, and failure to maintain the right balance is usually due to failure of supervision rather than to shortcomings of the drugs.

SUBARACHNOID BLOCKADE

Subarachnoid blockade has a very limited role to play in labor and vaginal delivery. It is usually a last-minute analgesic maneuver for delivery when circumstances have made continuous epidural blockade impossible or inappropriate. Subarachnoid analgesia produces intense motor block within the segmental distribution of its influence. This property is desirable if forceps delivery is planned. However, if spontaneous delivery is desired, the block will violate two of the five desiderata for ideal analgesic conditions in labor set out at the beginning of this chapter. First, the muscular integrity of the birth passages is disturbed, because the pelvic floor is rendered atonic and patulous by blockade of the upper sacral segments. Second, the expulsive powers are diminished if blockade rises to affect the abdominal segments.

Choice of agents for spinal analgesia in labor and delivery depends to a great degree on when the block is induced. A long-lasting agent such as dibucaine or tetracaine is indicated if spinal block is started before the cervix is fully dilated. A shorter acting agent such as lidocaine is indicated for a short period of perineal analgesia after the cervix is fully dilated and when delivery is imminent. Table 9.4 outlines the agents and doses that are suitable and their approximate duration of action.

CONTINUOUS EPIDURAL ANALGESIA FOR LABOR AND VAGINAL DELIVERY

Continuous epidural analgesia, when properly administered, is the only technique that can offer quiet and gentle progress through all the painful stages of labor

Table 9.4
Choice of Analgesic Agent for Subarachnoid Analgesia in Vaginal Delivery

Stage of Labor	Segments to be Anesthetized	Agent	Dose	Duration with Epinephrine Wash
			mg	hrs
Late first stage	T_{10}–S_5	Dibucaine	4–5	3½
	T_{10}–S_5	Tetracaine	5–6	2½
Second stage	T_{10}–S_5	Tetracaine	4–6	2½
	T_{10}–S_5	Lidocaine	30–40	1½
or				
"Saddle block"	S_1–S_5	Tetracaine	3	2½
	S_1–S_5	Lidocaine	25–30	1½

and delivery without undue risk and without the need for systemic analgesics.

Bupivacaine in labor. Bupivacaine has earned a place as the most reliable and least offensive amide local anesthetic for epidural analgesia in labor and delivery. Scanlon and his associates[14] used neurobehavioral tests to assess the effect of absorbed bupivacaine on the newborn after 3 hours of epidural analgesia with a cumulative maternal dose of 112 mg of bupivacaine. They found that umbilical vein concentrations of 110 ± 20 ng/ml at delivery were apparently innocuous to the infant. On the evidence available, it seems extremely unlikely that these very low concentrations of local anesthetic can possibly have any immediate or long-term adverse effects on the infant.

First-stage labor pain is quickly relieved by bupivacaine in 0.25 or 0.5 per cent concentration after lumbar injection, and segmental skin analgesia usually develops in 5 to 7 minutes.

However, perineal analgesia is achieved much more slowly, and a period of 20 minutes is usually needed to obtain satisfactory conditions for episiotomy and forceps delivery. The very dilute solution of 0.125 per cent bupivacaine with 1/400,000 epinephrine has been recommended by Van Steenberge and his colleagues.[25, 30] The three strengths of 0.5, 0.25 and 0.125 per cent bupivacaine will be discussed in turn.

0.5 per cent bupivacaine. Excellent analgesia for labor and delivery is provided by 0.5 per cent bupivacaine. Approximately 15 to 30 mg of bupivacaine are needed to give segmental blockade from T10 to L2 for first-stage labor pain. However, this mass of drug is contained in a volume of only 3 to 5 ml of 0.5 per cent bupivacaine, and these very small volumes are apt to give spotty anesthesia and missed segments.[31, 32] Hence, many practitioners give larger volumes to ensure an evenly distributed and homogeneous area of blockade. As a consequence the cumulative total number of milligrams of bupivacaine tends to be considerably higher than it need be.

Dose requirements for 0.5 per cent bupivacaine are 4 to 8 ml during labor and 10 to 12 ml for delivery. Epinephrine 1/300,000 to 1/200,000 may be omitted if the practitioner has strong feelings against its use in labor, but the author believes the result will be less effective blockade and larger cumulative dosage.

0.25 per cent bupivacaine. One important feature of weak solutions of bupivacaine must be appreciated for their successful use. It is this: Although satisfactory perineal analgesia is difficult to obtain with a single lumbar injection, in time, repeated lumbar injections will gradually spread downwards to involve the sacral segments. Repeated small injections at intervals of approximately 90 minutes show an increasing degree of caudal spread, until an appreciable amount of sacral anesthesia is often present by the third injection. At that stage a relatively small reinforcing dose given in the sitting or semi-sitting position will usually provide satisfactory analgesia for episiotomy and forceps delivery. Therefore, 0.25 per cent bupivacaine is useful in labors where analgesia is likely to be needed for 3 hours or more.

Bupivacaine in 0.25 per cent solution with 1/200,000 epinephrine gives good first-stage pain relief in doses of 6 to 8 ml, that is, 15 to 20 mg of bupivacaine. A final dose of 10 to 12 ml (25 to 30 mg) is usually sufficient for satisfactory perineal anesthesia, provided it has been preceded by two or three smaller doses.

0.125 per cent bupivacaine. Van Steenberge and his associates[25, 30] have attempted to reduce maternal uptake to a minimum by using a solution of 0.125 per cent bupivacaine with 1/400,000 epinephrine. They had successful results with the following dose regimen in 465 of 500 deliveries (93 per cent success rate):

	Volume (ml)	Dose of Bupivacaine (mg)
Induction dose	10	12.5
Top-up dose (when pain returned)	10	12.5
Final perineal dose	15	18.75

With this regimen maternal blood levels of bupivacaine were extremely low, and umbilical vein concentrations at birth were barely perceptible with a mean level of 40 ng of bupivacaine per ml. Others have had mixed degrees of success with this regimen. Bramwell and Bromage (unpublished data) found that 49 of 51 patients had completely satisfactory analgesia for labor and delivery. Success depended on close supervision and on the willingness to administer additional top-up doses immediately if any discomfort arose during the course of labor. In this respect, the regimen is demanding and likely to prove unsatisfactory unless supervision is close and continuous.

Figure 9.4 summarizes the mean regression lines for cumulative dosage plotted against hours of analgesia in a personally conducted series of cases using 0.5, 0.25 or 0.125 per cent bupivacaine with epinephrine 1/400,000 to 1/200,000. Minimal dose requirements were used, and satisfactory analgesia was obtained throughout labor and delivery in over 95 per cent of cases. It can be seen that cumulative dosage was related to concentration of bupivacaine, as indeed one might expect. Substantially larger cumulative doses of 0.5 per cent bupivacaine were required than were required of the two weaker solutions. The difference in cumulative dose between the 0.25 and the 0.125 per cent solution was not spectacular. The impression was formed that the 0.25 per cent solution was more convenient for routine use. The saving of dosage with the 0.125 per cent solution did not seem to justify its greater inconvenience.

Chloroprocaine in labor. Chloroprocaine can be administered in large doses if necessary during labor without running the risk of placental transfer and fetal depression. The transient action of chloroprocaine requires frequent top-up doses, and in prolonged labors this makes for unnecessary disturbance of the patient and increased likelihood of tachyphylaxis. Some anesthesiologists like to use chloroprocaine at the outset, in order to take advantage of its rapid action and assess blockade quickly in early labor. Chloroprocaine in 1.5 to 2.0 per cent concentration and volumes of 5 to 8 ml is adequate for

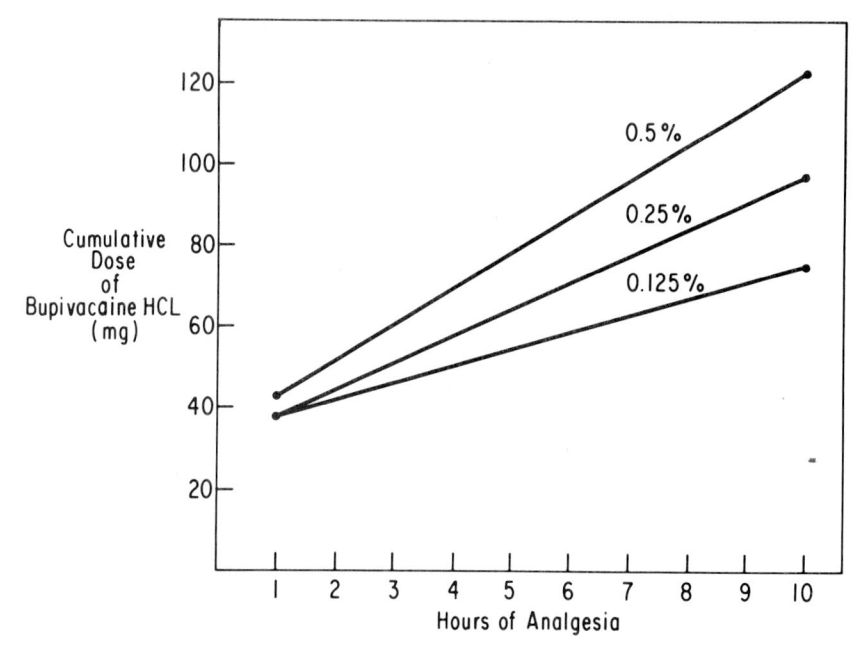

Figure 9.4. Bupivacaine for epidural analgesia in labor and delivery. Mean regression lines for cumulative dosage of bupivacaine 0.5 per cent, 0.25 per cent with 1/200,000 epinephrine and 0.125 per cent with 1/400,000 epinephrine.

first-stage pain relief, while the 3 per cent solution in doses of 10 to 15 ml gives excellent analgesia for episiotomy and forceps delivery within about 10 minutes of injection.

CONCLUSION

In conclusion, the attributes of available local anesthetics have been reviewed with a view to matching their qualities to the specific requirements of pain relief for abdominal and vaginal delivery. At the time of writing, bupivacaine and chloroprocaine in various concentrations appear to be the most appropriate agents for routine use in the United States.

References

1. Usubiaga JE, La Iuppa M, Moya F, et al.: Passage of procaine hydrochloride and paraaminobenzoic acid across the human placenta. Am J Obstet Gynecol 100:918, 1968.
2. de Jong RH: *Physiology and Pharmacology of Local Anesthesia.* Charles C Thomas, Springfield, Ill., 1970, p 196.
3. Bromage PR: A comparison of bupivacaine and tetracaine in epidural analgesia for surgery. Can Anaesth Soc J. 16:37, 1969.
4. Tucker GT, Boyes RN, Bridenbaugh PO, et al.: Binding of anilide-type local anesthetics in human plasma. I. Relationships between binding, physicochemical properties, and anesthetic activity. Anesthesiology 33:287, 1970.
5. Tucker GT, Boyes RN, Bridenbaugh PO, et al.: Binding of anilide-type local anesthetics in human plasma. II. Implications in vivo, with special reference to transplacental distribution. Anesthesiology 33:304, 1970.
6. Morishima HO, Daniel SS, Finster M, et al.: Transmission of mepivacaine hydrochloride (Carbocaine) across the human placenta. Anesthesiology. 27: 147, 1966.
7. Scanlon JW, Brown WU, Weiss JB, et al.: Neurobehavioral responses of newborn infants after maternal epidural anesthesia. Anesthesiology 40: 121, 1974.
8. Brown WU, Bell GC, Jurie AO, et al.: Newborn blood levels of lidocaine and mepivacaine in the first postnatal day following maternal epidural anesthesia. Anesthesiology 42:698, 1975.
9. Fujimori M, Nishimura K: Methemoglobinemia due to local anesthetics (a preliminary report). Far East J Anaesth 4:4, 1964.
10. Lund PC, Cwik JC: Propitocaine (Citanest®) and

methemoglobinemia. Anesthesiology 26:569, 1965.
11. Scott DB: Discussion—Citanest® and methemoglobinemia. In Citanest, S Wiedling, ed. Universitetsforlaget I Aarhus, Copenhagen, 1965, p 199.
12. Shnider SM, Way EL: Plasma levels of lidocaine (Xylocaine) in mother and newborn following obstetrical conduction anesthesia: Clinical applications. Anesthesiology 29:951, 1968.
13. Fox GS, Houle GL: Transmission of lidocaine hydrochloride across the placenta during caesarean section. Can Anaesth Soc J 16:135, 1969.
14. Scanlon JW, Ostheimer GW, Lurie AO, et al.: Neurobehavioral responses and drug concentrations in newborn after maternal epidural anesthesia with bupivacaine. Anesthesiology 45:400, 1976.
15. Bromage PR: A comparison of the hydrochloride salts of lidocaine and prilocaine for epidural analgesia. Br J Anaesth 37:753, 1965.
16. Bromage PR: Improved conduction blockade in surgery and obstetrics: Carbonated local anesthetics. Can Med Assoc J 97:1377, 1967.
17. Bromage PR, Burfoot MF, Crowell DE, et al.: Quality of epidural blockade. III. Carbonated local anaesthetic solutions. Br J Anaesth 39:197, 1967.
18. Poppers P, Covino B, Boyes N: Epidural block with etidocaine for labour and delivery. Acta Anaesth Scand (Suppl) 60:89, 1975.
19. Moir DD: Recent advances in pain relief in childbirth. II. Regional anaesthesia. Br J Anaesth 43: 849, 1971.
20. Bromage PR, Datta S, Dunford LA: Etidocaine: An evaluation in epidural analgesia for obstetrics. Can Anaesth Soc J 21:535, 1974.
21. Phillips G: A double-blind trial of bupivacaine (Marcaine) and etidocaine (Duranest) in extradural block for surgical induction of labour. Br J Anaesth 47:1305, 1975.
22. Hargrove L: Discussion. III. Obstetric analgesia. Acta Anaesth Scand (Suppl) 60:110, 1975.
23. Lund PC, Cwik JC, Gannon RT, et al.: Etidocaine for caesarean section—effects on mother and baby. Br J Anaesth 49:457, 1977.
24. Telivuo L: A new long-acting local anaesthetic for pain relief after thoracotomy. Ann Chir Gynaecol Fenn 52:513, 1963.
25. Geerinckx K, Vanderick G, Van Steenberge AL, et al.: Bupivacaine 0.125% in epidural block analgesia during childbirth: Maternal and foetal plasma concentrations. Br J Anaesth 46:939, 1974.
26. Bonica JJ: Principles and Practice of Obstetric Analgesia and Anaesthesia. Volume I: Fundamental Considerations. F. A. Davis, Philadelphia, 1967, p 556.
27. Clark RB, Thompson DS, Thompson CH: Prevention of spinal hypotension associated with cesarean section. Anesthesiology 45:670, 1976.
28. McGuinness GA, Merkow AJ, Kennedy, RL, et al.: Epidural anesthesia with bupivacaine for cesarean section: Neonatal blood levels and neurobehavioral responses. Anesthesiology. 49:270, 1978.
29. Magno R, Berlin A, Karlsson K, et al.: Anesthesia for cesarean section. IV. Placental transfer and neonatal elimination of bupivacaine following epidural analgesia for elective cesarean section. Acta Anaesth Scand 20:141, 1976.
30. Vanderick G, Geerinckx K, Van Steenberge AL, et al.: Bupivacaine 0.125% in epidural block analgesia during childbirth: Clinical evaluation. Br J Anaesth 46:838, 1974.
31. Ducrow M: The occurrence of unblocked segments during continuous lumbar epidural analgesia for relief of pain in labour. Br J Anaesth 43: 1172, 1971.
32. Bromage PR: Unblocked segments in epidural analgesia for relief of pain in labour. Br J Anaesth 44:676, 1972.

CHAPTER 10

Inhalation Analgesia and Anesthesia for Vaginal Delivery

Sheila E. Cohen, M.B., Ch.B., F.F.A.R.C.S.

Since James Simpson first administered ether to a woman in labor in 1847, almost every known inhalation anesthetic agent has been used for the relief of pain in labor. Few, however, have retained a secure position in the obstetric anesthetist's armamentarium. Inhalation analgesia or anesthesia is used in approximately one-third of all vaginal deliveries in the United States, making it the most common form of pain relief for this procedure.[1] This chapter will discuss the role of inhalation agents in modern obstetric practice and their effects, both beneficial and adverse, on the mother, the fetus and the process of labor. Detailed consideration of individual anesthetic agents will be restricted to those of most relevance to current anesthetic practice.

It is important to define the terms inhalation analgesia and inhalation anesthesia. **Inhalation analgesia** describes the administration of subanesthetic concentrations of inhalation agents to provide analgesia for the first and second stages of labor, either alone or as a supplement to regional or local anesthesia. The object of this technique is for the mother to remain awake throughout, to be cooperative and to maintain protective laryngeal reflexes while achieving analgesic levels of the agent. The anesthetic is usually administered via a mask or mouthpiece, either by an anesthetist or by the patient herself. The term **inhalation anesthesia** describes the practice of administering inhalation agents with the intention of producing unconsciousness for the purpose of performing cesarean section, vaginal delivery with forceps or vacuum extraction, or in cases where uterine relaxation is required.

INDICATIONS FOR INHALATION ANALGESIA

Inhalation analgesia provides a degree of pain relief which, although not comparable with that obtained with regional anesthesia, is satisfactory for a significant percentage of parturients. Many women elect not to have regional anesthesia because of fear of needles and spinal headaches or because they believe regional anesthesia will render them unable to participate in the delivery. In such cases the choice of analgesic techniques for the first stage of labor falls among inhalation agents, narcotics or other systemic drugs and paracervical block. Although narcotics are easily administered, they have the potential for causing neonatal respiratory and neurobehavioral depression. The high incidence of fetal bradycardia after paracervical block has caused many to consider this technique undesirable. Thus, inhalation techniques may provide an acceptable alternative, particularly when labor is progressing rapidly.

When a brief period of analgesia is required during the second stage of labor in the absence of, or to supplement, regional or local anesthesia, inhalation agents may again be useful. In recent years ketamine in low doses has also been used in this circumstance.[2] Although effective and without adverse fetal effects, ketamine is associated with a high incidence of amnesia for delivery, which many patients consider unsatisfactory. The use of ketamine in obstetrics is discussed in chapter 7.

The majority of obstetric anesthetics in this country, and perhaps in the world, are administered by personnel who have had no formal anesthesia training. A 1970 survey of obstetric practice by the American College of Obstetrics and Gynecology[1] revealed that in only 12 per cent of hospitals was anesthesia for vaginal delivery administered most frequently by an anesthesiologist. Although nurse anesthetists provided care for an additional 25 per cent of parturients, other personnel—including the obstetrician, delivery room nurse and house officer—administered the remainder of anesthetics. The survey further reported that only 8 per cent of hospitals in the United States had 24-hour coverage provided by anesthesiologists, and only 16 per cent had 24-hour coverage by nurse anesthetists. Strenuous attempts are being made to improve this situation, but it is likely that a major problem still exists, and the reality of present limitations in personnel must be faced. Thus, there is a great need for an analgesic method which is simple to administer and which has a high degree of safety for both mother and fetus. Inhalation analgesia in some respects fulfills these requirements; it has been widely used by nurse anesthetists and obstetric nurses in the United States and by midwives in the United Kingdom.[3]

INDICATIONS FOR INHALATION ANESTHESIA

Because the risk of aspiration of vomitus is significantly lower with regional anesthesia or inhalation analgesia, the author does not recommend the use of general anesthesia for vaginal delivery unless there is a specific indication. If acute fetal distress occurs during the second stage of labor and operative vaginal delivery is indicated, general anesthesia may be the most satisfactory technique because of the rapidity with which it can be instituted. If regional techniques are contraindicated (see chapter 8) and inhalation analgesia or low-dose ketamine is inadequate to allow a safe controlled delivery, general anesthesia may be necessary. Likely the most common indication for general anesthesia for vaginal delivery is the necessity for uterine relaxation. Intrauterine manipulations for internal podalic version, complete breech extraction, manual removal of the placenta and replacement of an inverted uterus are most easily performed under general anesthesia with halothane or enflurane. In addition, uterine relaxation might be necessary for relief of a tetanic uterine contraction or during a breech delivery when the uterus has clamped down before delivery of the head.

INHALATION ANALGESIA AND ANESTHESIA: GENERAL CONSIDERATIONS

Maternal Safety

Perhaps the greatest pitfall of inhalation techniques is their apparent simplicity. The ease of administration using devices which the patient holds herself may lead busy attendants to neglect her, with perhaps disastrous results. This is particularly hazardous because anesthesia is induced with great ease in the parturient for a variety of reasons. Physiologic changes in pregnancy include a reduction in functional residual capacity and an increase in alveolar ventilation, both of which lead to a more rapid equilibration of alveolar and inspired anesthetic concentrations. This results in more rapid induction of anesthesia and fluctuations of anesthetic level in response to changes in inspired concentration.[4] Pregnancy is also associated with reduced anesthetic requirements. In one study, MAC was decreased 32 per cent for methoxyflurane, 25 per cent for halothane, and 40 per cent for isoflurane.[5] Narcotics given in labor will further reduce MAC and thus contribute to the risk of unexpected loss of consciousness.

Therefore, the major risk from inhalation analgesia is inadvertent anesthetic overdose with loss of protective reflexes. Vomiting or silent regurgitation may then occur, resulting in immediate respiratory obstruction and asphyxia or delayed development of aspiration pneumonitis. Maternal deaths due to anesthesia make up 5 to 15 per cent of all maternal deaths in the United States, with approximately half of these due to aspiration.[6,7] In the state of Indiana during a 7-year period (1967-1974) 14 of 154 maternal deaths were directly related to anesthesia, and, of those, 10 women died of pulmonary failure due to aspiration of gastric fluid.[8]

In the United Kingdom, aspiration was also responsible for about 50 per cent of maternal anesthetic deaths, with the majority occurring either during induction or recovery from anesthesia.[9] When examining these statistics it is often unclear whether inhalation agents had been administered with the intention of producing general anesthesia or only analgesia, and in many instances there is no mention of endotracheal intubation. Also, it should not be assumed that inhalation anesthesia is necessarily more dangerous than regional anesthesia, as it must be remembered that the former method is used more frequently than the latter. If regional techniques were to be used on such a wide scale, it is possible that the number of deaths resulting from cardiovascular collapse or respiratory paralysis might be as great. Risk also relates as much to the training and skill of the person administering the anesthetic as to the technique itself.

The pregnant woman must always be regarded as being at risk from acid aspiration syndrome, whenever analgesia or anesthesia is undertaken (see chapter 19). The presence of a large volume of gastric juice or a dangerously low gastric pH cannot be excluded in any parturient, regardless of the time of last food intake or the onset of labor.[10] Routine administration of oral antacids to every parturient before induction of general anesthesia has therefore been recommended. It is likely that the over-all safety of inhalation analgesia and anesthesia would be increased if all patients were to receive 15 to 30 ml of antacid every 3 hours throughout labor. This practice is now becoming routine in many obstetric units.

Because the risk of aspiration can never be completely avoided, routine endotracheal intubation is indicated whenever general anesthesia is induced in the parturient.[11] This includes those situations in which inhalation analgesia is converted to anesthesia, for whatever reason.

In addition to the physiologic changes of pregnancy described above, there is a higher metabolic rate and increased oxygen consumption, predisposing the parturient to the rapid development of hypoxia in the event of respiratory depression or airway obstruction. Hypercapnea and acidosis may also develop extremely quickly in such circumstances, with these changes being exaggerated in the obese parturient who has additional derangements of pulmonary function. Hypoxia and hypercapnea are not usually encountered in healthy patients during the course of uneventful inhalation analgesia for labor.

Effects on the Fetus and Neonate

Placental transfer of all inhalation agents occurs rapidly, because these agents are highly lipid-soluble, un-ionized, and of fairly low molecular weight. Anesthetic levels rise rapidly in the fetal brain, and, in general, the degree of fetal and neonatal depression is directly proportional to the depth and duration of maternal anesthesia.[12] Neonatal depression may be a result of drug effect or of physiologic changes, such as hypoventilation or hypotension, induced in the mother. **Deep** halothane anesthesia has been shown to be associated with fetal acidosis,[13, 14] probably as a result of maternal hypotension which occurs in such cases (Figure 10.1) as well as fetal cardiovascular depression. Prolonged general anesthesia with nitrous oxide has also been associated with an increased number of depressed infants.[15, 16] This seems to correlate with the finding of

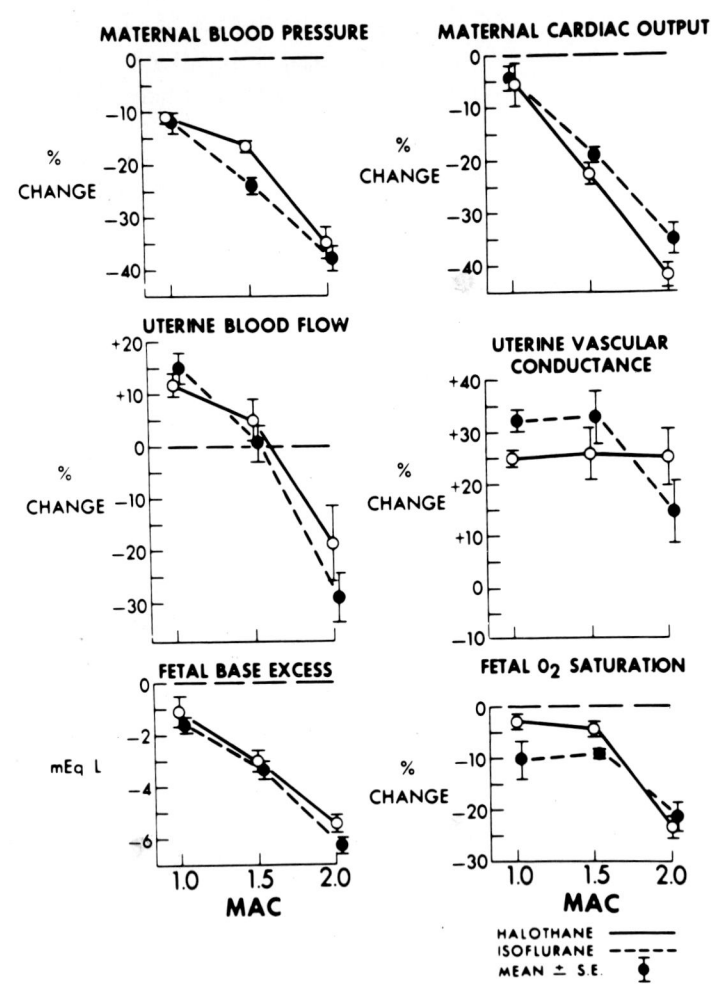

Figure 10.1. Changes from control values in mean maternal blood pressure, cardiac output, uterine blood flow, uterine vascular conductance, fetal arterial base excess and fetal arterial O$_2$ saturation at 1.0, 1.5 and 2.0 MAC halothane and isoflurane. Values represent means of results obtained at 15, 30, 60 and 90 minutes. (Reprinted by permission from Palahniuk RJ, Shnider SM: Maternal and fetal cardiovascular and acid-base changes during halothane and isoflurane anesthesia in the pregnant ewe. Anesthesiology 41:462, 1974.)

a nitrous oxide concentration ratio for umbilical artery to umbilical vein of 89 per cent at 36 minutes found by Stenger et al.[16] and with similar findings by Marx et al.,[17] who recorded 87 per cent equilibration in the fetal tissues after 15 to 19 minutes (Figure 10.2). Stenger et al. found a very wide maternal artery to uterine vein (umbilical vein) gradient for nitrous oxide early in the anesthetic. Fetal concentrations apparently approach maternal as the anesthetic is continued (Figure 10.3). Moya[18] found that the proportion of neonates with Apgar scores of less than 6 delivered after maternal cyclopropane anesthesia increased dramatically from 15 per cent after 6 minutes of anesthesia to over 60 per cent after 20 minutes of anesthesia (Figure 10.4).

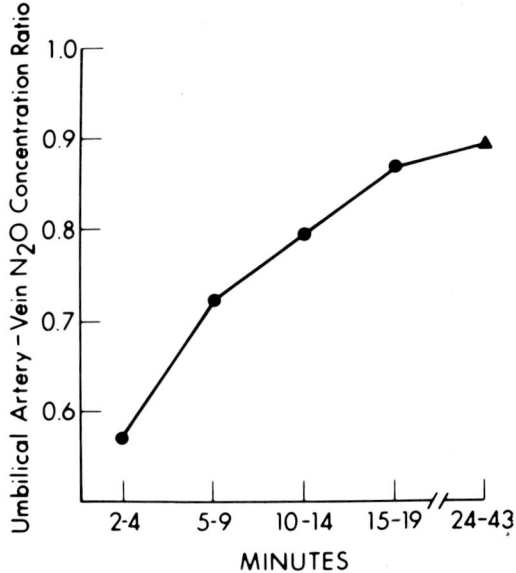

Figure 10.2. Umbilical artery blood nitrous oxide concentration—expressed as the ratio of umbilical vein blood N_2O concentration in relation to duration of N_2O administration. Reprinted by permission from Marx GF: Newer aspects of general anesthesia for cesarean section. NY State J Med 71: 1084, 1971. (Drawn from data in Marx GF, Joshi CW, Orkin LR: Placental transmission of nitrous oxide. Anesthesiology 32:429, 1970.)

Analgesic concentrations of anesthetic agents, on the other hand, have been claimed by Moya,[18] Shnider et al.,[19] and many other workers to be free from the effect of neonatal depression even if continued for a prolonged period (Figure 10.4). Clark and associates[20] agreed with these findings but demonstrated that, when prolonged methoxyflurane analgesia was followed by anesthesia with the same agent and nitrous oxide for delivery, the incidence of neonatal depression was increased. This was associated with higher umbilical vein levels of methoxyflurane measured at delivery.

When used in low concentrations, inhalation agents provide a considerable advantage for the fetus over systemic narcotics, as termination of hypnotic effect is not dependent on metabolism, and excretion is effected by the lungs. As long as the infant is breathing and circulation is adequate, depression from inhalation agents should progressively diminish in the period immediately after birth. Even if neonatal depression does occur, artificial ventilation can be instituted with the expectation of rapid improvement.

Effects on Labor

Most of the inhalation agents used in obstetric anesthesia cause dose-related depression of uterine contractility and tone. This is discussed fully in chapter 4. Uterine relaxation may prolong labor and, of more importance, may result in increased blood loss following delivery. Halothane, ether and chloroform lead to profound myometrial depression, which is considerably greater in the pregnant than in the non-pregnant state.[21] Naftalin et al.[22, 23] noted a dose-related decrease in resting tension in both pregnant and non-pregnant human myometrium exposed in vitro to halothane. Studies by Munson and Embro[24] of isolated human uterine muscle demonstrated that halothane, enflurane and

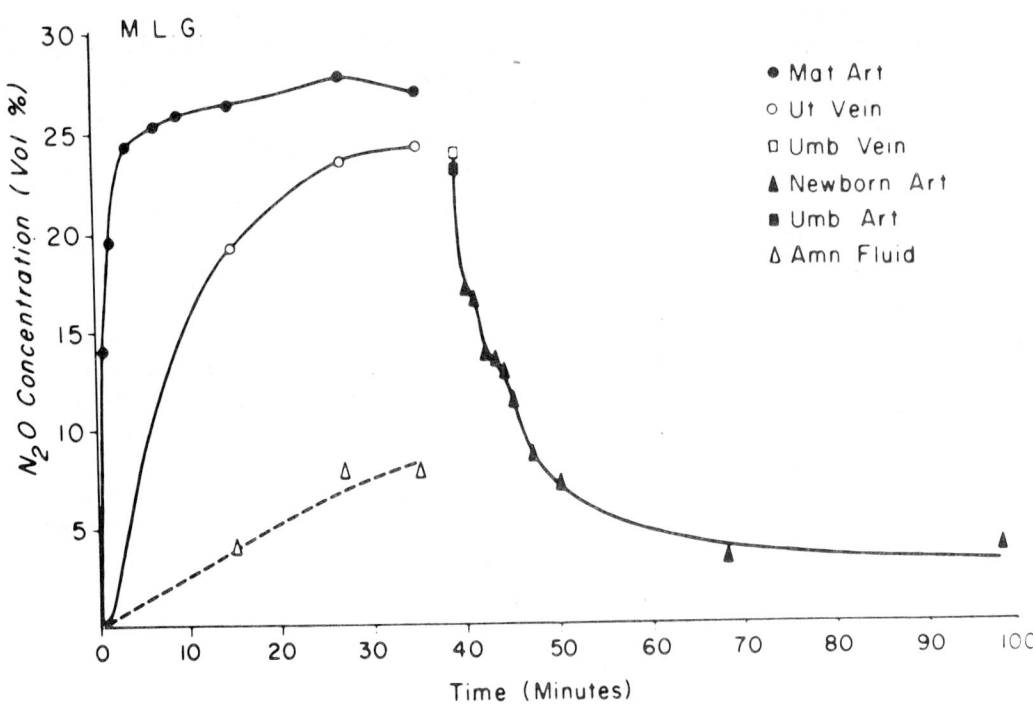

Figure 10.3. Serial concentrations of nitrous oxide during a prolonged anesthetic for a cesarean section. Note very wide maternal artery-uterine vein (umbilical vein) gradient for nitrous oxide early in the anesthetic. Fetal concentrations apparently approach maternal as the anesthetic is continued. (Reprinted by permission from Stenger VG, Blechner JN, Prystowsky H: A study of prolongation of obstetric anesthesia. Am J Obstet Gynecol 103:901, 1969.)

isoflurane are equally depressant when used in equipotent concentrations. Clinically, methoxyflurane and fluroxene in anesthetic concentrations are potent uterine depressants, whereas cyclopropane in low concentrations and nitrous oxide even in high concentrations seem to have little effect on uterine contractility. Clinical experience demonstrates the safety in this respect of analgesic concentrations of methoxyflurane and other agents commonly used for obstetric analgesia. Marx et al.[25] demonstrated in vivo that oxytocics are capable of counteracting the depression of uterine contractility caused by low concentrations of anesthetic halogenated agents, but they are unable to do so when profound depression is present.

Environmental Pollution

Recent epidemiologic evidence suggests that the operating room may be an environmentally hazardous occupational location.[26] There is an increased incidence of spontaneous abortion in female anesthetists, an increase in certain congenital abnormalities in their offspring and a slightly higher incidence of certain malignancies among female anesthetists. Exposure to trace concentrations of inhalation anesthetics may be the cause of these problems. Although many scavenging systems have been designed to reduce pollution in the operating room, all self-administration devices currently in use may result in pollution of the environment from expired air

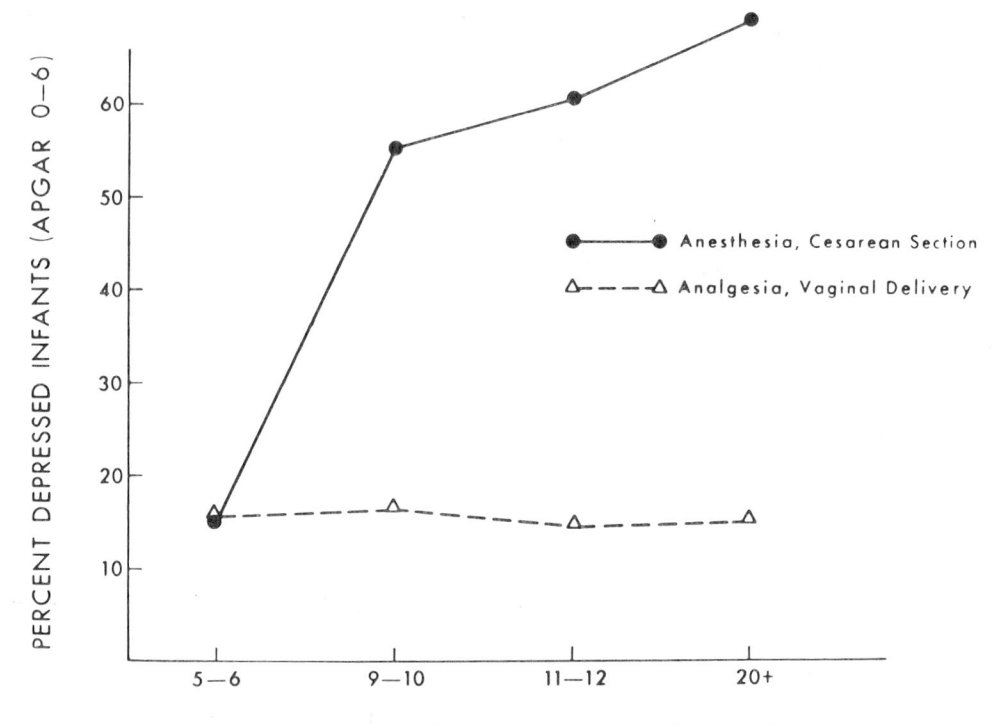

INHALATION ANALGESIA AND ANESTHESIA FOR VAGINAL DELIVERY

Figure 10.4. Neonatal effects of cyclopropane analgesia for vaginal delivery and cyclopropane anesthesia for elective cesarean section depending on duration of administration of agent to mother before birth. (Redrawn from Moya, F: Relationship of anesthesia to mortality in elective cesarean section. NY State J Med 62:2169, 1962; and Shnider SM, Moya F, Thorndike V, et al.: Clinical and biochemical studies of cyclopropane analgesia in obstetrics. Anesthesiology 24:11, 1963.)

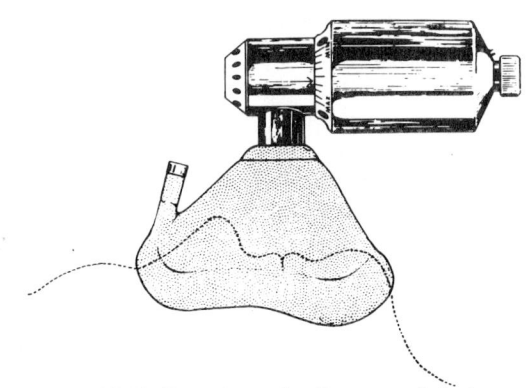

Figure 10.5. Drawing of a Cyprane inhaler.

containing inhalation agents. This problem is under investigation.

Apparatus

Inhalation analgesics may be administered either from a standard anesthetic machine or a flow-over vaporizer. When nitrous oxide is used for self-administered analgesia, it is usually combined with oxygen by a blender apparatus in varying concentrations depending on the requirements of the patient. Volatile anesthetics are administered via several types of vaporizers. Some are hand-held (Cyprane (Figure 10.5), Duke and Penthrane Analgizer (Figure 10.6)), and some precision vaporizers are attached to the anesthetic machine (Pentomatic) and allow the concommitant use of oxygen and nitrous oxide. A vaporizer used for inhalation analgesia must be capable of delivering a reliable concentration or range of concentrations of anesthetic vapor. These concentrations should be safe and should not be significantly altered by the patient's min-

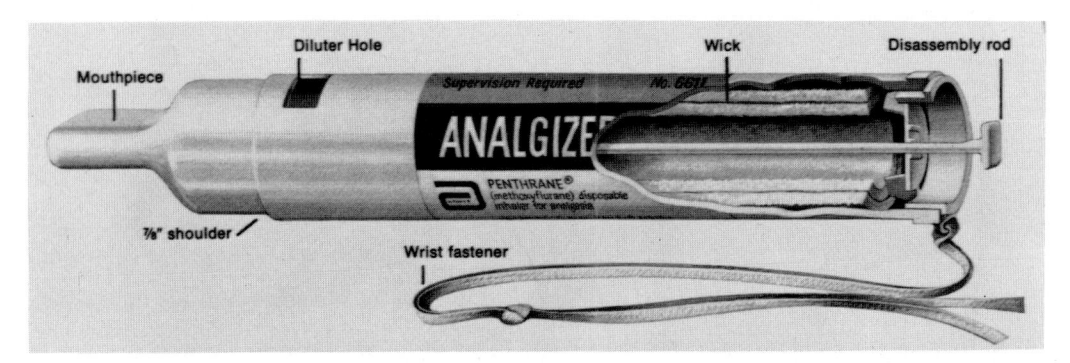

Figure 10.6. Penthrane Analgizer.

ute ventilation, peak flow or variations in room temperature. These considerations are especially important because of the wide variations in minute ventilation which occur during labor. Some devices incorporate a fail-safe device, requiring the patient to occlude a hole in the inhaler in order to obtain a higher anesthetic concentration or to generate a negative pressure to initiate gas flow. These mechanisms assume that the patient will be unable to operate them if excessively anesthetized, and that deepening of anesthesia will cause the mouthpiece or mask to fall from the face. Patients may, however, learn to circumvent these intended safety mechanisms by such ingenious maneuvers as holding on to the mouthpiece with their teeth or by propping the inhaler against the pillow.

The Penthrane Analgizer is a simple, light-weight, disposable device which is probably more convenient than the traditional Cyprane or Duke inhalers. It delivers a range of approximately 0.3 to 0.9 per cent of methoxyflurane, with the higher concentration obtained by occlusion of a hole in the side of the inhaler. Concentration falls with time, as the agent is exhausted and as the temperature falls. Marx and coworkers[27] found this apparatus to be effective and convenient to use because of its small size and light weight. There was a high degree of patient acceptance, and it was safe for mother and fetus. Others, however, have found the Cyprane inhaler to be more acceptable when used with methoxyflurane.[28] This might be explained by the higher concentration (up to 1.15 per cent) obtainable with the latter device. Such high concentrations, if inhaled for prolonged periods, may inadvertently produce general anesthesia, with all its attendant risks. Both studies found that patients prefer a mask to a mouthpiece, as it enables them to breathe through either their mouth or their nose. The analgizer has the added safety feature of being unaffected by changes in position; in some of the older devices this had caused flooding of the system and delivery of a high concentration of anesthetic vapor. The analgizer is designed to contain a maximum of 15 ml of methoxyflurane, a dose which, it has been suggested, is free from problems of nephrotoxicity. Unfortunately, refilling of the device cannot be prevented, and a case of renal failure has occurred following the use of an analgizer which was refilled seven times for analgesia before delivery and three more times for removal of a retained placenta.[29] A disadvantage of this device is that supplemental oxygen cannot be added to the inspired mixture. Also it is not temperature-compensated, so that, as with any hand-held vaporizer, a rise in temperature may occur during use, thus increasing the delivered concentration of anesthetic.

Nitrous oxide may be administered by an anesthetist, using a conventional anesthetic machine, or by the patient herself on demand. Several favorable reports evaluating apparatuses designed to deliver a pre-mixed concentration of nitrous oxide and oxygen have appeared in the American literature.[30, 31] However, these units have not gained wide acceptance, perhaps because they are rather unwieldy. In the United Kingdom, a pre-mixed container of 50 per cent nitrous oxide and 50 per cent oxygen, marketed under the name of Entonox, is very widely used. It is delivered from a single cylinder fitted with a reducing valve. This connects to a mask, which operates only when a negative pressure opens the valve. A possible danger of this mixture is that if the cylinder is allowed to reach −7°C, separation of the two gases occurs, allowing pure oxygen then pure nitrous oxide to be delivered as the cylinder is progressively emptied. This can be avoided by adequate mixing and warming of the cylinder. Recommendations for the use of nitrous oxide-oxygen apparatuses in obstetric analgesia, including specifications as to desired limits of accuracy, flow resistance and safety features, are included in a report by the subcommittee of the Medical Research Council in England.[32]

TECHNIQUES OF INHALATION ANALGESIA

Inhalation analgesics are administered either *intermittently*—only during contractions—or *continuously*—during and between uterine contractions. With either technique the anesthetist should first instruct the patient in the proper use of the equipment. The anesthetist must remain in verbal contact with the patient and provide continuous reassurance and encouragement. Rather than using a fixed concentration of anesthetic, the concentration

Table 10.1
Intermittent Inhalation Analgesia: A Suggested Technique

1. Administer 15 to 30 ml of antacid.
2. Check blood pressure.
3. Start intravenous infusion with indwelling catheter.
4. If the contractions are regular, initiate the inhalation analgesic 30 seconds before the onset of a contraction.
5. If the contractions are irregular, initiate the inhalation analgesic with the onset of the contraction.
6. Begin with $N_2O:O_2$ 70:30 per cent or methoxyflurane 0.5 per cent or a combination of the above.
7. During the first stage of labor apply the face mask or analgizer and have the patient take three deep breaths and then take three to four normal breaths.
8. During the second stage of labor, the technique is modified by the patient bearing down forcefully after the third deep breath and maintaining her expulsive effort as long as she is able. After another deep breath, the patient should bear down again. This sequence should be continued until the contraction ends or she becomes drowsy.
9. Remain in verbal contact with the patient and be reassuring. If the patient becomes confused, drowsy, excited or uncooperative, the inspired concentration should be lowered.
10. Remove the mask between contractions and instruct the patient to relax in a comfortable position and breathe normally.
11. Because this technique does not provide complete analgesia, the obstetrician should infiltrate the perineum with local anesthetic or perform a pudendal block for delivery.

must be regulated according to the anesthetist's clinical judgment and the patient's response. If the patient becomes confused, drowsy, excited or uncooperative, the inspired concentration should be lowered quickly. Otherwise the patient may lose her laryngeal reflexes, vomit or passively regurgitate and aspirate.

Intermittent Analgesia (Table 10.1)

There is a time lag between the initiation of inhalation analgesia and the maximum analgesic effect called *latency of analgesia*. The latency of analgesia is shortened by a high inspired concentration, increased alveolar ventilation and low lipid solubility of the agent. Unfortunately, there is only a brief interval between the onset of a uterine contraction and the perception of pain. If possible, the patient or anesthetist should time the uterine contractions so that administration of the analgesic agent is started about 30 seconds **before** the onset of the contraction. An adequate gas tension will then be achieved in the brain by the time the contraction becomes painful. If this is not possible, the latency of analgesia may be shortened by using a higher concentration for a brief period of time (30 to 60 seconds) and starting the administration at the onset of the contraction. When this is done, careful attention must be paid to the patient's level of consciousness and signs of excitement. If the patient takes three to six deep breaths at the onset of administration, the increased alveolar ventilation will also shorten the latency of analgesia.

The inhalation analgesics may also be self-administered. The technique is the same as when intermittent analgesia is administered by an anesthetist. The patient should have an experienced attendant to ensure instruction early in labor in the proper use of the equipment, to ascertain later that she is bearing down effectively and, most importantly, to monitor any change in the level of consciousness.

Continuous Technique (Table 10.2)

This technique offers the advantage of a more stable and more effective level of analgesia. Although the continuous technique may be used in a labor room during the first stage of labor, it is most commonly used in the delivery room shortly before birth. During the expulsive stage of labor, contractions are usually very frequent and the interval between the onset of a contraction and the perception of pain is only

Table 10.2
Continuous Inhalation Analgesia: A Suggested Technique

1. Administer 15 to 30 ml of antacid.
2. Check blood pressure.
3. Start intravenous infusion with indwelling catheter.
4. Initiate inhalation analgesia when the patient becomes uncomfortable during either the late first stage or, more commonly, the second stage of labor.
5. Begin with N_2O 40 per cent or methoxyflurane 0.3 per cent, or a mixture of N_2O 30 per cent and methoxyflurane 0.2 per cent and oxygen.
6. Use these low concentrations initially and gradually increase them until the maximum concentration is reached at which the patient is cooperative, oriented and comfortable.
7. With each expulsive effort instruct the patient to take three deep breaths and then bear down.
8. Remain in verbal contact with the patient and be reassuring. If the patient becomes confused, drowsy, excited or uncooperative, immediately lower the inspired concentration.
9. The obstetrician should infiltrate the perineum with a local anesthetic or perform a pudendal block for added analgesia.

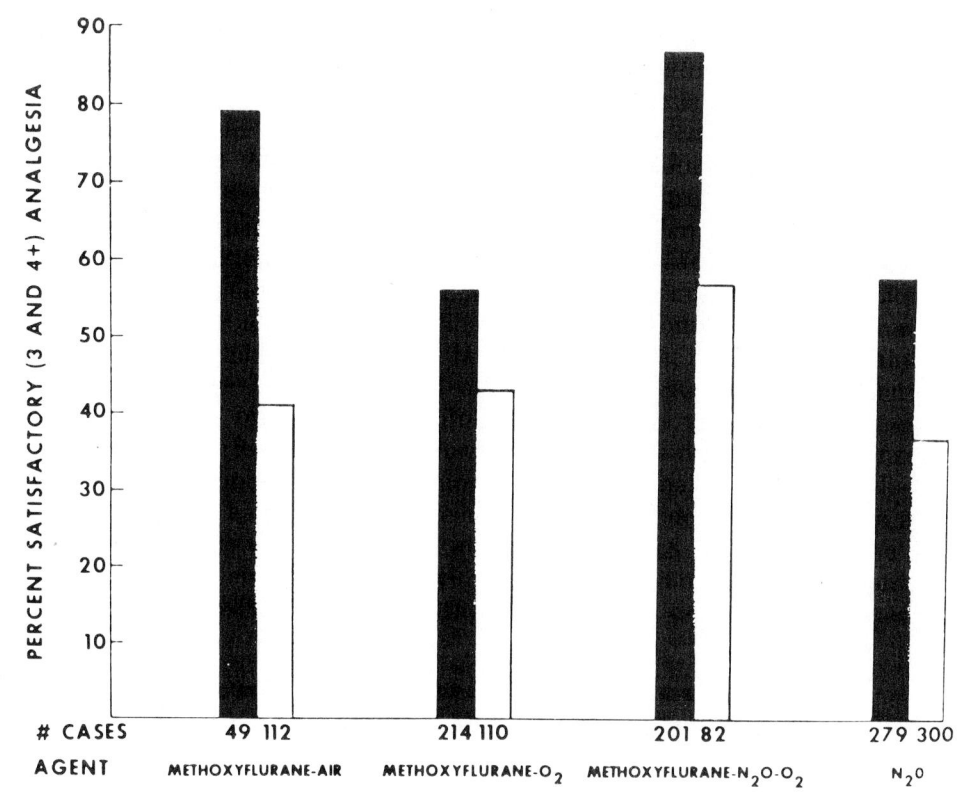

Figure 10.7. Comparison of continuous and intermittent techniques of inhalation analgesia.

5 to 10 seconds. Because the parturient must push with each contraction, precluding inhalation of anesthetic, the intermittent technique is less effective (Figure 10.7). When using the continuous technique, a low concentration of the inhalation analgesic is administered initially, then the concentration is gradually increased until the maximum concentration is reached at which the patient is analgesic and remains oriented and cooperative. The anesthetist must remain in continuous verbal contact with the patient and lower the concentration of the agent if the patient becomes confused, drowsy or uncooperative. Analgesia is improved if the patient takes two to three deep breaths before each expulsive effort and during crowning of the fetal head. To assure more effective pain relief during delivery and repair of the episiotomy, inhalation analgesia can be supplemented with a pudendal block or local infiltration of the perineum.

TECHNIQUES OF GENERAL ANESTHESIA

A "standard" obstetric general anesthetic technique has gained enormous popularity because of its maternal safety and relatively low depressant effects on the newborn. This technique is outlined in Table 10.3 and is similar to that used for general anesthesia for cesarean section. When uterine relaxation is necessary, halothane is currently the most popular agent. Here again, induction of anesthesia should be effected with oxygen inhalation, a small dose of a non-depolarizing relaxant, thiopental and succinylcholine admin-

Table 10.3
General Anesthesia for Vaginal Delivery: A Suggested Technique*

1. Pre-medicate the patient with 30 to 60 ml of oral antacid within 1 hour of induction.
2. Start intravenous infusion with a large-bore plastic cannula.
3. Pre-oxygenate the patient for 3 minutes if possible. Use high flow rates (greater than 6 L per minute).
4. Administer atropine 0.4 mg or glycopyrrolate 0.2 mg and curare 3 mg intravenously within 5 minutes of induction of anesthesia.
5. When delivery is imminent and forceps are to be applied, administer thiopental 4 mg/kg and succinylcholine 1.5 mg/kg at the start of uterine contraction. An assistant should apply cricoid pressure until the trachea is sealed by the cuff of the endotracheal tube.
6. If uterine relaxation is not necessary, administer N_2O 5 L per minute + O_2 5 L per minute. Use muscle relaxant as necessary.
7. If uterine relaxation is necessary, administer halothane 1 per cent and oxygen 99 per cent. When spontaneous ventilation resumes, halothane concentration may be increased to 3 per cent if necessary. Controlled ventilation with high concentrations of halothane should be used with extreme caution, with careful and constant monitoring of maternal heart sounds and blood pressure and only if uterine hypertonus is resulting in fetal jeopardy. Halothane should be discontinued after delivery of the infant and uterine tone restored with intravenous infusion of oxytocin drip and uterine massage.
8. Extubate the patient when she is fully awake.

* General anesthesia is not the preferred technique for routine vaginal delivery. Its use should be reserved for situations in which anesthesia is necessary but regional techniques are either contraindicated or inadequate. Some examples are acute fetal distress during the second stage of labor, intrauterine manipulations requiring uterine relaxation or an uncontrollable patient whose physical activity may damage the newborn during delivery.

istration, endotracheal intubation and then, solely for the purpose of uterine relaxation, halothane and oxygen should be administered. Because the patient is paralyzed, great caution must be exercised not to overdose the patient with halothane. Immediately after the intrauterine manipulation and delivery, halothane can be discontinued, the patient hyperventilated with nitrous oxide and oxygen or oxygen alone, the uterus massaged and an intravenous drip of oxytocin administered. Excessive uterine bleeding is unusual.[33]

INDIVIDUAL AGENTS

The ideal inhalation agent for use in obstetrics should be an excellent analgesic with little hypnotic effect, thus minimizing the risk of aspiration at analgesic concentrations. It should also be non-flammable, excreted wholly by the lungs and have no effect on uterine contractility. Of course, no single agent exists with all these properties. Only those most often used in modern obstetric practice will be considered here.

Nitrous Oxide

Various concentrations of nitrous oxide have been administered either by continuous or intermittent inhalation to provide pain relief in labor. A report of a large clinical trial in Great Britain[3] showed little difference in analgesic effect between intermittent inhalation of 50 per cent and 70 per cent nitrous oxide, except in abnormal labors in which the higher concentration was slightly superior. Approximately 70 per cent of women considered their relief in the first and second stages of labor to be complete or good, and 90 per cent said that use of the agent "helped them." Although both concentrations in this study proved safe for the mother and the baby, 3 per cent of parturients receiving 70 per cent nitrous oxide lost consciousness, as compared with only 0.4 per cent of those receiving 50 per cent nitrous oxide. As there was considerable variability in the mother's response to nitrous oxide, the authors emphasized the need for careful supervision.

As nitrous oxide has a very low blood solubility, concentrations in the brain rise and fall rapidly. Theoretical calculations of the kinetics of nitrous oxide distribution during intermittent administration for labor suggest that the optimal method of delivery is achieved by administration of a 50 per cent mixture for 50 seconds **before** the start of each contraction, continuing for a period equal to half the time between contractions.[33] In this way, the highest nitrous oxide brain levels will coincide with the maximum intensity of pain, but the patient will be awake between contractions. Intermittent inhalation of 50 per cent nitrous oxide is equivalent to breathing a 26.8 per cent concentration of nitrous oxide continuously until equilibrium occurs.[34] If nitrous oxide is inhaled continuously, a mean concentration of 41.2 per cent is necessary to provide adequate analgesia while maintaining consciousness.[35] Because the onset of contractions is often unpredictable, intermittent administration seldom is begun before the uterine contraction starts, and maximum analgesic effectiveness is not achieved. Consequently continuous analgesia is more reliable.

Nitrous oxide administered in analgesic concentrations appears to cause minimal maternal cardiovascular or respiratory depression and does not affect uterine con-

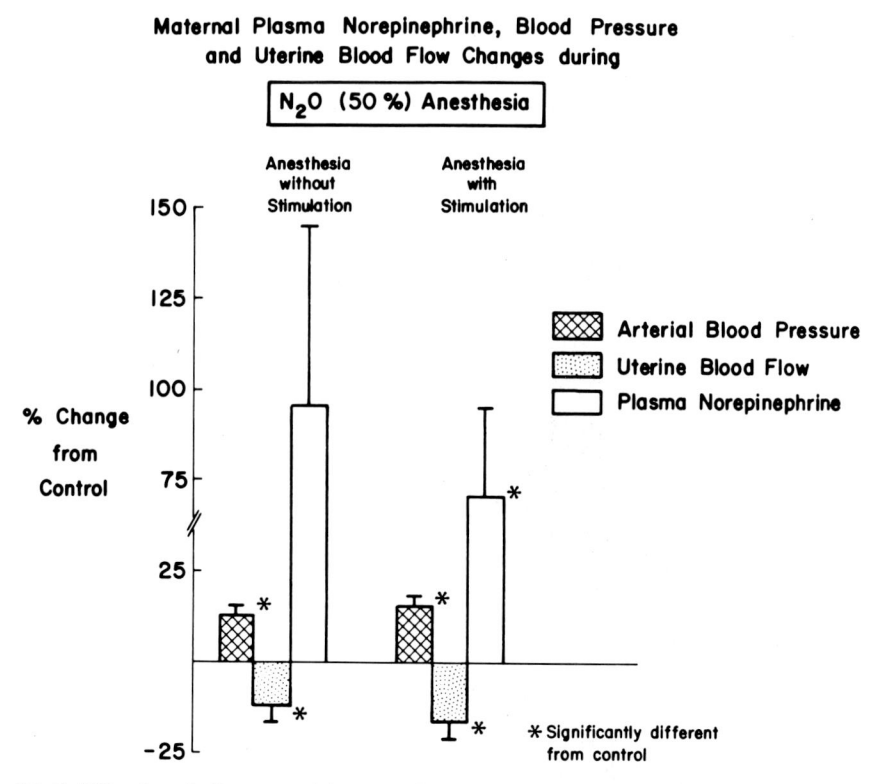

Figure 10.8. Effects of nitrous oxide anesthesia, with and without noxious stimulation, on maternal plasma norepinephrine, blood pressure and uterine blood flow in the pregnant ewe.

tractility. Occasionally, restlessness may occur during nitrous oxide administration, resulting in an uncooperative patient. This complication is less common with methoxyflurane or trichloroethylene.[36] Although accepted as safe for the fetus when used for obstetric analgesia, nitrous oxide has been implicated as contributing to fetal deterioration when anesthesia was prolonged during cesarean section.[16] In studies of pregnant ewes, Palahniuk and Cumming[37] found a significant decrease in fetal pH after only a brief period of anesthesia when a thiopental induction was followed by 70 per cent nitrous oxide. There was a fall in fetal PaO_2 after induction of anesthesia, and uterine blood flow was reduced by 18 to 30 per cent. Although the fetus seemed to be most susceptible to the changes following induction of anesthesia, further deterioration occurred and was thought to be related to reduced uterine perfusion related to light anesthesia and increased endogenous maternal catecholamines. Indeed, Shnider et al.[38] showed that noxious stimulation of a pregnant ewe during $N_2O:O_2$ anesthesia was associated with an increase in maternal blood pressure, a decrease in uterine blood flow and an increase in plasma norepinephrine of 71 per cent from the awake control state (Figure 10.8). By contrast noxious stimulation during $N_2O:O_2$ anesthesia that was supplemented with either 0.5 per cent halothane or 1 per cent enflurane did not increase plasma catecholamines or adversely affect uterine blood flow. In fact, uterine blood flow rose 20 per cent from control during $N_2O:O_2$ halothane anesthesia.

Diffusion hypoxia in the neonate after maternal administration of nitrous oxide is a theoretical cause of neonatal depression, if high concentrations of the agents are administered over a prolonged period. Reid,[39] however, was unable to demonstrate this when he measured alveolar nitrous oxide levels in the newborn.

Methoxyflurane

Methoxyflurane has been widely adopted as an obstetric inhalation analgesic agent and has tended to replace trichloroethylene for this purpose. Both of these agents are good analgesics at low concentrations, and both have high blood and fat solubilities. Major et al.[40] and Rosen et al.[36] concluded that methoxyflurane was a more satisfactory analgesic than trichloroethylene and was accompanied by a lower incidence of restlessness. They suggested that a concentration of 0.35 per cent methoxyflurane administered intermittently was ideal for use in obstetrics. Jones et al. found methoxyflurane to be a superior analgesic to nitrous oxide when both agents were administered either continuously[35] or intermittently[41] and found nausea and vomiting to occur significantly less frequently with methoxyflurane. A comparison of methoxyflurane with parenteral agents suggested the former to be more satisfactory and claimed various advantages for its use, including a shortening of labor.[42] Shnider and co-workers[19] reported that methoxyflurane 0.2 to 0.5 per cent and nitrous oxide 40 to 60 per cent, when administered individually, produced satisfactory analgesia in 67 per cent and 61 per cent of parturients, respectively. When the two agents were combined and given in lesser concentrations than when used alone, the incidence of satisfactory analgesia increased to 88 per cent.

No evidence of increased risk of fetal depression was found in the above reports, and Clark et al.[20] demonstrated that, even with prolonged use of low concentrations of methoxyflurane, maternal and fetal blood levels remained low. However, high concentrations used for prolonged periods were associated with increased blood levels of the agent and a greater number of infants with low Apgar scores. Although the high blood solubility of methoxyflurane enables satisfactory intermittent administration without the cyclical variation in brain level seen with nitrous oxide,[33] theoretically, a progressive accumulation of methoxyflurane should occur with prolonged administration. An explanation for the absence of such accumulation in the conscious parturient is suggested by the observation that, as labor progresses, the patient regulates uptake of the agent by reducing ventilation or using the inhaler for a shorter period of time.[43] Intermittent rather than continuous inhalation tends to prevent blood levels from rising, because some excretion of the agent occurs between contractions. Of course, if the patient inhales continuously or hyperventilates, higher blood levels must be expected.

All these trials confirm the efficacy of low concentrations of methoxyflurane for use in obstetric analgesia, with little effect on uterine contractility and a high degree of maternal safety. Although additional analgesia or anesthesia may be required for delivery, this agent has proved most useful for the first stage of labor.

RENAL EFFECTS OF METHOXYFLURANE

The potential nephrotoxicity of methoxyflurane, secondary to high levels of its metabolic products, inorganic fluoride and oxalic acid, has been well established.[44] There are many reports of increased concentrations of maternal and neonatal inorganic fluoride after the use of methoxyflurane in parturients, but renal failure is extremely rare. Cousins and Mazze[45] demonstrated that a serum inorganic fluoride level of over 80 μmol/L was associated with polyuric renal failure, and levels over 50 μmol/L were associated with subclinical renal toxicity and evidence of decreased concentrating ability. Creasser et al.[46] reported a mean peak maternal serum inorganic fluoride level of 22 μmol/L following awake analgesia for vaginal delivery, although two individuals had values over 50 μmol/L. Similarly, Young et al.[47] found maternal peak inorganic fluoride to be increased to 11 μmol/L following methoxyflurane administration for vaginal delivery or cesarean section; the lower fluoride levels in this series can be explained by a shorter period of administration. Considerable individual variation in metabolism occurs, and further increases might be expected in those patients taking drugs which are enzyme inducers. Although maternal blood urea nitrogen (BUN), serum creatinine and serum uric acid increased significantly 24 hours and 48 hours after delivery, values were still within normal limits.[46, 48] Oxalate excretion also increased significantly within the 2 days after delivery. The minimal amount of inorganic fluoride does not inhibit plasma cholinesterase activity.[49]

Neonatal levels of serum inorganic fluoride are also raised at time of delivery after methoxyflurane analgesia; mean values of 14.6 μmol/L and 5.3 μmol/L were obtained in the studies mentioned above, although they decreased over succeeding days.[46, 47] The presence of fluoride in the newborn may result from passive diffusion across the placenta during labor, and the fetus is also probably capable of metabolizing methoxyflurane. Although these levels do not approach the range known to be toxic in adults, little is known about the nephrotoxic potential of this ion in the newborn. In the only study to date, Clark et al.[50] measured neonatal BUN, creatinine, uric acid and osmolality after maternal methoxyflurane analgesia. They were not able to demonstrate renal impairment. The possibility of other effects of fluoride ion in the neonate, such as enzyme inhibition, or effects on the central nervous system should be considered, although little is known at this time.

In summary, it seems advisable to limit the use of methoxyflurane to a relatively small total dose, such as 15 ml, for labor and delivery. Even so, patients with pre-existing renal impairment (such as those with toxemia) and those taking enzyme-inducing agents or nephrotoxic drugs may still be at risk. If dosage limits are observed and patients carefully selected, the use of methoxyflurane in low concentrations for relatively short periods seems to be free from hazard.

Halothane

The use of halothane in obstetric anesthesia is still controversial. Although the uterine relaxant effect of the agent even at low concentrations is well established, its use in concentrations of less than 0.8 per cent for cesarean section[33] or vaginal delivery[51] has not been associated with increased blood loss. When used for cesarean section, it has proved superior to 70 per cent nitrous oxide, particularly when the effects on the fetus are considered. This probably results from the ability to use a higher percentage of inspired oxygen and improved uterine blood flow due to the inhibition of endogenous norepinephrine secretion by halothane.[38] Half per cent halothane is considered preferable to 0.8 per cent, however, as the incidence of hypotension with the greater concentration is unacceptably high. Halothane is not used to provide analgesia during labor, because the patient is likely to become unconscious before satisfactory analgesic levels have been obtained. There are other specific indications for its use, such as when rapid, profound uterine relaxation is needed.

Enflurane and Isoflurane

There are several reports detailing the use of enflurane in obstetric practice. Coleman and Downing[52] administered low doses to supplement anesthesia with 50 per cent nitrous oxide and a muscle relaxant for cesarean section. No adverse effects were noted on the neonate, nor was blood loss excessive.[22] When used for vaginal delivery some investigators found that enflurane, like halothane, produced little analgesic effect unless administered in concentrations which resulted in unconsciousness.[53, 54] On the other hand, Rolbin et al.[55] reported that enflurane (0.25 to 1.25 per cent) was an effective analgesic for delivery. In a study comparing continuous analgesia with either nitrous oxide or enflurane, the obstetricians rated enflurane superior to nitrous oxide. Enflurane causes a dose-related depression of uterine contractility. In high doses, e.g. 3 per cent, it may produce increased postpartum uterine blood loss.[25] Thus, enflurane and halothane share many characteristics, and indications for their use in obstetric anesthesia are similar. Perhaps the only advantage of enflurane as compared to halothane is that its effects are more rapidly reversible because of its lower blood solubility. Enflurane is metabolized to inorganic fluoride, although to a much lesser extent than methoxyflurane. Its use in patients with renal impairment should be avoided and other agents chosen in preference.

At the time of this writing, isoflurane is still unavailable for clinical practice. At equipotent concentrations its effect on uterine contractility is similar to that of halothane and enflurane.[24] Hicks et al.[56] reported that continuous analgesia with isoflurane (0.2 to 0.7 per cent) was equianalgesic to 40 per cent nitrous oxide when administered for more than 10 minutes prior to delivery.

Other Agents

Cyclopropane achieved great popularity in obstetric practice because it enabled rapid induction of anesthesia, caused little uterine relaxation and, in analgesic concentrations, did not adversely affect the fetus. It was not usually associated with hypotension, perhaps because its administration resulted in a high level of circulating catecholamines. In recent years it has been replaced by non-flammable agents. Other disadvantages of cyclopropane are the high incidence of vomiting and cardiac arrhythmias associated with its administration.

Trichloroethylene was also extensively used to provide obstetric analgesia and is still recommended by Crawford[57] for cesarean section. Its main drawback is the inability to use it in a closed circuit, because of its interaction with soda lime to form toxic products. There are also reports of overdose and cardiac arrest associated with its unsupervised use in self-administration inhalers. It is no longer commercially available in the United States.

References

1. National Study of Maternity Care Survey of Obstetric Practice and Associated Services in Hospitals in the United States. A report of the Committee on Maternal Health of the American College of Obstetricians and Gynecologists, Chicago, 1970.
2. Akamatsu TJ, Bonica JJ, Rehmet R, et al.: Experiences with the use of ketamine for parturition. 1. Primary anesthetic for vaginal delivery. Anesth Analg Curr Res 53:284, 1974.
3. Report by M.R.C. Committees Sir Dugald Biard, chairman. Clinical trials of different concentrations of oxygen and nitrous oxide for obstetric analgesia. Br Med J 1:709, 1970.
4. Bonica JJ: Physiology of pregnancy. In *Principles and Practice of Obstetric Analgesia and Anesthesia*. F. A. Davis, Philadelphia, 1972, p 21.
5. Palahniuk RJ, Shnider SM, Eger EI II: Pregnancy decreases the requirement for inhaled anesthetic agents. Anesthesiology 41:82, 1974.
6. Bonica JJ: Anesthetic deaths. In *Principles and Practice of Obstetric Analgesia and Anesthesia*. F. A. Davis, Philadelphia, 1972, p 751.
7. Merrill RB, Hingson RA: Study of incidence of maternal mortality from aspiration of vomitus during anesthesia occurring in major obstetrical hospitals in the United States. Anesth Analg 30: 121, 1951.
8. Bond VK, Ragan WD: Maternal mortality in Indiana as related to anesthesia. In *Abstracts of Scientific Papers*, Annual Meeting, Society for Obstetric Anesthesia and Perinatology, Seattle, 1977, p 13.
9. Arthure H, Tomkinson J, Organe G, et al.: *Report on Confidential Enquiries into Maternal Deaths in England and Wales 1967-1969*. Department of Health and Social Security, Reports on Health and Social Subjects, 1. Her Majesty's Stationery Office, London, 1972.
10. Roberts RB, Shirley MA: Reducing the risk of acid aspiration during cesarean section. Anesth Analg Curr Res 53:859, 1974.
11. Smiler BG, Goldberger R, Sivak BJ, et al.: Routine endotracheal intubation in obstetrics. Am J Obstet Gynecol 103:947, 1969.
12. Moya F: Volatile inhalation agents and muscle relaxants in obstetrics. Acta Anaesth Scand (Suppl) 25:368, 1966.
13. Palahniuk RJ, Shnider SM: Maternal and fetal cardiovascular and acid-base changes during halothane and isoflurane anesthesia in the pregnant ewe. Anesthesiology 41:462, 1974.
14. Cosmi EV, Marx GF: The effect of anesthesia on the acid-base status of the fetus. Anesthesiology 30:238, 1969.
15. Finster M, Poppers PJ: Safety of thiopental used for induction of general anesthesia in elective cesarean section. Anesthesiology 29:190, 1968.
16. Stenger VG, Blechner JN, Prystowsky H: A study of prolongation of obstetric anesthesia. Am J Obstet Gynecol 103:901, 1969.
17. Marx GF, Joshi CW, Orkin LR: Placental transmission of nitrous oxide. Anesthesiology 32:429, 1970.
18. Moya F: General anesthesia. In *Obstetrical Anesthesia: Current Concepts and Practice*, SM Shnider, Ed. Williams & Wilkins, Baltimore, 1969, p 88.
19. Shnider SM, Steffenson JL, Margolis AJ: Methoxyflurane analgesia in obstetrics. Obstet Gynecol 33:594, 1969.
20. Clark RB, Cooper JO, Brown WE, et al.: The effect of methoxyflurane on the foetus. Br J Anaesth 42: 286, 1970.
21. Munson ES: Uterine activity and anesthesia. In *Obstetrical Anesthesia: Current Concepts and Practice*, SM Shnider, Ed. Williams & Wilkins, Baltimore, 1969, p 29.
22. Naftalin NJ, Phear WPC, Goldberg AH: Halothane and isometric contractions of isolated pregnant rat myometrium. Anesthesiology 42:458, 1975.
23. Naftalin NJ, McKay DM, Phear WPC, et al.: The effects of halothane on pregnant and nonpregnant human myometrium. Anesthesiology 46:15, 1977.
24. Munson ES, Embro WJ: Enflurane, isoflurane, and halothane and isolated human uterine muscle. Anesthesiology 46:11, 1977.
25. Marx GF, Kim YI, Lin CC, et al.: Postpartum uterine pressures under halothane or enflurane anesthesia. Obstet Gynecol 51:695, 1978.
26. Ad Hoc Committee on the Effect of Trace Anesthetics on the Health of Operating Room Personnel: A national study. Anesthesiology 41:321, 1974.
27. Marx GF, Chen LK, Tabora JA: Experiences with a disposable inhaler for methoxyflurane analgesia during labour: Clinical and biochemical results. Can Anaesth Soc J 16:66, 1969.
28. Enrile LL, Roux JF, Wilson R, et al.: Methoxyflurane (Penthrane) inhalation in labor. Obstet Gynecol 41:860, 1973.
29. Mazze RI: Personal Communicaton.
30. Hanisch EC, Sankawa H, Gauert WB, et al.: Clinical and mechanical evaluation of an A.E. gas

machine for obstetric analgesia and anesthesia. Anesth Analg Curr Res 50:190, 1971.
31. Wilson RD, Priano LL, Allen CR, et al.: Demand analgesia and anesthesia in obstetrics. South Med J 65:556, 1972.
32. Cole PV, Crawford JS, Doughty AG, et al.: Specifications and recommendations for nitrous oxide/oxygen apparatus to be used in obstetric analgesia. Anaesthesia 25:317, 1970.
33. Waud BE, Waud DR: Calculated kinetics of distribution of nitrous oxide and methoxyflurane during intermittent administration in obstetrics. Anesthesiology 32:306, 1970.
34. Latto LP, Molloy MJ, Rosen M: Arterial concentrations of nitrous oxide during intermittent patient-controlled inhalation of 50% nitrous oxide in oxygen (Entonox) during the first stage of labour. Br J Anaesth 45:1029, 1973.
35. Jones PL, Rosen M, Mushin WW, et al.: Methoxyflurane and nitrous oxide as obstetric analgesics. I. A comparison by continuous administration. Br Med J 3:255, 1969.
36. Rosen M, Mushin WW, Jones PL, et al.: Field trial of methoxyflurane, nitrous oxide, and trichloroethylene as obstetric analgesics. Br Med J 3:263, 1969.
37. Palahniuk RJ, Cumming M: Foetal deterioration following thiopentone-nitrous oxide anaesthesia in the pregnant ewe. Can Anaesth Soc J 24:361, 1977.
38. Shnider SM, Wright RG, Levinson G, et al.: Plasma norepinephrine and uterine blood flow changes during endotracheal intubation and general anesthesia in the pregnant ewe. In *Abstracts of Scientific Papers,* Annual Meeting, Society for Obstetrical Anesthesia and Perinatology, Memphis, 1978, p 48.
39. Reid DHS: Diffusion anoxia at birth. Lancet 1:757, 1958.
40. Major V, Rosen M, Mushin WW: Methoxyflurane as an obstetric analgesic: A comparison with trichloroethylene. Br Med J 2:1554, 1966.
41. Jones PL, Rosen M, Mushin WW, et al.: Methoxyflurane and nitrous oxide as obstetric analgesics. II. A comparison by self-administered intermittent inhalation. Br Med J 3:259, 1969.
42. Barber IJ, Barnett HA, Williams CH: Comparison of methoxyflurane and parenteral agents for obstetric analgesia. Anesth Analg 48:209, 1969.
43. Latto IP, Rosen M, Molloy MJ: Absence of accumulation of methoxyflurane during intermittent self-administration for pain relief in labour. Br J Anaesth 44:391, 1972.
44. Mazze RI, Trudell RJ, Cousins MJ: Methoxyflurane metabolism and renal dysfunction: Clinical correlation in man. Anesthesiology 35:247, 1971.
45. Cousins MJ, Mazze RI: Methoxyflurane nephrotoxicity—a study of dose response in man. JAMA 225:1611, 1973.
46. Creasser CW, Stoelting RK, Krishna G, et al.: Methoxyflurane metabolism and renal function after methoxyflurane analgesia during labor and delivery. Anesthesiology 41:62, 1974.
47. Young SR, Stoelting RK, Bond VK, et al.: Methoxyflurane biotransformation and renal function following methoxyflurane administration for vaginal delivery or cesarean section. Anesth Analg Curr Res 55:415, 1976.
48. Clark RB, Beard AG, Thompson DS, et al.: Maternal and neonatal plasma inorganic fluoride levels after methoxyflurane analgesia for labor and delivery. Anesthesiology 45:88, 1976.
49. Palahniuk RJ, Cumming M: Plasma fluoride levels following obstetrical use of methoxyflurane. Can Anaesth Soc J 22:291, 1975.
50. Clark RB, Beard AG, Thompson DS: Renal function in newborns and mothers exposed to methoxyflurane analgesia for labor and delivery. In *Abstracts of Scientific Papers,* Annual Meeting, American Society of Anesthesiologists, San Francisco, 1976, p 247.
51. Stallabras P: Halothane and blood loss at delivery. Acta Anaesth Scand (Suppl) 25:376, 1966.
52. Coleman AJ, Downing JW: Enflurane anesthesia for cesarean section. Anesthesiology 43:354, 1975.
53. Westmoreland RT, Evans JA, Chastain GM: Obstetric use of enflurane (Ethrane). South Med J 67:527, 1974.
54. Devoghel JC: Enflurane (Ethrane) in obstetrics. Acta Anaesthesiol Belg 2:283, 1974.
55. Rolbin SH, Wright RG, Shnider SM, et al.: Enflurane analgesia for vaginal delivery. In *Abstracts of Scientific Papers,* Annual Meeting, Society for Obstetric Anesthesia and Perinatology, Memphis, 1978, p 53.
56. Hicks JS, Shnider SM, Cohen H: Isoflurane (Forane) analgesia in obstetrics. In *Abstracts of Scientific Papers,* Annual Meeting, American Society of Anesthesiologists, Chicago, 1975, p 99.
57. Crawford JS, Davies P: A return to trichloroethylene for obstetric anaesthesia. Br J Anaesth 47:482, 1975.

SECTION THREE

COMPLICATED OBSTETRICS

CHAPTER 11

Pre-term Labor
Part 1: Pharmacologic Therapy for Pre-term Labor
Part 2: Anesthetic Considerations in Pre-term Labor

Ermelando V. Cosmi, M.D., L.D.*

PART 1: PHARMACOLOGIC THERAPY FOR PRE-TERM LABOR

The incidence of pre-term labor ranges from 5 to 13 per cent of all deliveries, depending on the population, the criteria for screening and the methods used for quantitating uterine activity and cervical dilation and effacement and for statistical processing of data. Pre-term delivery is a major cause of perinatal mortality and morbidity, the incidence increasing with decreasing gestational age and birth weight. Despite continual efforts to understand the mechanisms underlying initiation of labor and the voluminous literature that has accumulated on the subject, the problem of pre-term labor remains a mystery. Many factors have been alleged to be responsible for the initiation of labor. Oxytocin,[1-7] catecholamines,[8-12] estrogen,[13-18] progesterone[16, 18, 19] and prostaglandins[12, 16,] [18, 20-26] have all individually been implicated. A fetal role has been also suggested.[27-36] Some of the factors associated with pre-term labor are cervical and uterine abnormalities,[37-39] multiple gestation,[40, 41] previous pre-term delivery and abortion,[42-45] fetal malformations,[46] medical and obstetric complications (e.g. preeclampsia, eclampsia, diabetes,[47, 48] polyhydramnios,[48] premature rupture of membranes,[49] abruptio placentae,[48] placental malformations,[50] infectious disorders[51]) and socio-biologic variables (e.g. parity, age, weight, height, employment during pregnancy and smoking habits[48, 52-54]). However, all these factors seem to be predisposing rather than causative, inasmuch as they may operate in pregnancies carried out to term. In fact, a significant number of pregnant women go into pre-term labor without identifiable causal or associated factors.

In many cases there is a lack of information on the true incidence of pre-term delivery and on the etiologic factors. One reason for this lack of information has

---
* Supported in part by Consiglio Nazionale delle Richerche (Italia) Grant No. 77.01560.65, by the Program Project from the National Heart and Lung Institute, National Institutes of Health (HL'16137), and by the National Science Foundation (U.S.A.)

been the confusion in the terminology. Initially, the term "prematurity" was used to define infants with a birth weight of 2,500 gm or less, later to denote infants born before the completion of the thirty-seventh week of gestation from the first day of the last menstrual period.[48, 55] It became apparent, however, that birth weight was a poor determinant of gestational age, the most striking example being the large pre-term infants of diabetic mothers. Also, about 25 per cent of the small infants born are not premature but rather victims of intrauterine growth retardation.[56-59] Thus, the terms "premature infant" and "premature labor" have been replaced more appropriately by "low birth weight infants," meaning infants weighing less than 2,500 gm, "pre-term infants," meaning those delivered less than 37 completed weeks from the first day of the last menstrual period, and "pre-term labor."[48, 60]

In recent years various biophysical and biochemical methods have been developed to assess gestational age and fetal maturity, thereby decreasing the iatrogenic induction of labor and allowing proper timing of delivery, especially in the presence of placental insufficiency and poor intrauterine fetal growth. Gestational age and fetal growth can be estimated quite accurately (in about 70 per cent of cases) by serial ultrasonic cephalometry[61-65] and abdominometry[66, 67] (see chapter 23). Fetal pulmonary maturity can be determined by a variety of laboratory tests, among which the lecithin/sphingomyelin ratio[68-70] and the foam or shake test[71, 72] are the most widely used. However, there are conditions—notably diabetes, maternal hypertension, toxemia, and renal diseases—in which these tests fail to accurately predict fetal lung maturity.[73-76] Maternal urinary or serum estriol[77-81] and, to a lesser extent, human placental lactogen levels[82-85] have been used not only to detect fetal jeopardy in the case of placental insufficiency but also as a criterion for testing the adequacy of fetal growth. However, the possibility of false positive tests exists[66, 67, 69, 73-79, 85-88] and is of great concern because it could lead to the iatrogenic pre-term delivery of a small-for-gestational-age infant.

Thus, in recent years the main emphasis in the management of pre-term labor has been placed on preventive measures (e.g. prevention and treatment of infectious diseases, treatment of medical problems, diminished activity and bed rest) and on attempting to suppress uterine activity and accelerate fetal lung maturity. Various drugs have been tested both in animals and humans for the purposes of inhibiting uterine contractions and accelerating fetal lung maturity. However, the usefulness of certain drugs may be limited by their troublesome side effects on both mother and fetus and possible long-term consequences in the infant. Furthermore, their use may pose special problems to the anesthesiologist and perinatologist in cases of preexisting maternal cardiovascular and metabolic disturbances. There also exists the possibility of drug interaction when other drugs have been previously administered.

The effects of the most commonly used drugs for the prevention and treatment of pre-term labor will be reviewed in this chapter. These include β-adrenergic drugs, diazoxide, methylxanthines, ethanol and prostaglandin inhibitors (Figure 11.1). The anesthetic management of the patient with a pre-term delivery will then be discussed.

Prevention and Treatment

β-ADRENERGIC AGENTS

The inhibitory effects of β-adrenergic agents on uterine contractility have been well documented both **in vitro**[89-91] and **in vivo**.[92-98] The first agent to be used clinically was isoxsuprine (Vasodilan) administered intravenously to the mother in a dose of 0.5 mg/min.[92, 99, 100] Subsequently, several investigators have used other

PRE-TERM LABOR

Drugs

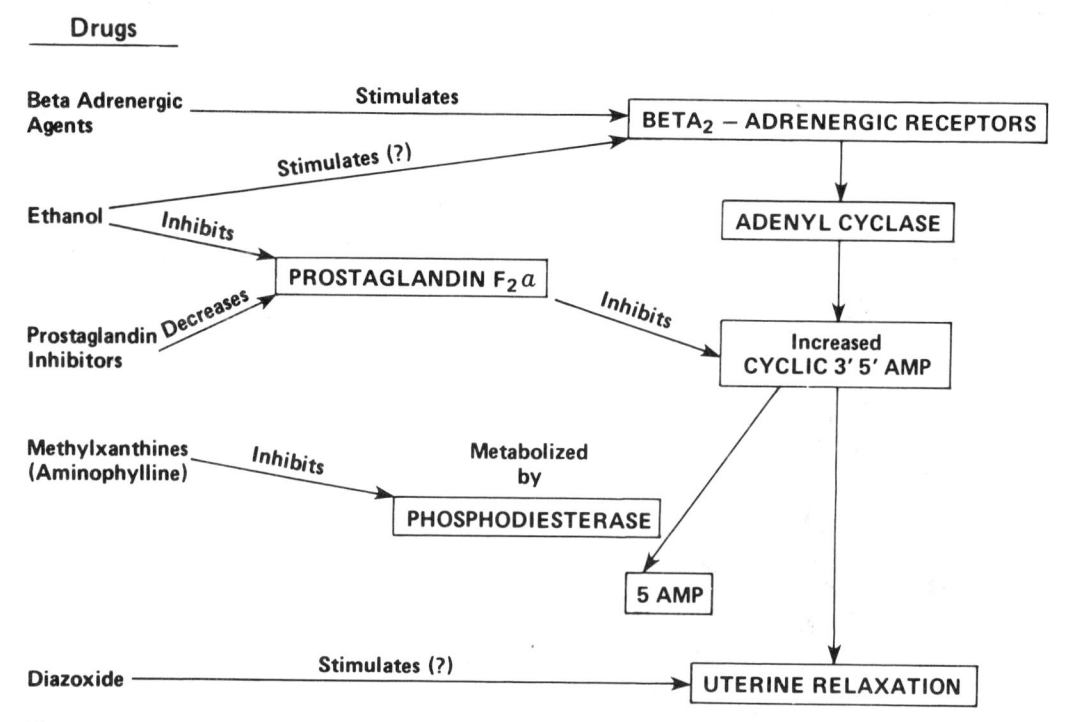

Figure 11.1. Principal site of pharmacologic action of drugs used to inhibit uterine contractility and stop pre-term labor.

agents, including orciprenaline (Alupent) (20 to 40 µg/min),[101, 102] p-hydroxy phenyl isopropylarterenol (Cc-25) (Figure 11.2), nylidrine hydrochloride[104] and the methanesulfonamide derivates of isoxsuprine.[105] However, the usefulness of many of these drugs has been limited by their cardiovascular side effects, such as hypotension and tachycardia, congestive heart failure, restlessness, palpitation and metabolic side effects, such as maternal and fetal hyperglycemia, ketosis and acidemia[92, 100, 106–110] (Table 11.1).

New agents have been developed during the last few years acting predominantly on β_2 receptors in smooth muscles—e.g. uterus, bronchi, peripheral vessels—and possessing less β_1 activity—e.g. cardiac and metabolic action (Table 11.2). Among these agents, fenoterol (Partusisten), a derivate of orciprenaline (0.5 to 9 µg/min),[111–114] ritodrine, a derivate of isoxsuprine (50 to 600 µg/min),[95–97, 115–117] terbutaline (Brethine) (10 to 25 µg/min[118–120]), salbutamol (Ventolin) (1.8 to 76 µg/min)[121–123] and hexoprenaline (0.38 µg/min)[124, 125] have been found to inhibit uterine contractions effectively, prevent premature labor and produce fewer cardiovascular and metabolic side effects in the mother and the fetus. The reported success rate in postponing delivery with the use of these agents is variable, depending on the selection of the patients and the criteria defining pre-term labor. Success rate also appears to vary depending on the agent employed, the individual dosage and the duration of treatment. The best reported figures in postponing delivery for a week or more are with the use of terbutaline,[119] ritodrine[116] and fenoterol,[126] with a success rate of about 80 per cent. However, the reliability of most studies is hampered by the lack of a sufficient number of patients and the absence of a control series. Placebo administration has itself been asso-

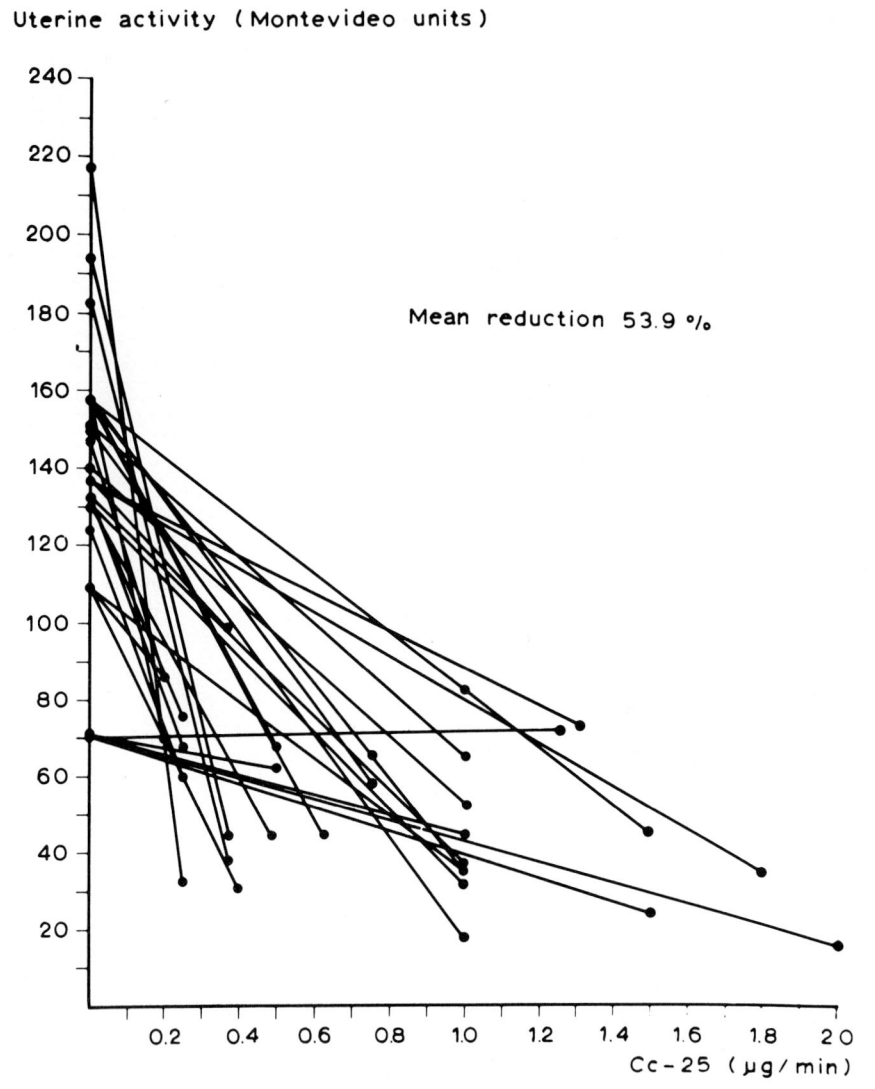

Figure 11.2. The influence of Cc-25 on uterine activity measured with the transabdominal open-tip catheter in seven pregnant women. The mean reduction of the intensity calculated on 23 determinations was 53.9 per cent. (Reprinted by permission from Eskes TKAB: The influence of β-mimetic catecholamines upon uterine activity in human pregnancy and labor. In *Uterine Contraction: Side Effects of Steroidal Contraceptives,* JB Josimovich, ed. John Wiley & Sons, New York, 1973, p 277.)

ciated with a variable success of up to 73 per cent.[127] This raises the question of whether prolongation of pregnancy is the result of the β-stimulant therapy or the conservative treatment, e.g. bed rest, sedation, psychological support. Thus, adequately controlled studies are necessary to determine the usefulness of β-stimulants. There is one reported double-blind, placebo-controlled, multicenter study of ritodrine in pre-term labor with intact membranes. Pregnancy was prolonged beyond the treatment period (7 days) in 77 per cent of patients receiving ritodrine compared with 48 per cent of those under placebo treatment.[115]

Recently, attempts to accelerate fetal lung maturity and prevent respiratory distress syndrome (RDS) in the newborn by antepartum administration of glucocorticoids to the mother have stimulated further interest in the use of β-stimulants. The rationale is to further inhibit pre-term uterine contractions in order to allow time to obtain the desired effect of corticosteroids. A significantly lower incidence of RDS in pre-term infants whose mothers received a β-adrenergic drug in conjunction with glucocorticoid therapy has been reported.[128-130] Preliminary reports also indicate that β-stimulants alone, administered to the mother prior to delivery, may

Table 11.1
Side Effects of Drugs Used to Stop Labor

Maternal	Fetal and Neonatal
β-Adrenergic agents	
Hypotension	Tachycardia
Tachycardia	Hyperglycemia
Congestive heart failure	Increased free fatty acids
Arrhythmias (atrial and ventricular)	Fetal asphyxia with large doses due to maternal hypotension or increased uterine vascular resistance resulting in decreased uterine blood flow
Anxiety, nervousness	
Nausea and vomiting	
Headache	
Hyperglycemia	Decreased incidence of respiratory distress syndrome (?)
Metabolic (lactic) acidosis	
Diazoxide	
Hypotension	Tachycardia
Myocardial ischemia	Hyperglycemia
Tachycardia (atrial)	Displaces bilirubin from albumin with potential for kernicterus
Hyperglycemia	
Increased sodium retention	
Aminophylline	
Hypotension	Increased beat-to-beat variability
Tachycardia	Hyperglycemia
Arrhythmias (atrial and ventricular)	Decreased apnea of prematurity (?)
Skeletal muscle tremors	Accelerates lung maturity (?)
Nausea and vomiting	
Headache	
Hyperglycemia	
Increased plasma free fatty acids	
Ethanol	
Central nervous system depression with:	Fetal and neonatal depression
Hypoventilation	Fetal and neonatal hypotension
Hypotension	Neonatal respiratory depression
Disorientation and agitation	Hypotonia
Increased gastric secretion and acidity	Metabolic acidosis
Nausea and vomiting	Hypoglycemia
Hypoglycemia	Temperature instability
Metabolic acidosis	Gastric irritation and vomiting
	Fetal alcohol syndrome (withdrawal syndrome)
Prostaglandin inhibitors	
Gastrointestinal irritation	Premature closure of the ductus arteriosus
Inhibition of platelet function	
Reduced Factor XII	
Depresses immune system	

Table 11.2
Selective β-Adrenergic Receptor* Stimulation

	β_1	β_2
Uterine muscle	No effect	Relaxation
Cardiovascular		
Blood vessels	?	Vasodilation
Heart rate	Increase	No effect
Heart muscle (strength of contraction)	Stimulation	No effect
Cardiac output	Increase	?
Respiratory		
Bronchial muscle	No effect	Relaxation
Secretions	No effect	Slight increase
Central nervous system	?	Stimulation
Gastrointestinal	?	Relaxation
Metabolic	Increased blood; Glucose, lactic acid, free fatty acids	?

* All β-agonists when given systemically have combined β_1 and β_2 effects.

reduce the incidence of RDS in the newborn infant.[131-135] This last observation has been supported by experiments on the rabbit fetus where the administration of isoxsuprine seems to promote the release of pulmonary surfactant from type II alveolar cells.[136, 137] Nevertheless, it is not known whether these beneficial effects are an indirect result of uterine relaxation and possibly increased uterine blood flow or are a direct result of the effect of isoxsuprine on the fetus. Furthermore, it has not been clearly determined what pharmacologic doses are needed to obtain the desired effect on fetal lung maturation and whether or not β-stimulants produce undesirable responses in the fetus.

Because β-stimulants have also been used to treat fetal asphyxia due to uterine hyperactivity[95, 109, 138-149] and placental insufficiency,[150] it is necessary to determine the efficacy of each drug and the possible side effects on the mother and fetus in the likelihood that their use will come into general clinical application.

Studies in pregnant animals, mainly sheep and monkeys, have helped to clarify some of the beneficial and untoward effects that β-stimulants may exert on the mother and fetus. The author's studies on pregnant sheep have shown that orciprenaline, isoxsuprine, fenoterol and ritodrine can effectively inhibit spontaneous or induced uterine contractions but that they may produce untoward effects, especially when high doses are used and/or the fetus is already acidotic.[151-154] The intravenous infusion of orciprenaline to the pregnant ewe, in doses of up to 0.2 μg/kg/min, suppressed uterine contractions within a few minutes after the start of infusion, irrespective of whether they were spontaneous or induced by synthetic oxytocin (Figure 11.3). After the infusion was discontinued uterine contractions returned to pre-infusion levels within 30 minutes or less. Within 1 minute from the start of the infusion, orciprenaline produced an increase in maternal heart rate (about 40 per cent above control). Fetal tachycardia also appeared 1 to 2 minutes after the maternal cardiovascular changes commenced, but it was of smaller magnitude than maternal tachycardia. Uterine artery blood flow tended to increase slightly after cessation of uterine contractions. This last effect was observed even when orciprenaline was administered to the mother while the uterus was quiescent. This is consonant with the radioangiographic findings of

Wallenburg et al.[155] of accelerated intervillous spurts of blood after intravenous infusion of orciprenaline to the pregnant monkey. The maternal and fetal arterial PO_2, pH, PCO_2 and base deficit remained within normal limits during the infusion. However, the mother developed a slight metabolic acidosis, which was directly related to the dose and the duration of the infusion. The maternal and fetal cardiovascular changes were related to the dose used. When the drug was given to the mother in higher doses there was a pronounced maternal and fetal tachycardia, a fall of maternal diastolic pressure and a decrease of uterine artery blood flow. These changes persisted for longer periods (30 minutes or more) after the infusion had been completed and were accompanied by fetal hypoxia and acidosis. The effect of orciprenaline on the fetal acid-base status was more pronounced in the previously acidotic fetus.

After the intravenous infusion of fenoterol (0.1 to 0.4 μg/kg/min) and ritodrine (2.5 to 6 μg/kg/min) to the ewe, the author and his colleagues have observed effects similar to those of orciprenaline on uterine contractions, maternal and fetal cardiovascular function and acid-base status.[151-154] When these drugs were given to the ewe in small doses they caused a prompt inhibition of uterine contractions, maternal tachycardia (about 30 per cent above control), a slight decrease in diastolic pressure (less than 10 per cent from control), slight variations in uterine artery flow and fetal tachycardia, with no significant changes in the maternal and fetal acid-base status. However, the inhibitory effect on uterine contractions was more prompt and long-lasting, whereas the maternal and fetal cardiovascular effects were less pronounced than those of orciprenaline. Nevertheless, when fenoterol and ritodrine were administered to the ewe in high doses, they produced marked maternal and fetal cardiovascular changes with deterioration of fetal oxygenation and acid-base status, especially when the fetal condition was already compromised. Under the same experimental conditions isoxsuprine was not as effective in inhibiting uterine contractions. The high doses (38

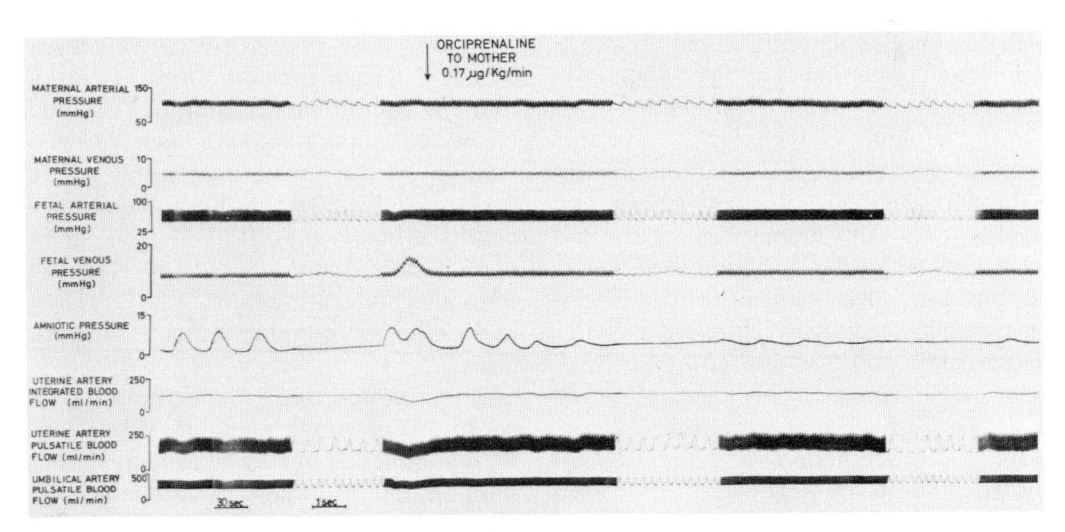

Figure 11.3. A section of continuous recording representing the typical response of the ewe and fetus to orciprenaline during induced labor. (Reprinted by permission from Cosmi EV, Condorelli S: Valutazione degli effetti esercitati da alcuni farmaci beta-stimolanti sulla madre e sul feto. Acta Anaesth (Ital) 24:17, 1973.)

μg/kg/min) required to suppress uterine contractions caused fetal asphyxia secondary to reductions in uterine artery blood flow and maternal blood pressure.[151-153] Thus, despite inhibition of uterine activity, asphyxia developed in fetuses whose mothers received large doses of β-stimulants or when their condition was already compromised or both.

These dose-dependent effects on uterine blood flow have also been observed by Siimes and Creasy,[156] Ehrenkranz et al.[157-159] and Brennan et al.[160] after the intravenous infusion of ritodrine and isoxsuprine to the pregnant sheep, and by Caritis et al.[161] after the intravenous infusion of terbutaline to the pregnant baboon. However, in these studies fetal asphyxia did not develop despite large doses of β-stimulant. Ehrenkranz et al.[157-159] have also observed that fenoterol, ritodrine and salbutamol have a greater inhibitory effect on uterine activity and less cardiovascular side effects on the ewe and fetus than does isoxsuprine. Furthermore, Brennan et al.[160] found that fenoterol produces maternal cardiovascular changes of lesser magnitude than do ritodrine and salbutamol.

All β-stimulants produced maternal acidemia and maternal and fetal hyperglycemia which were dose-related.[157-161] These metabolic changes are compatible with the knowledge that β-stimulants initiate glycogenolysis, gluconeogenesis and lipolysis[162-166] and increase glucagon and insulin blood levels.[167-169] Increased maternal and fetal blood concentrations of glucose, lactate, pyruvate, free fatty acids, acetoacetate and β-hydroxybutyrate with relative acidemia, have been observed after the infusion of ritodrine,[150] fenoterol[170] and salbutamol[166,171] to pregnant women. These findings dictate increased concern regarding the use of β-stimulants, particularly in diabetic women, because they may cause maternal and fetal acidosis.

The fetal cardiovascular and metabolic changes observed both in animals[151-154, 157-161] and humans[92, 95, 96, 100, 106-116, 138-141, 150, 172-175] suggest that β-stimulants cross the placenta. The placental transfer of catecholamines has been documented both in animals[153, 154, 176-179] and humans.[180-182]

The maternal and fetal cardiovascular and metabolic changes may persist for variable periods after the administration of β-stimulants, depending on the agent, the dose and the duration of treatment. The reported elimination half-life of β-stimulants varies from up to 3 minutes for epinephrine and isoproterenol to 5 to 12 hours for ritodrine, terbutaline and salbutamol.[183-187]

The relaxing effect on smooth muscles and the metabolic effects of β-stimulants have been attributed to the activation of adenyl cyclase, an enzyme located within the plasma membrane of the target cell which catalyzes the conversion of adenosine triphosphate to cyclic adenosine monophosphate, thereby increasing its intracellular concentration[188-194] (Figure 11.1). Another theory put forward to explain smooth muscle relaxation is the hyperpolarization of the muscle cell membrane.[195] It has recently been suggested that the continued exposure of the target tissue to β-stimulants may cause desensitization of the membrane-bound adenyl cyclase and, therefore, limit their therapeutic effectiveness.[194, 196-198] This could explain some of the failure to stop preterm uterine contractions after repeated and prolonged administration of β-stimulants.

Attempts have been made to prevent the cardiovascular and metabolic side effects of β-stimulants by the simultaneous administration of β-blockers with contradictory results. Eskes et al.[199] found that pronethanol and propranolol prevent the cardiovascular side effects of β-stimulants without interfering with their utero-inhibitory effect. On the other hand, Barden and Stander[107] found that propranolol reverses the cardio-acceleratory effect of isoxsuprine, but that it may also reverse its uterine inhibitory effects. McDevitt et al.[200] made a similar observation with the simultaneous use of salbutamol and practolol. In the pregnant sheep it was found that propranolol reverses both the uterine and the cardiovascular effects of ritodrine and prevents maternal and fetal hyperglycemia.[156, 157] Practolol partially reversed the cardiovascular response without affecting uterine inhibition.[156] It has also been found that propranolol crosses the ovine placenta in moderate amounts[201, 202] and that it may produce fetal acidosis.[203] Its duration of action in the fetus was three times longer than in the ewe.[202] Metoprolol was also found to cross the ovine placenta.[204] These effects on the animal fetus have been confirmed in the human fetus where it was found that the administration of propranolol for the treatment of maternal hypertension and tachycardia causes fetal hypoxia, delayed onset of breathing at birth and neonatal hypoglycemia secondary to its placental transfer.[205-208] The plasma drug level in the infant 4 hours after birth was twice that found at birth.[208] Other studies have reported hypoglycemia associated with propranolol administration in children.[209] These results indicate that the combined administration of β-stimulants and β-blockers should be used cautiously and only when indicated.

In summary, effectiveness with which β-stimulants inhibit uterine contractility is related to the agent and the dose used. Although small doses of β-stimulants have no untoward effects on the mother and fetus, high doses may be detrimental to the fetus, especially when its condition is already compromised. Well controlled studies are needed to determine the long-term effects on newborn infants, especially when they are exposed to prolonged and repeated administrations of β-stimulants during gestation.

Relative contraindications to the use of β-stimulants include placenta praevia, premature detachment of a normally inserted placenta, diabetes mellitus, hyperthyroidism, heart disease and consumption of monoamine oxidase inhibitors.[109, 210]

DIAZOXIDE

Diazoxide (Hyperstat), a benzothiadiazine structurally related to thiazide diuretics but devoid of chloriuretic and natriuretic activity, is a potent smooth muscle relaxant.[211] Studies *in vitro*[212, 213] and *in vivo*[214-217] indicate that diazoxide effectively suppresses uterine activity and that, if hypotension does not occur, the drug does not exert untoward effects on the fetus and newborn infant.[214, 215] It has also been used for the treatment of maternal hypertension without apparent adverse effects on the mother, fetus or neonate, providing severe hypotension does not occur.[218, 219]

In subhuman primates it was found that diazoxide suppresses uterine activity more effectively than orciprenaline and ritodrine.[217, 220] However, in both the pregnant baboon[216, 220] and sheep[221, 222] it was also found that, even in recommended doses (i.e. 5 mg/kg), diazoxide causes maternal tachycardia and hypotension and maternal and fetal hyperglycemia without significant changes in the utero-placental blood flow and fetal cardiovascular function and acid-base status. These effects were related to dose and method of administration. They were more pronounced when diazoxide was administered in high doses (up to 15 mg/kg) as a bolus intravenous injection than when it was administered as a slow intravenous infusion in doses of 0.06 to 0.08 mg/kg/min over a 4-hour period.[220, 222]

Diazoxide has been found to cross the placenta in both the sheep[221] and the monkey.[216] The concentration in the fetus increased after the completion of the infusion to the mother. Likewise maternal and fetal hyperglycemia attained higher concentrations after the infusion was discontinued, thereby indicating that the drug has a long half-life. The reported physiologic half-life of diazoxide varies from 3 to 12 hours, and the biologic half-life varies from 22 to 32 hours.[211, 223] The hyperglycemic effect frequently reported has been attributed to decreased insulin secretion,[211, 224-229] enhanced epinephrine release,[211, 224, 226, 230] inhibition of glucose uptake by tissues[230] and increased hepatic glucose production.[211, 230]

Because 90 per cent of the drug in the serum is bound to albumin[211] it is possible that high levels of diazoxide in the fetus may compete with bilirubin for binding to albumin, thereby causing hyperbilirubinemia and predisposing the pre-term newborn infant to kernicterus.

After several weeks of oral administration of diazoxide to pregnant women there have been reports of neonatal alopecia, hypertrichosis lanuginosa and decreased bone age.[231]

METHYLXANTHINES

Methylated xanthines, especially theophylline, have been used as central nervous system stimulants for the treatment of congestive heart failure, smooth muscle relaxants for the treatment of bronchial asthma[232-240] and, recently, for the prevention of apnea of prematurity. Theophylline produces a synergistic relaxing effect when used with β-stimulants which has been attributed to its blocking action on cyclic nucleotide phosphodiesterase (Figure 11.1), the enzyme responsible for the catabolism of cyclic adenosine monophosphate.[237, 241-245, 248-252] It has also been found that aminophylline inhibits the activity of the non-pregnant human uterus[246] and oviduct.[247]

Preliminary clinical trials in the author's delivery suite indicate that aminophylline effectively relaxes the human myometrium (Figure 11.4). The effective dose range of aminophylline varied from patient to patient. Uterine inhibition was achieved at the rate of 1.78 mg/min in a few patients, whereas in the majority a dose rate as high as 12.9 mg/min was required. When aminophylline was given as a loading dose followed by intravenous infusion, the inhibitory effect was more prompt and pronounced. Both maternal and fetal heart rate were not significantly affected by the administration of small doses of aminophylline. However, fetal beat-to-beat variability tended to increase. In more than 70 per cent of patients delivery was postponed for more than 72 hours. In the remainder, progressive cervical changes and rupture of membranes occurred despite the inhibition of uterine contractions. Nausea, vomiting, palpitation, tachycardia, tremor and headache occasionally occurred with high doses of aminophylline, which necessitated reducing the dosage (Table 11.1).

Patients unsuccessfully treated with isoxsuprine subsequently responded to aminophylline therapy. In the experimental animal (Figure 11.5) and in some patients, the author has found that the uteroinhibitory effect of aminophylline was enhanced by the previous or subsequent infusion of ritodrine.

However, it should be stressed that patients with either ruptured membranes or well established labor did not respond to this treatment, despite intermittent infusions of isoxsuprine or ritodrine and aminophylline.

All infants were in good clinical condition at birth and free of apnea during the neonatal period.

The combined use of β-stimulants and aminophylline in the author's experience did not result in a higher incidence of side effects in the mother. Owing to wide in-

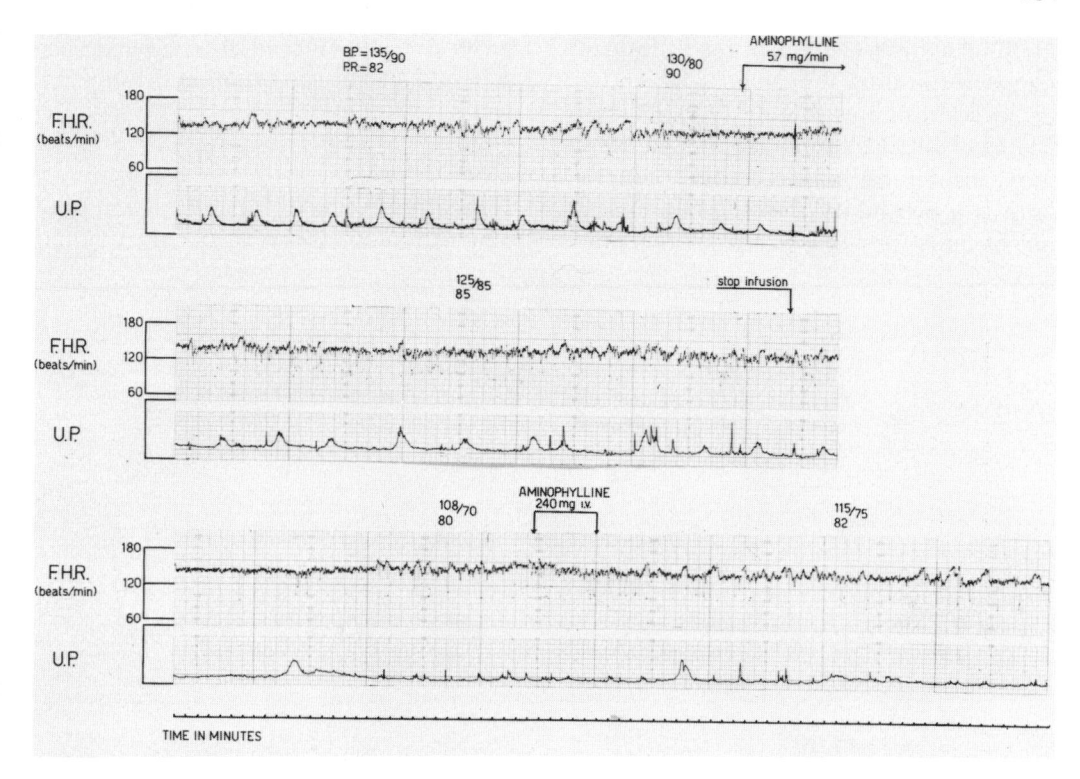

Figure 11.4. Effects of aminophylline on uterine contractility and fetal heart rate. Continuous recordings of uterine contractions (*U.P.*) by external tocometry and fetal heart rate (*F.H.R.*) by ultrasonic flow detector in a primigravida at 31 weeks' gestation. Above the tracing are given the values of maternal blood pressure (*B.P.*), measured indirectly by an external sphygmomanometer, and maternal pulse frequency (*P.R.*).

dividual variations in the rate of metabolism[233, 234] and the narrow margin between therapeutic and toxic blood levels,[234, 235] aminophylline treatment should preferably be instituted on the basis of blood level determinations in order to achieve optimal therapeutic effectiveness and minimize side effects. It is generally accepted that the therapeutic serum concentrations are between 10 and 20 µg/ml, and the concentrations greater than 20 µg/ml are associated with the frequent incidence of side effects.[233, 234, 253–255]

Further studies are needed to define the immediate effects of aminophylline on the mother and fetus and the long-term effects on the newborn infant. Known metabolic effects of xanthines include increased plasma levels of free fatty acids[256–258] and glucose[258, 259] and stimulation of glucagon and insulin release.[260] These effects could have serious implications, especially if one considers that the elimination half-life of aminophylline is on the order of 4[261] to 11 hours[253] in the adult and 14 to 57 hours in the premature newborn infant.[262, 263]

The author believes that aminophylline may also prove to be useful for the prevention of apnea of prematurity. The administration of methylxanthines to premature newborn infants has been found to effectively reduce apneic attacks,[264–269] although the mechanism of this effect has not been established. An increased sensitivity of the medullary respiratory center to CO_2 has been suggested.[264–267, 270] In the sheep fetus the author has found that the intravenous or intracarotid administration of aminophylline in doses of 10 to 20 mg/kg induces regular respiratory movements which last for several minutes (Figure 11.6). This indicates a direct stimulation on the respiratory center by aminophylline. Finally, there is a possibility that the administration of aminophylline to the mother may accelerate fetal lung maturity, as indicatated by recent preliminary studies in pregnant rabbits.[271, 272]

ETHANOL

The use of ethanol for the treatment of premature labor was advocated by Fuchs

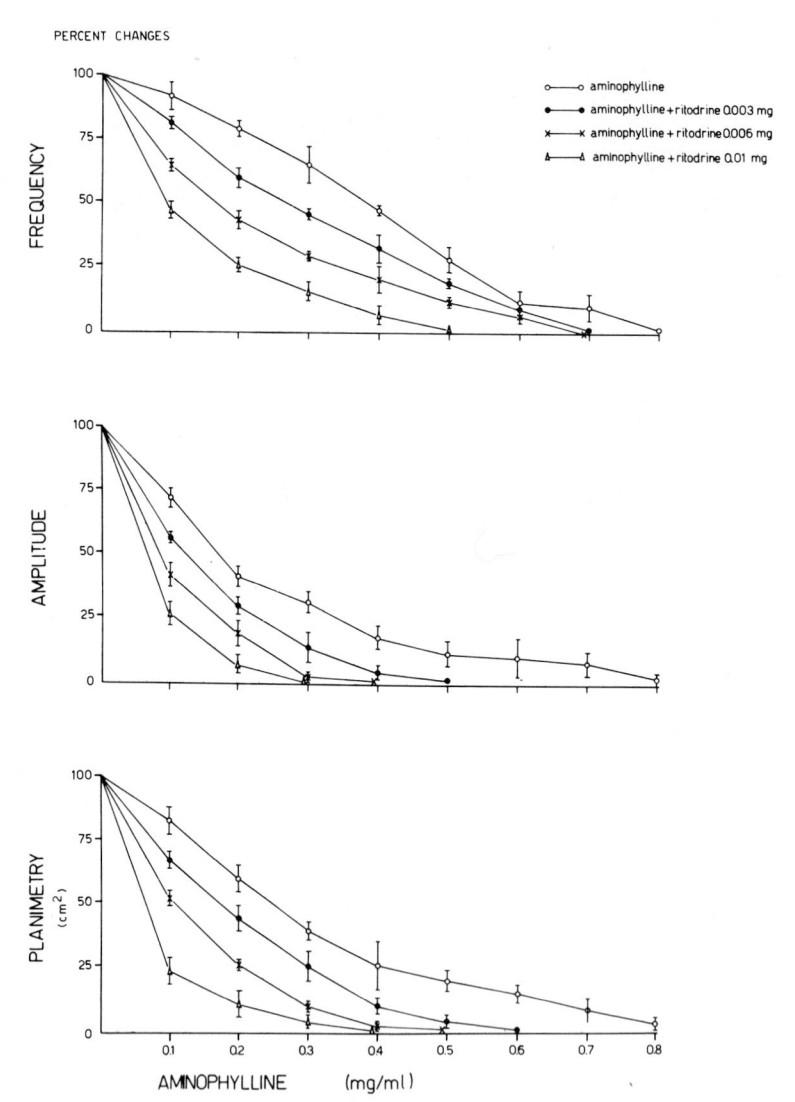

Figure 11.5. Dose response curves of the isometric myograms of uterine muscles of non-pregnant rats in relation to aminophylline and to aminophylline + ritodrine added to the bathing media in increasing concentrations. Mean values ± S.E. of the means for frequency, amplitude and contractility (the area between the resting and developed tensions per unit time calculated by compensating polar planimetry over an interval of at least 30 minutes).

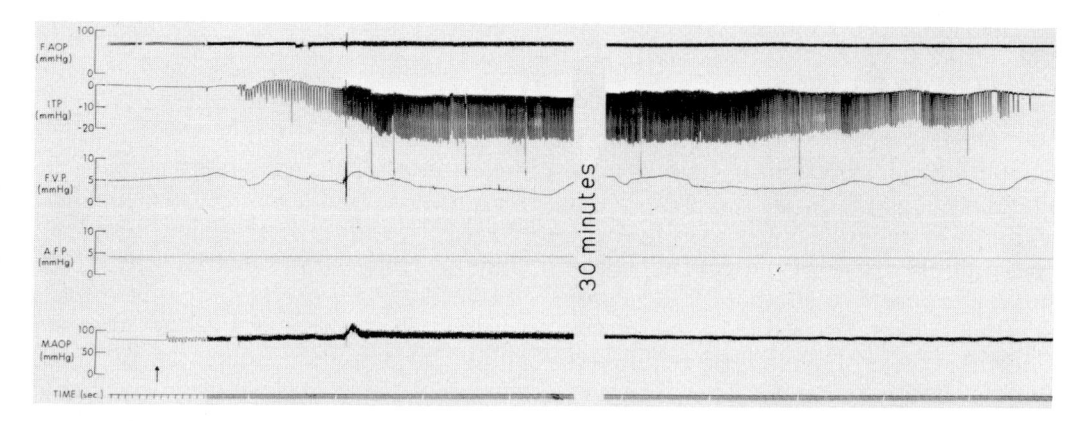

Figure 11.6. Effect of intracarotid injection of 10 mg/kg of aminophylline (marked with the *arrow* at the bottom of the tracing) on aortic pressure (*F.AOP*), intratracheal pressure (*ITP*) and venous pressure (*F.V.P.*) of the fetal lamb in utero, on amniotic fluid pressure (*A.F.P.*) and on maternal aortic pressure (*M.AOP*).

in 1965.[273] Studies **in vivo** and **in vitro** have shown that alcohol inhibits uterine contractions.[3, 274, 275] Various mechanisms have been suggested to explain its inhibitory effect, such as: (1) inhibition of release of vasopressin and oxytocin from the neurohypophysis[3, 274]; (2) epinephrine release through sympathetic activation[276]; (3) inhibition of prostaglandin synthesis or release[276, 277]; (4) direct effect on myometrial cells[276]; (5) a non-competitive antagonism of oxytocin on the uterus[278] (Figure 11.1).

However, contradictory results have been reported after its use. Some authors report that ethanol effectively suppresses uterine activity without interfering with fetal homeostasis,[279–280] whereas others[127, 281] have found that ethanol does not prevent pre-term delivery and may cause neonatal depression. A recent study indicates that ethanol is less effective than β-stimulants in delaying pre-term delivery.[117]

Animal experiments have not helped clarify this controversy. In pregnant sheep Dilts[282] did not encounter adverse effects on the mother and fetus, whereas in pregnant monkeys Horiguchi et al.[283] found that ethanol is not a very effective inhibitor of uterine contractions, even when administered in high doses, and that it may cause maternal respiratory depression and maternal and fetal hypotension and acidosis (Table 11.1). Fetal hypotension and acidosis have been reported also by Mann et al.[284] in the pregnant sheep; moreover, they found that ethanol readily crosses the placenta, attaining high concentrations in the fetus which remain in the blood stream for several hours during the post-infusion period. The rapid placental transfer of ethanol has been well documented in both monkeys[283, 285] and humans.[286–288]

These latter findings are of special concern because of the reduced rate of ethanol clearance in the newborn infant, especially in pre-term infants, compared to adults.[288–290] In fact, newborn infants delivered during or after unsuccessful ethanol treatment may have high blood concentrations of ethanol, which could cause central nervous system depression with subsequent respiratory and circulatory changes, gastric irritation with vomiting, temperature instability, hypoglycemia[288] and alteration of bone marrow structure.[291] Because ethanol-induced hypoglycemia is probably due to inhibition of hepatic gluconeogenesis[292, 293] and is related inversely to the hepatic stores of glycogen,[292] harmful effects can be expected in the pre-term infant whose glycogen stores may be scanty. A withdrawal syndrome, "fetal alcohol syndrome," which is similar to narcotic withdrawal syndrome, has also been reported in the neonate following acute and chronic exposure to ethanol.[294-296] Side effects may also be expected in the mother when high doses of ethanol are required to suppress uterine activity. These may include alteration of respiration, increased gastric secretion with nausea and vomiting and hypotension.[284, 297] Possible interactions of ethanol with pharmacologic agents should also be considered. Additive hypotensive and central nervous system depressant effects can be produced by the concurrent administration of hypnotics, phenothiazines, antihistamines, reserpine, methyldopa, hydralazine or diuretics.[298]

Thus, the beneficial and the untoward effects of ethanol on the mother, fetus and newborn infant should be weighed carefully before considering its use for the management of pre-term labor.

PROSTAGLANDIN INHIBITORS

The several observations that prostaglandins may play an important role in the onset of labor prompted the suggestion that non-steroidal anti-inflammatory drugs and other inhibitors of prostaglandin synthesis could be useful for the management of pre-term labor.[299, 300] Two established inhibitors, indomethacin and aspirin, have been reported to abolish uterine contractions **in vitro**,[301, 302] prevent induced abortion,[303, 304] delay the onset of term labor[305] and delay the onset of labor and suppress premature uterine contractions both in animals[306-309] and humans.[310-312] Indomethacin was found to suppress uterine activity even in the presence of ruptured membranes where treatment with β-stimulants was unsuccessful.[311-314] Non-steroidal anti-inflammatory drugs have also been used as a complementary therapy to β-stimulants.[310, 311] Their mechanism of action seems to be mediated both by inhibition of prostaglandin synthesis and cyclic adenosine monophosphate phosphodiesterase[302, 315] and by increased efflux of calcium ion from the myometrial cells[302] (Figure 11.1).

Although some investigators have reported no untoward effects on the newborn infant after the use of prostaglandin inhibitors for the management of pre-term labor,[310, 311, 313, 314] there is considerable evidence that serious side effects may occur in the fetus and newborn. These drugs traverse the placenta and produce profound circulatory effects in the fetus, including constriction of the ductus arteriosus, an increase in pulmonary vascular smooth muscle development associated with an increase in pulmonary arterial pressure and the syndrome of persistent pulmonary hypertension of the newborn.[316] They may also result in gastrointestinal irritation, maternal and neonatal hemorrhage as a result of inhibition of platelet aggregation and reduced Factor XII activity[317] and retarded intrauterine fetal growth.[318-321]

The premature closure of the ductus has been documented in the animal fetus after the administration of indomethacin to the mother.[318, 321, 322] The sensitivity of the ductus to indomethacin increased as pregnancy approached term.[321] After delivery newborn rats developed cyanosis and dyspnea with respiratory acidosis.[318] In the human fetus, the premature closure of the ductus in utero has been observed in association with salicylate ingestion during pregnancy.[323, 324] In addition, closure of the ductus has been produced in pre-term infants with oral and rectal doses of indomethacin and aspirin.[325, 326] The premature closure of the ductus in utero would be hazardous to the fetus because it produces cardiovascular changes which are comparable to those occurring during severe hypoxia and acidosis.[322]

It has been suggested that when indomethacin and sodium salicylate are administered before 33 weeks of gestation there is less likelihood of inducing closure of the ductus.[312,321] In rhesus monkeys it was found that fenoprofen produces fewer maternal and fetal side effects, while suppressing uterine activity as effectively as indomethacin.[309] Paracetamol (acetaminophen, an antipyretic analgesic) and mefenamic acid also seem to produce fewer side effects than indomethacin and aspirin.[327,328] It is noteworthy that psychotropic drugs, including monoamine oxidase inhibitors and tricyclic antidepressants,[300,329,330] seem to inhibit prostaglandin synthesis; therefore, their concomitant use with indomethacin or aspirin could precipitate the side effects of the latter in the fetus.

Summary

In conclusion, various drugs are presently available or are under experimental trial which may be useful for the prevention of pre-term labor and delivery. Their successful use depends on the proper selection of patients and timely institution of treatment.

PART 2: ANESTHETIC CONSIDERATIONS

Anesthetic Management for Pre-term Labor: General Considerations

The pre-term infant, in contrast to the fully mature one, has special requirements and risks. His soft, poorly calcified cranial bones and fragile dura mater make him more susceptible to intracranial hemorrhage during spontaneous vaginal delivery. Consequently, a slow, well controlled delivery, with minimal maternal pushing, a generous episiotomy and outlet forceps are usually used to protect the small premature head. Thus, adequate anesthesia is mandatory. In a Canadian study of 10 university teaching hospitals[331] the perinatal death rate for premature infants was 440 per 1000 when no anesthesia was administered as compared to 140 per 1000 when conduction anesthesia was administered. These differences probably reflect a large number of precipitous or poorly controlled deliveries with subsequent injury of the fetal head.

In selecting an analgesic technique it must be remembered that the pre-term fetus and newborn is particularly susceptible to the depressant effects of transplacentally acquired systemic medications and local and general anesthetic agents as a result of: (1) less protein available for drug binding[332] (2) increased levels of bilirubin[333,334] which may compete with the drug for protein binding; (3) increased likelihood that the drug may attain high concentrations in the central nervous system because of poorly developed blood-brain barrier[335]; (4) higher incidence of asphyxia during labor and delivery[332,336]; and (5) decreased ability to metabolize and excrete drugs.

However, the capability of the fetus to metabolize drugs is greater than originally thought. In contrast to fetuses of other species, liver microsomes of human fetuses have significant amounts of cytochrome P-450, detectable as early as the fourteenth week of gestation[337-339] and catalyze the oxidation of various drugs.[340,341] For example, the human fetus, even pre-term, has the capability of metabolizing both ester- and amide-type local anesthetics.[342-346] In fact, recent findings in sheep indicate that pre-term fetuses are more **resistant** to toxic reactions than term fetuses. Teramo et al.[347,348] administered lidocaine to pre-term sheep fetuses either by continuous intravenous infusion or by bolus injection and found that as long as fetal arterial concentration of lidocaine remained below 7 µg/ml there were no fetal cardiovascular changes. On the other hand, concentrations of lidocaine of 11.6 µg/ml produced transient episodes of hypertension associated initially with tachycardia. Immediately before the onset of hypertension and tachycardia, epileptiform high-voltage activity was recorded in the electroencephalogram (Figure 11.7). Only with the bolus injection of 30 to 50 mg of lidocaine did they observe an initial fetal bradycardia and hypotension[347] (Figure 11.8). The amounts of lidocaine necessary to produce convulsive episodes were dependent on fetal gestational age, i.e. younger fetuses required far more lidocaine than older fetuses[348] (Figure 11.9). Gestational age also influenced the fetal cardiovascular response, i.e. increases in blood pressure and heart rate in response to lidocaine were greater with advancing gestational age. Teramo et al. have suggested that the greater toxicity of local anesthetics in the older fetuses could be related to an increased propensity of the drug to enter the neural tissues or to the increased number and sensitivity of individual neurons. Thus, toxic reactions in the fetus are not only related to blood levels of local anesthetics but also to gestational age.

However, as mentioned previously, preterm fetuses may still be at great risk of developing toxic reactions to local anesthetics and increased depression after maternally administered narcotic, sedative and general anesthetic drugs because of low protein-binding capacities,[342, 349–355]

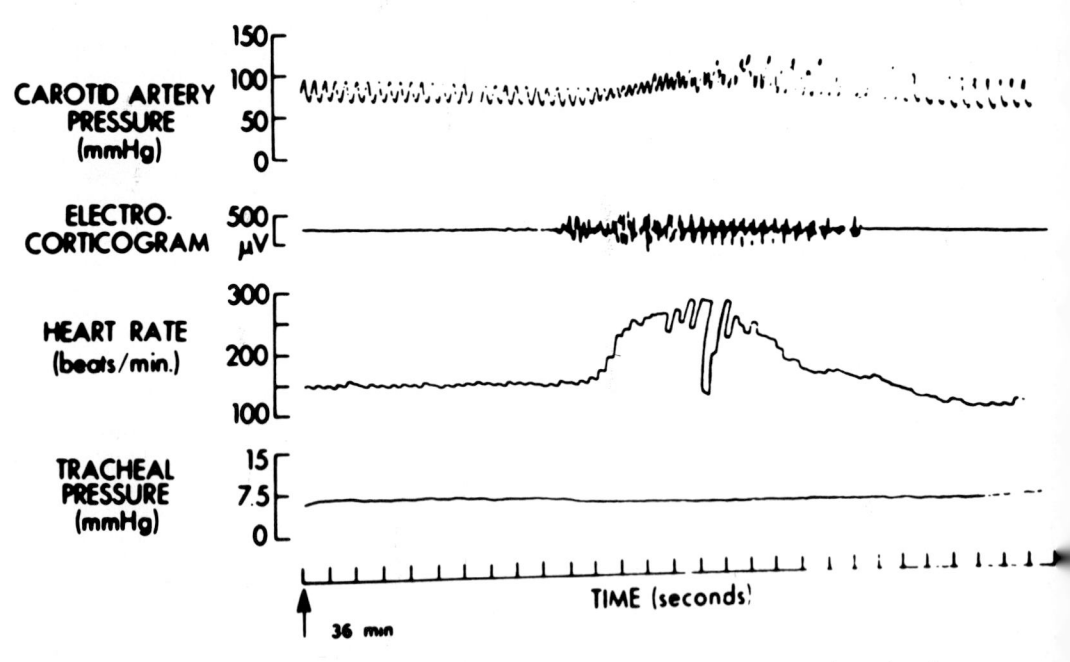

Figure 11.7. Fetal arterial pressure, electrocorticogram, heart rate and tracheal pressure during one epileptiform burst following fetal infusion of 1.98 mg/min^{-1}/kg^{-1} of lidocaine. The epileptiform activity precedes increases in blood pressure and heart rate by approximately 2 seconds. The fetus had been paralyzed with succinylcholine. *Thirty-six minutes* indicates the time from the beginning of the infusion. (Reprinted by permission from Teramo K, Benowitz N, Heymann MA, et al.: Effects of lidocaine on heart rate, blood pressure, and electrocorticogram in fetal sheep. Am J Obstet Gynecol 118:935, 1974.)

PRE-TERM LABOR

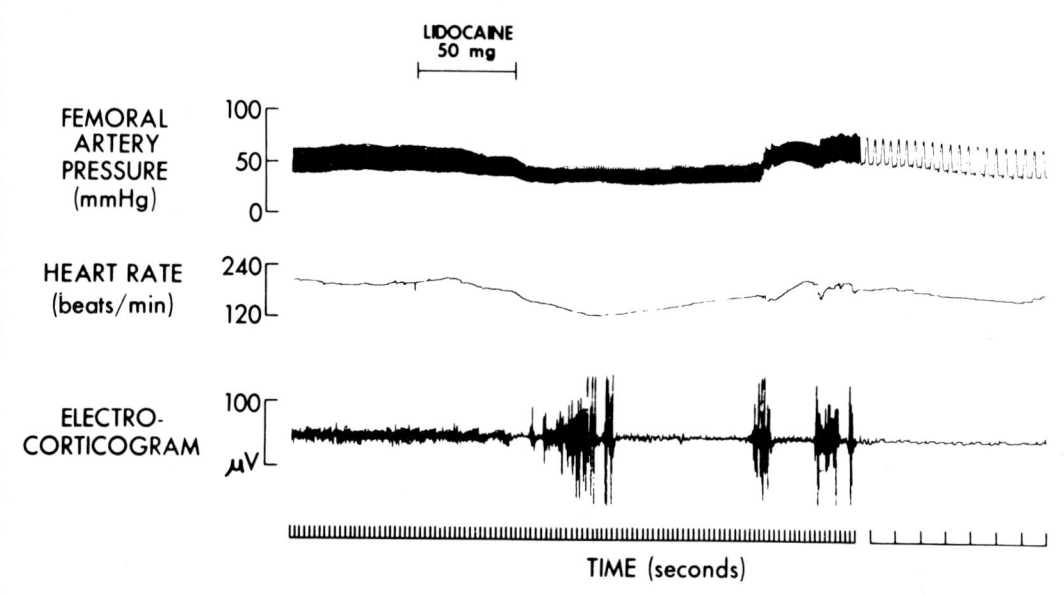

Figure 11.8. Effect of 50 mg (22.2 mg/kg) of lidocaine injected as a bolus into the femoral vein of the fetal lamb in utero. (Reprinted by permission from Teramo K, Benowitz N, Heymann MA, et al.: Effects of lidocaine on heart rate, blood pressure, and electrocorticogram in fetal sheep. Am J Obstet Gynecol 118:935, 1974.)

poorly developed blood-brain barrier[335] and a higher incidence of asphyxia during labor and delivery.[332, 336] In fact, asphyxia (1) reduces the protein-binding capacity[352, 356, 357]; (2) increases ionization and, therefore, "trapping"[353, 354, 357-360]; (3) enhances the myocardial depressant effects of local anesthetics[361-364]; and (4) increases the blood-brain barrier permeability.[365, 366]

Often utero-inhibitory agents have been given to the mother immediately prior to the administration of anesthesia. Patients treated or under treatment with utero-inhibitory drugs may pose special problems for both the mother and the fetus, because of possible interactions with anesthetic agents. For example, ethanol produces central nervous system depression and also increased gastric acid secretion. β-mimetics produce generalized vasodilation, hypotension and increased cardiac irritability. Many of the effects of these drugs may be present even after discontinuation of therapy.

All of these considerations—that is, the special need of the pre-term infant for anesthesia combined with the increased risks to the mother and neonate of many anesthetic drugs and techniques—must be carefully weighed in the choice of anesthetic technique.

Prior to administration of any anesthetic or analgesic the residual side effects of any drugs used to stop labor should be assessed. Table 11.1 outlines possible side effects of special interest to the anesthesiologist. Hypotension and tachycardia are usually transient following discontinuation of intravenous β-mimetics. The effects of ethanol may last many hours. Ideally, anesthesia is deferred until all potential serious side effects disappear. If, however, emergency delivery is necessary, fluids and small doses of intravenous ephedrine may be administered prior to anesthesia to correct hypotension. Oral antacids should be used to neutralize gastric acidity associated with ethanol.

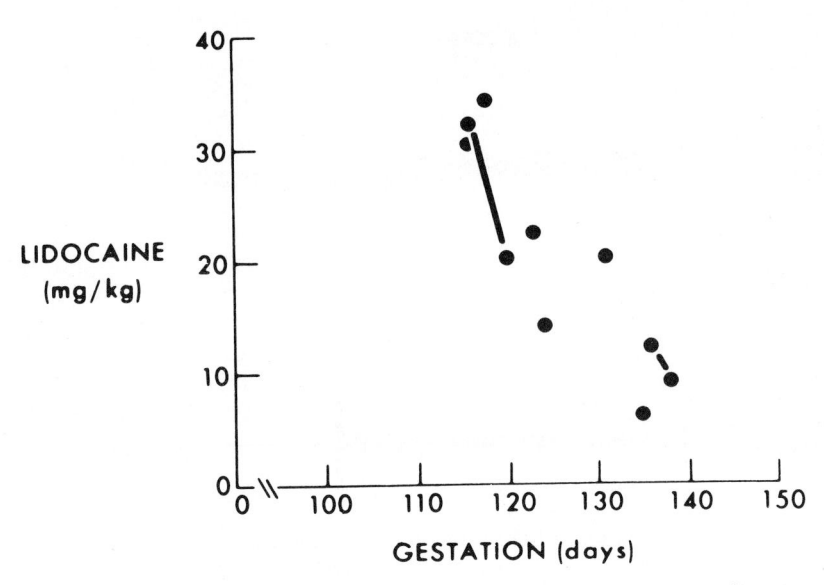

Figure 11.9. Correlation between the convulsive dose of lidocaine (mg/fetal weight) and gestational age in the lamb fetus. *Points* connected with a *line* represent data from the same fetus. (Reprinted by permission from Teramo K, Benowitz N, Heymann MA, et al.: Gestational differences in lidocaine toxicity in the fetal lamb. Anesthesiology 44:133, 1976.)

During labor, systemic medication should either be avoided or given in the smallest dose possible. During the latent phase emotional support and reassurance are usually sufficient. If analgesia is necessary during the active phase, continuous lumbar epidural is the anesthetic of choice. Minimal doses of local anesthetic can be used to provide segmental analgesia during the first stage and then extended to provide perineal relaxation for forceps delivery during the second stage. Chloroprocaine is rapidly metabolized and bupivacaine is highly protein-bound, so fetal toxicity is minimal with either agent. If delivery is imminent, a saddle block most rapidly provides maximum perineal relaxation and analgesia. Pudendal nerve block combined with nitrous analgesia may also be satisfactory.

For cesarean section either lumbar epidural or spinal anesthesia is preferred so as to avoid the potential neonatal central nervous system depression associated with general anesthesia.

After delivery the pre-term neonate often requires extensive resuscitation as outlined in chapter 26. These infants have a high incidence of birth asphyxia, respiratory distress, hypovolemia, hypoglycemia, anemia and temperature instability.

References

1. Caldeyro-Barcia R, Sica-Blanco Y, Poseiro JJ, et al.: A quantitative study of the action of synthetic oxytocin on the pregnant human uterus. J Pharmacol Exp Ther 121:18, 1957.
2. Caldeyro-Barcia R, Fuchs A-R, Csapo A, et al.: Effects of oxytocin on uterine contractility. In *Initiation of Labor*, JM Marshall and WM Burnett, eds, Publication No 1390. United States Public Health Service, Bethesda, 1963, p 29.
3. Fuchs A-R, Wagner G: The effect of ethyl alcohol on the release of oxytocin in rabbits. Acta Endocrinol 44:593, 1963.
4. Turnbull AC, Anderson ABM: Induction of labor. Part II. Intravenous oxytocin infusion. J Obstet Gynaecol Br Commonw 74:24, 1968.
5. Turnbull AC, Anderson ABM: Induction of labor. Part III. Results with amniotomy and oxy-

tocin "titration." J Obstet Gynaecol Br Commonw 75:32, 1968.
6. Chard T, Boyd NRH, Forsling ML, et al.: The development of a radioimmunoassay for oxytocin: The extraction of oxytocin from plasma, and its measurement during parturition in human and goat blood. J Endocrinol 48:223, 1970.
7. Chard T, Hudson CN, Edwards CRW, et al.: Release of oxytocin and vasopressin by the human foetus during labour. Nature (Lond) 234:352, 1971.
8. Rudzik AD, Miller JW: The effect of altering the catecholamine content of the uterus on the rate of contractions and the sensitivity of the myometrium to relaxin. J Pharmacol 138:88, 1962.
9. Zuspan FP, Cibils LA, Pose SV: Myometrial and cardiovascular responses to alterations in plasma epinephrine and norepinephrine. Am J Obstet Gynecol 84:841, 1962.
10. Cibils LA, Zuspan FP: Pharmacology of the uterus. Clin Obstet Gynecol 11:34, 1968.
11. Nakanishi H, McLean J, Wood C, et al.: The role of sympathetic nerves in control of the nonpregnant and pregnant human uterus. J Reprod Med 2:20, 1969.
12. Walker M, Lawrence CB: Changes in catecholamines and prostaglandins at parturition in sheep. J Endocrinol 71:50P, 1976.
13. Jung H: Hormonal control of the conduction of impulse in the myometrium. J Obstet Gynaecol Br Commonw 69:1040, 1962.
14. Marshall JM: Regulation of activity in uterine smooth muscle. Physiol Rev (Suppl 5) 42:213, 1962.
15. Masson GM, Klopper A: Changes in plasma oestriol concentration associated with the onset of labour. J Obstet Gynaecol Br Commonw 79:970, 1972.
16. Liggins GC, Fairclough RJ, Grieves SA, et al.: The mechanism of initiation of parturition in the ewe. Recent Progr Horm Res 29:111, 1973.
17. Tamby Raja RL, Anderson ABM, Turnbull AC: Endocrine changes in premature labour. Br Med J 2:67, 1974.
18. Csapo AI, Pohanka O, Kaihola HL: Progesterone deficiency and premature labour. Br Med J 1:137, 1974.
19. Luukkainen T, Csapo AI: Effect of progesterone on pregnancy. Nature 192:329, 1961.
20. Karim SMM: Appearance of prostaglandin $F_{2\alpha}$ in human blood during labour. Br Med J 4:618, 1968.
21. Liggins GC, Grieves SA: Possible role for prostaglandin $F_{2\alpha}$ in parturition in sheep. Nature (Lond) 232:629, 1971.
22. Williams KI: Prostaglandin synthesis by the pregnant rat uterus at term and its possible relevance in parturition. Br J Pharmacol 47:628P, 1973.
23. Currie WB, Thornburn GD: Induction of premature parturition in goats by prostaglandin $F_{2\alpha}$ administered into the uterine vein. Prostaglandins 4:201, 1973.
24. Gustavii B: Release of lysosomal acid phosphatase into the cytoplasm of decidual cells before the onset of labour in humans. Br J Obstet Gynaecol 82:177, 1975.
25. Schultz FM, Schwarz BE, MacDonald PC, et al.: Initiation of human parturition. II. Identification of phospholipase A_2 in fetal chorioamnion and uterine decidua. Am J Obstet Gynecol 123:650, 1975.
26. Haning RV, Barrett DA, Alberino SP, et al.: Interrelationships between maternal and cord prolactin, progesterone, estradiol, 13,14-dihydro-15-keto-prostaglandin F and cord cortisol at delivery with respect to initiation of parturition. Am J Obstet Gynecol 130:204, 1978.
27. Liggins GC, Kennedy PC, Holm LW: Failure of initiation of parturition after electrocoagulation of the pituitary of the fetal lamb. Am J Obstet Gynecol 98:1080, 1967.
28. Drost M, Holm LW: Prolonged gestation in ewes after foetal adrenalectomy. J Endocrinol 40:293, 1968.
29. Liggins GC: Premature parturition after infusion of corticotrophin or cortisol into foetal lambs. J Endocrinol 42:323, 1968.
30. Liggins GC: The foetal role in the initiation of parturition in the ewe. In *Foetal Autonomy*, Ciba Foundation Symposium. J & A Churchill, London, 1969, p 218.
31. Honnebier WJ, Swaab DF: The influence of anencephaly upon intrauterine growth of fetus and placenta and upon gestation length. J Obstet Gynaecol Br Commonw 80:577, 1973.
32. Murphy BEP: Does the human fetal adrenal play a role in parturition? Am J Obstet Gynecol 115:521, 1973.
33. Cawson MJ, Anderson ABM, Turnbull AC, et al.: Cortisol, cortisone and 11-deoxycortisol levels in human umbilical and maternal plasma in relation to the onset of labour. J Obstet Gynaecol Br Commonw 81:737, 1974.
34. Rees LH, Jack PMB, Thomas AL, et al.: Role of foetal adrenocorticotrophin during parturition in sheep. Nature 253:274, 1975.
35. Nwosu U, Wallach EE, Boggs TR, et al.: Possible role of the fetal adrenal glands in the etiology of postmaturity. Am J Obstet Gynecol 121:366, 1975.
36. Challis JRG, Kendall JZ, Robinson JS, et al.: The regulation of corticosteroids during late pregnancy and their role in parturition. Biol Reprod 16:57, 1977.
37. Fenton AN, Singh BP: Pregnancy associated with congenital abnormalities of the female reproductive tract. Am J Obstet Gynecol 63:744, 1952.
38. Savarese MFR, Chang IW: Incompetent cervical os: A collective review of the literature with a report of thirty new cases. Obstet Gynecol Surv 19:201, 1964.
39. Forssman L: Post-traumatic intrauterine synechiae and pregnancy. Obstet Gynecol 26:710, 1965.
40. Bender S: Twin pregnancy: A review of 472 cases. J Obstet Gynaecol Br Emp 59:510, 1952.

41. McKeown T, Record RG: Observations on foetal growth in multiple pregnancy in man. J Endocrinol 8:386, 1952.
42. Klinger A: Demographic consequences of the legalization of induced abortion in Eastern Europe. Int J Gynaecol Obstet 8:680, 1970.
43. Czeizer A, Bognar Z: Mortality and morbidity of legal abortions. Lancet 2:209, 1971 (Letter).
44. Papaevangelou G, Vrettos AS, Papadatos C, et al.: The effect of spontaneous and induced abortion on prematurity and birthweight. J Obstet Gynaecol Br Commonw 80:418, 1973.
45. Richardson JA, Dixon G: Effects of legal termination on subsequent pregnancy. Br Med J 1:1303, 1976.
46. Ratten GJ, Beischer NA, Fortune DW: Obstetric complications when the fetus has Potter's syndrome. Am J Obstet Gynecol 115:890, 1973.
47. Turner RC, Oakley NW, Beard RW: Human fetal plasma growth hormone prior to the onset of labour: Effects of stress, glucose, arginine and maternal diabetes. Biol Neonate 22:169, 1976.
48. Turnbull AC, Anderson ABM: Preterm labor. In Reviews in Perinatal Medicine, EM Scarpelli and EV Cosmi, eds, vol II. Raven Press, New York, 1978, p 103.
49. Gillibrand PN: Premature rupture of the membranes and prematurity. J Obstet Gynaecol Br Commonw 74:678, 1967.
50. Brody S, Frenkel DA: Marginal insertion of the cord and premature labor. Am J Obstet Gynecol 65:1305, 1953.
51. Baird D: Infection of the urinary tract during pregnancy. Part IV. J Obstet Gynaecol Br Emp 42:774, 1935.
52. Fedrick J: Antenatal identification of women at high risk of spontaneous pre-term birth. Br J Obstet Gynaecol 83:351, 1976.
53. Illsley R, Thompson B: Social characteristics identifying women at risk for premature delivery. In Prevention of Handicap through Antenatal Care, AC Turnbull and FP Woodford, eds. Associated Scientific Publishers, Amsterdam, 1976, p 149.
54. Anderson ABM, Laurence KM, Davies K, et al.: Fetal adrenal weight and the causes of premature delivery in human pregnancy. J Obstet Gynaecol Br Commonw 78:481, 1971.
55. World Health Organization: Public Health Aspects of Low Birthweight, Technical Report Series 271. World Health Organization, Geneva, 1961.
56. Lubchenco LO: Assessment of gestational age and development at birth. Pediatr Clin North Am 17:129, 1970.
57. Lugo G, Cassady G: Intrauterine growth retardation. Am J Obstet Gynecol 109:620, 1971.
58. Weingold AB: Intrauterine growth retardation: Obstetric aspects. J Reprod Med 14:244, 1975.
59. Cook LN: Intrauterine and extrauterine recognition and management of deviant fetal growth. Pediatr Clin North Am 24:431, 1977.
60. Paul RH: Management of the threatened premature delivery. In Perinatal Intensive Care, S Aladjem and AK Brown, eds. C. V. Mosby, St Louis, 1977, p 208.
61. Campbell S, Dewhurst CJ: Diagnosis of the small-for-dates fetus by serial ultrasonic cephalometry. Lancet 2:1002, 1971.
62. Hamilton LA Jr, Szujewski PF, Patel MK: Combined sonographic and biochemical estimation of fetal maturity in high-risk pregnancy. Obstet Gynecol 41:837, 1973.
63. Bartolucci L: Biparietal diameter of the skull and fetal weight in the second trimester: An allometric relationship. Am J Obstet Gynecol 122:439, 1975.
64. Poll V: Precision of ultrasonic fetal cephalometry. Brit J Obstet Gynaecol 83:217, 1976.
65. Drumm JE: The prediction of delivery date by ultrasonic measurement of fetal crown-rump length. Br J Obstet Gynaecol 84:1, 1977.
66. Campbell S, Wilkin D: Ultrasonic measurement of fetal abdominal circumference in estimation of fetal weight. Br J Obstet Gynaecol 82:689, 1975.
67. Kurjac A, Breyer B: Estimation of fetal weight by ultrasonic abdominometry. Am J Obstet Gynecol 125:962, 1976.
68. Gluck L, Kulovich MV, Borer RC Jr, et al.: Diagnosis of the respiratory distress syndrome by amniocentesis. Am J Obstet Gynecol 109:440, 1971.
69. Condorelli S, Cosmi EV, Scarpelli EM: Determinazione del grado di maturità polmonare del feto in utero mediante il dosaggio dei fosfolipidi del liquido amniotico. La Clin Ostet Ginecol (Ital) 73:228, 1971.
70. Bhagwanani SG, Fahmy D, Turnbull AC: Prediction of neonatal respiratory distress by estimation of amniotic fluid lecithin. Lancet 1:159, 1972.
71. Clements JA, Platzker ACG, Tierney DF, et al.: Assessment of the risk of the respiratory distress syndrome by a rapid test for surfactant in amniotic fluid. N Engl J Med 286:1077, 1972.
72. Wagstaff TI, Bromham DR: A comparison between the lecithin/sphingomyelin ratio and the "shake test" for the estimation of surfactant in amniotic fluid. J Obstet Gynaecol Br Commonw 80:412, 1973.
73. Aubry RH, Rourke JE, Almanza R, et al.: The lecithin/sphingomyelin ratio in a high-risk obstetric population. Obstet Gynecol 47:21, 1976.
74. Morrison JC, Whybrew WD, Bucovaz ET, et al.: The lecithin/sphingomyelin ratio in cases associated with fetomaternal disease. Am J Obstet Gynecol 127:363, 1977.
75. Dahlenburg GW, Martin FIR, Jeffrey PE, et al.: Amniotic fluid lecithin/sphingomyelin ratio in pregnancy complicated by diabetes. Br J Obstet Gynaecol 84:294, 1977.
76. Gabbe SG, Lowensohn RI, Mestman JH, et al.: Lecithin/sphingomyelin ratio in pregnancies complicated by diabetes mellitus. Am J Obstet Gynecol 128:757, 1977.

77. Magendantz HG, Klausner D, Ryan KJ, et al.: Estriol determinations in the management of high-risk pregnancies. Obstet Gynecol 32:610, 1968.
78. Masson GM: Plasma oestriol in retarded intrauterine fetal growth. J Obstet Gynaecol Br Commonw 80:423, 1973.
79. Duenhoelter JH, Whalley PJ, MacDonald PC: An analysis of the utility of plasma immunoreactive estrogen measurements in determining delivery time of gravidas with a fetus considered at high risk. Am J Obstet Gynecol 125:889, 1976.
80. Biezenski JJ, Millner SN: Correlation between morning urine estriol concentration and 24-hour estriol excretion. Obstet Gynecol 48:678, 1976.
81. Sakakini J Jr, Buster JE, Killam AP: Serum unconjugated estriol levels in the third trimester and their relationship to gestational age. II. Am J Obstet Gynecol 127:452, 1977.
82. Soler NG, Nicholson HO, Malins JM: Serial determinations of human placental lactogen in the last half of normal and complicated pregnancies. Am J Obstet Gynecol 120:214, 1974.
83. Kelly AM, England P, Lorimer JD, et al.: An evaluation of human placental lactogen levels in hypertension of pregnancy. Br J Obstet Gynaecol 82:272, 1975.
84. Stroobants WLA, Van Zanten AK, De Bruijn HWA, et al.: Serial human placental lactogen estimations in serum and placental weight-for-dates. Br J Obstet Gynaecol 82:899, 1975.
85. Spellacy WN, Cruz AC, Gelman SR, et al.: Fetal movements and placental lactogen levels for fetal-placental evaluation: A preliminary report. Obstet Gynecol 49:113, 1977.
86. Curzen P, Varma R: A comparison of serum cystine aminopeptidase and urinary estrogen excretion as placental function tests. Am J Obstet Gynecol 115:929, 1973.
87. Hensleigh PA, Cheatum SG, Spellacy WN: Oxytocinase and human placental lactogen for prediction of intrauterine growth retardation. Am J Obstet Gynecol 129:675, 1977.
88. Crane JP, Kopta MM, Welt SI, et al.: Abnormal fetal growth patterns: Ultrasonic diagnosis and management. Obstet Gynecol 50:205, 1977.
89. Bygdeman M, Eliasson R: The effect of isoxsuprine on the motility pattern of the isolated human myometrium. Experientia 19:650, 1963.
90. Landesman R, Wilson K: The relaxant effect of adrenergic compounds on isolated gravid human myometrium. Am J Obstet Gynecol 100:969, 1968.
91. Sullivan SF, Marshall JM: Quantitative evaluation of effects of exogenous amines on contractility of human myometrium in vitro. Am J Obstet Gynecol 107:139, 1970.
92. Hendricks CH, Cibils LA, Pose SV, et al.: The pharmacology control of excessive uterine activity with isoxsuprine. Am J Obstet Gynecol 82:1064, 1961.
93. Wansbrough H, Nakanishi H, Wood C: The effect of adrenergic receptor blocking drugs on the human uterus. J Obstet Gynaecol Br Commonw 75:189, 1968.
94. Krapohl AJ, Anderson JM, Evans TN: Isoxsuprine suppression of uterine activity. Obstet Gynecol 32:178, 1968.
95. Gamissans O, Esteban-Altirriba J, Maiques V: Inhibition of human myometrial activity by a new β-adrenergic drug (DU-21220). J Obstet Gynaecol Br Commonw 76:656, 1969.
96. Baumgarten K, Frölich H, Seidl A, et al.: A new β-sympathomimetic preparation for intravenous and oral inhibition of uterine contractions. Eur J Obstet Gynecol 2:69, 1971.
97. Landesman R, Wilson KH, Coutinho EM, et al.: The relaxant action of ritodrine, a sympathomimetic amine, on the uterus during term labor. Am J Obstet Gynecol 110:111, 1971.
98. Csapo AI, Herczeg J, Pitkanen Y, et al.: The effects of isoxsuprine on uterine contractility. Obstet Gynecol 46:58, 1975.
99. Bishop EH, Woutersz TB: Isoxsuprine, a myometrial relaxant. Obstet Gynecol 17:442, 1961.
100. Shenker L: Effect of isoxsuprine on fetal heart rate and fetal electrocardiogram. Obstet Gynecol 26:104, 1965.
101. Eskes TKAB, Seelen JC, Van Gent I: The effect of betamimetic adrenergic drugs on the activity of pregnant human uterus tested with the intrauterine pressure method. Arzneim Forsch 16:762, 1966.
102. Baillie P, Meehan FP, Tyack AJ: Treatment of premature labour with orciprenaline. Br Med J 4:154, 1970.
103. Stolte L, Eskes TKAB, Seelen JC, et al.: Epinephrine derivates and the activity of the human uterus. I. The inhibiting effects of p-hydroxyphenylisopropylarterenol(CC-25) upon uterine activity in human pregnancy. Am J Obstet Gynecol 92:865, 1965.
104. Gummerus M: Prevention of premature birth with Nylidrin and Verapamil. Z Geburtshilfe Perinatol, 179:261, 1975.
105. Landesman R, Wilson K, Zlatnik FJ: The myometrial relaxant properties of isoxsuprine and 2 methanesulfonamido derivatives. Obstet Gynecol 28:775, 1966.
106. Barden TP, Stander RW: Myometrial and cardiovascular effects of two methanesulfonamidophenethanolamines. Am J Obstet Gynecol 96:1069, 1966.
107. Barden TP, Stander RW: Myometrial and cardiovascular effects of an adrenergic blocking drug in human pregnancy. Am J Obstet Gynecol 101:91, 1968.
108. Unbehaun V: Effects of sympathomimetic tocolytic agents on the fetus. J Perinat Med 2:17, 1974.
109. Durán-Sánchez P, Esteban-Altirriba J: Betamimetic drugs in obstetrics. In *Reviews in Perinatal Medicine*, EM Scarpelli and EV Cosmi, eds, vol I. University Park Press, Baltimore, 1976, p 295.
110. Elliott HR, Abdulla U, Hayes PJ: Pulmonary oedema associated with ritodrine infusion and

betamethasone administration in premature labour. Br Med J 2:799, 1978.
111. Weidinger H, Wiest W: The treatment of late abortion and of threatened premature birth with Th 1165a combined with Isoptin. Z Geburtshilfe Perinatol 177:233, 1973.
112. Künzel W, Reinecke J: Der Einfluss von Th1165a auf die Gaspartialdrucke und auf kardiovaskulare Parameter von Mutter und Fetus. Zugleich eine quantitative Analyse der Wehentätigkeit. Z Geburtshilfe Perinatol 177:81, 1974.
113. Mosler KH, Linka F, Dornhöfer W, et al.: Tocolytic therapy in obstetrics. J Perinat Med 2:3, 1974.
114. Lipshitz J, Baillie P: The effects of the fenoterol hydrobromide (Partusisten) aerosol on uterine activity and the cardiovascular system. Br J Obstet Gynaecol 83:864, 1976.
115. Wesselius De Casparis A, Thiery M, Yo Le Sian A, et al.: Results of a double-blind, multicentre study with ritodrine in premature labour. Br Med J 3:144, 1971.
116. Renaud R, Irrmann M, Gandar R, et al.: The use of ritodrine in the treatment of premature labour. J Obstet Gynaecol Br Commonw 81:182, 1974.
117. Lauersen NH, Merkatz IR, Tejani N, et al.: Inhibition of premature labor: A multicenter comparison of ritodrine and ethanol. Am J Obstet Gynecol 127:837, 1977.
118. Andersson K-E, Gengtsson LPh, Ingemarsson I: Terbutaline inhibition of midtrimester uterine activity induced by prostaglandin $F_{2\alpha}$ and hypertonic saline. Br J Obstet Gynaecol 82:745, 1975.
119. Ingemarsson I: Effect of terbutaline on premature labor: A double-blind placebo-controlled study. Am J Obstet Gynecol 125:520, 1976.
120. Åkerlund M, Andersson K-E: Vasopressin response and terbutaline inhibition of the uterus. Obstet Gynecol 48:528, 1976.
121. Liggins GC, Vaughan GS: Intravenous infusion of salbutamol in the management of premature labor. J Obstet Gynaecol Br Commonw 80:29, 1973.
122. Korda AR, Lyneham RC, Jones WR: The treatment of premature labour with intravenously administered salbutamol. Med J Aust 1:744, 1974.
123. Lunell NO, Joelsson I, Björkam U, et al.: The use of salbutamol in obstetrics. Acta Obstet Gynecol Scand 55:333, 1976.
124. Lipshitz J, Baillie P, Davey DA: A comparison of the uterine $beta_2$-adrenoreceptor selectivity of fenoterol, hexoprenaline, ritodrine and salbutamol. S Afr Med J 50:1969, 1976.
125. Lipshitz J, Baillie P: Uterine and cardiovascular effects of $beta_2$-selective sympathomimetic drugs administered as an intravenous infusion. S Afr Med J 50:1973, 1976.
126. Richter R: Evaluation of success in treatment of threatening premature labor by betamimetic drugs. Am J Obstet Gynecol 127:482, 1977.
127. Castrén O, Gummerus M, Saarikoski S: Treatment of imminent premature labour: A comparison between the effects of nylidrin chloride and isoxsuprine chloride as well as of ethanol. Acta Obstet Gynecol Scand 54:95, 1975.
128. Liggins GC, Howie RN: A controlled trial of antepartum glucocorticoid treatment for prevention of the respiratory distress syndrome in premature infants. Pediatrics 50:515, 1972.
129. Caspi E, Schreyer P, Weinraub Z, et al.: Prevention of the respiratory distress syndrome in premature infants by antepartum glucocorticoid therapy. Br J Obstet Gynaecol 83:187, 1976.
130. Dluholuchý S, Babic J, Taufer I: Reduction of incidence and mortality of respiratory distress syndrome by administration of hydrocortisone to mother. Arch Dis Child 51:420, 1976.
131. Castrén O, Gummerus M, Saarikoski S, et al.: Zur Wirkung der Beta-sympathikomimetika während der Geburt auf die Adaptation des Neugeborenen. Geburtshilfe Frauenheilkd 32:943, 1972.
132. Kero P, Hirvonen T, Välimäki I: Prenatal and postnatal isoxsuprine and respiratory distress syndrome. Lancet 2:198, 1973.
133. Boog G, Ben Brahim M, Gandar R: Beta-mimetic drugs and possible prevention of respiratory distress syndrome. Br J Obstet Gynaecol 82:285, 1975.
134. Cabero L, Quílez M, Escribano I, et al.: Sindrome de distress respiratorio en casos de amenaza de parto prematuro tratados con betamimeticos. Clin Invest Ginecol Obstet (Spain) 3:169, 1976.
135. Van Iddekinge B, Hughes EA: The effect of intrauterine fetal transfusion and a β-sympathomimetic substance on the lecithin/sphingomyelin ratio in human amniotic fluid. Br J Obstet Gynaecol 84:669, 1977.
136. Wyszogrodski I, Taeusch HW, Avery ME: Isoxsuprine-induced alterations of pulmonary pressure-volume relationships in premature rabbits. Am J Obstet Gynecol 119:1107, 1974.
137. Enhorning G, Chamberlain D, Contreras C, et al.: Isoxsuprine-induced release of pulmonary surfactant in the rabbit fetus. Am J Obstet Gynecol 129:197, 1977.
138. Caldeyro-Barcia R, Magaña JM, Castillo JB, et al.: A new approach to the treatment of acute intrapartum fetal distress. In *Perinatal Factors Affecting Human Development*, Scientific Publication 185. Pan American Health Organization, Washington DC, 1969, p 248.
139. Cosmi EV, Gozzi G, Lauri A, et al.: L'impiego di metaproterenolo nel trattamento della sofferenza fetale. Acta Anaesth (Ital) (Suppl 2) 19:33, 1970.
140. Cosmi EV: Nuovo trattamento della sofferenza fetale e neonatale. Acta Anaesth (Ital) (Suppl) 21:33, 1970.
141. Zilianti M, Aller J: Action of orciprenaline on uterine contractility during labor, maternal cardiovascular system, fetal heart rate, and acid-base balance. Am J Obstet Gynecol 109:1073, 1971.
142. Moneta E, Romanini C, Oliva C, et al.: Experience with a new beta-mimetic drug in obstetrics:

Ritodrine. In *Treatment of Foetal Risks*, Proceedings of the International Symposium, K Baumgarten and A Wesselius De Casparis, eds. University of Vienna, 1973, p 32.
143. Renaud R, Brettes P, Irrmann M, et al.: A double-blind cross-over trial to assess the effect of ritodrine on uterine blood flow in normal and pathological pregnancies (a preliminary report). In *Treatment of Foetal Risks*, Proceedings of the International Symposium, K Baumgarten and A Wesselius De Casparis, eds. University of Vienna, 1973, p 53.
144. Humphrey M, Chang A, Gilbert M, et al.: The effect of intravenous ritodrine on the acid-base status of the fetus during the second stage of labour. Br J Obstet Gynaecol 82:234, 1975.
145. Klöck FK, Chantraine H: Möglichkeiten und Grenzen der intrauterine Reanimation. Z Geburtshilfe Perinatol 179:401, 1975.
146. Fischer WM: Uterusmotilitätsstörungen, akuter "fetal distress" und die Anwendung von Betamimetika während der Geburt. In *Th 1165a (Partusisten) bei der Behandlung in der Geburtshilfe und Perinatologie*, Symposium at Reisenburg, 1973, H Jung and FK Klöch, eds. Georg Thieme Verlag, Stuttgart, 1975, p 74.
147. Lippert TH, De Grandi PB, Fridrich R: Actions of the uterine relaxant, fenoterol, on uteroplacental hemodynamics in human subjects. Am J Obstet Gynecol 125:1093, 1976.
148. Brettes JP, Renaud R, Gandar R: A double-blind investigation into the effects of ritodrine on uterine blood flow during the third trimester of pregnancy. Am J Obstet Gynecol 124:164, 1976.
149. Lipshitz J: Use of a β_2-sympathomimetic drug as a temporizing measure in the treatment of acute fetal distress. Am J Obstet Gynecol 129:31, 1977.
150. Miller FC, Nochimson DJ, Paul RH, et al.: Effects of ritodrine hydrochloride on uterine activity and the cardiovascular system in toxemic patients. Obstet Gynecol 47:50, 1976.
151. Cosmi EV, Condorelli S: Effects of beta-stimulant agents on the cardiovascular system and acid-base status of the mother and foetus. In *Treatment of Foetal Risks*, Proceedings of the International Symposium, K Baumgarten and A Wesselius De Casparis, eds. University of Vienna, 1973, p 67.
152. Cosmi EV, Condorelli S: Valutazione degli effetti esercitati da alcuni farmaci beta-stimolanti sulla madre e sul feto. Acta Anaesth (Ital) 24:17, 1973.
153. Cosmi EV: Drugs, anesthetics, and the fetus. In *Reviews in Perinatal Medicine*, EM Scarpelli and EV Cosmi, eds, vol I. University Park Press, Baltimore, 1976, p 191.
154. Cosmi EV: Effects of beta-stimulants on maternal and fetal cardiovascular function and acid-base status, and on fetal breathing. In *Recent Advances on Beta-mimetic Drugs in Obstetrics*, A Bompiani, EV Cosmi, B Fischetti, F Gasparri, and C Romanini, eds. Società Editrice Universo Publ, Rome, 1977, p 17.
155. Wallenburg HCS, Mazer J, Hutchinson DL: Effects of a beta-adrenergic agent (metaproterenol) on uteroplacental circulation: An angiographic study in the pregnant rhesus monkey. Am J Obstet Gynecol 117:1067, 1973.
156. Siimes ASI, Creasy RK: Effect of ritodrine on uterine activity, heart rate, and blood pressure in the pregnant sheep: Combined use of alpha or beta blockade. Am J Obstet Gynecol 126:1003, 1976.
157. Ehrenkranz RA, Walker AM, Oakes GK, et al.: Effect of ritodrine infusion on uterine and umbilical blood flow in pregnant sheep. Am J Obstet Gynecol 126:343, 1976.
158. Ehrenkranz RA, Walker AM, Oakes GK, et al.: Effect of fenoterol (Th1165a) infusion on uterine and umbilical blood flow in pregnant sheep. Am J Obstet Gynecol 128:177, 1977.
159. Ehrenkranz RA, Hamilton LA Jr, Brennan SC, et al.: Effects of salbutamol and isoxsuprine on uterine and umbilical blood flow in pregnant sheep. Am J Obstet Gynecol 128:287, 1977.
160. Brennan SC, McLaughlin MK, Chez RA: Effects of prolonged infusion of β-adrenergic agonists on uterine and umbilical blood flow in pregnant sheep. Am J Obstet Gynecol 128:709, 1977.
161. Caritis SN, Morishima HO, Stark RI, et al.: Effects of terbutaline on the pregnant baboon and fetus. Obstet Gynecol 50:56, 1977.
162. Arnold A, McAuliff JP, Colella DF, et al.: The β-2 receptor mediated glycogenolytic responses to catecholamines in the dog. Arch Int Pharmacodyn 176:451, 1968.
163. Innes IR, Nicherson M: Norepinephrine, epinephrine, and the sympathomimetic amines. In *The Pharmacological Basis of Therapeutics*, ed 5. LS Goodman and A Gilman, eds, Macmillan, New York, 1975, chap 24.
164. Goldenberg R, Joffe BI, Bersohn I, et al.: Metabolic responses to selective β-adrenergic stimulation in man. Postgrad Med J 51:53, 1975.
165. Kusaka M, Ui M: Activation of the Cori cycle by epinephrine. Am J Physiol 232 (2):E145, 1977.
166. Lunell NO, Joelsson I, Larsson A, et al.: The immediate effect of a β-adrenergic agonist (salbutamol) on carbohydrate and lipid metabolism during the third trimester of pregnancy. Acta Obstet Gynecol Scand, 56:475, 1977.
167. Gerich JE, Langois M, Noacco C, et al.: Adrenergic modulation of pancreatic glucagon secretion in man. J Clin Invest 53:1441, 1974.
168. Massara F, Fassio V, Camanni F, et al.: Salbutamol-induced increase in plasma insulin in man. Hormone Metab Res, 7:94, 1975.
169. Kaneto A, Miki E, Kosaka K: Effect of beta$_1$ and beta$_2$ adrenoreceptor stimulants infused intrapancreatically on glucagon and insulin secretion. Endocrinology 97:1166, 1975.
170. Unbehaun V, Conradt A, Schlotter CM, et al.: Changes in metabolism during infusion of Th1165a. Z Geburtshilfe Perinatol 178:118, 1974.
171. Chapman MG: Salbutamol-induced acidosis in pregnant diabetics. Br Med J 1:639, 1977.
172. Barden TP: Effect of ritodrine on human uterine motility and cardiovascular responses in term

labor and the early postpartum state. Am J Obstet Gynecol 112:645, 1972.
173. Nochimson DJ, Riffel HD, Yeh S-Y, et al.: The effects of ritodrine hydrochloride on uterine activity and the cardiovascular system. Am J Obstet Gynecol 118:523, 1974.
174. Bieniarz J, Ivankovich A, Scommegna A: Cardiac output during ritodrine treatment in premature labor. Am J Obstet Gynecol 118:910, 1974.
175. Dawson AM, Davies HJ: The effect of intravenous and oral salbutamol on fetus and mother in premature labour. Br J Obstet Gynaecol 84:348, 1977.
176. Condorelli S, Cosmi EV: Passaggio placentare di alcune amine adrenergiche: Studio sugli ovini. Acta Anaesth (Ital) 21:539, 1970.
177. Cosmi EV, Mazzoni P, Marzetti L, et al.: Efectos de la orciprenalina y norepinefrina sobre el sistema cardiovascular y el equilibrio acido-basico del feto de oveja. In *El Feto de Riesgo Elevado*, International Symposium, J Gonzales-Merlo, and J Esteban-Altirriba, eds. Editorial Eco, Barcelona, 1970, p 305.
178. Morgan CD, Sandler M, Panigel M: Placental transfer of catecholamines in vitro and in vivo. Am J Obstet Gynecol 112:1068, 1972.
179. Parvez S, Parvez H: Placental transfer of ^{3}H-epinephrine and its metabolites to the fetal heart during variable hormonal treatments. Hormone Res 5:321, 1974.
180. Sandler M: Transmission of ^{14}C-noradrenaline across the human placenta. J Clin Pathol 16:389, 1963.
181. Sandler M, Ruthven CRJ, Wood C: Metabolism of ^{14}C-norepinephrine and ^{14}C-epinephrine and their transmission across the human placenta. Int J Neuropharmacol 3:123, 1964.
182. Zuspan FP, Whaley WH, Nelson GH, et al.: Placental transfer of epinephrine. I. Maternal-fetal metabolic alterations of glucose and nonesterfied fatty acids. Am J Obstet Gynecol 95:284, 1966.
183. Post LC: Pharmacokinetics of beta-adrenergic agonists in preterm labor. In *Proceedings of the Fifth Study Group of the Royal College of Obstetricians and Gynaecologists*, 1977.
184. Conolly ME, Davies DS, Dollery CT, et al.: Metabolism of isoprenaline in dog and man. Br J Pharmacol 46:458, 1972.
185. Kadar D, Tang HY, Conn AW: Isoproterenol metabolism in children after intravenous administration. Clin Pharmacol Ther 16:789, 1974.
186. Eskes TKAB: The influence of β-mimetic catecholamines upon uterine activity in human pregnancy and labor. In *Uterine Contraction—Side Effects of Steroidal Contraceptives*, JB Josimovich, ed. John Wiley & Sons, New York, 1973, p 283.
187. Brittain RT: Pharmacology of recent beta-adrenoreceptor stimulants. Proc R Soc Med 65:759, 1972.
188. Sutherland EW, Rall TW: The relations of adenosine-3',5'-phosphate and phosphorylase to the actions of catecholamines and other hormones. Pharmacol Rev 12:265, 1960.
189. Robinson GA, Butcher RW, Sutherland EW: Cyclic AMP. Ann Rev Biochem 37:149, 1968.
190. Marshall JM, Kroeger EA: Adrenergic influences on uterine smooth muscle. Trans R Soc Lond (Ser B) 265:135, 1973.
191. Sullivan A, Zaimis E: The effect of isoprenaline on cyclic AMP concentrations in skeletal muscle. J Physiol 231:102P, 1973.
192. Steer ML, Atlas D, Levitzki A: Inter-relations between β-adrenergic receptors, adenylate cyclase and calcium. N Engl J Med 292:409, 1975.
193. Lefkowitz RJ: Heterogeneity of adenylate cyclase-coupled β-adrenergic receptors. Biochem Pharmacol 24:583, 1975.
194. Lefkowitz RJ: β-adrenergic receptors: Recognition and regulation. N Engl J Med 295:323, 1976.
195. Kroeger EA, Marshall JM: Beta-adrenergic effects on rat myometrium: Mechanisms of membrane hyperpolarization. Am J Physiol 225:1339, 1973.
196. Mukherjee C, Caron MG, Lefkowitz RJ: Catecholamine-induced subsensitivity of adenylate cyclase associated with loss of β-adrenergic receptors. Proc Nat Acad Sci USA 72:1945, 1975.
197. Mickey J, Tate R, Lefkowitz RJ: Subsensitivity of adenylate cyclase and decreased β-adrenergic receptor binding after chronic exposure to (−)-isoproterenol in vitro. J Biol Chem 250:5727, 1975.
198. Kebabian JW, Zatz M, Romero JA, et al.: Rapid changes in rat pineal β-adrenergic receptor: Alterations in [3H] alprenolol binding and adenylate cyclase. Proc Nat Acad Sci USA 72:3735, 1975.
199. Eskes TKAB, Stolte L, Seelen J, et al.: Epinephrine derivates and the activity of the human uterus. II. The influence of pronethanol and propranolol on the uterine and systemic activity of p-hydroxy-phenylisopropyl arterenol (Cc-25). Am J Obstet Gynecol 92:871, 1965.
200. McDevitt DG, Wallace RJ, Roberts A, et al.: The uterine and cardiovascular effects of salbutamol and practolol during labour. Br J Obstet Gynaecol 82:442, 1975.
201. Joelsson I, Barton MD, Daniel S, et al.: The response of the unanesthetized sheep fetus to sympathomimetic amines and adrenergic blocking agents. Am J Obstet Gynecol 114:43, 1972.
202. Van Petten GR, Willes RF: β-adrenoreceptive responses in the unanesthetized ovine foetus. Br J Pharmacol 38:572, 1970.
203. Joelsson I, Barton MD: The effect of blockade of the beta receptors of the sympathetic nervous system of the fetus. Acta Obstet Gynecol Scand, 48:75, 1969.
;204. Van Petten GR: Cardiovascular effects of metoprolol in the pregnant ewe and fetus. Proc West Pharmacol Soc 19:470, 1976.
205. Tunstall ME: The effect of propranolol on the onset of breathing. Br J Anaesth 41:792, 1969.
206. Reed RL, Cheney CB, Fearon RE, et al.: Propran-

olol therapy throughout pregnancy: A case report. Anesth Analg 53:214, 1974.
207. Gladstone GR, Hordorf A, Gersony WM: Propranolol administration during pregnancy: Effects on the fetus. J Pediatr 86:962, 1975.
208. Cottrill CM, McAllister RG Jr, Gettes L, et al.: Propranolol therapy during pregnancy, labor, and delivery: Evidence for transplacental drug transfer and impaired neonatal drug disposition. J Pediatr 91:812, 1977.
209. McBride JT, McBride MC, Viles PH: Hypoglycemia associated with propranolol. Pediatrics 51:1085, 1973.
210. Leading article: Delaying premature labour. Lancet 2:875, 1974.
211. Koch-Weser J: Diazoxide. N Engl J Med 294:1271, 1976.
212. Daniel EE, Nash CW: The effects of diuretic and non-diuretic benzothiadiazine and of structurally related diuretic drugs on active ion transport and contractility in smooth muscles. Arch Int Pharmacodyn 158:139, 1965.
213. Landesman R, Wilson KH: The relaxant effect of diazoxide on isolated gravid and nongravid human myometrium. Am J Obstet Gynecol 101:120, 1968.
214. Landesman R, Adeodato de Souza J, Coutinho EM, et al.: The inhibitory effect of diazoxide in normal term labor. Am J Obstet Gynecol 103:430, 1969.
215. Barden TP, Keenan WJ: Effects of diazoxide in human labor and the fetus-neonate. Obstet Gynecol 37:631, 1971.
216. Morishima HO, Cohen H, Brown WU, et al.: The inhibitory action of diazoxide on uterine activity in the subhuman primate: Placental transfer and effect on the fetus. J Perinat Med 1:13, 1973.
217. Wilson KH, Lauersen NH, Raghvan KS, et al.: Effects of diazoxide and beta adrenergic drugs on spontaneous and induced uterine activity in the pregnant baboon. Am J Obstet Gynecol 118:499, 1974.
218. Finnerty FA Jr: Treatment of acute hypertension in pregnancy. Obstet Gynecol Dig, 12:30, 1970.
219. Morris JA, Arce JJ, Hamilton CJ, et al.: The management of severe preeclampsia and eclampsia with intravenous diazoxide. Obstet Gynecol 49:675, 1977.
220. Morishima HO, Caritis SN, Yeh M-N, et al.: Prolonged infusion of diazoxide in the management of premature labor in the baboon. Obstet Gynecol 48:203, 1976.
221. Nuwayhid B, Brinkman CR III, Katchen B, et al.: Maternal and fetal hemodynamic effects of diazoxide. Obstet Gynecol 46:197, 1975.
222. Caritis SN, Morishima HO, Stark RI, et al.: The effect of diazoxide on uterine blood flow in pregnant sheep. Obstet Gynecol 48:464, 1976.
223. Symchowicz S, Winston L, Black J, et al.: Diazoxide blood levels in man. J Pharm Sci, 56:915, 1967.
224. Tabachnick IIA, Gulbenkian A, Seidman F: The effect of a benzothiadiazine, diazoxide, on carbohydrate metabolism. Diabetes 13:408, 1964.
225. Kvam DC, Stanton HC: Studies on diazoxide hyperglycemia. Diabetes 13:639, 1964.
226. Graber AL, Porte D Jr, Williams RH: Clinical use of diazoxide and mechanism for its hyperglycemic effect. Diabetes 15:143, 1966.
227. Seltzer HS, Crout JR: Obliteration of insulin secretion by diazoxide and its reversal by tolbutamide. Diabetes 15:523, 1966.
228. Loubatières A, Mariani MM, Alric R: The action of diazoxide on insulin secretion, medullo-adrenal secretion, and the liberation of catecholamines. Ann NY Acad Sci 150:226, 1968.
229. Fajans SS, Floyd JC Jr, Thiffault CA, et al.: Further studies on diazoxide suppression of insulin release from abnormal and normal islet tissue in man. Ann NY Acad Sci 150:261, 1968.
230. Altszuler N, Hampshire J, Moraru E: On the mechanism of diazoxide-induced hyperglycemia. Diabetes 26:931, 1977.
231. Milner RE, Chouksey SK: Effects of fetal exposure to diazoxide in man. Arch Dis Child 47:537, 1972.
232. Maselli R, Casal GL, Ellis EF: Pharmacologic effects of intravenously administered aminophylline in asthmatic children. J Pediatr 76:777, 1970.
233. Jenne JW, Wyze E, Roods FS, et al.: Pharmacokinetics of theophylline: Application to adjustment of the clinical dose of aminophylline. Clin Pharmacol Ther 13:349, 1972.
234. Mitenko PA, Ogilvie RI: Rational intravenous doses of theophylline. N Engl J Med 289:600, 1973.
235. Nicholson DP, Chick TW: A reevaluation of parenteral aminophylline. Am Rev Resp Dis 108:241, 1973.
236. Mitenko PA, Ogilvie RI: Bioavailability and efficacy of a sustained-release theophylline tablet. Clin Pharmacol Ther 16:720, 1974.
237. Svedmyr N: The role of the theophyllines in asthma therapy. Scand J Resp Dis (Suppl) 101:125, 1977.
238. Paterson JW: Discussion: International symposium on salbutamol. Postgrad Med J 47 (Suppl):120, 1971.
239. Larsson S, Thiringer G, Svedmyr N: On development of bronchial beta$_2$-receptor tolerance. Scand J Resp Dis (Suppl) 101:91, 1977.
240. Jenne JW, Chick TW, Strickland RD, et al.: Subsensitivity of beta responses during therapy with a long-acting beta$_2$ preparation. J Allergy Clin Immunol 59:383, 1977.
241. Svedmyr K, Mellstrand T, Svedmyr N: A comparison between effects of aminophylline, proxyphylline and terbutaline in asthmatics. Scand J Resp Dis (Suppl) 101:139, 1977.
242. Triner L, Overwag NIA, Nahas GG: Cyclic 3',5'-AMP and uterine contractility. Nature 225:282, 1970.
243. Triner L, Nahas GG, Vulliemoz Y, et al.: Cyclic

AMP and smooth muscle function. Ann NY Acad Sci 185:458, 1971.
244. Polson JB, Krzanowski JJ, Fitzpatrick DF, et al.: Studies on the inhibition of phosphodiesterase-catalyzed cyclic AMP and cyclic GMP breakdown and relaxation of canine tracheal smooth muscle. Biochem Pharmacol 27:254, 1978.
245. Miech RP, Lohman SM: Metabolism and pharmacodynamics of theophylline. In *New Directions in Asthma*, M Stein, ed. American College of Chest Physicians Publications, Park Ridge, Ill., 1975, p 377.
246. Coutinho EM, Vieira Lopes AC: Inhibition of uterine motility by aminophylline. Am J Obstet Gynecol 110:726, 1971.
247. Maia H Jr, Coutinho EM: Cyclic AMP and oviduct contractility. In *Physiology and Genetics of Reproduction*, part B, EM Coutinho and F Fuchs, eds. Plenum Press, New York, 1974, p 167.
248. Assael BM, Caccamo ML, Gerna M, et al.: Effect of exchange transfusion on elimination of theophylline in premature neonates. J Pediatr 91:331, 1977.
249. Polacek I, Daniel EE: Effects of α- and β-adrenergic stimulation on the uterine motility and adenosine 3',5'-monophosphate level. Can J Physiol Pharmacol 49:988, 1971.
250. Verma SC, McNeill JH: Isoproterenol-induced relaxation, phosphorylase activation and cyclic adenosine monophosphate levels in the polarized and depolarized rat uterus. J Pharmacol Exp Ther 198:539, 1976.
251. Lohmann SM, Miech RP, Butcher FR: Effects of isoproterenol, theophylline and carbachol on cyclic nucleotide levels and relaxation on bovine tracheal smooth muscle. Biochim Biophys Acta, 499:238, 1977.
252. Meisheri KD, McNeill JH: Cyclic nucleotide levels in spontaneously contracting rat uterine strips. Proc West Pharmacol Soc 20:139, 1977.
253. Chrzanowski FA, Niebergall PJ, Mayock RL, et al.: Kinetics of intravenous theophylline. Clin Pharmacol Ther 22:188, 1977.
254. Loren M, Miklich DR, Chai H, et al.: Aminophylline bioavailability and the cross-time stability of plasma theophylline levels. J Pediatr 90:473, 1977.
255. Fixley M, Shen DD, Azarnoff DL: Theophylline bioavailability: A comparison of the oral absorption of a theophylline elixir and two combination theophylline tablets to intravenous aminophylline. Am Rev Resp Dis 115:955, 1977.
256. Bellet S, Kershbaum A, Aspe J: The effect of caffeine on free fatty acids. Arch Intern Med 116:750, 1965.
257. Avogaro P, Capri C, Pais M, et al.: Plasma and urine cortisol behavior and fat mobilization in man after coffee ingestion. Isr J Med Sci 9:114, 1973.
258. Oberman Z, Harell A, Herzberg M, et al.: Changes in plasma cortisol, glucose and free fatty acids after caffeine ingestion in obese women. Isr J Med Sci 11:33, 1975.
259. Aranda JV, Dupont C: Metabolic effect of theophylline in the premature neonate. J Pediatr 89:833, 1976.
260. Leach FN, Ashworth MA, Barson AJ, et al.: Insulin release from human fetal pancreas in tissue culture. J Endocrinol 59:65, 1973.
261. Mitenko PA, Ogilvie RI: Pharmacokinetics of intravenous theophylline. Clin Pharmacol Ther 14:509, 1973.
262. Aranda JV, Sitar DS, Parsons WD, et al.: Pharmacokinetic aspects of theophylline in premature newborns. N Engl J Med 295:413, 1976.
263. Neese AL, Soyka LF: Development of a radioimmunoassay for theophylline application to studies in premature infants. Clin Pharmacol Ther 21:633, 1977.
264. Kuzmko JA, Paala J: Apnoeic attacks in the newborn treated with aminophylline. Arch Dis Child 48:404, 1973.
265. Uauy R, Shapiro DL, Smith B, et al.: Treatment of severe apnea in prematures with orally administered theophylline. Pediatrics 55:595, 1975.
266. Shannon DC, Gotay F, Stein IM, et al.: Prevention of apnea and bradycardia in low-birth-weight infants. Pediatrics 55:589, 1975.
267. Bednarek FJ, Roloff DW: Treatment of apnea of prematurity with aminophylline. Pediatrics 58:335, 1976.
268. Giacoia G, Jusko WJ, Menke J, et al.: Theophylline pharmacokinetics in premature infants with apnea. J Pediatr 89:829, 1976.
269. Aranda JV, Gorman W, Bergsteinsson H, et al.: Efficacy of caffeine in treatment of apnea in the low-birth-weight infant. J Pediatr 90:467, 1977.
270. Richmond GH: Action of caffeine and aminophylline as respiratory stimulants. J Appl Physiol 2:16, 1949.
271. Brinkman CR III, Nuwayhid B, Assali NS: Renal hypertension and pregnancy in sheep. I. Behavior of uteroplacental vasomotor tone during mild hypertension. Am J Obstet Gynecol 121:931 1975.
272. Karotkin EH, Kido M, Cashore WJ, et al.: Acceleration of fetal lung maturation by aminophylline in pregnant rabbits. Pediatr Res 10:722, 1976
273. Fuchs F: Treatment of threatened premature labor with alcohol. J Obstet Gynaecol Br Commonw 72:1011, 1965.
274. Fuchs A-R, Coutinho EM, Xavier R, et al.: Effect of ethanol on the activity of the nonpregnant human uterus and its reactivity to neurohypophyseal hormones. Am J Obstet Gynecol 101:997 1968.
275. Wilson KH, Landesman R, Fuchs A-R, et al.: The effect of ethyl alcohol on isolated human myometrium. Am J Obstet Gynecol 104:436, 1969.
276. Fuchs A-R, Fuchs F: Possible mechanism of the inhibition of labor by ethanol. In *Uterine Contraction: Side Effects of Steroidal Contraceptives*, JB Josimovich, ed. Wiley-Interscience New York, 1973, p 287.
277. Karim SMM, Sharma SD: The effect of ethyl alcohol on prostaglandins E_2 and $F_{2\alpha}$ induce

uterine activity in pregnant women. J Obstet Gynaecol Br Commonw 78:251, 1971.
278. Martell CD, Higgins GC: The effect of ethanol on the myometrial response to oxytocin in women at term. J Obstet Gynaecol Br Commonw 77:976, 1970.
279. Mehra P, Raghavan KS, Devi PK, et al.: Effect of alcohol on premature labour. Int J Gynaecol Obstet 8:160, 1970.
280. Zlatnik FJ, Fuchs F: A controlled study of ethanol in threatened premature labor. Am J Obstet Gynecol 112:610, 1972.
281. Graff G: Failure to prevent premature labor with ethanol. Am J Obstet Gynecol 110:878, 1971.
282. Dilts PV Jr: Effect of ethanol on maternal and fetal acid-base balance. Am J Obstet Gynecol 107:1018, 1970.
283. Horiguchi T, Suzuki K, Comas-Urrutia AC, et al.: Effect of ethanol upon uterine activity and fetal acid-base state of the rhesus monkey. Am J Obstet Gynecol 109:910, 1971.
284. Mann LI, Bhakthavathsalan A, Liu M, et al.: Placental transport of alcohol and its effect on maternal and fetal acid-base balance. Am J Obstet Gynecol 122:837, 1975.
285. Idänpään-Heikkilä JE, Fritchie GE, Ho BT, et al.: Placental transfer of C^{14}-ethanol. Am J Obstet Gynecol 110:426, 1971.
286. Idänpään-Heikkilä J, Jouppila P, Åkerblom HK, et al.: Elimination and metabolic effects of ethanol in mother, fetus, and newborn infant. Am J Obstet Gynecol 112:387, 1972.
287. Waltman R, Iniquez ES: Placental transfer of ethanol and its elimination at term. Obstet Gynecol 40:180, 1972.
288. Cook LN, Shott RJ, Andrews BF: Acute transplacental ethanol intoxication. Am J Dis Child 129:1075, 1975.
289. Wagner L, Wagner G, Guerrero J: Effect of alcohol on premature newborn infants. Am J Obstet Gynecol 108:308, 1970.
290. Seppala M, Raiha NCR, Tamminen U: Ethanol elimination in a mother and her premature twins. Lancet 1:1188, 1971.
291. Lopez R, Montoya MF: Abnormal bone marrow morphology in the premature infant associated with maternal infusion of alcohol. J Pediatr 79:1008, 1971.
292. Madison LL, Lochner A, Wulff J: Ethanol-induced hypoglycemia. I. Mechanism of suppression of hepatic gluconeogenesis. Diabetes 16:252, 1967.
293. Potter DE, Wilson LM, Ellis S: Suppression of isoproterenol-induced hyperglycemia by ethanol (38230). Proc Soc Exp Biol Med 146:972, 1974.
294. Nichols MM: Acute alcohol withdrawal syndrome in a newborn. Am J Dis Child 113:714, 1967.
295. Tenbrinck MS, Buchin SY: Fetal alcohol syndrome. Report of a case. JAMA 232:1144, 1975.
296. Pierog S, Chandavasu O, Wexler I: Withdrawal symptoms in infants with the fetal alcohol syndrome. J Pediatr 90:630, 1977.
297. Johnstone RE, Reier CE: Acute respiratory effects of ethanol in man. Clin Pharmacol Ther 14:501, 1973.
298. Finnegan L: Clinical effects of pharmacologic agents on pregnancy, the fetus, and the neonate. Ann NY Acad Sci 281:74, 1976.
299. Ramwell PW, Shaw J: The biological significance of the prostaglandins. Ann NY Acad Sci 180:10, 1971.
300. Tothill A, Bamford D, Draper J: Inhibition of prostaglandin release and the control of threatened abortion. Lancet 2:381, 1971.
301. Vane JR, Williams KI: Prostaglandin production contributes to the contractions of the rat isolated uterus. Br J Pharmacol 45:146P, 1972.
302. Hargrove JL, Nesbitt D, Gaspar MJ, et al.: Indomethacin induces rat uterine contractions in vitro and alters reactivity to calcium and acetylcholine. Am J Obstet Gynecol 124:25, 1976.
303. Waltman R, Tricomi V, Palav AB: Aspirin and indomethacin: Effect on instillation/abortion time of mid-trimester of hypertonic saline induced abortion. Prostaglandins 3:47, 1973.
304. Niebyl JR, Blake DA, Burnett LS, et al.: The influence of aspirin on the course of induced midtrimester abortion. Am J Obstet Gynecol 124:607, 1976.
305. Lewis RB, Schulman JD: Influence of acetylsalicyclic acid, an inhibitor of prostaglandin synthesis, on the duration of human gestation and labour. Lancet 2:1159, 1973.
306. Novy MJ, Cook MJ, Manaugh L: Indomethacin block of normal onset of parturition in primates. Am J Obstet Gynecol 118:412, 1974.
307. Challis JRG, Davies IJ, Ryan KJ: The effects of dexamethasone and indomethacin on the outcome of pregnancy in the rat. J Endocrinol 64:363, 1975.
308. Lau IF, Saksena SK, Chang MC: Effects of indomethacin and prostaglandin $F_{2\alpha}$ on parturition in the hamster. Prostaglandins 10:1011, 1975.
309. Johnson WL, Harbert GM, Martin CB: Pharmacologic control of uterine contractility: In vitro human and in vivo monkey studies. Am J Obstet Gynecol 123:364, 1975.
310. Mosler KH, Dornhofer W: The inhibitor of premature labor by β-adrenergic sympathomimetics and prostaglandin antagonists in managing premature onset of labour. Naunyn-Schmiedebergs Arch Pharmakol (Suppl) 277:R48, 1973.
311. Zuckerman H, Reiss U, Rubinstein I: Inhibition of human premature labor by indomethacin. Obstet Gynecol 44:787, 1974.
312. Wiqvist N, Lundstrom V, Green K: Premature labor and indomethacin. Prostaglandins 10:515, 1975.
313. Zuckerman H, Reiss U, Atad J, et al.: The effect of indomethacin on plasma levels of prostaglandin $F_{2\alpha}$ in women in labour. Br J Obstet Gynaecol 84:339, 1977.

314. Wiqvist N: Endogenous prostaglandins in normal pregnancy and labor. Pharmac Ther B, 1:297, 1975.
315. Beatty CH, Bocek RM, Young MK, et al.: Effect of indomethacin on cyclic AMP phosphodiesterase activity in myometrium from pregnant rhesus monkeys. Prostaglandins 11:713, 1976.
316. Levin DL, Fixler DE, Morriss FC, et al.: Morphologic analyses of the pulmonary vascular bed in infants exposed in utero to prostaglandin synthetase inhibitors. J Pediatr 921:478, 1978.
317. Smith ID, Shearman RP: Prostaglandin inhibitors in the perinatal period. In *Reviews in Perinatal Medicine*, EM Scarpelli and EV Cosmi, eds, vol II. Raven Press, New York, 1978, p 199.
318. Sharpe GL, Thalme B, Larsson KS: Studies on the closure of the ductus arteriosus. XI, Ductal closure in utero by a prostaglandin synthetase inhibitor. Prostaglandins 8:363, 1974.
319. Collins E, Turner G: Maternal effects of regular salicyclate ingestion in pregnancy. Lancet 2:335, 1975.
320. Turner G, Collins E: Fetal effects of regular salicyclate ingestion in pregnancy. Lancet 2:338, 1975.
321. Sharpe GL, Larsson KS, Thalme B: Studies on closure of the ductus arteriosus. XII. In utero effect of indomethacin and sodium salicyclate in rats and rabbits. Prostaglandins 9:585, 1975.
322. Heymann MA, Rudolph AM: Effects of acetylsalicyclic acid on the ductus arteriosus and circulation in fetal lambs in utero. Circ Res 38:418, 1976.
323. Arcilla RA, Thilenius OG, Ranniger K: Congestive heart failure from suspected ductal closure in utero. J Pediatr 75:74, 1969.
324. Kohler HG: Intrauterine cardiac failure associated with premature closure of the ductus arteriosus. Arch Dis Child 42:335, 1967.
325. Friedman WF, Hirschklau MJ, Printz MP, et al.: Pharmacologic closure of patent ductus arteriosus in the premature infant. N Engl J Med 295:526, 1976.
326. Heymann MA, Rudolph AM, Silverman NH: Closure of the ductus arteriosus in premature infants by inhibition of prostaglandin synthesis. N Engl J Med 295:530, 1976.
327. Waltman R, Tricomi V, Palav A: The effect of analgesic drugs on the installation/abortion time of hypertonic saline induced midtrimester abortion. Prostaglandins 7:411, 1974.
328. Waltman R, Tricomi V: Pentazocine, mefenamic acid and hypertonic-saline abortion. Lancet 2:468, 1974.
329. Lee RE: The influence of psychotropic drugs on prostaglandin-biosynthesis. Prostaglandins 5:63, 1974.
330. Krupp PJ, Wesp M: Inhibition of prostaglandin synthetase by psychotropic drugs. Experientia 31:330, 1975.
331. Ontario Perinatal Mortality Study Committee: *Second Report of the Perinatal Mortality Study in Ten University Teaching Hospitals*, Three reports. Department of Health, Toronto, 1967. (Sec. 1, 1961, Suppl. to 2nd Report, Tables 108–124, 1967.)
332. Cook LN: Intrauterine and extrauterine recognition and management of deviant fetal growth. Pediatr Clin North Am 24:431, 1977.
333. Boggs TR, Hardy JB, Frazier TM: Correlation of neonatal serum total bilirubin concentration and developmental status at age eight months. J Pediatr 71:553, 1967.
334. Chez RA, Fleischman AR: Fetal therapeutics: Challenges and responsibilities. Clin Pharmacol Ther 14:754, 1973.
335. Himwich WA: Physiology of the neonatal central nervous system. In *Physiology of Perinatal Period*, U Stave, ed. Appleton-Century-Crofts, New York, 1970, p 725.
336. Douglas Jones M Jr, Battaglia FC: Intrauterine growth retardation. Am J Obstet Gynecol 127:540, 1977.
337. Rane A, Sjöqvist F, Orrenius S: Cytochrome P-450 in human fetal liver microsomes. Chem Biol Interactions 3:305, 1971.
338. Yaffe SJ, Juchau MR: Perinatal pharmacology. Annu Rev Pharmacol 14:219, 1974.
339. Alvares AP, Schilling G, Levin W, et al.: Cytochromes P-450 and b5 in human liver microsomes. Clin Pharmacol Ther 10:655, 1969.
340. Pelkonen O, Vorne M, Arvela P, et al.: Drug metabolizing enzymes in human fetal liver and placenta in early pregnancy. Scand J Clin Lab Invest (Suppl) 27:116, 1971.
341. Rane A, Sjöqvist F, Orrenius S: Drugs and fetal metabolism. Clin Pharmacol Ther 14:666, 1973.
342. Vallner JJ: Binding of drugs by albumin and plasma protein. J Pharm Sci 66:447, 1977.
343. Magno R, Berlin A, Karlsson K, et al.: Anesthesia for cesarean section. IV. Placental transfer and neonatal elimination of bupivacaine following epidural analgesia for elective cesarean section. Acta Anaesth Scand 20:141, 1976.
344. Shnider SM, Way EL: The kinetics of transfer of lidocaine (Xylocaine) across the human placenta. Anesthesiology 29:944, 1968.
345. Meffin P, Long GL, Thomas J: Clearance and metabolism of mepivacaine in the human neonate. Clin Pharmacol Ther 14:218, 1973.
346. Brown WU Jr, Bell GB, Lurie AO, et al.: Newborn blood levels of lidocaine and mepivacaine in the first postnatal day following maternal epidural anesthesia. Anesthesiology 42:698, 1975.
347. Teramo K, Benowitz N, Heymann MA, et al.: Effects of lidocaine on heart rate, blood pressure, and electrocorticogram in fetal sheep. Am J Obstet Gynecol 118:935, 1974.
348. Teramo K, Benowitz N, Heymann MA, et al.: Gestational differences in lidocaine toxicity in the fetal lamb. Anesthesiology 44:133, 1976.
349. Burt RAP: The foetal and maternal pharmacology of some of the drugs used for the relief of pain in labour. Br J Anaesth 43:824, 1971.
350. Scott DB: Analgesia in labour. Br J Anaesth 49:11, 1977.

351. Mather LE, Long GJ, Thomas J: The binding of bupivacaine to maternal and foetal plasma proteins. J Pharm Pharmacol 23:359, 1971.
352. Tucker GT, Mather LE: Pharmacokinetics of local anaesthetic agents. Br J Anaesth 47:213, 1975.
353. Thomas J, Long G, Moore G, et al.: Plasma protein binding and placental transfer of bupivacaine. Clin Pharmacol Ther 19:426, 1976.
354. Ralston DH, Shnider SM: The fetal and neonatal effects of regional anesthesia in obstetrics. Anesthesiology 48:34, 1978.
355. Covino BG: Local anesthesia (Review). N Engl J Med 286:975, 1035, 1972.
356. Tucker GT: Plasma binding and disposition of local anesthetics. Int Anesthesiol Clin 13:33, 1975.
357. Shnider SM, Way EL: Plasma levels of lidocaine (Xylocaine) in mother and newborn following obstetrical conduction anesthesia: Clinical applications. Anesthesiology 29:951, 1968.
358. Brown WU Jr, Bell GC, Alper MH: Acidosis, local anesthetics, and the newborn. Obstet Gynecol 48:27, 1976.
359. Dodson WE: Neonatal drug intoxication: Local anesthetics. Pediatr Clin North Am 23:399, 1976.
360. Biehl D, Shnider SM, Levinson G, et al.: Placental transfer of lidocaine: Effects of fetal acidosis. Anesthesiology 48:409, 1978.
361. Asling JH, Shnider SM, Margolis AJ, et al.: Paracervical block anesthesia in obstetrics. II. Etiology of fetal bradycardia following paracervical block anesthesia. Am J Obstet Gynecol 107:626, 1970.
362. Rosefsky JB, Petersiel ME: Perinatal deaths associated with mepivacaine paracervical block anesthesia in labor. N Engl J Med 278:530, 1968.
363. Anderson KE, Gennser G, Nilsson E: Influence of mepivacaine on isolated human foetal hearts at normal or low pH. Acta Physiol Scand (Suppl) 353:34, 1970.
364. Morishima HO, Heymann MA, Rudolph AM, et al.: Transfer of lidocaine across the sheep placenta to the fetus: Hemodynamic and acid-base responses of the fetal lamb. Am J Obstet Gynecol 122:581, 1975.
365. Lending M, Slobody LB, Mestern J: Effect of hyperoxia, hypercapnia and hypoxia on blood-cerebrospinal fluid barrier. Am J Physiol 200:959, 1961.
366. Evans CAN, Reynolds JM, Reynolds ML, et al.: The effect of hypercapnia on a blood-brain barrier mechanism in foetal and new-born sheep. J Physiol 255:701, 1976.

CHAPTER 12

Anesthesia for Abnormal Positions, Presentations and Multiple Births

Gershon Levinson, M.D.
Sol M. Shnider, M.D.

The presenting part is that portion of the fetus that is felt through the cervix on vaginal examination. The presenting part determines the **presentation. Position** refers to the relation of an arbitrarily chosen portion of the fetus (occiput, chin, sacrum) to the left or right side of the mother. At delivery, approximately 90 per cent of single gestation fetuses present as a cephalic presentation, either occiput transverse or anterior. All other positions (persistent occiput posterior, face, brow) and presentations (breech, shoulder) are considered abnormal. Compared to single gestation vertex deliveries, multiple gestations and single gestations with abnormal positions and presentations are associated with a higher risk of maternal, fetal and neonatal morbidity and mortality.[1-14] Management of these parturients involves several unique problems for the anesthesiologist and obstetrician.

PERSISTENT OCCIPUT POSTERIOR

Early in labor it is not unusual for the occiput to be in the transverse or posterior position. During descent, or later during the active phase, the occiput usually undergoes normal internal rotation and comes to lie beneath the symphysis pubis. If this rotation does not occur, the persistent occiput posterior results in a more prolonged and painful labor than the occiput anterior position. The head does not fit well into the pelvis, resulting in prolonged or arrested descent and cervical dilation. The occiput exerts increasing pressure on the posterior sacral nerves, resulting in severe back pain. Spontaneous delivery requires more uterine and abdominal work. Cervical and perineal lacerations and postpartum bleeding are common.[15] Although spontaneous delivery can occur, especially in the multipara with a large pelvis, usually manual or forceps rotation and extraction are performed. A prolonged second stage or a difficult mid-forceps rotation is associated with increased birth trauma, intracranial hemorrhage and birth asphyxia.[16]

Anesthetic Considerations

If the vertex is known to be in the occiput posterior position during the first stage of labor and the parturient requests anesthesia, regional techniques which paralyze the perineal muscles are ideally avoided until spontaneous internal rotation occurs. Analgesia is best provided with a segmental lumbar epidural block. If despite an adequate T10–L1 block severe back pain persists, the epidural may be extended to the sacral segments with dilute local anesthetic solutions, e.g. bupivacaine 0.125 to 0.25 per cent or chloroprocaine 1 to 2 per cent. This differential block should not produce relaxation of the levator ani muscles which play an important role in producing internal rotation.

For delivery, if spontaneous rotation has not occurred and mid-forceps rotation is planned, it is ideal that complete analgesia and perineal relaxation be provided. Using a saddle block or caudal block or extending the existing lumbar epidural block to the perineum with 3 per cent chloroprocaine should provide the optimal conditions for an atraumatic delivery, thus minimizing maternal and neonatal morbidity. Mid-forceps delivery without adequate anesthesia is attended by increased fetal and maternal morbidity (lacerations and head trauma). In contrast, mid-vacuum application and delivery can be carried out safely with minimal or no anesthesia.

BREECH PRESENTATION

In approximately 3.5 per cent of pregnancies the breech rather than the vertex presents first.[17] There are three main types of breech presentations: frank, complete and incomplete (Figure 12.1). A frank breech is one in which the lower extremities are flexed at the hips and extended at the knees so that the feet are against the face. A complete breech is one in which the fetal lower extremities are flexed at both the hips and knees so that the buttocks with the feet along side them present at the cervix. Incomplete breech presentation is one in which one or both fetal lower extremities are extended and one or both feet present in the vagina or introitus.

This type is also referred to as a single or double footling breech presentation. Frank breech is present in about 60 per cent of breech deliveries, incomplete breech in about 30 per cent and complete breech in approximately 10 per cent.

Etiology

All causes of breech presentation are unknown, but several associated abnormalities are thought to predispose to this presentation. During the first 35 weeks of pregnancy the fetus constantly changes its presentation, probably as a result of intrauterine fetal activity. It is believed that as the fetus approaches term it tends to accommodate to the shape of the uterine cavity, assuming a longitudinal lie with a vertex presentation. Breeches are more common in premature than full-term fetuses.[6, 7, 18] When the fetus is premature, its smaller size requires less accommodation, and thus breech presentation is more frequent. Other factors that may interfere with the normal process of accommodation between the fetal head, uterine cavity and maternal pelvis include placenta praevia, uterine anomalies, pelvic tumors, fetal congenital anomalies—especially hydrocephalus and anencephaly—and uterine relaxation associated with great parity, multiple fetuses and polyhydramnios.[18]

Obstetric Management

The diagnosis of breech presentation is usually made by manual examination. There is a growing trend now to deliver all breeches by cesarean section. Consequently, the leading cause for primary elective cesarean section in many maternity units is breech presentation. Many obstetricians, however, believe it is safe to deliver selected breeches vaginally.[10, 13, 18, 19] Their indications for cesarean section are listed in Table 12.1.

In many centers external version prior to the expected date of confinement is

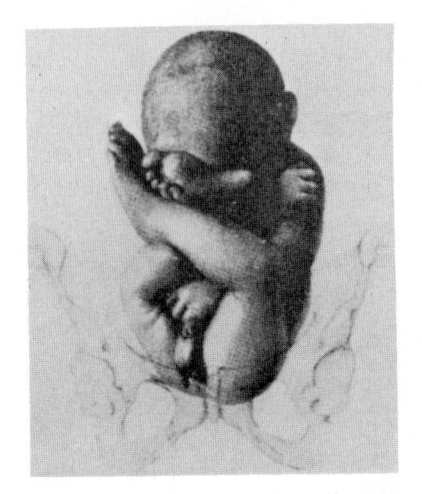

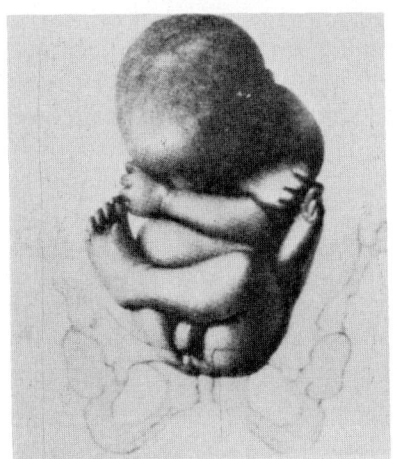

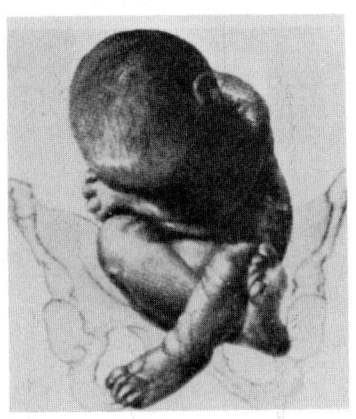

Figure 12.1. Types of breech presentation. *Upper left,* frank breech; *upper right,* complete breech; *lower,* incomplete breech. (Reprinted by permission from Pritchard JA, MacDonald PC: *Williams Obstetrics*, ed. 15. Appleton-Century-Crofts, New York, 1976.)

Table 12.1
Breech Presentation: Indications for Cesarean Section

Prematurity (infant less than 2500 gm)
Large infant (greater than 3600 gm)
Contracted or borderline pelvis
Abnormal first or second stage of labor
Elderly primipara
Hyperextension of the head
Prolapse of umbilical cord
Other obstetric complications not specific to breech presentation

attempted to convert a breech to a vertex presentation. Anesthesia is not recommended for this procedure lest it mask injury and possible rupture of the uterus.

METHODS OF BREECH DELIVERY

Breeches are delivered vaginally in one of four ways. During **spontaneous breech delivery** the entire infant is expelled by the mother without any traction or manipulation by the obstetrician other than support of the infant. **Partial breech extraction**—also called **assisted breech delivery**—refers to spontaneous delivery of the fetus as far as the umbilicus, with the obstetrician extracting the remainder of the body with or without forceps application to the aftercoming head. When the entire body of the infant is extracted with intrauterine manipulation by the obstetrician, the delivery is termed **total breech** *extraction*. ***Breech decomposition and extraction*** refers to the intrauterine conversion of a frank into an incomplete breech by flexion of the fetal knee(s) and extending the hips prior to extraction.

MATERNAL, FETAL AND NEONATAL HAZARDS

Breech deliveries are associated with increased maternal morbidity. Compared to vertex presentations there is greater likelihood of cervical lacerations, perineal injury, shock due to intrapartum and postpartum hemorrhage, retained placenta and infection.[18]

Neonatal prognosis is significantly worse in breech deliveries. Trauma to the term breech during vaginal delivery is 12 times higher than in vertex presentations.[6-8] The perinatal mortality rate, corrected for prematurity and congenital anomalies, is almost four times higher.[7] With vaginal delivery, pre-term breech infants have twice the rate of neurologic abnormalities at 1 year of age compared to vertex presentations.[20] Pre-term infants undergoing spontaneous breech delivery have a higher mortality rate than if delivered with Piper forceps. Large newborns (more than 3,500 g) delivered vaginally have an increased neonatal mortality rate.

There are several reasons for the increased perinatal morbidity and mortality associated with breech presentations. These infants are more likely to suffer asphyxia from cord compression and intracranial hemorrhage from head trauma. Intrauterine manipulation may further increase fetal trauma and cord compression. During spontaneous breech delivery, the uncontrolled expulsion of the fragile fetal head can result in tentorial tears and brain damage.

Prolapse of the umbilical cord is a significant cause of increased fetal mortality. The gestational age of the baby has no effect on the incidence of cord prolapse, but the type of breech presentation does. The incidence of cord prolapse is 0.5 per cent in vertex deliveries, 0.5 per cent with frank breech presentations and 10 per cent with incomplete or complete breech presentations.[18] The cause of increased frequency of prolapse of the umbilical cord is believed due to failure of the presenting part to fill the lower uterine segment.

Anesthetic Considerations in Breech Delivery

If the breech is to be delivered by elective primary cesarean section, either regional or general anesthesia may be used (see chapter 17). With either spinal or epidural anesthesia difficulty extracting the infant through the uterine incision may be encountered. If uterine hypertonus is the primary cause, the anesthesiologist must be prepared to induce general anesthesia rapidly. Following endotracheal intubation halothane should be administered to relax the uterus. If emergency cesarean section is to be performed for fetal distress or prolapsed umbilical cord, general anesthesia is usually indicated.

If the breech is to be delivered vaginally, an anesthesiologist must also be immediately available. Not only may he be required to provide adequate analgesia for labor and delivery but he must also be prepared to provide perineal or uterine relaxation or sufficient anesthesia for emergency cesarean section rapidly. Preanesthetic preparations for breech presentations are listed in Table 12.2.

For vaginal breech delivery, partial breech extraction is the method of choice. At the end of the second stage of labor the parturient must be able to expel the fetus until the umbilicus is seen, whereupon the obstetrician can extract the arms and deliver the aftercoming head manually or with Piper forceps. Labor is often managed with narcotics and tranquilizers and the delivery managed with perineal infiltration of local anesthetic or pudendal block.

Table 12.2
Pre-anesthetic Preparations for Breech or Multiple Deliveries

Type and cross-match for 2 units of blood
Start intravenous with 16- or 18-gauge plastic indwelling catheter
Administer no food or fluids by mouth
Administer oral antacid every 4 hours
Monitor fetal heart rate continuously
Prepare for possible rapid induction of general anesthesia
Prepare to resuscitate newborn

Inhalation analgesia, if needed, may be administered by an anesthesiologist.

These techniques, on occasion, do not provide adequate analgesia or perineal muscle relaxation for delivery of the aftercoming head. Rapid induction of general anesthesia with thiopental, succinylcholine, endotracheal intubation and nitrous oxide may be necessary and will provide optimal operating conditions. Halothane is not necessary for the application of Piper forceps. Rarely, however, the lower uterine segment contracts and traps the aftercoming head and halothane must be added to relax the uterus and facilitate delivery.

Some obstetricians avoid major regional anesthesia because of concern over prolonging the first or second stages of labor, decreasing the ability of the mother to push effectively and thereby increasing the incidence of total breech extraction with its associated high fetal mortality. On the other hand, many find that spinal, epidural or caudal anesthesia offer significant advantages.

Regional anesthesia allows for an alert, cooperative patient who, with proper coaching, can push effectively. It provides better pain relief compared to other methods of analgesia and provides maximal perineal relaxation for delivery of the aftercoming head. In addition, if there is a shortage of trained personnel, the anesthesiologist is more likely to be available for infant resuscitation. The incidence of complete breech extraction is not increased with regional anesthesia, although the second stage is lengthened slightly.[21,22] Major regional anesthesia compared with no anesthesia, minor perineal local nerve blocks or general anesthesia is not associated with an increased incidence of neonatal depression (Table 12.3).[21-27]

If uterine relaxation is required for complete breech extraction, halothane anesthesia with rapid endotracheal intubation may be the preferred technique. However, if a major regional anesthetic has been used for labor, intrauterine manipulation can often be performed safely and easily between contractions. If general anesthesia is to be used to provide uterine relaxation for intrauterine manipulation, then a rapid intravenous induction of anesthesia and endotracheal intubation with application of cricoid pressure is recommended. Ketamine should not be used because in doses greater than 1 mg/kg it increases uterine tone.[28] After intubation with thiopental and succinylcholine, halothane will provide uterine relaxation with rapid onset and reversibility. The parturient is especially susceptible to overdosage with inhalational anesthetics, and utmost caution must be exercised during controlled ventilation with potent agents.

Table 12.3
Anesthesia for Breech Presentation (Infants over 2500 gm and No Antepartum Obstetric or Medical Complications)*

	Number of Patients	Neonatal Depression at 1 Minute of Age	
		Moderate Depression	Severe Depression
		%	
Vaginal delivery and no epidural	79	42	20
Vaginal delivery with epidural	47	40	6

* Adapted by permission from J. S. Crawford: J Obstet Gynecol Br Commonw 81:867, 1974.

ABNORMAL POSITIONS, PRESENTATIONS AND MULTIPLE BIRTHS

FACE OR BROW POSITIONS OR SHOULDER PRESENTATION

Most infants with cephalic presentation and a face or brow position are delivered by cesarean section because of cephalopelvic disproportion. Either regional or general anesthesia may be used. Similarly, most infants in a transverse lie with a shoulder presentation are delivered by elective cesarean section. Occasionally, internal podalic version and extraction (Figures 12.2 and 12.3) are performed and the baby delivered vaginally as a breech presentation. Under these circumstances the intrauterine manipulation is best performed under general endotracheal halothane anesthesia (Table 10.3).

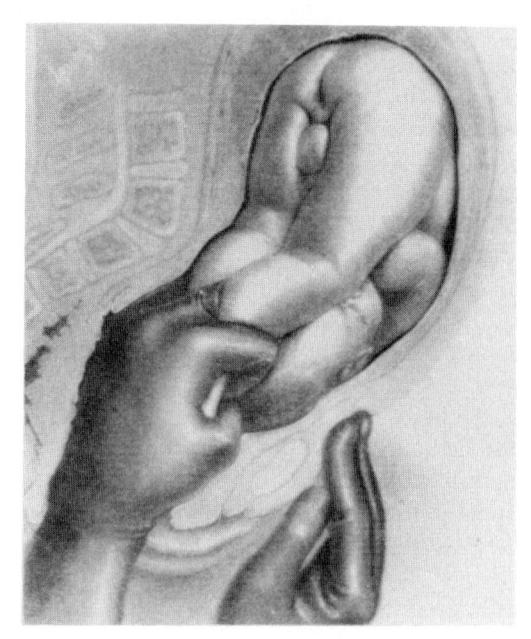

Figure 12.3. Internal podalic version. Upward pressure on head is made as downward traction is exerted on feet. (Reprinted by permission from Pritchard JA, MacDonald PC: *Williams Obstetrics*, ed. 15. Appleton-Century-Crofts, New York, 1976.)

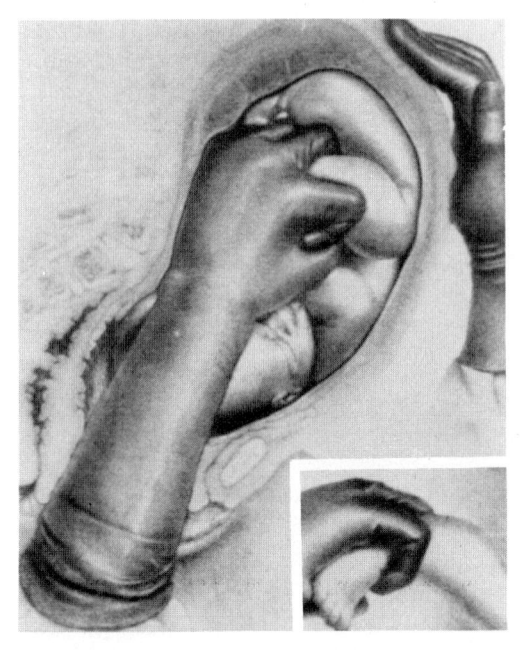

Figure 12.2. Internal podalic version. If at all possible, both feet are grasped, because this technique makes the turning much easier. (Reprinted by permission from Pritchard JA, MacDonald PC: *Williams Obstetrics*, ed. 15. Appleton-Century-Crofts, New York, 1976.)

MULTIPLE GESTATIONS

The incidence of twin gestation in the United States is approximately 1 in 90 births.[29, 30] The incidence of twins is higher in blacks and lower in Orientals. Triplets occur in 1 in 9,800 and quadruplets in 1 in 70,000 births.

Twin gestations may be single ovum (monozygous, identical twins) or double ovum (polyzygous). Heredity, maternal age and increasing parity influence the incidence of double-ovum twinning.[29, 30] Approximately 30 per cent of twins are monozygotic.[30, 31]

Maternal, Fetal and Neonatal Hazards

THE MOTHER

Preeclampsia-eclampsia, anemia, premature labor, prolonged labor and antepartum and postpartum hemorrhage are more common in multiple gestations.[32-33] Despite the fact that maternal blood volume increases earlier in pregnancy and reaches levels approximately 40 per cent greater than in single gestation, anemia occurs more frequently and is more severe in multiple gestations.[39] The larger uterus predisposes the parturient to more severe supine hypotension. The increase in uterine distension due to multiple gestation also leads to a more frequent occurrence of nausea and vomiting, dyspnea, leg edema and varicosities.[38] Blood loss during twin delivery is twice that of single gestation and manual extraction of the placenta is required twice as often.[37] Maternal mortality is two to three times higher in multiple gestations.

THE FETUS

There are two circumstances in monozygotic twinning which pose special hazards to the fetuses. An anastomosis may be present between the two vascular systems, resulting in transfusion of blood from one fetus to the other. In such cases one twin may receive most of the blood and become polycythemic with cardiomegaly and heart failure, while the other twin becomes anemic and hypovolemic. In extreme cases one twin may not receive enough blood to survive. The other hazard of monozygotic twins involves being monoamniotic; this occurs in up to 4 per cent of identical twins and is associated with an increased fetal mortality (50 per cent chance of intrauterine death) due to intertwining and occlusion of the umbilical vessels.

THE NEONATE

Prematurity occurs six to 10 times more frequently in multiple gestations compared to single births.[5, 35, 36] Approximately 60 per cent of twins are premature. The etiology of prematurity is not known but has been attributed to overdistension of the uterus and an increased incidence of maternal complications such as preeclampsia-eclampsia. Fetal growth is independent of the number of fetuses in the uterus until 28 weeks gestation, at which point a progressive weight lag develops when compared with single gestations. The neonatal death rate is higher in infants of multiple gestations, due mostly to prematurity. However, mature twins also have a higher mortality than mature single births; this is most likely due to a higher incidence of other factors, such as congenital anomalies, prolapse of umbilical cord, abnormal presentations and neonatal intracranial and visceral hemorrhage.

The second twin is likely to be more depressed and asphyxiated and require resuscitation more frequently than the first.[32, 36, 40-43] The most significant risk factor in the second twin is the period of hypoxemia caused either by contraction of the uterus or by premature separation of the placenta after the first infant is delivered.

Obstetric Management

Any combination of presentations of the fetuses can occur but the commonest are both vertex or one vertex and one breech (Table 12.4). Rarely, interlocking and interference with engagement or delivery of one infant by his twin may occur. Duration of labor is often shorter in multiple gestations because of the small fetal size and frequent effacement of the cervix before

Table 12.4
Presentation of Fetuses in Twin Delivery

	Approximate Per Cent of Deliveries
Both vertex	39
Vertex and breech	37
Both breech	10
Longitudinal and shoulder	8
Both shoulder	6

the onset of contractions. On the other hand, labor may be prolonged in some cases due to dysfunctional uterine contractions associated with an overdistended uterus.

Anesthetic Considerations

The major considerations in regard to choice of anesthesia for multiple gestations are the frequent occurrence of prematurity and breech presentation. The anesthesiologist may have to rapidly provide anesthesia for version, extraction, breech delivery, cesarean section or midforceps delivery. Therefore an early preoperative evaluation and preparation of the parturient is essential. As described previously for a singleton breech delivery (Table 12.2), a large intravenous cannula should be placed, blood should be crossmatched, oral antacids should be administered and personnel and equipment to resuscitate both infants should be available. Continuous fetal heart rate monitoring of both infants is recommended. If this is not feasible, after delivery of the first infant, the second infant should also have continuous monitoring for immediate recognition of acute fetal asphyxia.

Many obstetricians prefer pudendal block or local infiltration with or without inhalation analgesia. These techniques may provide adequate analgesia for delivery with minimum depression of the neonates. However, they do not provide analgesia during the first stage of labor and for many woman, do not provide satisfactory analgesia during the second stage. These techniques do not provide adequate perineal or uterine relaxation if they are necessary. The authors and others believe that if analgesia is required, continuous epidural is ideal.[44-46] Continuous regional blockade eliminates the need for administration of maternal narcotics and sedatives. Avoiding narcotics is of particular value in pre-term infants. Reduced perinatal mortality for both mature and preterm twin infants whose mothers received conduction anesthesia (when compared with general anesthesia or local or no anesthesia) has been reported.[5] With regional anesthesia, the first stage is not significantly prolonged, and the interval between the delivery of the first and second twin may be shortened.[44] Forceps deliveries, which are more frequent with multiple gestations, are easier to accomplish with the good perineal relaxation found under epidural anesthesia. Even for version and extraction, some experts prefer conduction anesthesia, although most advise general anesthesia for uterine relaxation if intrauterine manipulations are necessary. When internal podalic version and complete extraction are performed under regional anesthesia, manipulations should be made between contractions. The anesthesiologist must be prepared for rapid induction of general anesthesia and uterine relaxation with halothane should difficulties arise.

Segmental lumbar epidural anesthesia with 2 per cent chloroprocaine or 0.25 per cent bupivacaine provides complete pain relief but still assures adequate strength in the abdominal muscles so the mother may push and thereby assist with delivery. Some prefer a double-catheter technique—one catheter in the lumbar epidural space to provide pain relief during labor and a second catheter in the caudal canal for perineal analgesia and relaxation. The double-catheter technique provides maximum anesthesia with the least amount of drug (see chapter 8).

With major conduction anesthesia, the parturient with a multiple gestation is at greater risk of hypotension. The larger gravid uterus produces more aortocaval compression and, together with the sympathetic block, increases the incidence and severity of maternal hypotension. Also, patients with sympathetic blockade will not vasoconstrict or maintain blood pressure in response to the increased blood loss at delivery. Left uterine displacement during labor and delivery and adequate fluid and blood replacement are essential.

On occasion, a cesarean section may be indicated. Either regional or general anesthesia may be used, the evidence available not favoring one method over the other. The choice of anesthesia for cesarean delivery of multiple gestation depends on the preference and experience of the anesthesiologist, the obstetrician and the patient.[47]

References

1. Cruikshank DP, White CP: Obstetric malpresentations: Twenty years' experience. Am J Obstet Gynecol 116:1097, 1973.
2. Powers WF: Twin pregnancy: Complications and treatment. Obstet Gynecol 42:795, 1973.
3. Rementeria JL, Janakammal S, Hollander M: Multiple births in drug-addicted women. Am J Obstet Gynecol 122:958, 1975.
4. Scholtes G: Problems in twin pregnancy (German: Zum Problem der Zwillingsschwangerschaft). Arch Gynaekol 210:188, 1971.
5. Aaron JB, Halperin J: Fetal survival in 376 twin deliveries. Am J Obstet Gynecol 69:794, 1955.
6. Hall JE, Kohl S: Breech presentation: A study of 1,456 cases. Am J Obstet Gynecol 72:977, 1956.
7. Morgan HS, Kane SH: An analysis of 16,327 breech births. JAMA 187:262, 1964.
8. Potter MG Jr, Heaton CE, Douglas GW: Intrinsic fetal risk in breech delivery. Obstet Gynecol 15:158, 1960.
9. Abrams IF, Bresnan MJ, Zuckerman JE, et al: Cervical cord injuries secondary to hyperextension of the head in breech presentations. Obstet Gynecol 41:369, 1973.
10. Bird CC, McElin TW: A six-year prospective study of term breech deliveries utilizing the Zatuchni-Andros prognostic scoring index. Am J Obstet Gynecol 121:551, 1975.
11. Brenner WE, Bruce RD, Hendricks CH: The characteristics and perils of breech presentation. Am J Obstet Gynecol 118:700, 1974.
12. Rovinsky JJ, Miller JA, Kaplan S: Management of breech presentation at term. Am J Obstet Gynecol 115:497, 1973.
13. Zatuchni GI, Andros GJ: Prognostic index for vaginal delivery in breech presentation at term. Am J Obstet Gynecol 93:237, 1965.
14. Sokol RJ, Roux JF: Computer diagnosis of labor progression. VI. Fetal stress and labor in the occipitoposterior position. Am J Obstet Gynecol 122:253, 1975.
15. Cannell DE: The management of the occiput posterior. Am J Obstet Gynecol 60:496, 1950.
16. Pritchard JA, MacDonald PC: *Williams Obstetrics*, ed 15. Appleton-Century-Crofts, New York, 1976, pp 666–698.
17. Greenhill JP, Friedman EA: *Biological Principles and Modern Practice of Obstetrics*. W.B. Saunders, Philadelphia, 1974, p 598.
18. Pritchard JA, MacDonald PC: *Williams Obstetrics*, ed 15. Appleton-Century-Crofts, New York, 1976, pp 889–902.
19. Morley GW: Breech presentation: A 15 year review. Obstet Gynecol 30:745, 1967.
20. Bonica JJ, Nace FM: Breech delivery. In *Principles and Practice of Obstetric Analgesia and Anesthesia*, JJ Bonica, ed, chapter 70 F. A. Davis, Philadelphia, 1969.
21. Crawford JS: An appraisal of lumbar epidural blockade in patients with singleton fetus presenting by the breech. J Obstet Gynaecol Br Commonw 81:867, 1974.
22. Bowen-Simpkins P, Fergusson ILC: Lumbar epidural block and the breech presentation. Br J Anaesth 46:420, 1974.
23. Daily HI, Rogers SF: Saddle block anesthesia in breech delivery. Surg Gynecol Obstet 105:630, 1957.
24. Sears RT: Use of spinal analgesia in forceps and breech deliveries. Br Med J 1:755, 1959.
25. Boyson WA, Simpson JW: Breech management with caudal anesthesia. Am J Obstet Gynecol 79:1121, 1960.
26. Gunther RE, Harer WB: Single-injection caudal anesthesia. Am J Obstet Gynecol 92:305, 1965.
27. Salvatore CA, Cicivizzo E, Turath S: Breech delivery with saddle block anesthesia. Obstet Gynecol 26:261, 1965.
28. Galloon S: Ketamine and the pregnant uterus. Can Anaesth Soc J 20:141, 1973.
29. Guttmacher AF: The incidence of multiple births in man and some of the other unipara. Obstet Gynecol 2:22, 1953.
30. Gedda L: *Twins in History and Science*. Charles C Thomas, Springfield, Ill., 1961.
31. Guttmacher AF, Kohl SG: The fetus of multiple gestations. Obstet Gynecol 12:528, 1958.
32. Bender S: Twin pregnancy: A review of 472 cases. J Obstet Gynaecol Br Emp 59:510, 1952.
33. Kotsalo K: Observations on the premature separation of the normally implanted placenta. Acta Obstet Gynaecol Scand 37:155, 1958.
34. Graves LR, Adams JQ, Schreier PC: The fate of the second twin. Obstet Gynecol 19: 246, 1962.
35. Friedman EA, Sachtleben M: The effect of uterine overdistension on labor. I. Multiple pregnancy. Obstet Gynecol 23:164, 1964.
36. Little WA, Friedman EA: The twin delivery: factors influencing second twin mortality. A review. Obstet Gynecol Surv 13:611, 1958.
37. Pritchard JA, Baldwin RM, Dickey JC, et al.: Blood volume changes in pregnancy and the puerperium. Red blood cell loss and changes in apparent blood volume during and following vaginal delivery, cesarean section, plus total hysterectomy. Am J Obstet Gynecol 84:1271, 1962.

38. Pritchard JA, MacDonald PC: *Williams Obstetrics*, ed 15. Appleton-Century-Crofts, New York, 1976, pp 529–550.
39. Rovinsky JJ, Jaffin H: Cardiovascular hemodynamics in pregnancy. I. Blood and plasma volumes in multiple pregnancy. Am J Obstet Gynecol 93:1, 1966.
40. Corston J McD: Twin survival: A comparison of mortality rates of the first and second twin. Obstet Gynecol 10:181, 1957.
41. Camilleri AP: In defense of the second twin. J Obstet Gynaecol Br Emp 70:258, 1963.
42. MacDonald RR: Management of the second twin. Br Med J 1:518, 1962.
43. Wyshak G, White C: Birth hazard of the second twin. JAMA 186:869, 1963.
44. Crawford JS: An appraisal of lumbar epidural blockade in labour in patients with multiple pregnancy. J Obstet Gynaecol Br Commonw 82:929, 1975.
45. James FM III, Crawford JS, Davies P, et al.: Lumbar epidural analgesia for labor and delivery of twins. Am J Obstet Gynecol 127:176, 1977.
46. Abouleish E: Caudal analgesia for quadruplet delivery. Anesth Analg 55:61, 1976.
47. Craft JB, Levinson G, Shnider SM: Anaesthetic considerations in caesarean section for quadruplets. Can Anaesth Soc J 25:236, 1978.

CHAPTER 13

Anesthesia for the Pregnant Cardiac Patient

Dennis Thomas Mangano, Ph.D., M.D.

The pregnant patient with heart disease challenges the anesthesiologist's skills. Pregnancy and labor each impose demands on the circulation, and anesthesia during delivery may compromise an already stressed cardiovascular system. To avoid such a compromise the anesthesiologist must be aware of the nature and progression of heart disease during pregnancy, the normal physiology of labor, delivery and the puerperium, the cardiovascular effects of various anesthetic regimens and the therapies used to manage acute complications. This chapter will discuss the clinical manifestations, pathophysiology and anesthetic considerations of serious cardiovascular diseases occurring during pregnancy. The first section covers the over-all incidence, morbidity and mortality of heart disease. Cardiovascular changes during pregnancy are summarized and anesthetic guidelines are presented. The second, third and fourth sections describe rheumatic heart disease, congenital heart disease and several other significant cardiovascular diseases. For each disease the clinical manifestations, pathophysiology and anesthetic considerations are discussed. The final section reviews the effects of cardiac therapeutics on the fetus.

GENERAL CONSIDERATIONS

Over the past 25 years the incidence of heart disease during pregnancy has declined from 3.6 per cent to the present figure of approximately 1.6 per cent (Figure 13.1).[1-8] Rheumatic heart disease, despite the declining incidence, still accounts for most cases. The incidence of congenital heart disease in pregnant patients has been increasing because a greater number of women with congenital heart lesions now reach the childbearing age due to improvements in medical and surgical therapy.[1,4,9] Maternal mortality with rheumatic heart disease and pregnancy varies from less than 1 per cent in asymptomatic patients to 17 per cent in patients with mitral stenosis complicated by atrial fibrillation (Table 13.1).[8] Congenital diseases are associated with a large range of mortality; however, several congenital diseases have a high incidence of maternal and fetal mortality regardless of their stage of progression. These are primary pulmonary hypertension, dominant right-to-left shunt (Eisenmenger's syndrome, tetralogy of Fallot), severe aortic stenosis and coarctation of the aorta. These diseases, as well as diseases which have a significant rate of occurrence, will be discussed in detail.

Cardiovascular Changes during Pregnancy and Parturition

The cardiovascular changes associated with pregnancy and parturition which were discussed in chapter 1 are briefly summarized here.[10-15] The cardiovascular

ANESTHESIA FOR THE PREGNANT CARDIAC PATIENT

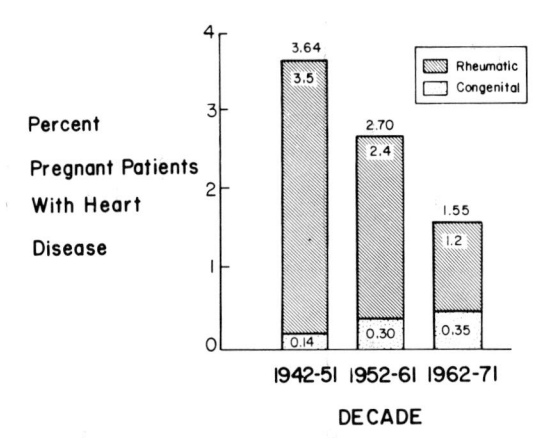

Figure 13.1. Incidence and distribution of heart disease during pregnancy over three decades. (Data were drawn from a review of more than 50,000 cases reported by Szekely P, and Snaith L. In *Heart Disease and Pregnancy*, Churchill Livingstone, London, 1974.)

system is progressively stressed during pregnancy and parturition (Figures 13.2 to 13.5).[10-16] During labor, pain and apprehension increase and precipitate a progressive increase in stroke volume and cardiac output to 45 per cent over pre-labor values.[14] Additional stresses are imposed by uterine contraction causing, in effect, an autotransfusion. With each uterine contraction, central blood volume and cardiac output increase by 10 to 25 per cent.[15] This acute preload stress is well tolerated by the normal heart but may represent the deciding physiologic stress in a diseased heart which has become increasingly compromised during pregnancy and labor. After delivery the central blood volume increases; obstruction of the vena cava and aorta are relieved and result in a marked increase in stroke volume (up to 80 per cent of pre-labor values). Systemic vascular resistance decreases.[14] These changes, along with those induced by hemorrhage or the administration of oxytocic drugs, may cause a rapid decompensation in patients with a compromised cardiovascular system.

An Overview of Anesthetic Considerations

Anesthesia for the pregnant patient with heart disease requires an understanding of the type, severity and progression of the disease in the context of the normal cardiovascular adaptations to pregnancy. The anesthesiologist's assessment of the patient's tolerance to pain during labor and surgery, the autotransfusion of uterine contraction and the post-delivery changes induced by relief of vena caval obstruction, oxytocic agents and hemorrhage must each be considered to determine the best anesthetic regimen.

The pre-anesthetic detection of a symptomatic history either at rest or with exercise is of paramount importance, because such a history correlates directly with morbidity and mortality.[4,17,18] Physical examination plus consultation with the primary physician and cardiologist should also be used to define the severity of the disease. Cardiac medications needed prior to pregnancy should usually be continued throughout pregnancy, labor and delivery.

For most diseases, no one anesthetic technique is exclusively indicated or contraindicated. The primary concern is to avoid and/or treat specific pathophysiologic changes which exacerbate the disease process. These pathophysiologic changes will be delineated for each disease, and the recommended anesthetic considerations will be discussed.

The decision to use invasive techniques (e.g. a radial arterial line or thermodilution pulmonary artery catheter) depends on the severity and progression of disease. Most asymptomatic patients who have not evidenced disease progression and who have no signs of impaired right or left ventricular performance will have an uneventful course and do not require invasive monitoring. Exceptions are patients, even if asymptomatic, with primary pulmonary hypertension, right-to-left shunt, dissect-

Table 13.1
Incidence and Mortality of Rheumatic and Congenital Heart Disease in Pregnancy

	Distribution	Mortality Maternal	Fetal Mortality	References
	%	%	%	
Rheumatic heart disease (75%)				
Mitral stenosis	90	1–17	3.5	1, 3, 4, 38, 54
Mitral insufficiency	6.5			
Aortic insufficiency	2.5			
Aortic stenosis	1.0			
	100			
Congenital heart disease (25%)				
Ventricular septal defect	7–26	7–40	2–16	9, 48, 51–53, 55
Atrial septal defect	8–38	1–12	1–12	1, 4, 7, 9, 48, 55
Patent ductus arteriosus	6–20	5–6	17	4, 9, 50, 55
Tetralogy of Fallot	2–15	4–12	36–59	1, 4, 9, 55, 58, 59, 61, 62
Eisenmenger's syndrome	2–4	12–33	30–54	1, 2, 4, 52, 53, 57, 59
Coarctation of the aorta	4–18	3–9	10–20	4, 52, 64, 65
Aortic stenosis	2–10		22	1, 4, 54, 55
Pulmonic stenosis	8–16		4	1, 4, 55, 72
Primary pulmonary hypertension	1–2	53	7	1, 4, 49, 52, 56

ing aortic aneurysm, severe aortic stenosis or coarctation of the aorta. In patients with severe heart disease, a full hemodynamic profile—including cardiac output, vascular resistance, central venous pressure (CVP) and pulmonary capillary wedge (PCW) pressure—is desirable. Based on these measurements a therapeutic plan should be designed for handling each of the acute complications which may occur with that disease. It is well recognized that placement of a pulmonary artery catheter is time consuming, requires expertise and may have associated morbidity and even mortality. Nonetheless, the author believes that in patients with severe cardiac disease the information derived from pulmonary artery catheterization is worth the risk.

The hemodynamic aberrations seen during labor and delivery may continue after delivery. Thus, patients with symptomatic heart disease who have had a complicated labor and delivery period should be monitored in an intensive care unit.

Treatment of complications which occur during an anesthetic course may involve the use of electrocardioversion or pharmacologic agents such as digoxin, propranolol, lidocaine, metaraminol, sodium nitroprusside and phentolamine. These drugs may have untoward fetal effects. Their use or non-use depends on the seriousness of maternal impairment and whether that impairment will result in severe fetal morbidity which will outweigh the morbidity associated with the therapy. The author's philosophy is to correct immediately any severe maternal impairment, even though the therapy may cause fetal morbidity.

Finally, it should be clearly understood that there exist few well controlled studies addressing the effects of anesthetics and therapeutics on pregnant patients with heart disease. However, the physiologic changes occurring during pregnancy, the pathophysiology of these disease processes and the effects of anesthetics on pregnant patients without cardiovascular disease are well documented. The anesthetic and therapeutic considerations and recommendations stated in this chapter have been synthesized from these mostly

ANESTHESIA FOR THE PREGNANT CARDIAC PATIENT

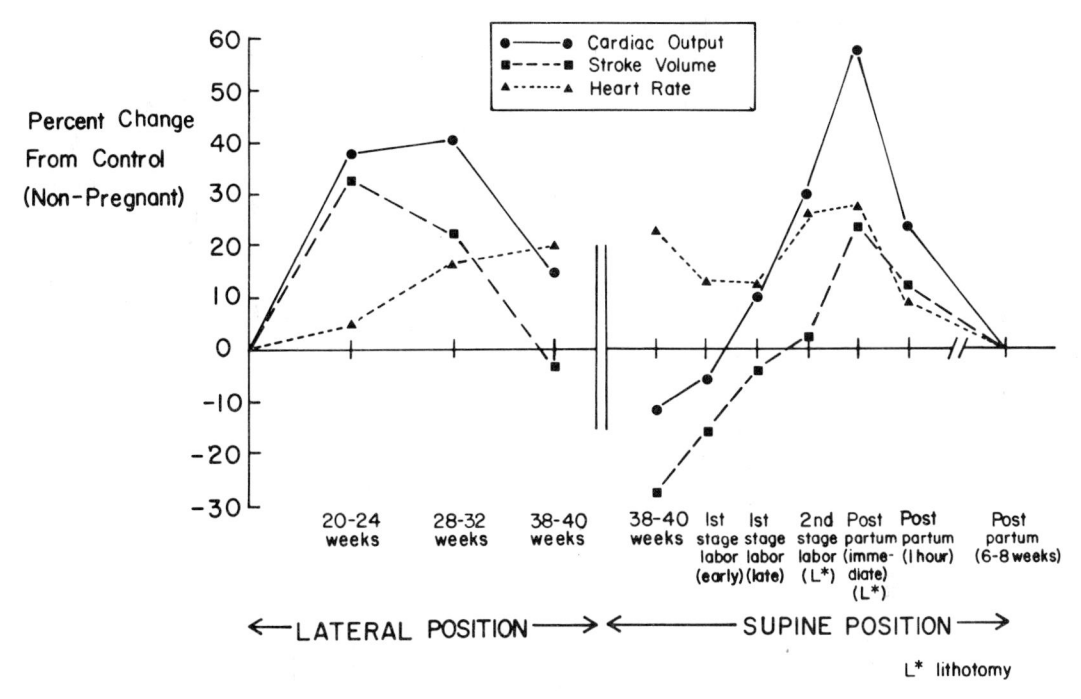

Figure 13.2. Maternal cardiovascular changes during pregnancy and labor from studies on patients in the lateral and supine positions. (Based on data reported by Ueland K, Hansen J: Maternal cardiovascular dynamics. II. Posture and uterine contractions. Am J Obstet Gynecol 103:1, 1969; Ueland K, Hansen J: Maternal cardiovascular dynamics. III. Labor and delivery under local and caudal analgesia. Am J Obstet Gynecol 103:8, 1969; Ueland K, Novy M, Peterson E, et al. Maternal cardiovascular dynamics. IV. The influence of gestational age on the maternal cardiovascular response to posture and exercise. Am J Obstet Gynecol 104:156, 1969.)

independent bodies of information and represent the opinions of this author.

RHEUMATIC HEART DISEASE

Rheumatic fever is a diffuse inflammatory disease affecting the heart, joints and subcutaneous tissues following group-A β-hemolytic streptococcal infection. Acute rheumatic fever is evidenced by a history of a streptococcal infection and a subsequent clinical picture which usually includes recurrent migratory polyarthritis with or without carditis. Polyarthritis tends to be self-limited, but the carditis can progressively and permanently damage valves or heart muscle. Although the prophylactic administration of antibiotics generally prevents the sequelae of rheumatic fever, rheumatic heart disease continues to commonly cause death in the United States and in many other countries.[17-21] Left or right ventricular failure, atrial dysrhythmias, systemic or pulmonary embolism and infective endocarditis may complicate rheumatic heart disease during pregnancy (Table 13.2). Although the incidence of these complications during pregnancy has progressively decreased, they still occur in 15 per cent of patients.

Mitral Stenosis

Rheumatic fever usually first occurs in 6- to 15-year-old children. If carditis occurs, mitral insufficiency ensues followed in about 5 years by mitral stenosis. Symptoms usually do not appear for another 15 years. Pulmonary congestion, pulmonary hypertension and right ventricular failure develop 5 to 10 years after the occurrence of symptoms.[22, 23] On average, symptoms appear at 31 years and proceed in 7 years to total incapacity.[24] Without surgical correction 20 per cent of totally incapacitated

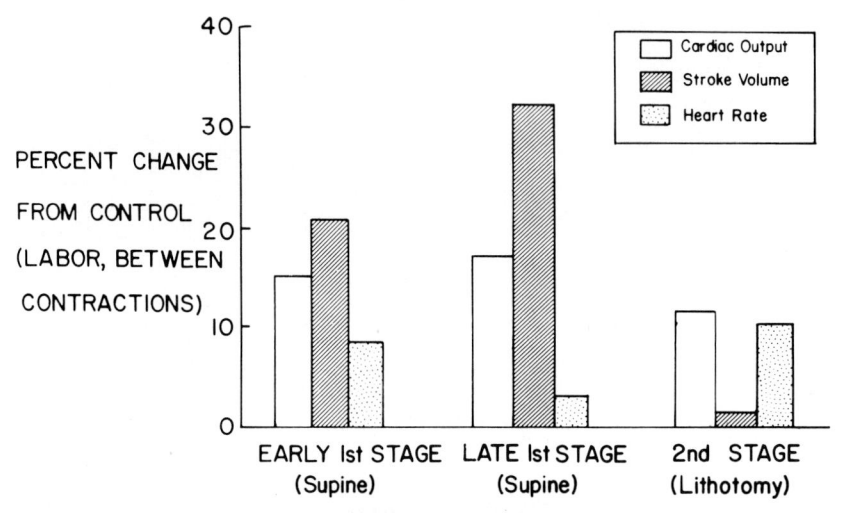

Figure 13.3. Effects of uterine contractions on cardiac output, stroke volume and heart rate during labor. Values represent per cent increases from control measurements in late pregnancy. (Redrawn from Ueland K, Hansen J: Maternal cardiovascular dynamics. III. Labor and delivery under local and caudal analgesia. Am J Obstet Gynecol 103:8, 1969.)

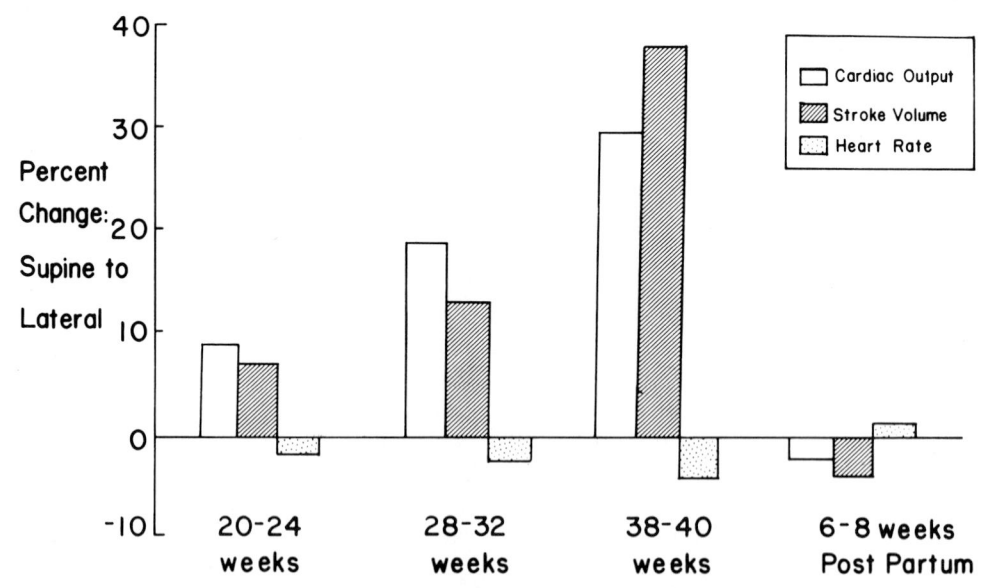

Figure 13.4. Per cent change in cardiac output, stroke volume and heart rate when the pregnant woman turns from supine to lateral position. (Redrawn from Ueland K, Hansen J: Maternal cardiovascular dynamics. II. Posture and uterine contractions. Am J Obstet Gynecol 103:1, 1969.)

ANESTHESIA FOR THE PREGNANT CARDIAC PATIENT

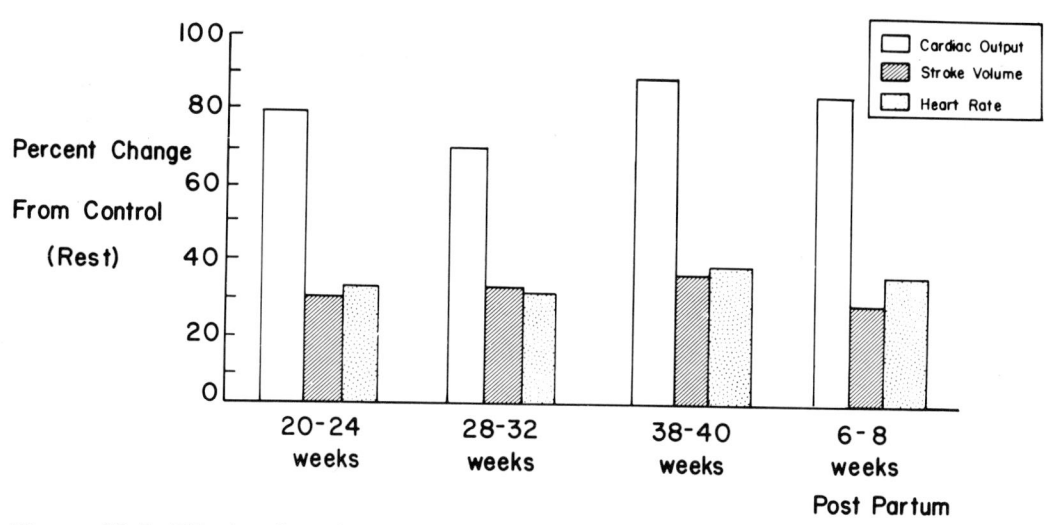

Figure 13.5. Effects of moderate exercise on cardiac output, stroke volume and heart rate during pregnancy. (Redrawn from Ueland K, Novy M, Peterson E, et al. Maternal cardiovascular dynamics. IV. The influence of gestational age on the maternal cardiovascular response to posture and exercise. Am J Obstet Gynecol 104:156, 1969.)

Table 13.2
Pregnant Patients with Rheumatic Heart Disease*

Major Complications	Incidence
	%
Left or right ventricular failure	8.5
Atrial dysrhythmias	6.5
Systemic or pulmonary embolism	1.6
Infective endocarditis	0.4

*Data adapted from Szekely P, Snaith L: *Heart Disease and Pregnancy*. Churchill Livingstone, London, 1974.

patients die in 6 months, 50 per cent in 5 years, 75 per cent in 10 years and 90 per cent in 15 years.[24-27]

Clinical manifestations. The initial symptoms are fatigue and dyspnea on exertion with progression to paroxysmal nocturnal dyspnea, orthopnea and dyspnea at rest. Hemoptysis with rupture of broncho-pulmonary varices and pulmonary or systemic arterial embolization occur infrequently. When mitral stenosis is severe, supraimposition of stresses such as atrial fibrillation, pulmonary embolism, infection or pregnancy may precipitate rapid decompensation.

Physical examination may reveal a presystolic or mid-diastolic murmur which, if faint, will only be heard when the patient lies on her left side. The intensity of the murmur correlates poorly with the degree of stenosis, perhaps because other hemodynamic effects (e.g. depressed cardiac output) reduce flow through the valve. In addition to this murmur an opening snap may be heard at the base of the heart along the left sternal border. Atrial fibrillation occurs in approximately one-third of patients with severe mitral stenosis.

Radiologic studies are normal early in the course of mitral stenosis, but left atrial and right ventricular enlargement occurs as the disease progresses. Severe mitral stenosis may produce generalized pulmonary edema.

The electrocardiogram shows a broadened P-wave in lead V1, signifying left atrial enlargement. Right axis deviation signifies right ventricular enlargement. Cardiac catheterization commonly shows capillary wedge pressures of 25 to 30 mm Hg (normal is 0 to 12 mm Hg) occurring when the mitral valve orifice area is less than 2 cm^2. There is an associated increase in pulmonary vascular resistance. Severe mitral stenosis is consistent with valvular diastolic pressure gradients in excess of 25 mm Hg (normal is 5 mm Hg or less).[18]

Pathophysiology. The decrease in mitral valve orifice area impairs left ventricular filling. Although the left atrium initially may overcome this obstruction, ventricular filling is eventually decreased; left atrial volume and pressure, pulmonary venous pressure and pulmonary capillary wedge pressure then rise. Transudation of fluid into the pulmonary interstitial space occurs, pulmonary compliance decreases and the work of breathing rises, producing progressive dyspnea on exertion. With pulmonary hypertension, pulmonary artery medial thickening and fibrosis result, and pulmonary vascular resistance becomes permanently elevated. Right ventricular hypertrophy, dilation and failure then occur, leading to tricuspid insufficiency with hepatic and peripheral congestion. Atrial fibrillation, tachycardia or increased metabolic demands (e.g. pregnancy and labor) may exacerbate the above processes.[28-30] With pregnancy an anatomically moderate stenosis can become functionally severe.[7] Pregnant patients with mitral stenosis have an increased incidence of pulmonary congestion (25 per cent), atrial fibrillation (7 per cent) and paroxysmal atrial tachycardia (3 per cent).[4] Left ventricular dysfunction is uncommon (15 per cent) with pure mitral stenosis,[18] and its presence suggests an associated element of mitral or aortic insufficiency.

Anesthetic considerations. Asymptomatic patients without evidence of pulmonary congestion have minimally increased risk and do not require additional invasive monitoring but should be attended with caution. On the other hand, patients with marked symptoms may be at significant risk, and radial artery and pulmonary artery monitoring is recommended. The following considerations should be noted (Table 13.3):

1. Neither sinus tachycardia nor atrial fibrillation with a rapid ventricular response is tolerated well. Digoxin therapy used to control atrial fibrillation prior to pregnancy should be continued (with readjustment of dose, if necessary) to maintain ventricular rates below 110 beats per minute (bpm). Development of atrial fibrillation with a rapid ventricular response may dramatically decrease cardiac output and produce pulmonary edema.[27] The treatment is cardioversion starting with 25 watt-seconds of energy. The fetal safety of cardioversion has been documented.[31, 32] If cardioversion is unavailable, or if time (minutes) allows, propranolol 0.2 to 0.5 mg intravenously every 3 minutes may be used to lower the rate below 110 bpm. Propranolol administration should be discontinued when a total dose of 0.1 mg/kg is given or evidence of heart failure occurs (increasing PCW). Digitalization is used in stable situations where prolonged but not immediate (seconds to minutes) ventricular rate control is necessary. Digoxin, 0.50 mg intravenously is given over 10 minutes followed by 0.25 mg intravenously every 2 hours to achieve a full digitalizing dose. Each dose has an effect in 15 minutes with a full effect in 1 to 2 hours.

Sinus tachycardia in excess of 140 bpm

Table 13.3
Mitral Stenosis: Anesthetic Considerations

1. Prevent rapid ventricular rates.
2. Minimize increases in central blood volume.
3. Avoid marked decreases in systemic vascular resistance.
4. Prevent increases in pulmonary artery pressure.

or causing decreased cardiac output or increased PCW should be corrected immediately by reversing a precipitating event (pain, light general anesthesia, hypercarbia, acidosis) or by administering propranolol as described above.

2. Marked increases in central blood volume are poorly tolerated. Overtransfusion, Trendelenburg position, or autotransfusion via uterine contraction can precipitate right heart failure, pulmonary hypertension, pulmonary edema or atrial fibrillation. Increases in CVP or PCW may be used to assess increases in central blood volume.

3. Marked decreases in systemic vascular resistance may not be tolerated. With severe stenosis, decreases in systemic vascular resistance are compensated by increases in heart rate (stroke volume is fixed). This response is limited and marked increases in heart rate may lead to decompensation. The author recommends that, if necessary, systemic vascular resistance be maintained with an intravenous infusion of metaraminol (10 mg in 250 ml of saline). Because ephedrine may increase heart rate, it is not recommended.

4. Exacerbation of pulmonary hypertension and right ventricular failure can be precipitated by multiple factors. Any degree of hypercarbia, hypoxia, acidosis, lung hyperinflation or increased lung water can elevate pulmonary vascular resistance. If pulmonary hypertension and right ventricular compromise persist, inotropic support with dopamine (3 to 8 $\mu g/kg/min$) and pulmonary vasodilation with low-dose sodium nitroprusside (0.1 to 0.5 $\mu g/kg/min$) are recommended. Higher doses of nitroprusside may produce undesirable vasodilation and elevated maternal and fetal cyanide levels (see final section). Prolonged mechanical ventilation may be required if hemodynamic or pulmonary complications occur.

Anesthesia for vaginal delivery and cesarean section. The author recommends segmental lumbar epidural anesthesia for labor and vaginal delivery. This eliminates the pain and tachycardia that attend uterine contractions. Perineal analgesia blocks the urge to push and thereby prevents exertion, fatigue and the deleterious effect of a Valsalva maneuver. Fetal descent is accomplished by the uterine contractions per se, and delivery is facilitated with vacuum extraction or outlet forceps. Hypotension may be prevented by continuous left uterine displacement and judicious fluid infusion. Prophylactic ephedrine and rapid hydration should be avoided. If hypotension occurs metaraminol is the preferred vasopressor.

Either regional or general anesthesia may be used for cesarean section. A continuous lumbar epidural block is preferred to spinal anesthesia because epidural anesthesia produces more controllable hemodynamic changes. The anesthetic level should be established slowly by titration of local anesthetic through the epidural catheter. Epinephrine is omitted from the local anesthetic because of the potential for tachycardia and peripheral vasodilation.

As with regional anesthesia for vaginal delivery, a blood pressure reduction associated with decreased pulmonary capillary wedge pressure may be cautiously treated with fluid infusion to re-establish normal filling pressures. If pulmonary capillary wedge pressure remains normal or if pulmonary artery monitoring is not possible, hypotension should be corrected by infusion of metaraminol.

If general anesthesia is used, drugs which produce tachycardia, such as atropine, pancuronium, meperidine and ketamine, should be avoided. Patients with mild disease may be managed with an intravenous thiopental induction, intubation and light general anesthesia. Those with moderate or severe stenosis may be unduly stressed by this regime and a slow induction with halothane or intravenous fentanyl is recommended. If significant right or left ventricular compromise exists, fentanyl is preferred to halothane. With either technique tachycardia may follow endotracheal intubation or surgical incision; it should be treated by increasing the anesthetic depth or with propranolol. A halothane or fentanyl induction increases the risk of maternal aspiration or neonatal depression, but the author believes that the benefits outweigh these hazards.

Mitral stenosis may produce pulmonary dysfunction. The usual assessment of respiratory adequacy (arterial blood gases, pulmonary mechanics, chest roentgenogram) must be made on weaning from controlled ventilation. Intensive care unit monitoring in the post-operative period may be necessary.

Mitral Insufficiency

Mitral insufficiency is the second most common valvular defect in pregnancy.[4, 22] Left ventricular volume work is chronically increased. This is usually tolerated well, and patients with insufficiency may remain asymptomatic for 30 to 40 years. However, congestive failure follows, and with symptoms, a rapid downhill course occurs with a 5-year mortality rate of 50 per cent. Other complications occurring during the fourth or fifth decade are atrial fibrillation, systemic embolization and bacterial endocarditis.[22, 33, 34]

Because complications usually occur late in life—after the childbearing age—most patients with mitral regurgitation tolerate pregnancy well. However, Szekely and Snaith[4] reported a 5.5 per cent incidence of pulmonary congestion during pregnancy. In addition, they reported a 4.3 per cent incidence of atrial tachycardia, a 2.8 per cent incidence of pulmonary embolism and an 8.5 per cent incidence of infective endocarditis.

Clinical manifestations. The principal symptoms of advanced mitral insufficiency are those of left ventricular failure. The cardinal sign is a pansystolic murmur of blowing quality, loudest at the cardiac apex, referred to the left axilla or the infrascapular area. Atrial fibrillation occurs in approximately one-third of patients. With mild mitral insufficiency the electrocardiogram is normal, but advanced mitral insufficiency produces signs of left ventricular hypertrophy and, at times, right ventricular hypertrophy. Roentgenographic findings in mild mitral insufficiency are normal. However, severe mitral insufficiency causes left ventricular and especially left atrial enlargement. Late sequellae associated with mitral insufficiency include pulmonary congestion, pulmonary hypertension and right ventricular enlargement.[18, 22]

Pathophysiology. With mitral insufficiency there is regurgitation of blood from the left ventricle through the incompetent mitral valve into the left atrium. With chronic mitral insufficiency, the left atrium adapts to this increased blood volume by dilating and increasing its compliance. When left atrial pressure rises, pulmonary venous and pulmonary capillary wedge pressures also rise, causing pulmonary congestion and edema. With progressive left ventricular failure, pulmonary hypertension and right ventricular compromise will occur. Left atrial pressure does not increase until late in the course of the disease; thus, the left atrium protects the pulmonary venous, capillary and arterial beds from pressure overload. Left ventricular dilation occurs as well because of the increase in preload afforded by the hypervolemic left atrium. Forward ejection of blood through the aortic valve can be impaired by as much as 50 to 60 per cent and depends on the ratio of resistance through the aortic valve to that through the insufficient mitral valve. Reduction of left ventricular afterload can then play an important role in decreasing the amount of regurgitant blood flow and increasing forward cardiac output.

The chronically compromised left ventricle may not tolerate the increase in intravascular volume associated with pregnancy, and pulmonary congestion may occur.[35] Changes in systemic resistance may play an important role. The decreased peripheral resistance of pregnancy may improve forward flow at the expense of regurgitant flow.[36] In contrast, pain, apprehension, uterine contractions or surgical stimulation associated with labor and delivery may increase systemic vascular resistance by augmenting sympathetic activity. The resultant decrease in forward flow and increase in regurgitant flow may precipitate acute left ventricular failure and pulmonary congestion.[35] It should be noted that the murmurs of mitral and aortic insufficiency may decrease during pregnancy.[37]

Anesthetic considerations. Asymptomatic patients with mild mitral insufficiency and an unchanging murmur throughout pregnancy may be approached in a routine but cautious fashion. In symptomatic patients radial artery and pulmonary artery monitoring is desirable. Table 13.4 gives the principal anesthetic considerations.

1. Large increases in systemic vascular resistance can cause acute decompensation of the left ventricle. Treatment consists of left ventricular afterload reduction with low doses of sodium nitroprusside (0.1 to 0.5 µg/kg/min) or phentolamine (0.1 to 1.0 µg/kg/min).

2. Myocardial depressants are not well tolerated. Because left ventricular impairment usually accompanies mitral insufficiency, even minimal myocardial depression may result in significant compromise.

3. Atrial fibrillation can cause left ventricular decompensation. The preferred treatment is direct current countershock as outlined in the section on mitral stenosis.

4. Bradycardia is not tolerated well. Forward stroke volume may be limited, and cardiac output will principally depend on heart rate. Maintenance of normal to slightly elevated heart rates is advocated.

5. The amount of regurgitant flow correlates with: (1) the intensity of the insufficiency murmur and (2) the size of the v-wave in the pulmonary capillary wedge pressure tracing. Both can be useful parameters in assessing the amount of ventricular failure with chronic insufficiency. Pulmonary capillary wedge pressure is a poor measure of left atrial volume or left ventricular end-diastolic volume since the left atrium is very compliant. However, minor changes in pressure indicate changes in left ventricular end-diastolic volume. On the other hand, with acute mitral insufficiency, the left atrium will be less compliant, and changes in pulmonary capillary wedge pressures correlate with changes in left atrial and left ventricular end-diastolic pressures. The anesthetic considerations in regard to pulmonary hypertension and right ventricular compromise are delineated in the section on mitral stenosis and apply here as well.

6. Afterload reduction may be useful therapy. Left ventricular failure may benefit from afterload reduction with small amounts of sodium nitroprusside or phentolamine, combined with dopamine to give left ventricular inotropic support.

Anesthesia for vaginal delivery and cesarean section. For labor and vaginal delivery, lumbar epidural analgesia is recommended. This technique will prevent the peripheral vasoconstriction associated

Table 13.4
Mitral Insufficiency: Anesthetic Considerations

---

1. Prevent peripheral vasoconstriction.
2. Avoid myocardial depressants.
3. Treat acute atrial fibrillation immediately.
4. Maintain a normal or slightly elevated heart rate.
5. Monitor pulmonary capillary wedge pressure and intensity of murmur.

---

with the pain of labor and will increase the forward flow of blood. This latter advantage also applies to regional versus general anesthesia for cesarean section. However, regional anesthesia will increase venous capacitance and may require administration of intravenous fluids to maintain the filling volume of the enlarged left ventricle. Constant left uterine displacement and a 10° Trendelenburg position should be used to maintain venous return. The positive inotropic and chronotropic effects of ephedrine are especially useful in preventing and treating hypotension.

Nitrous oxide-relaxant anesthesia may be dangerous because of the associated peripheral vasoconstriction. However, when combined with sodium nitroprusside to prevent peripheral vasoconstriction, this technique may be useful in patients with compromised ventricular function, because this approach avoids myocardial depression and maintains an elevated heart rate. However, in patients without severe ventricular compromise, halothane or enflurane may be added to the nitrous oxide.

Aortic Insufficiency

A 7- to 10-year latent period after an acute attack of rheumatic fever usually precedes the development of aortic regurgitation with associated widened pulse pressure, decreased systemic diastolic pressure and bounding peripheral pulses.[18, 22] The disease usually remains asymptomatic for another 7 to 10 years. Patients presenting with (1) left ventricular enlargement, (2) electrocardiographic evidence of ventricular hypertrophy and (3) a large peripheral pulse pressure have a 33 per cent chance of developing heart failure, angina or death within 1 year, 50 per cent within 2 years, 65 per cent within 3 years and 87 per cent within 6 years.[22] Patients with one or two of these signs have a 10 per cent chance of developing heart failure, angina or death over a 10-year period, and patients with none of these signs have uneventful courses over the same period.[17, 18, 20]

Because symptoms usually develop during the fourth or fifth decades of life, most patients with dominant aortic insufficiency have uneventful pregnancies. However, heart failure complicates 3 to 9 per cent of such patients during pregnancy.[1, 4, 7, 38]

Clinical manifestations. The symptoms of aortic insufficiency relate to left ventricular failure. Moderately severe insufficiency produces a widened pulse pressure with diastolic blood pressures below 60 mm Hg.[17, 18, 22] Systolic pressure is commonly less than 160 mm Hg. An early blowing diastolic murmur is usually heard along the left sternal border in the second, third or fourth intercostal space. Duration of the diastolic murmur depends on the severity of aortic insufficiency. The electrocardiogram in severe insufficiency displays increased QRS amplitude, depressed ST segments, inverted T-waves and a horizontal axis. Atrial fibrillation suggests concomitant mitral valve disease or myocardial failure with moderately severe aortic insufficiency. Chest roentgenogram will reveal left ventricular dilation.

Pathophysiology. With aortic insufficiency left ventricular volume overload occurs. This volume depends on the area of the regurgitation orifice, the diastolic pressure gradient between aorta and left ventricle and the duration of diastole.[39] With chronic volume overload, the left ventricle becomes eccentrically distended and compliance increases. Left ventricular end-diastolic pressure remains normal for several years. The left ventricle usually tolerates this chronic increase in left ventricular volume work and can become markedly distended without evidencing cardiac failure. However, once failure begins, forward stroke volume decreases, end-diastolic volume precipitously increases and left ventricular end-diastolic pressure rises above normal. Pulmonary capillary congestion and signs of pulmonary edema follow.[18, 40]

The decrease in systemic vascular resistance and the increase in heart rate during pregnancy may reduce both the regurgitant flow and the intensity of the murmur of insufficiency.[37, 41] On the other hand, the increase in intravascular volume seen throughout pregnancy and the increases in systemic vascular resistance with the stress of labor and delivery can lead to left ventricular dysfunction.

Anesthetic considerations. Asymptomatic patients without signs of pulmonary congestion have minimally increased risk. Symptomatic patients with an increased murmur intensity, decreased diastolic blood pressure, increased peripheral pulse pressure or signs of pulmonary congestion are at increased risk and may benefit from radial artery and pulmonary artery catheterization. The following should be considered (Table 13.5):

1. *Systemic vascular resistance increases can precipitate left heart failure.* This should be corrected by titration with a vasodilator such as sodium nitroprusside or phentolamine. Usually, less than 0.5 μg/kg/minute of nitroprusside is necessary.

2. *Bradycardia is poorly tolerated.* Bradycardia increases the duration of ventricular diastole and, consequently, the amount of blood regurgitated across the aortic valve. Heart rates should be maintained between 80 and 100 bpm.

Table 13.5
Aortic Insufficiency: Anesthetic Considerations

1. Avoid marked increases in systemic vascular resistance.
2. Maintain a normal or slightly elevated heart rate.
3. Avoid myocardial depressants.
4. Monitor arterial diastolic pressure, pulmonary capillary wedge pressure and intensity of murmur.

3. *Myocardial depressants exacerbate left ventricular failure.* Aortic insufficiency usually produces left ventricular impairment. If myocardial reserve is small, minimal myocardial depression may result in failure.

4. *Decreasing diastolic blood pressure, increasing arterial pulse pressure or increasing intensity or duration of the aortic murmur indicate left ventricular compromise.* Pulmonary capillary wedge pressure elevation is a late sign, and even small elevations may suggest significant left ventricular failure.

5. *Afterload reduction may be useful therapy.* Left ventricular failure may benefit from afterload reduction with small amounts of sodium nitroprusside or phentolamine, combined with dopamine to give left ventricular inotropic support.

Anesthesia for vaginal delivery and cesarean section. For aortic insufficiency the anesthetic management is comparable to that of mitral insufficiency. (See preceding section.) Continuous lumbar epidural analgesia will prevent peripheral vasoconstriction and is recommended for vaginal delivery. For cesarean section regional or general anesthesia, as previously described, may be used.

Aortic Stenosis

Aortic stenosis appears as the dominant valve lesion in 0.5 to 3 per cent of parturients.[1, 4, 7, 38] This relative rarity results from the 35- to 40-year latent period between acute rheumatic fever and symptoms of severe stenosis: congestive failure, syncope and angina. Most patients become symptomatic in their fifth or sixth decade.[42] Progressive decompensation follows the appearance of symptoms, with a 50 per cent mortality within 5 years. Sudden death occurs in 3 to 10 per cent of these patients.[17, 18, 22, 43] Asymptomatic pregnant patients with aortic stenosis are not at increased risk,[4] although they have reduced hemodynamic responses to the demands of pregnancy and exercise.[44] Symptomatic aortic stenosis markedly increases maternal and fetal morbidity and mortality.[1, 4, 7]

Clinical manifestations. The cross-sectional area of the aortic valve orifice in normal adults is 2.6 to 3.5 cm^2.[45] A 25 to 50 per cent decrease in area results in a loud aortic systolic murmur. Narrowing to less than 1 cm^2 markedly increases left ventricular end-diastolic pressures. Areas below 0.75 cm produce exertional dyspnea, angina pectoris and syncope.[18, 45, 46] The principal physical finding is a systolic ejection murmur loudest in the second right intercostal space adjacent to the sternum and radiating into the neck. Intensity of the murmur may not correlate with the degree of stenosis. A low cardiac output or decreased velocity of ejection decreases the intensity of the murmur. The electrocardiogram in severe aortic stenosis shows left ventricular hypertrophy and occasionally a left bundle branch block. Radiographs may show left ventricular enlargement, post-stenotic dilation of the aorta and, in older adults, calcification of the aortic valve. Catheterization findings are usually normal when the aortic valve orifice area exceeds 1 cm^2. Smaller areas usually produce a systolic pressure gradient between the aorta and left ventricle. A gradient of 50 mm Hg or more indicates severe stenosis, except in patients with congestive heart failure where reduced left ventricular stroke volume may produce only 30 mm Hg gradients even with severe aortic stenosis.[17, 18]

Anesthetic considerations. The appearance of symptoms, evidence of left ventricular failure or progression of stenosis suggest monitoring via radial artery and pulmonary artery catheters. The following considerations should be noted (Table 13.6):

1. Decreases in systemic vascular resistance are poorly tolerated. In normal patients increases in stroke volume and heart rate usually compensate for a decrease in systemic vascular resistance. Aortic stenosis relatively fixes stroke volume, and patients with stenosis must rely on elevation of heart rate to maintain blood pressure. However, elevations of heart rate above 140 bpm will decrease diastolic filling and cardiac output. Vascular resistance should be maintained during anesthesia by using light levels or by using a vasoconstrictor (e.g. metaraminol).

2. Bradycardia is poorly tolerated for the reasons outlined above.

3. Decreases in venous return and left ventricular filling are poorly tolerated. Because of the increased and fixed afterload, left ventricular stroke volume will be maintained only if the end-diastolic volume is adequate. Marked decreases in ventricular filling will decrease stroke volume and cardiac output.

Anesthesia for vaginal delivery and cesarean section. These patients usually tolerate the hemodynamic effects of pain and stress. When possible avoid sympathetic blockade; if regional anesthesia is necessary, a gradually administered continuous epidural technique is indicated. Because hypotension is poorly tolerated, maternal blood pressure should be sustained with left uterine displacement, fluids and metaraminol or ephedrine. For labor and vaginal delivery, systemic medication, inhalation analgesia and pudendal nerve block anesthesia are suggested. For cesarean section, general anesthesia with the standard nitrous oxide-relaxant technique is recommended. Halogenated anesthetics, with their potential for undue myocardial de-

Table 13.6
Aortic Stenosis: Anesthetic Considerations

1. Avoid decreases in systemic vascular resistance.
2. Avoid bradycardia.
3. Maintain venous return and left ventricular filling.

pression, should be avoided when evidence of severe left ventricular compromise exists. Signs or symptoms of ventricular ischemia associated with hypotension indicate the need to elevate or maintain systemic vascular resistance with metaraminol.

CONGENITAL HEART DISEASE

The major categories of congenital heart disease are: left-to-right shunt (ventricular septal defect, atrial septal defect, patent ductus arteriosus), right-to-left shunt (tetralogy of Fallot, Eisenmenger's syndrome) and congenital valvular and vascular lesions (coarctation of the aorta, aortic stenosis, pulmonary stenosis).

Left-to-Right Shunt

VENTRICULAR SEPTAL DEFECT

Ventricular septal defect (VSD) occurs in 7 per cent of adults with congenital heart disease. The size of the VSD and the degree of pulmonary hypertension determine the course of patients with VSD.[9, 18, 48] The VSD in most adult patients is small, with a minimal left-to-right shunt, insignificant pulmonary hypertension and no symptoms. Pregnancy is usually uneventful[9] but rarely may be complicated by bacterial endocarditis or congestive heart failure.[9, 38, 49]

The few patients with uncorrected large VSD's usually display growth retardation, recurrent respiratory infection, pulmonary hypertension, and left and right ventricular compromise.[50] Their mortality during pregnancy is between 7 and 40 per cent.[4, 7, 51-53] Severe right ventricular failure with shunt reversal (Eisenmenger's syndrome) is the major complication. Operative correction of the VSD before pregnancy does not increase maternal or fetal morbidity or mortality during pregnancy.[4, 9, 54]

Clinical manifestations. A small VSD produces a mild pansystolic murmur in the fourth or fifth left intercostal space, a normal chest roentgenogram and a right bundle branch pattern on the electrocardiogram. Intracardiac pressures are normal with minimal left-to-right shunting. A moderate to large VSD produces loud pansystolic murmurs with expiratory splitting of the second heart sound and evidence of left ventricular enlargement. Eventually, right ventricular enlargement occurs. Right ventricle oxygen saturation is increased as a result of the left-to-right shunt. Right ventricular end-diastolic pressure, pulmonary artery pressure and left ventricular end-diastolic pressure are increased. A moderate VSD usually decreases pulmonary vascular resistance; a large VSD usually increases it. Prolonged elevation of pulmonary vascular resistance causes bi-directional and eventually right-to-left shunting with concomitant cyanosis and clubbing.

Pathophysiology. The left-to-right shunt associated with a small VSD initially increases pulmonary blood flow and secondarily decreases pulmonary vascular resistance, thus preserving normal pulmonary artery pressures. The increase in left ventricular volume work is well tolerated. With a larger VSD, the greater left-to-right shunt markedly increases pulmonary blood flow, but pulmonary vascular resistance cannot compensate for this increased flow and pulmonary hypertension develops. The increase in left ventricular volume work leads to left ventricular dysfunction, elevation of pulmonary capillary wedge pressure and exacerbation of the pulmonary hypertension. Right ventricular failure follows, with eventual equalization of right and left ventricular pressures, and bi-directional or reverse shunting with peripheral cyanosis follows.[52, 53]

With pregnancy, elevations in heart rate, cardiac output and intravascular volume may increase the left-to-right shunt, exacerbate pulmonary hypertension and cause left and right ventricular failure. Elevation of vascular resistance with stress associated with labor and surgical stimulus increases right and left ventricular dysfunction. Bi-directional shunting or right-to-left shunting may result. If right ventricular afterload is increased as much as left afterload is increased, then there may be no increase in shunting.

Anesthetic considerations. A small VSD in an asymptomatic patient with normal ventricular function does not require specialized monitoring. Symptoms, abnormal ventricular function or a large VSD indicate monitoring via radial and pulmonary artery catheters. The following should be considered (Table 13.7):

1. Systemic vascular resistance increases may not be tolerated.

2. Marked increases in heart rate are poorly tolerated. An increased systemic vascular resistance or heart rate may increase the left-to-right shunt. Pulmonary hypertension and ventricular failure may follow. Therefore, adequate anesthesia is essential to prevent the sympathetic response that attends pain during labor and delivery, endotracheal intubation and surgical stimulation. Vasodilation with low doses of sodium nitroprusside or phentolamine (0.1 to 0.5 μg/kg/min) may be needed to reduce shunting and improve cardiac output.

3. With pulmonary hypertension and right ventricular compromise, marked decreases in systemic vascular resistance may not be well tolerated. With a marked decrease in systemic vascular resistance, a right-to-left shunt and hypoxia will occur. Pressure decreases consequent to regional anesthesia should be corrected.

4. Factors which increase pulmonary vascular resistance should be avoided in patients with pulmonary hypertension and evidence of right ventricular compromise. These factors are discussed in the sections on mitral stenosis and primary pulmonary hypertension.

Anesthesia for vaginal delivery and cesarean section. For labor and vaginal delivery continuous lumbar epidural anesthesia permits control of systemic resistance and painful stimuli. For cesarean section, either regional or general anesthesia may be used. If regional anesthesia is selected, a continuous lumbar epidural technique will ensure slower changes in systemic resistance and allow more time for correction of pressure changes. General anesthesia which combines inhalation and narcotic techniques may best minimize increases in systemic vascular resistance and myocardial depression. Addition of a vasodilator may be necessary.

Peripheral cyanosis in the presence of an elevated cardiac output indicates an imbalance between the pulmonary and systemic resistances with right-to-left shunt as the most probable cause. One hundred per cent oxygen should be delivered. The systemic vascular resistance should be increased by lightening anesthesia or by administering small amounts of metaraminol. Peripheral cyanosis associated with a depressed cardiac output indicates right and/or left ventricular failure. Therapy includes an increase in oxygen delivery, withdrawal of anesthesia and use of an inotrope such as dopamine.

ATRIAL SEPTAL DEFECT

Atrial septal defect (ASD) occurs in 17.5 per cent of adults with congenital heart disease and is the most common congenital

Table 13.7
Anesthetic Considerations: Ventricular Septal Defect

1. Avoid marked increases in systemic vascular resistance.
2. Avoid marked increases in heart rate.
3. With pulmonary hypertension, avoid marked decreases in systemic vascular resistance.
4. With pulmonary hypertension, avoid marked increases in pulmonary vascular resistance.

heart lesion.[4, 9, 50, 55] ASD is consistent with prolonged longevity.[8, 49] Cardiac dysrhythmia, pulmonary hypertension, right ventricular failure and left ventricular failure are commonly not seen until the fourth or fifth decades. Most women with uncorrected ASD tolerate pregnancy well, even when pulmonary blood flow is increased.[4, 9] However, the risk of left ventricular failure during pregnancy is increased.[1, 7, 56] Maternal and fetal mortality range between 1 and 12 per cent.[1, 4, 7, 56, 57]

Clinical manifestations. Physical examination reveals fixed expiratory splitting of the second heart sound and a systolic ejection murmur at the upper left sternal border whose intensity varies with the degree of left-to-right shunt.[18] The electrocardiogram usually exhibits right axis deviation with an osteum secundum defect. Chest roentgenogram may show right heart enlargement, pulmonary artery prominence and increased pulmonary vascular markings. Cardiac catheterization of the parturient usually reveals normal pulmonary artery, right ventricular and right atrial pressures even with moderate right ventricular dilation.

Pathophysiology. The left-to-right shunting increases right ventricular preload, right ventricular volume work and pulmonary blood flow. However, a compensatory decrease in pulmonary vascular resistance keeps pulmonary artery pressures normal until the fourth or fifth decade. The increase in right and left atrial blood volume eventually causes right and left atrial distension and associated supraventricular dysrhythmias, particularly atrial fibrillation. The chronically elevated pulmonary blood flow causes pulmonary vascular changes, leading to increased pulmonary vascular resistance, and pulmonary hypertension. Right ventricular failure may occur with prolonged increase in volume work, particularly when pressure work increases secondary to pulmonary hypertension.

Pregnancy accelerates these changes by increasing blood volume and cardiac output with consequent increases in left-to-right shunt, right ventricular volume work, pulmonary blood flow and left ventricular volume work. Pulmonary hypertension and right and left ventricular dysfunction may follow. Left atrial distension may precipitate supraventricular dysrhythmias. Supraventricular dysrhythmias are particularly hazardous because incomplete emptying of the left atrium occurs and left atrial volume and pressure increase and exacerbate the left-to-right shunt.

Anesthetic considerations. Most asymptomatic patients without evidence of pulmonary hypertension or right ventricular compromise do not require unusual care. Symptoms, pulmonary hypertension or right ventricular failure indicate radial artery, pulmonary artery and right atrial pressure monitoring. The following considerations should be noted (Table 13.8):

1. Supraventricular dysrhythmias are poorly tolerated and may increase left-to-right shunt. Medications (digoxin, quinidine, etc.) given to control chronic supraventricular dysrhythmias should be continued and adjusted throughout pregnancy and the puerperium. The acute onset of supraventricular dysrhythmias should be treated with direct current cardioversion or propranolol if right ventricular failure or systemic hypotension occur. Digitalization is recommended if these complications are absent.

2. Increased systemic vascular resistance may not be tolerated.

3. Marked decreases in pulmonary vascular resistance are poorly tolerated. An increase in peripheral resistance or a decrease in pulmonary resistance may increase the left-to-right shunt and cause systemic hypotension.

4. Increases in pulmonary vascular resistance exacerbate pre-existing pulmonary hypertension, and right ventricular failure may occur.

Table 13.8
Anesthetic Considerations: Atrial Septal Defect

1. Prevent or immediately treat supraventricular dysrhythmias.
2. Avoid increases in systemic vascular resistance.
3. Avoid decreases in pulmonary vascular resistance.
4. With pulmonary hypertension, avoid further increases in pulmonary vascular resistance.

Anesthesia for vaginal delivery and cesarean section. For labor, vaginal delivery and cesarean section segmental continuous lumbar epidural anesthesia avoids the hazard of increases in systemic vascular resistance. General anesthesia may be used if the above considerations are borne in mind.

PATENT DUCTUS ARTERIOSUS

Patent ductus arteriosus (PDA) constitutes 15 per cent of all congenital heart disease.[4] Early surgical intervention presently makes this a rarely significant finding during pregnancy. Patients with a small ductus usually have a benign clinical course until the fourth or fifth decade of life, when left or right ventricular failure may occur. However, a ductus of large internal diameter (greater than 1 cm) may produce growth retardation, respiratory infection, congestive heart failure and pulmonary hypertension during childhood and early adult life. Even without congestive heart failure prior to pregnancy, maternal mortality from ventricular failure is 5 to 6 per cent in un-operated pregnant patients.[4, 9]

Clinical manifestations. A patent ductus arteriosus produces a continuous murmur, enveloping the second heart sound with late systolic accentuation, terminating in late or mid-diastole, and radiating to the first left intercostal space. A large ductus enlarges the left ventricle and widens the arterial pulse pressure. The electrocardiogram can be normal (with a small ductus) or demonstrate left or right ventricular hypertrophy (with a large ductus). The chest roentgenogram can appear normal (with a small ductus) or can demonstrate left ventricular, left atrial or pulmonary artery enlargement. Right ventricular enlargement is seen with severe pulmonary hypertension.

Pathophysiology. The left-to-right shunt of aortic blood via the ductus to the pulmonary artery increases central circulatory flow at the expense of peripheral flow. Both length and cross-section of the ductus determine resistance to flow and hence the amount of left-to-right shunt. A small internal diameter (less than 1 cm) generally permits a small left-to-right flow. A secondary decrease in pulmonary vascular resistance prevents the increase in pulmonary artery flow from producing pulmonary hypertension. Both the left and right ventricles tolerate this small increase in flow.

A ductus with a moderate internal diameter (1 to 2 cm) permits a significant increase in pulmonary blood flow. Pulmonary hypertension ultimately results from the inability of the pulmonary vasculature to compensate for the increased flow. Left ventricular volume work is increased, and left ventricular failure eventually ensues. With failure, elevation of left ventricular end-diastolic pressure further exacerbates the pulmonary hypertension. Progressive medial hypertrophy and intimal fibrosis increase pulmonary resistance, and right ventricular failure follows.

A large internal diameter (greater than 2 cm) telescopes the temporal development of the above changes. Severe pulmonary hypertension with right ventricular failure may eventually produce a right-to-left shunt and peripheral cyanosis (Eisenmenger's syndrome).

The increased intravascular volume associated with pregnancy can increase shunting, pulmonary hypertension and left ventricular volume work. In addition, the increased heart rate and stroke volume will increase myocardial oxygen demand and may compromise left ventricular function during stressful periods, such as uterine contractions. The decrease in systemic vascular resistance, seen throughout pregnancy and particularly during the postpartum period, can lead to shunt reversal and cyanosis, particularly in patients with a large ductus.

Anesthetic considerations. Asymptomatic patients with normal hemodynamics and no evidence of ventricular dysfunction do not require unusual care. Evidence of left ventricular failure, pulmonary hypertension, right ventricular failure, or reversal of the left-to-right shunt indicates monitoring via an arterial line and a pulmonary artery catheter with the following considerations noted (Table 13.9):

1. Increases in systemic vascular resistance may not be tolerated. Proportionate increases in pulmonary vascular resistance may not occur and left-to-right shunt may increase.

2. Marked increases in blood volume may be poorly tolerated. Acute hypervolemia may precipitate failure by increasing left ventricular volume work and oxygen consumption.

3. Marked decreases in systemic vascular resistance or increases in pulmonary resistance may lead to reverse shunting in patients with pre-existing pulmonary hypertension and right ventricular compromise. See the section on Eisenmenger's syndrome.

4. Patients with left ventricular failure may not tolerate additional myocardial depression.

Anesthesia for vaginal delivery and cesarean section. Use of a continuous epidural technique for labor, vaginal delivery and cesarean section prevents increases in systemic vascular resistance associated with pain. In addition, decreases in systemic vascular resistance may reduce left-to-right shunt. If general anesthesia is selected for cesarean section, increases in systemic vascular resistance should be rapidly treated by deepening anesthesia or use of a vasodilating agent such as sodium nitroprusside or phentolamine.

Right-to-Left Shunt

TETRALOGY OF FALLOT

Tetralogy of Fallot constitutes 15 per cent of all congenital heart disease and is the most common cyanotic congenital heart disease.[18, 55] This anomaly is characterized by right ventricular outflow obstruction, VSD, right ventricular hypertrophy and overriding aorta. In the past, few women demonstrated tetralogy of Fallot during pregnancy, because most died before the childbearing age. However, antibiotic therapy and palliative or corrective surgery have increased the number of parturients presenting with corrected or uncorrected tetralogy of Fallot.[9, 50, 55]

Pregnancy increases the morbidity and mortality of uncorrected tetralogy of Fallot, particularly in patients with a history of syncope, polycythemia, decreased arterial oxygen saturation (less than 80 per cent) and right ventricular hypertension.[1, 5, 7, 52, 58–60] Left heart failure, bacterial endocarditis and cerebral thrombosis are increased. Most complications develop immediately postpartum when systemic vascular resistance is lowest, thereby exacerbating the right-to-left shunt. In partu-

Table 13.9
Anesthetic Considerations: Patent Ductus Arteriosus

1. Avoid increases in systemic vascular resistance.
2. Avoid marked increases in blood volume.
3. With pulmonary hypertension, avoid marked decreases in systemic vascular resistance or increases in pulmonary vascular resistance.
4. With left ventricular failure, avoid myocardial depressants.

rients with uncorrected tetralogy of Fallot 40 per cent suffer from heart failure and 12 per cent die.[1] The fetal death rate is 36 per cent. Patients undergoing pulmonary valvulotomy during pregnancy are not at increased risk, but fetal mortality approaches 50 per cent.[61, 62] Maternal mortality is not increased in patients with a corrected tetralogy of Fallot, but fetal mortality can be as high as 25 per cent.[1, 54, 58]

Clinical manifestations. Uncorrected tetralogy of Fallot causes cyanosis, clubbing and a systolic thrill at the left sternal border near the second or third intercostal space. The degree of pulmonary hypertension and pulmonary blood flow determine the loudness of the thrill. The electrocardiogram suggests right ventricular hypertrophy. Chest roentgenogram demonstrates an enlarged heart but sparse peripheral pulmonary vasculature. Catheterization reveals decreased pulmonary artery pressure and significant right-to-left shunt.

Pathophysiology. The increased resistance to right ventricular outflow promotes right-to-left shunting via the ventricular septal defect. Shunting and, therefore, cyanosis depend on the size of the VSD, the obstruction to outflow from the right ventricle and the ability of the right ventricle to overcome that obstruction. The obstruction may result from a fixed pulmonic stenosis or dynamic infundibular hypertrophy. If infundibular hypertrophy exists, then increases in myocardial contractility or decreases in right ventricular volume may increase outflow obstruction (see the section on asymmetric septal hypertrophy). If significant hypertrophy does not exist, then maintenance of right ventricular contractility is important for preservation of pulmonary blood flow and peripheral oxygenation. Regardless of the type of right ventricular outflow obstruction, decreases in systemic vascular resistance may exacerbate shunting and produce cyanosis.

Labor and postpartum changes may compromise these patients. The stress of labor may increase pulmonary vascular resistance and consequently increase the right-to-left shunt. Decreases in systemic vascular resistance noted throughout pregnancy and after delivery may increase the right-to-left shunt and produce cyanosis. Finally, patients with infundibular obstruction may be particularly at risk during labor, when increases in contractility may be highest.

Anesthetic considerations. If the tetralogy has not been corrected, then special considerations are warranted, including radial artery and central venous pressure monitoring. Patients with corrected tetralogy of Fallot may suffer from residual right ventricular failure and also require special considerations (see the section on primary pulmonary hypertension). In the absence of symptoms or right ventricular compromise the usual anesthetic considerations can be applied. The following considerations should be noted (Table 13.10):

1. Decreases in systemic vascular resistance, blood volume or venous return are not well tolerated. A fall in systemic vascular resistance increases the right-to-left shunt. A fall in blood volume or a decrease in venous return will decrease the ability of the right ventricle to perfuse the lungs. With right ventricular compromise high central blood volumes are necessary for maintenance of right ventricular output.

2. Myocardial depressants may not be well tolerated. In patients with right ventricular compromise, even small amounts of myocardial depression may not be tol-

Table 13.10
Anesthetic Considerations: Tetralogy of Fallot

1. Avoid decreases in systemic vascular resistance.
2. Avoid decreases in blood volume.
3. Avoid decreases in venous return.
4. Avoid myocardial depressants.

erated, and inotropic support with dopamine may be necessary.

Anesthesia for vaginal delivery and cesarean section. For labor and vaginal delivery these patients are likely to be most safely managed with systemic medication, inhalation analgesia, paracervical or pudendal block anesthesia. Epidural or spinal anesthesia should be used with extreme caution. To avoid decreases in systemic vascular resistance and venous return, volume infusion and continuous left uterine displacement are recommended. Ephedrine should be administered cautiously, because it may produce a marked increase in pulmonary vascular resistance.

For cesarean section a general anesthetic technique is preferred. If the patient does not present with infundibular obstruction, light planes of anesthesia should be well tolerated, and nitrous oxide-relaxant (and narcotic after the delivery) may be most efficacious. However, if the patient does present with infundibular stenosis, increases in myocardial contractility or heart rate and decreases in ventricular volume will not be well tolerated, and an inhalation anesthetic, such as halothane or enflurane, might be most efficacious. Maintenance of normal or slightly elevated right ventricular filling pressure and systemic vascular resistance is advocated (see the section on asymmetric septal hypertrophy).

Increasing peripheral cyanosis occurring in patients without infundibular obstruction usually indicates a decrease in systemic vascular resistance or increased right ventricular compromise. Treatment consists of delivering the maximum concentration of oxygen and decreasing the anesthetic depth. Increasing peripheral cyanosis in patients with a history of significant infundibular obstruction is usually precipitated by tachycardia, increased myocardial contractility or decreased right ventricular volume. Treatment consists of increasing the depth of halothane or enflurane anesthesia, increasing venous return and central blood volume and decreasing contractility and heart rate by titration of propranolol.

EISENMENGER'S SYNDROME

Eisenmenger's syndrome consists of pulmonary hypertension and a right-to-left or bi-directional shunt with peripheral cyanosis.[9, 18] The shunt may be atrial, ventricular or aortopulmonary. The incidence of Eisenmenger's syndrome has been reported to be approximately 3 per cent of all patients with congenital heart disease; it is commonly found with left-to-right shunt reversal during the end stages of patent ductus arteriosus, ventricular septal defect and atrial septal defect.[55] Most patients with Eisenmenger's syndrome have a particularly poor prognosis, and survival beyond the age of 40 is uncommon. This condition is not amenable to surgical correction; high pulmonary artery pressures with fixed vascular resistance are not reversed by surgical intervention.[9, 48, 55]

Maternal and fetal prognoses depend on the severity of pulmonary hypertension.[2, 48] Maternal mortality has been reported to be between 12 and 33 per cent and fetal mortality between 30 and 54 per cent.[52, 53, 57, 59]

Clinical manifestations. Clinical manifestations of Eisenmenger's syndrome are dependent on the degree of pulmonary hypertension and right-to-left shunt.[2, 18] The type of murmur detected is a function of the specific right-to-left defect (for example a systolic ejection murmur with ASD, or a holosystolic murmur with VSD). The electrocardiogram usually demonstrates right ventricular hypertrophy with right axis deviation, and the chest roentgenogram usually demonstrates increased pulmonary artery markings with a prominent right ventricle.

Pathophysiology. The degree of right-to-left shunt depends on the severity of pulmonary hypertension and the size of the right-to-left circulatory communication. In addition, the relationship between the pulmonic and systemic vascular resistance plays an important role. Increases in pulmonary vascular resistance or decreases in systemic vascular resistance exacerbate the right-to-left shunt and produce peripheral cyanosis. The third factor which affects the degree of shunt is the contractile state of the right ventricle. Progressive right ventricular dysfunction will decrease pulmonary blood flow and increase shunt.

Pregnancy is not tolerated well. In patients with Eisenmenger's syndrome the typical fall in pulmonary vascular resistance during pregnancy is not seen since the resistance is fixed. However, the decrease in systemic vascular resistance does occur, and, consequently, the right-to-left shunt markedly increases.[7, 52, 63] Increases in heart rate and stroke volume will increase right ventricular oxygen consumption and, in the presence of relatively desaturated blood, may produce right ventricular compromise with increased right-to-left shunt.[18, 63]

Diuresis is usually seen in the post-delivery period and may increase hematocrit and thus decrease blood viscosity and pulmonary blood flow. Adequate crystalloid replacement and maintenance of hematocrit below 55 per cent are advocated.

Anesthetic considerations. All patients with Eisenmenger's syndrome are at markedly increased risk and should be monitored with radial arterial and central venous catheters. The following considerations should be noted (Table 13.11):

1. Decreases in systemic vascular resistance or venous return are not well tolerated. See the section on tetralogy of Fallot.

2. Elevations of pulmonary vascular resistance are not well tolerated. Even minimal hypercarbia, acidosis or hypoxia should be avoided; if they do occur, they should be treated aggressively. See the section on primary pulmonary hypertension.

Anesthesia for vaginal delivery and cesarean section. The anesthetic management of patients with Eisenmenger's syndrome is essentially identical to that previously outlined for patients with tetralogy of Fallot.

Other Congenital Heart Diseases

COARCTATION OF THE AORTA

Coarctation of the aorta represents approximately 8 per cent of all cases of congenital heart disease in adults.[55] The incidence of this disease in the pregnant population has been steadily decreasing, because most cases are surgically corrected in early childhood. With corrected lesions maternal and fetal morbidity and mortality are not increased.[7, 64, 65] The maternal mortality for patients with uncorrected coarctation of the aorta has been reported to be between 3 and 9 per cent, and fetal mortality may be as high as 20 per cent.[4, 7, 64, 65] The incidence of congenital heart disease in the offspring is also elevated and is between 3 and 5 per cent.[4, 9] The principal risks to the mother with coarctation of the aorta are left ventricular failure, aortic rupture and infective endocarditis

Clinical manifestations. Physical examination usually reveals a significant difference in blood pressures obtained in the upper and lower extremities or in the right and left upper extremities. Other findings with significant stenosis include an increase in intensity of the aortic component of the second heart sound, a medium-pitched systolic blowing murmur (heard best between the scapulae), a ventricular heave and a laterally displaced point of

Table 13.11
Anesthetic Considerations: Eisenmenger's Syndrome

1. Avoid decreases in systemic vascular resistance.
2. Avoid decreases in venous return.
3. Avoid increases in pulmonary vascular resistance, e.g. hypercarbia, acidosis, hypoxia.

maximal impulse. Late in the course, the electrocardiogram will demonstrate signs of left ventricular hypertrophy, and the chest roentgenogram will demonstrate left ventricular enlargement and a characteristic "three" sign in the aortic knob. Cardiac catheterization is indicated in complicated cases and is useful in assessing the severity of the disease.

Pathophysiology. Coarctation, like aortic stenosis, represents a fixed obstruction to left ventricular ejection. Thus, stroke volume tends to be limited, and increases in cardiac output are achieved primarily through increases in heart rate. Because of increased left ventricular afterload, ventricular pressure work increases and concentric hypertrophy occurs. Patients with mild coarctation tolerate this well and progression to ventricular dilation and failure occurs late in the course. With severe coarctation these complications will be precipitated much earlier. In addition to these ventricular changes, pathologic changes in the arterial wall at the site of coarctation will occur and serve as the nidus for dissection and rupture.

Both left ventricular compromise and vascular wall damage can be exacerbated by pregnancy. Because stroke volume is limited, the increased intravascular volume and increased metabolic demand seen in pregnancy can be accommodated only by increases in heart rate. During periods of high demand (labor) or acute increases in intravascular volume (uterine contraction), supranormal heart rates may not be able to compensate for limited stroke volume, and left ventricular failure will occur. With respect to vascular wall damage, there is evidence that anatomic changes in the aortic intima and media can be precipitated by pregnancy.[64,65] With increased heart rate and contractility seen with stress, the rate of ejection of blood from the left ventricle will increase and may cause aortic dissection and rupture. Finally, systemic arterial dilation seen during pregnancy and immediately after delivery may not be tolerated because stroke volume is fixed.

Anesthetic considerations. Asymptomatic patients without left ventricular enlargement or dysfunction can be approached in the usual fashion. Other patients may be at markedly increased risk and should be monitored with radial artery and pulmonary artery catheters. The following considerations should be noted (Table 13.12):

1. Decreases in systemic vascular resistance are not well tolerated. Because stroke volume is fixed, compensation for decreases in systemic vascular resistance is limited, and hypotension may result. Maintenance of systemic vascular resistance in a normal to slightly elevated range with either metaraminol or "light" anesthesia is recommended. Particular caution should be given to the period immediately after delivery.

2. Decreases in heart rate are not well tolerated. In the presence of a fixed stroke volume, cardiac output is primarily determined by heart rate. Vagal stimulants, medications or anesthetics which either decrease the heart rate or depress the sinus node should be avoided. Bradycardia should be treated by removing the precipitant cause and, if necessary, administering atropine or isoproterenol.

3. Decreases in left ventricular filling are not well tolerated. In the presence of a fixed obstruction to left ventricular emptying, adequate stroke volume will require high end-diastolic volumes. Venous return must be maintained, hypovolemia avoided and atrial dysrhythmias promptly treated.

Table 13.12
Anesthetic Considerations: Coarctation of the Aorta

1. Avoid decreases in systemic vascular resistance.
2. Avoid bradycardia.
3. Maintain left ventricular filling.

Anesthesia for vaginal delivery and cesarean section. The anesthetic management of these patients is similar to those with rheumatic aortic stenosis as previously described. For vaginal delivery systemic medication, inhalation analgesia or pudendal nerve block are recommended. For cesarean section, light general anesthesia using a nitrous oxide-relaxant technique is advocated. Increased levels of heart rate, contractility and vascular resistance can be maintained with this technique. In addition, if the possibility of aortic dissection exists, the anesthetic considerations listed in the section on dissecting aneurysm of the aorta should be noted.

CONGENITAL AORTIC STENOSIS

Congenital aortic stenosis can be supravalvular, valvular or subvalvular.[66-68] The supravalvular lesion has been described in the maternal rubella syndrome,[69] and the narrowing occurs just distal to the coronary artery orifices. The subvalvular lesion may be diaphragmatic or muscular (such as asymmetric septal hypertrophy). However, the most common valvular form, as well as the most common congenital malformation of the heart, is the bicuspid aortic valve occurring in 1 to 2 per cent of the general population.[70] Unlike the supravalvular and subvalvular forms, the bicuspid form may not become clinically apparent until late in adult life. Studies by Bacon and Matthews[71] suggest that 20 to 30 per cent of patients with a congenitally bicuspid aortic valve eventually develop aortic stenosis, secondary to blood turbulence and fibrin deposition.

Mendelson[1], Ueland[54] and Szekely and Snaith[4] reported on 14 patients with congenital aortic stenosis complicating pregnancy. Ten of 14 pregnancies were uncomplicated. In the other four pregnancies one was terminated because of intractable heart failure, and three required aortic valvulotomy during pregnancy. Of these three patients, one had an uncomplicated postoperative course and an uneventful delivery, one had a miscarriage 10 days after operation, and the third patient delivered a child with congenital abnormalities who died at the age of 4 months. Thus, with congenital aortic stenosis, as with rheumatic aortic stenosis, the maternal morbidity and fetal mortality seem to be increased.

Aside from asymmetric septal hypertrophy (which is discussed later in this chapter), the pathophysiology and anesthetic considerations of congenital aortic stenosis are similar to those already described for rheumatic aortic stenosis (Table 13.6).

CONGENITAL PULMONIC STENOSIS

Isolated pulmonic stenosis constitutes approximately 13 per cent of all congenital heart disease.[55] The lesion may be valvular or subvalvular (infundibular stenosis).[72] The valvular lesion is usually non-progressive until late in adult life.[18] However, the subvalvular lesion, which has a different pathophysiology, can be progressive. The considerations for patients with subvalvular stenosis will be discussed in the section on asymmetric septal hypertrophy. Only valvular stenosis will be discussed here.

Mendelson[1] and Szekely and Snaith[4] reviewed a total of 71 patients with isolated pulmonic stenosis during pregnancy. There were no maternal deaths; however five of the 71 pregnancies were complicated by right heart failure, and there were three fetal deaths.

Clinical manifestations. In patients with severe right heart failure, decreased left ventricular output occurs and the symptoms of fatigue and syncope result. Auscultation reveals a pulmonic ejection click following the first heart sound and a systolic ejection murmur in the second left intercostal space. With increasing severity of pulmonic stenosis, the murmur has an increased duration and a late systolic accentuation; in addition, the pulmonic component of the second heart sound is delayed, with an expiratory splitting of the second heart sound. In mild pulmonic stenosis the electrocardiogram usually reveals a right bundle branch block. With severe stenosis, a predominant R-wave is seen in lead V1 which usually exceeds 20 mm in height[73]; it is usually correlated with a right ventricular systolic pressure of at least 80 mm Hg.[74] Right ventricular strain manifested by negative T-waves in the right precordial leads may occur as well. The characteristic radiologic finding is prominence of the left pulmonary artery. With severe stenosis right ventricular and atrial enlargement are usually seen

Pathophysiology. With progressive stenosis of the right ventricular outflow tract, pressure work increases and concentric hypertrophy occurs. The right ventricle seems to adapt readily to this situation. Right ventricular output is maintained until late in the course of the disease, notably when right ventricular systolic pressure exceeds approximately 80 mm Hg.[75] As right ventricular output decreases so does left ventricular preload and, therefore, cardiac output. Systemic vascular resistance increases in an effort to compensate for the decreased left ventricular output. However, as right ventricular failure progresses, further decreases in cardiac output are uncompensated, and symptoms of low cardiac output—such as fatigue and syncope—occur with exercise and later at rest.

Although patients with isolated pulmonary valvular stenosis have uneventful courses until late in life[18]—that is, after the childbearing years—their course may become complicated during the stressful periods of pregnancy, labor and delivery.[1,4] Right ventricular failure can be precipitated during pregnancy by both the increase in intravascular volume (increasing right ventricular preload, stroke work and oxygen consumption) and the increase in heart rate (increasing oxygen consumption). Furthermore, the decrease in systemic vascular resistance, which is usually seen during pregnancy, and especially after delivery, may counteract an important compensatory mechanism needed during low right ventricular output states.

Anesthetic considerations. Patients who are asymptomatic without progression of right ventricular compromise may be approached in the usual manner. Otherwise, radial artery and central venous pressure monitoring is advocated. The first sign of impending right ventricular failure may be subtle but progressive rise in end-diastolic pressure or CVP. In providing anesthesia the following considerations should be noted (Table 13.13):

1. Marked increases or decreases in right ventricular filling pressure are not well tolerated. Maintenance of the patient's right ventricular filling pressure in her usual range is necessary for effective contraction of her ventricle against the increased pulmonic resistance. Excessive volume transfusion may overdistend the right ventricle and produce further right ventricular failure. On the other hand, sudden drops in venous return, such as obstruction of the vena cava or acute hemorrhage, will decrease the effectiveness of right ventricular contraction.

2. Decreases in heart rate are not well tolerated. Right ventricular output will depend primarily on heart rate because stroke volume is limited. Maintenance of at least normal (90 to 110 bpm) heart rates, by choosing drugs with a positive chronotropic effect and using light anesthesia, is recommended.

3. Marked decreases in systemic vascular resistance may not be tolerated. With a low output state, systemic pressure is preserved by increases in vascular resistance. Maintenance of a normal to high systemic vascular resistance by light levels of general anesthesia or by the addition of a vasoconstrictor, such as ephedrine or metaraminol, is advocated.

4. Negative inotropes may not be well

tolerated. The contractile state of the right ventricle may be compromised, and further myocardial depression may result from negative inotropes such as halothane or enflurane. Likewise, use of medications or techniques with positive inotropic action is efficacious.

Anesthesia for vaginal delivery and cesarean section. For labor and vaginal delivery, techniques which reduce systemic vascular resistance and venous return should be used with extreme caution. These patients are probably best managed with systemic or inhalation analgesics and pudendal blocks.

If epidural, caudal or spinal anesthesia is chosen, prophylactic administration of intravenous fluids and ephedrine is recommended. Maintenance of a normal CVP is necessary. Decreases in systemic vascular resistance should be anticipated and immediately corrected with left uterine displacement and ephedrine or metaraminol.

For cesarean section general anesthesia using a nitrous oxide-relaxant technique is recommended. Maintenance of vascular resistance, heart rate and contractility is the goal. If signs of right ventricular failure develop (elevation of filling pressure), treatment consists of lightening the anesthetic level and administering an inotrope such as dopamine.

OTHER HEART DISEASES

Primary Pulmonary Hypertension

Primary pulmonary hypertension is a disease which particularly affects young women.[76-78] Maternal mortality is more than 50 per cent.[52, 79] Most deaths occur during the periods of labor and the puerperium, and the pattern is similar to that described in Eisenmenger's syndrome.[7, 9, 52, 56] There is speculation that amniotic fluid embolism might be a possible precipitating factor in the fulminant course of this disease during labor and the puerperium.[4]

Clinical manifestations. The principal symptoms of this disease, exertional dyspnea and fatigue, characteristically occur late in its natural course as differentiated from other causes of pulmonary hypertension. These symptoms are due to a low fixed cardiac output. The signs of this disease are dependent on the degree of pulmonary hypertension and right ventricular compromise. Usually, patients are acyanotic, have cool extremities with poor peripheral pulses and have a quiet precordium. Prominent A-waves in the deep jugular veins can be noted. Late in the disease, a systolic ejection murmur is heard over the pulmonary valve. In addition, evidence of tricuspid insufficiency can be detected. The electrocardiogram usually reveals right ventricular hypertrophy and right atrial enlargement. Chest roentgenogram shows a prominent main pulmonary artery and a slightly enlarged heart with a right atrial and right ventricular configuration. Late in the course of this disease the heart size may increase considerably. Cardiac catheterization demonstrates isolated pulmonary hypertension in the face of a normal pulmonary capillary wedge pressure.

Pathophysiology. Pulmonary hypertension is present when the pulmonary artery pressure exceeds 30/15 mm Hg or the mean pulmonary artery pressure exceeds 25 mm Hg.[78] With elevation of pulmonary pressure, morphologic changes occur in the pulmonary vasculature producing me-

Table 13.13
Anesthetic Considerations: Congenital Pulmonic Stenosis

1. Avoid marked increases in intravascular volume.
2. Avoid marked decreases in venous return.
3. Avoid bradycardia.
4. Avoid marked decreases in systemic vascular resistance.
5. Avoid myocardial depressants.

dial hypertrophy and intimal fibrosis. A large spectrum of changes can occur in this vasculature, and the reactivity of these vessels can be quite variable. With increasing pulmonary hypertension, right ventricular afterload and, therefore, right ventricular pressure work increase. The right ventricle hypertrophies and eventually fails, causing an elevated right ventricular end-diastolic pressure and a decreased cardiac output. This elevation of end-diastolic pressure is reflected by an elevation of central venous pressure, producing passive congestion of the liver and peripheral edema. With progression of the disease, the right ventricle will become dilated, and tricuspid insufficiency will occur. Characteristically, throughout this course, the pulmonary capillary wedge or left ventricular preload is not elevated. The left ventricle usually functions well; however, left ventricular output falls because of the failing right ventricle.

Anesthetic considerations. It is imperative that the degree of pulmonary hypertension and right ventricular failure be assessed before proceeding with an anesthetic plan. If possible, the reactivity of the pulmonary vasculature should be determined, for it may be responsive to pharmacologic vasodilation. Monitoring of radial artery and pulmonary artery pressure is recommended in all patients. The following considerations should be noted (Table 13.14):

1. Increases in pulmonary vascular resistance are not well tolerated. Hypercarbia, hypoxia, acidosis, lung hyperinflation, pharmacologic vasoconstrictors and stress can markedly elevate pulmonary vascular resistance and should be avoided.

2. Marked decreases in right ventricular volume are not well tolerated. Early correction of fluid and blood loss and avoidance of inferior vena caval obstruction are important for the maintenance of normal to slightly elevated CVP.

3. Marked decreases in systemic vascular resistance may not be well tolerated. Cardiac output is limited by a fixed right ventricular output. The patient may be unable to compensate for decreases in systemic vascular resistance.

4. Right ventricular contractility may be compromised, and negative inotropes may result in marked depression of ventricular function.

Anesthesia for vaginal delivery and cesarean section. In these patients pain, anxiety and stress are especially detrimental, because pulmonary vascular resistance may increase markedly. Adequate psychological support and analgesia are mandatory. For labor and vaginal delivery, intravenous narcotics, inhalation analgesia, paracervical and pudendal nerve blocks are recommended. It is recognized that neonatal depression from the narcotics may result, and use of neonatal naloxone should be anticipated. These techniques are preferred to major conduction anesthesia, for they are not associated with marked peripheral vasodilation and reduction in venous return. If a continuous epidural technique is used, a dermatome-by-dermatome titration of local anesthetic is recommended. Meticulous attention must be given to changes in venous capacitance and vascular resistance. Continuous intravenous titration of fluids is necessary. Correction of small decreases in systemic vascular resistance is not advocated, because the treatment might have a marked effect on the pulmonary vascular resistance. Only marked decreases in systemic vascular resistance should be corrected by titration of ephedrine.

For cesarean section general anesthesia

Table 13.14
Anesthetic Considerations: Primary Pulmonary Hypertension

1. Avoid increases in pulmonary vascular resistance.
2. Avoid marked decreases in venous return.
3. Avoid marked decreases in systemic vascular resistance.
4. Avoid myocardial depressants.

is preferred. The conventional rapid induction with thiopental, succinylcholine and endotracheal intubation may precipitate marked pulmonary hypertension and right ventricular failure. One suggested approach is an inhalation induction with halothane and oxygen. There is some evidence that use of an inhalation agent, such as halothane, may decrease pulmonary vascular resistance.[80] Intubation should not be performed until an adequate depth of anesthesia is achieved. To avoid possible hypoventilation and hypercarbia during induction, it is suggested that the patient be paralyzed with pancuronium immediately after loss of consciousness; ventilation can then be controlled. Hyperinflation of the lungs should be avoided, and a tidal volume of 5 to 10 ml/kg is recommended.

It is recognized that there is an increased risk of aspiration with this technique. Antacids should be administered prior to induction, and cricoid pressure should be applied continously until intubation is performed.

The most serious complication is right ventricular decompensation resulting from increases in pulmonary hypertension. An early sign is a subtle but progressive elevation of CVP even though other parameters are stable and normal. If this should occur, hypercarbia, hypoxia, acidosis and light anesthesia should be ruled out or corrected. If the situation persists, inotropes such as dopamine or isoproterenol should be titrated slowly. If these measures fail, pulmonary vasodilation with low-dose sodium nitroprusside or phentolamine (0.1 to 0.5 μg/kg/min) should be attempted.

Hypertensive Disorders

The incidence of hypertension during pregnancy from all causes is approximately 6 per cent, a quarter of these patients having pre-existent hypertension.[81-84] In addition to essential hypertension, the principal causes of hypertension are toxemia, renal disease and, more rarely, coarctation of the aorta and pheochromocytoma. Both maternal and fetal morbidity and mortality seem to be affected by the occurrence, degree, pattern and treatment of hypertension during pregnancy.[4, 81-90] With essential hypertension, patients whose blood pressure does not exceed 160/100 mm Hg before and during the first 20 weeks of pregnancy have, as a rule, an excellent prognosis.[81] In addition, those who demonstrate the characteristic fall in systolic blood pressure during the second trimester seem to have much lower fetal mortality (4.6 per cent) as compared with those who show no fall (16 per cent). Patients with essential hypertension who received antihypertensive drugs during pregnancy had a lower incidence of toxemia (6 per cent versus 18 per cent) and fetal mortality (9 per cent versus 24 per cent) in comparison with a similar group of patients who did not receive antihypertensive therapy but were managed with rest, sedation and salt restriction.[81]

The cardiovascular changes seen in patients with preeclampsia-eclampsia and essential hypertension have been studied and contrasted with those changes seen in normal pregnancy. Recent data seem to indicate that patients with preeclampsia or essential hypertension have a lower cardiac index and smaller increase in blood volume than patients with hypertension during pregnancy. Patients with toxemia have been shown to have increased sensitivity to the effects of catecholamines,[91] vasopressin[92] and angiotensin II.[93] As in normal pregnancy, patients with essential hypertension seem to have a marked increase in sensitivity to ganglionic blocking drugs which may precipitate severe hypotension. However, in patients with toxemia this sensitivity has not been demonstrated.[94, 95] A complete discussion of preeclampsia-eclampsia is found in chapter 14.

Clinical manifestations. The clinical

manifestations of hypertension will depend on its etiology. In general, symptoms of serious end organ involvement—such as transient cerebral ischemic attacks, left ventricular failure, angina or renal insufficiency—are indicative of long-standing or malignant hypertension and warrant special consideration. Especially noteworthy are signs of left ventricular hypertrophy or dilation which indicate more severe myocardial damage. These signs are a displaced point of maximal impulse, left ventricular heave on physical examination, left ventricular strain pattern (in addition to an excessive left ventricular voltage pattern) on electrocardiogram and an enlarged and "boot-shaped" heart on chest roentgenogram.

Pathophysiology. Hypertension affects nearly all organs of the body. Two pathophysiologic changes are noteworthy. First, with long-standing or severe hypertension arterial damage may occur and alter both the distribution of organ blood flow and its autoregulatory processes. There is evidence that these tissues may require higher perfusion pressures than normal in order to maintain tissue blood flow.[18, 96] Second, with increased systemic pressure, left ventricular pressure work progressively increases, and the ventricle concentrically hypertrophies. Ventricular dilation and cardiomegaly occur later in the disease process when significant myocardial compromise and failure occur.[17, 18]

Pregnancy can complicate the course of pre-existing hypertension, can uncover essential hypertension or can precipitate new forms of hypertension, such as toxemia.[4, 81-89] The mechanisms by which these changes occur are increases in intravascular volume, increases in cardiac demand (heart rate, stroke volume), acute increases in systemic vascular resistance with stress and changes in renal or endocrine function. The final result is left ventricular ischemia and failure with decreased cardiac output and decreased organ (including uterine) perfusion.

Anesthetic considerations. The continuation of antihypertensive medications is recommended. In patients with severe or malignant hypertension prior to delivery, blood pressure should be reduced to reasonable levels (160 to 180/100 to 110 mm Hg) with intravenous vasodilators such as hydralazine. These patients may be very sensitive to vasodilators, and slow titration is recommended. With left ventricular failure radial artery and pulmonary artery monitoring is recommended.

Anesthesia for vaginal delivery and cesarean section. For labor and vaginal delivery, regional anesthesia is recommended and is discussed fully in chapter 14. Because labor pains can exacerbate hypertension and its sequellae, a continuous lumbar epidural technique is advocated. Intravascular volume may be relatively decreased in these patients and sympathectomy may lead to severe hypotension. Hydration prior to administration of a block and correction of hypotension with left uterine displacement and small amounts of ephedrine (2.5 mg intravenously) are suggested.

For cesarean section either regional or general anesthesia is acceptable. With regional anesthesia, administration of 500 to 1,000 ml of crystalloid prior to the regional block is recommended. With general anesthesia, addition of a halogenated agent should prevent the acute rise in blood pressure associated with light planes of anesthesia. With severe or malignant hypertension associated with left ventricular dysfunction, radial artery and pulmonary capillary wedge pressure monitoring is advocated. Sodium nitroprusside or phentolamine may be necessary to treat an acute hypertensive crisis.

Cardiomyopathy of Pregnancy

The occurrence of left ventricular failure late in the course of pregnancy or during the first 6 months of the postpartum period without known etiology has been termed cardiomyopathy of pregnancy, peripartum cardiomyopathy, puerperal cardiomyopathy and postpartal heart disease.[4, 60, 97] It is not clear whether this condition is closely related to pregnancy or whether pregnancy exacerbates a pre-existing, latent myocardial disorder. The incidence of this disorder is increased in older multiparous women; in the presence of twins, toxemia, viral infection, poor nutrition and genetic disorders; and in members of the black race.[98] The long-term prognosis is highly variable. Mortality rates are between 15 and 60 per cent.[4, 82, 97] The occurrence of heart failure during subsequent pregnancies and the long-term survival seem to be dependent on the return of heart size to normal 6 months after the first episode of cardiomyopathy. Demakis and Rahimtoola[99] studied the clinical course of this disease in 27 women. All patients presented with left ventricular failure during the last month of pregnancy or within the first 5 months of the postpartum period. In 14 of the 27 patients heart size returned to normal within 6 months. However, in 13 patients cardiomegaly persisted beyond 6 months. Eleven of these 13 patients had chronic congestive heart failure and died after an average of 4.7 years.

Clinical manifestations. The clinical manifestations associated with this disorder are signs and symptoms of left or right ventricular failure.[4, 18] Pulmonary embolism or infarction may also occur.[100] The electrocardiogram demonstrates left ventricular hypertrophy, diffuse ST-T wave abnormalities or left ventricular conduction defects. The chest roentgenogram is consistent with either left, right or bi-ventricular failure.

Pathophysiology. Either left or right myocardial damage may be significant while the patient remains asymptomatic until a physiologic stress such as pregnancy occurs. With pregnancy a deleterious effect may be produced by several normal physiologic changes: the increase in preload associated with the stresses of uterine contraction or surgery and the increase in cardiac demand (heart rate, stroke volume, contractility). With progressive ventricular failure, end-diastolic volume increases (decreasing subendocardial blood flow), cardiac output decreases (decreasing coronary perfusion) and myocardial oxygen demand increases. Thus, a myocardial oxygen supply-demand imbalance occurs, leading to further ventricular compromise.

Anesthetic considerations. Patients presenting with ventricular failure (left or right) prior to delivery should be treated with bed rest, salt restriction, diuresis, digitalization and preload-afterload reduction as necessary. If ventricular failure persists at the time of delivery, monitoring with a radial arterial line and a pulmonary artery catheter is recommended. Acute increases in afterload occurring with endotracheal intubation or surgical incision can precipitate left ventricular failure and should be anticipated and controlled with a vasodilator.

Anesthesia for vaginal delivery and cesarean section. For labor and vaginal delivery regional anesthesia is recommended. With a continuous epidural technique, deleterious increases in afterload secondary to stress can be avoided. In addition, the resultant preload and afterload reduction may be efficacious in patients with ventricular compromise. A slow titration of the local anesthetic is suggested. Pre-hydration and prophylactic ephedrine should not be routinely used. Continuous fetal heart rate monitoring will help determine when the fall in blood pressure should be treated.

For cesarean section either regional or general anesthesia may be used. If general anesthesia is chosen, a nitrous oxide-relaxant technique is recommended in patients with marked ventricular failure. Afterload reduction with either sodium nitroprusside or phentolamine may be necessary. If regional anesthesia is chosen, a continuous epidural technique is recommended, be-

Dissecting Aneurysm of the Aorta

Although dissecting aneurysm of the aorta is more commonly found in men over 50 years of age, there has been a well recognized association between pregnancy and dissecting aneurysm of the aorta.[101] Up to 50 per cent of dissecting aneurysms in women less than 40 years old occurred in association with pregnancy.[101-103] Possible etiologic factors are syphilis, sepsis, Erdheim's medial necrosis, arteriosclerosis and coarctation of the aorta. The effect of pregnancy per se on the histologic changes in the aorta is controversial.[7, 102] However, pathologic changes occurring with pregnancy, such as hypertension, are known to influence the course of aortic dissection. The maternal mortality of patients with acute dissection of the aorta is similar to that of non-pregnant patients and depends on the extent of the process and the location of the intimal tear.[4] During pregnancy, maternal mortality ranging from 19 to 91 per cent has been reported.[2]

Clinical manifestations. An abrupt, excruciating pain is the most characteristic feature. Most commonly the pain begins in the thorax or abdomen and migrates posteriorly to the interscapular or lumbar areas.[17, 18] However, pain can also originate in the neck, extremities, or jaw. Painless dissection is most commonly seen in patients with Marfan's syndrome. Physical examination usually demonstrates hypertension and tachycardia; however, with dissection, hypotension may occur. If the ascending aorta is involved, a murmur of aortic insufficiency may be found; if the abdominal aorta is involved, a palpable tender aneurysm may be detected. Other findings include asymmetric pulses in the major vessels, focal neurologic signs or evidence of myocardial ischemia.

Pathophysiology. With aortic medial degeneration and the hydraulic stresses of pulsatile flow, dissection will occur. In approximately 70 per cent of patients the dissection originates in the ascending aorta; in the remainder it usually originates distal to the left subclavian artery.[18] Dissection may be localized or extend throughout the aorta. Proximal extension may involve the aortic valve (producing aortic insufficiency), the pericardium or the left pleural space. Distal extension may involve the femoral vessels. In addition, dissection may occur primarily in the anterior or posterior regions of the aorta. With posterior dissection, tamponade may occur and slow the dissection process; with anterior dissection, acute rupture with hemorrhage into a body cavity may occur.

Anesthetic considerations

The non-emergent situation. Patients with a history of aortic dissection which has been well controlled medically should continue to receive their medications throughout pregnancy, labor and delivery. Regional anesthesia for labor and delivery (vaginal or cesarean section) is recommended. Maintenance of both a pain-free state and normal to slightly decreased blood pressure (a systolic pressure between 90 and 110 mm Hg) is necessary. Continuous fetal heart rate monitoring should be employed to determine the acceptable degree of hypotension. If general anesthesia is selected for cesarean section, an inhalation technique with halothane is suggested, because hypertension and tachycardia will be less likely and the force of ventricular ejection of blood may be decreased.

Trimethaphan and propranolol are useful for control of hypertension and tachycardia. These drugs are recommended if hemodynamic control cannot be achieved by a quiet environment, reassurance, pain control with a regional anesthetic and mild sedation.

Rupture with severe hemorrhage should always be anticipated. Two large-bore intravenous catheters should be placed, at least 8 units of whole blood should be available and preparation for rapid intubation and resuscitation should be made.

The emergent situation. In patients presenting with progressive dissection requiring emergency surgical correction, all efforts should be made to expedite surgery. However, the induction of anesthesia is critical.

In patients who are normotensive to hypertensive, an inhalation induction with halothane is recommended. Control of blood pressure and minimization of the response to endotracheal intubation will help prevent hemodynamic decompensation prior to surgical control of the aorta. Immediately prior to induction, the surgical field should be prepped and draped, and the surgeon should be prepared to make an incision and cross-clamp the aorta if severe hypotension should occur with induction or intubation. Patients who are mildly to severely hypotensive may not be able to tolerate an inhalation agent, a barbiturate or even a narcotic prior to intubation. Rapid induction with succinylcholine with or without ketamine is recommended. Even with marked sympathetic stimulation, blood pressure elevation may not occur because of severe intravascular volume depletion. Immediate surgical control of the aorta is the only treatment.

After control of the aortic dissection classical cesarean section should be performed.

Asymmetric Septal Hypertrophy

Asymmetric septal hypertrophy (ASH), also known as idiopathic hypertrophic subvalvular stenosis (IHSS), is a cardiomyopathy characterized by a marked hypertrophy of the ventricle involving the interventricular septum and the outflow tract.[68,104-107] During ventricular systole constriction of the outflow tract occurs, producing obstruction to ventricular ejection. Typically, ASH is a disease of young adults, with the majority of patients being in their third and fourth decades.

Several authors have reported that pregnant patients with ASH have an increased risk of left ventricular failure and supraventricular dysrhythmias.[4,108,109] Brown et al.[108] reported on 12 patients; one developed left ventricular failure in her last month of pregnancy, and two developed atrial dysrhythmias in late pregnancy. Of the 12 patients, three died during the first postpartum year. On the other hand, Turner et al.[109] and Szekely and Snaith[4] reported on 13 patients with ASH during pregnancy and found that only one patient had a complicated pregnancy marked by episodes of supraventricular tachycardia without evidence of left ventricular failure. All patients had normal deliveries, and there was no evidence of an increased morbidity or mortality during the postpartum period. Thus, the course of patients with ASH during pregnancy is quite variable.

Clinical manifestations. The most frequent symptoms of patients with ASH are exertional dyspnea, angina pectoris and syncope.[110] Late in the course of the disease, symptoms of left ventricular failure occur as well. On physical examination the heart is usually enlarged with a left ventricular lift, a double apical impulse and a systolic murmur commencing late after the first heart sound and best heard at the apex.[18] The electrocardiogram is usually abnormal with evidence of left ventricular hypertrophy; in addition, a Wolff-Parkinson-White syndrome or abnormal Q-waves in the inferior or left precordial leads may be seen.[110] Chest roentgenogram usually displays an enlarged left ventricle.

Pathophysiology. Patients with ASH involving the left ventricle exhibit a marked hypertrophy of the entire left ventricle with a bulging of the ventricular myocardium in the septal region several centimeters below the aortic valve. The ventricular cavity is relatively small. With each systolic contraction the muscle about the outflow tract constricts and left ventricular ejection is obstructed. Progression of left ventricular hypertrophy eventually leads to ventricular failure.

Agents or events which increase myocardial contractility will exacerbate the left ventricular outflow obstruction and precipitate failure.[18] Decreases in systemic vascular resistance may also cause an increase in left ventricular ejection force and increase obstruction.[17,18] Decreases in left ventricular preload will decrease the size of the left ventricle cavity during systole and increase obstruction.[111] Thus, rapid atrial rates or loss of atrial kick is not well tolerated.[112]

During pregnancy the increase in intravascular volume is helpful in these patients, because it will cause left ventricular distension and decrease the amount of outflow obstruction. However, the decrease in systemic vascular resistance and the increase in heart rate and myocardial contractility seen throughout pregnancy may be deleterious and may precipitate left ventricular failure.

Anesthetic Considerations. In patients who are symptomatic or present with a hemodynamically significant atrial dysrhythmia, monitoring with an arterial line and a pulmonary artery catheter may be especially helpful. In addition, the following should be noted (Table 13.15):

1. Decreases in preload are not well tolerated. Maintenance of slight hypervolemia is recommended, because the increase in ventricular volume tends to decrease the amount of outflow obstruction.

2. Supraventricular tachycardia, atrial fibrillation or atrial flutter are not well tolerated. With these dysrhythmias ventricular filling will be decreased. Immediate treatment with direct current cardioversion or propranolol is advocated.

Table 13.15
Anesthetic Considerations: Asymmetric Septal Hypertrophy

1. Avoid decreases in blood volume and venous return.
2. Avoid or correct supraventricular tachycardia, atrial fibrillation and atrial flutter.
3. Avoid decreases in systemic vascular resistance.
4. Avoid increases in myocardial contractility.
5. Treat ventricular compromise with phenylephrine, intravenous fluids and propranolol.

3. Decreases in systemic vascular resistance are not well tolerated. Maintenance of a normal to a slightly elevated systemic resistance is advocated, because the degree of outflow obstruction will be minimized.

4. Increases in contractility may not be well tolerated. Increases in myocardial contractility may markedly increase outflow obstruction.

5. The treatment of ventricular failure with ASH is markedly different from the usual treatment of failure. Increasing afterload (metaraminol) and preload (intravenous fluids) and decreasing heart rate (propranolol) and contractility (propranolol and halothane) are efficacious.

Anesthesia for vaginal delivery and cesarean section. Anesthesia for labor and vaginal delivery is best provided with systemic or inhalation analgesics, paracervical and pudendal blocks. Major regional anesthetic techniques may reduce systemic vascular resistance and venous return, thereby increasing outflow obstruction. If these techniques are used, prophylactic administration of intravenous fluids, continuous left uterine displacement and, if necessary, metaraminol infusion may be used to maintain blood pressure. For cesarean section a general anesthetic with an inhalation agent, such as halothane, is recommended, because the degree of outflow obstruction may be reduced by the negative inotropic and chronotropic effects of halothane.

Coronary Artery Disease

Coronary artery disease occurring prior to or during pregnancy is uncommon and has been reported in approximately one in 10,000 pregnancies.[4] In 108 cases of acute myocardial infarction during pregnancy the maternal and fetal mortality were 35 and 37 per cent, respectively.[4,7,113-118] Seventy per cent of the patients who did succumb had a myocardial infarction during the last trimester. The clinical manifestations and pathophysiology are similar to those in the non-pregnant patient.[17,18]

Anesthetic Considerations. Patients with a history of crescendo angina, recent (6 weeks) myocardial infarction or congestive heart failure should be monitored with an arterial line and a pulmonary artery catheter. Patients maintained on nitrates or propranolol for treatment of angina should have their medications continued throughout pregnancy, labor, delivery and the puerperium.

Anesthesia for Vaginal Delivery and Cesarean Section. For labor and vaginal delivery, regional anesthesia is recommended. Regional anesthesia will minimize pain and stress, which could precipitate angina, and may decrease afterload and preload, which will be beneficial. However, severe decreases in afterload (producing systemic diastolic pressures below 50 mm Hg) or large increases in heart rate (greater than 120 beats per minute) can precipitate decreased diastolic filling of the coronary arteries and angina. Correction with metaraminol or propranolol, respectively, is advocated. Administration of nitroglycerin to treat angina in the presence of a sympathetic block may cause a further decrease in preload and cardiac output and may produce more ischemia.

For cesarean section either regional or general anesthesia may be used. The considerations for regional anesthesia are discussed above. For general anesthesia the most important consideration is to minimize the stress of intubation and surgery. If there is no evidence of congestive failure, an inhalation technique is recommended. If congestive failure is present and general anesthesia is selected, a nitrous oxide-relaxant technique with narcotic supplementation is suggested. Evidence of myocardial ischemia on the electrocardiogram (lead V5 preferably) should be approached by first "normalizing" blood pressure and heart rate, changing the anesthetic level or administering therapeutics (sodium nitroprusside, propranolol). With normalized vital signs but persistent evidence of ischemia, administration of sublingual nitroglycerine is suggested.

The rapid hemodynamic changes during the postpartum period can precipitate ischemia. An uneventful delivery does not ensure that the patient will have an uncomplicated course. Because of the marked changes in systemic vascular resistance and blood volume occurring during the postpartum period, the patient should be closely monitored, preferably in an intensive care unit.

Pregnancy after Valvular Surgery

There have been more than 700 cases of pregnancy after mitral valvulotomy and more than 150 cases after mitral and aortic valve replacement.[4,119-126]

MITRAL VALVULOTOMY

Patients with a previous mitral valvulotomy have increased maternal and fetal mortality, pulmonary embolization and atrial fibrillation (Table 13.16).[4,119-121] These complications seen to be related to residual right and left ventricular dysfunction, residual pulmonary hypertension and a dilated, compliant left atrium. Although these statistics are not as foreboding as those for patients with prosthetic valves (especially mitral valves), they are significantly higher than those for patients without heart disease and warrant special anesthetic considerations.

Anesthetic considerations

1. Assessment of the status of the valvulotomy should be made throughout pregnancy and prior to delivery. Changes in signs or symptoms with pregnancy and exercise are particularly important. Residual or new mitral stenosis or insufficiency may be present. If so, the previously discussed anesthetic considerations for these lesions should be applied (Tables 13.3 and 13.4).

2. Residual pulmonary hypertension may exist despite correction of the valvular lesion. Pulmonary hypertension may be subtle, and symptoms of associated low cardiac output may be precipitated only with exercise or stress. If symptoms or signs exist, the considerations listed under primary pulmonary hypertension also apply here (Table 13.14).

3. Residual right or left ventricular dysfunction may exist. Patients with corrected mitral valvular lesions have been shown to have decreased cardiac output and a decreased response of cardiac output with exercise. The considerations are those described under mitral stenosis and insufficiency (Tables 13.3 and 13.4).

4. Atrial fibrillation is associated with a marked increase in morbidity. The incidence of systemic embolization and left atrial failure (pulmonary edema with a depressed cardiac output) is increased. Maintenance and adjustment of medications such as digoxin or quinidine throughout pregnancy, labor and delivery are necessary. Treatment of acute atrial fibrillation is outlined in the sections on mitral stenosis and dysrhythmias.

5. The choice of anesthetic is dependent on the type and severity of residual disease involving the mitral valve, pulmonary artery and left and right ventricles. For a discussion of these considerations, see the sections on mitral stenosis and insufficiency.

MITRAL VALVE REPLACEMENT

More than 100 cases of pregnancy after mitral valve replacement have been reported.[4,7,122-126] Although maternal mortality is not significantly different from that associated with valvulotomy, maternal morbidity, fetal mortality and fetal malformations are significantly increased (Table 13.16).

In the non-pregnant population, mitral valve replacement is associated with a number of chronic, post-operative complications: thromboembolism, paravalvular regurgitation, ball or disc variance, hemolysis and endocarditis. In addition, these

Table 13.16
Maternal and Fetal Complications in Patients with Previous Valvular Surgery

Surgical Procedure	Maternal Mortality	Fetal Mortality	Maternal Morbidity (Emboli, Hemorrhage)	Incidence of Fetal Malformations	References
	%	%	%	%	
Mitral valvulotomy	2.3–5.5	5.5–16.5	6.6–8.0	1	4,119–121
Mitral valve replacement	1.2	41	36	20	4,122–126
Mitral and aortic valve replacement	0	87	Unknown	Unknown	4,122–126
Aortic valve replacement	0	14	21	2	4,122–126

patients typically have a low resting cardiac output, a subnormal increase in cardiac output with exercise, residual pulmonary vascular disease and some degree of right or left heart dysfunction.[127-131] Pregnancy aggravates these complications further because of increased intravascular volume, increased myocardial oxygen demand and increased risk of thromboembolism.

Anesthetic considerations

1. All patients should be assumed to have some degree of residual myocardial dysfunction and pulmonary hypertension. Occurrence or progression of any signs or symptoms during pregnancy especially with exercise or stress indicate that a considerable amount of residual myocardial damage exists. The anesthetic considerations listed in the previous section and in the sections on mitral valve disease will then apply here as well.

2. Pulmonary artery monitoring is recommended with symptomatic disease or with evidence of ventricular compromise, or pulmonary hypertension. Because the risk of endocarditis is increased in these patients, a strictly sterile technique must be used in the placement and maintenance of this catheter.

3. These patients are invariably anticoagulated. Usually coumarin anticoagulants are replaced with heparin during pregnancy.[132-136] One anesthetic approach is to continue the patient on heparin throughout labor and delivery, avoiding all forms of regional anesthesia, and using systemic medication, inhalation analgesia and general anesthesia if necessary. The second approach is to discontinue heparin immediately prior to labor and administer protamine until coagulation tests become normal. Regional anesthesia can then be conducted and heparin resumed 24 hours after removal of the epidural catheter.[136] Because experience with the latter technique is limited, the morbidity associated with this technique cannot truly be assessed at this time.

AORTIC VALVE REPLACEMENT

Patients with an aortic valve prosthesis have a lower incidence of complications than those with a mitral prosthesis (Table 13.16).[4,122-126] The reasons for this difference can be attributed to the difference in myocardial function and the more restricted use of anticoagulants in patients with aortic valve prostheses. Cardiac output at rest and in response to exercise is generally normal in patients with aortic valve prostheses, and ventricular function in general seems to be better.[137-139] However, abnormalities do exist and depend principally on the pre-operative myocardial status and the quality of valve function. The complications in non-pregnant patients include ball and disc variance, paravalvular regurgitation, hemolysis, endocarditis and thromboembolism. Compared to patients with mitral valve prostheses, however, the risk of thromboembolism, residual pulmonary hypertension or right ventricular compromise is not as great.

Anesthetic considerations

1. All patients should be assumed to have some degree of residual myocardial dysfunction. Symptoms or signs of left ventricular compromise, especially with stress or exercise, are indicative of increased risk, and the anesthetic considerations delineated under the sections on aortic insufficiency and stenosis should be applied (Tables 13.5 and 13.6).

2. Pulmonary artery monitoring is recommended with symptomatic disease or with evidence of left ventricular compromise.

3. If the patient is anticoagulated the anesthetic management should be modified as previously discussed.

Open-Heart Surgery during Pregnancy

Approximately 100 cases of cardiac surgery during pregnancy have been reported.[4,140-145] From these cases it seems that maternal mortality is no different from non-pregnant patients having open-heart surgery. The fetal mortality is, however, very high (33 to 50 per cent). Zitnik et al.[145] reviewed 21 cases and found no correlation of pump time, ischemic time or type of perfusate with maternal or fetal mortality.

Anesthetic considerations. Basic considerations for anesthetic management of pregnant patients undergoing non-obstetric operations are discussed in chapter 21. A detailed delineation of the anesthetic considerations for open-heart surgery is beyond the scope of this chapter. However, the following basic considerations should be noted.

1. The anesthetic considerations for the various cardiac lesions are particularly applicable for patients undergoing open-heart surgery.

2. The fetus should be monitored as fully as possible during the operative and post-operative periods (chapter 24).

3. Monitoring systemic vascular resistance as well as systemic blood pressure is recommended throughout the perioperative period, and particularly during cardiopulmonary bypass. Uterine blood flow is dependent on both uterine perfusion pressure and vascular resistance. Agents which increase systemic vascular resistance probably increase uterine vascular resistance as well and may result in decreased uterine blood flow in the face of an elevated systemic pressure. If continuous fetal heart rate monitoring indicates fetal distress during cardiopulmonary bypass and arterial pressure is low, perfusion pressure should be increased by increasing flow rate. If fetal distress occurs and vascular resistance is high, small doses of hydralazine are recommended.

Cardiac Dysrhythmias

Cardiac dysrhythmias are common during pregnancy even in patients without detectable organic heart disease. Most normal pregnant patients manifest some type of cardiac dysrhythmia during pregnancy, labor and delivery.[4,7,146-153] Fortunately, most of these dysrhythmias are benign. The more serious dysrhythmias are usually found in association with rheumatic heart disease and are considered here.

ATRIAL FIBRILLATION

Atrial fibrillation occurring during pregnancy is usually associated with advanced rheumatic mitral valve disease, primarily dominant mitral stenosis.[4,7] Patients with recent onset of atrial fibrillation during pregnancy have an increased mortality, an increased incidence of heart failure and embolization. Mendelson[1] reported on 117 pregnancies in which atrial fibrillation had occurred and found that the maternal mortality was 17 per cent and fetal mortality was 50 per cent; heart failure developed in 52 per cent of the cases. Szekely and Snaith[4] found that 62 per cent of the patients who developed atrial fibrillation during pregnancy had associated heart failure. In approximately half the cases heart failure developed before the onset of atrial fibrillation, and in the remaining half it developed 1 week to 6 months after the onset of atrial fibrillation. In addition, they found a high incidence of systemic (13 per cent) and pulmonary (18 per cent) embolization. These authors also reported that the incidence of atrial fibrillation after mitral valvulotomy was higher in pregnant (31 per cent) than in non-pregnant patients (16.5 per cent).[148]

Treatment. Patients who have had a history of atrial fibrillation and who have responded well to treatment should be maintained on this therapy (digitalis, propranolol, quinidine) throughout pregnancy; the doses of these drugs should be adjusted to achieve ventricular rates between 90 and 110 beats per minute. The effects of these drugs on the fetus are discussed in the following section. Patients without underlying heart disease who develop new atrial fibrillation during pregnancy, labor and delivery should be treated immediately if evidence of hypotension, left ventricular failure or myocardial ischemia exists. If these changes are profound, direct current cardioversion, starting with 100 watt-seconds, should be performed immediately. If electrocardioversion is unavailable or if more time permits (minutes), administration of propranolol should be instituted. Rapid digitalization will, as well, slow the ventricular response but will take a minimum of 15 to 30 minutes before significant slowing occurs and is not recommended for the acute life-threatening situation. However, if time does permit (hours), digitalization is the treatment of choice. When the patient is fully digitalized, restoration of a sinus rhythm can then be accomplished with quinidine or procainamide. In patients with advanced rheumatic heart disease who develop atrial fibrillation, rapid decompensation can occur, and immediate direct current cardioversion or propranolol administration is recommended.

ATRIAL FLUTTER

Atrial flutter is rarely seen in normal patients, and is less commonly found than atrial fibrillation. The atrial rate is usually between 280 and 320 beats per minute and a two-to-one block usually exists, resulting in a ventricular rate of about 150 beats per minute.

Treatment. There are few reports of atrial flutter during pregnancy.[1,4] The clinical implications and the general guidelines of therapy are similar to those of atrial fibrillation. However, several differences do exist. Treatment with direct current cardioversion usually requires less energy; 20 watt-seconds are often successful. Approximately 30 per cent of the patients will convert to atrial fibrillation, usually with a slower ventricular response. Atrial fibrillation is then treated as discussed above.

PAROXYSMAL ATRIAL TACHYCARDIA

Paroxysmal atrial tachycardia (PAT) can occur during pregnancy with or without underlying organic heart disease.[1,4] Szekely and Snaith[150] reported no increased incidence of morbidity when PAT was associated with structurally normal hearts. Mendelson[1] reported a 14 per cent incidence of heart failure and a 5.5 per cent mortality rate when PAT was associated with mitral stenosis. Szekely and Snaith[4] reported on pregnant patients with rheumatic heart disease who developed PAT. Eighty-five per cent of the PAT occurred during pregnancy, labor and delivery and 15 per cent occurred postpartum. Peak incidence occurred during the third trimester of pregnancy. Moderate to severe mitral stenosis was present in 90 per cent of the patients and mitral regurgitation in 10 per cent of the patients. All patients manifested cardiac enlargement. Eighty-eight per cent of the paroxysms lasting for more than 6 hours were associated with left ventricular failure, whereas paroxysms lasting less than 2 hours were not associated with ventricular failure.

Treatment of choice for life-threatening PAT during pregnancy is direct current countershock. If more time permits, any of the following treatment modalities can be instituted: edrophonium (5 to 10 mg intravenously), carotid sinus stimulation, propranolol or digoxin. Neosynephrine sometimes used to slow the heart reflexly should not be used in the pregnant patient.

OTHER DYSRHYTHMIAS

Other dysrhythmias occurring during pregnancy, such as heart block, bundle branch block, Wolff-Parkinson-White syndrome and ventricular dysrhythmias are uncommon but can precipitate significant complications, especially in the patient with underlying organic heart disease.[1,4,38,151-153] Treatment of these dysrhythmias is identical to that in the nonpregnant patient.[17,18]

EFFECTS OF CARDIAC THERAPEUTICS ON THE FETUS

A variety of medications (antiarrhythmics, vasopressors and vasodilators) as well as electrocardioversion are used to treat maternal cardiac disorders. The effects of these therapeutics on the fetus and uterine blood flow and contractility must be considered. Many of the drugs are discussed in more detail in the chapters on obstetric anesthesia and uterine blood flow (chapter 3), effects of anesthesia on uterine activity and labor (chapter 4), perinatal pharmacology (chapter 5) and choice of local anesthetics in obstetrics (chapter 9).

Antiarrhythmics

Lidocaine. High maternal blood levels of lidocaine (greater than 5 µg/ml) are associated with neonatal depression. The usual therapeutic level for suppression of ventricular dysrhythmias is 2 to 5 µg/ml[17] which is comparable to that found with conventional obstetric anesthesia. Very high blood levels of lidocaine—greater than 200 µg/ml in pregnant ewes—were found to cause a dose-related transient (2 to 3 minutes) decrease in uterine blood flow and a simultaneous increase in intrauterine pressure.[154] However, constant intravenous infusion (plasma level of 2 to 4 µg/ml) did not significantly change maternal or fetal hemodynamics or blood gases, uterine blood flow or tone.[155,156]

Propranolol. Propranolol crosses the placenta.[157] Interference with autonomic responses during labor[158] and depressant effects on the neonate have been reported.[159] Fetal bradycardia and hypoglycemia resolving over a prolonged period (3 days) have been associated with the administration of propranolol.[160] Decreased fetal hepatic metabolism may prolong the half-life of propranolol. In pregnant ewes, propranolol causes an impairment of the fetal response to anoxia.[161,162]

Vasopressors and Inotropes

Norepinephrine. In pregnant ewes during sympatholytic hypotension, norepinephrine restores maternal blood pressure to normal without increasing uterine blood flow.[163] In normotensive ewes uterine blood flow decreases despite a marked increase in maternal blood pressure.[164] Norepinephrine also produces an increase in uterine tonus, intensity and frequency of contraction.[165]

Metaraminol. In pregnant ewes with spinal hypotension, metaraminol will restore maternal blood pressure to normal and, on the average, will increase uterine blood flow to 70 to 80 per cent of normal.[166] Some reports indicate that maternal blood pressure and uterine blood flow are returned to normal, but fetal acidosis and hypoxia are not necessarily corrected.[167]

Phenylephrine, methoxamine, angiotensin II. In pregnant ewes with spinal hypotension, these drugs restore maternal blood pressure to normal but without increasing reduced uterine blood flow.[168] In normotensive ewes they also produce uterine vasoconstriction and decreased uterine blood flow.

Ephedrine. In hypotensive pregnant ewes ephedrine was found to restore maternal blood pressure to normal, increase uterine blood flow to 85 per cent of normal and correct fetal hypoxia and acidosis.[166,168,169] Comparison with metaraminol revealed that ephedrine caused less maternal bradycardia and a greater increase in uterine blood flow.[166]

Epinephrine. Despite increases in systemic blood pressure, epinephrine markedly decreases uterine blood flow.[164] In low doses epinephrine decreases uterine contractility and in high doses it increases uterine contractility.[170]

Isoproterenol. Isoproterenol causes a decrease in mean blood pressure and uterine blood flow. No direct vasodilation of gravid uterine vessels has been demonstrated.[171] Uterine contractions are inhibited by approximately 50 per cent when doses of 2 to 8 µg/min are administered.[172]

Dopamine. Differing effects of dopamine on uterine blood flow have been reported.[173-176] In normotensive sheep dopamine increased uterine blood flow despite an increase in uterine vascular resistance.[173] However, in pregnant ewes high doses of dopamine increased maternal cardiac output and blood pressure but decreased uterine blood flow and did not change renal blood flow.[174] Doses less than 10 µg/kg/min produced no significant change in maternal hemodynamics. In pregnant ewes with spinal hypotension and decreased uterine blood flow, dopamine in doses sufficient to maintain blood pressure at control values (20 to 40 µg/kg/min) further decreased uterine blood flow and increased uterine vascular resistance.[175] In hypotensive patients undergoing cesarean section, dopamine (2 to 10 µg/g, min) restored systolic pressure to 100 mm Hg without depression of Apgar scores. However, depression of maternal arterial PO$_2$ was found when compared to controls. Infants, as well, had a significantly lower PO$_2$ in umbilical arterial and venous blood than controls.[176]

Digoxin. Digoxin crosses the placental barrier in both the exteriorized and the intrauterine fetal lamb preparations, and the half-life is significantly longer in the ewe.[177-178] The amount which crossed the placenta was found to be small but could preserve cardiac function in these preparations. In this study[177] no toxicity was found. Observations on three women during their eleventh and twelfth weeks of pregnancy showed that less than 1 per cent of the administered digitoxin was detectable in the fetus.[179] On the other hand, one case report revealed that digitoxin may profoundly affect the fetus. A mother who injested 8.9 mg of digitoxin during her eighth month of pregnancy gave birth to an infant with digitalis intoxication who died shortly after birth.[180]

Vasodilators

Sodium nitroprusside. In pregnant ewes with phenylephrine-induced hypertension, sodium nitroprusside restores blood pressure to normal values but uterine blood flow remains depressed.[181] Furthermore, in ewes, prolonged administration may produce fetal death from cyanide toxicity.[182]

Hydralazine. In pregnant ewes hydralazine lowers blood pressure to control values during phenylephrine-induced hypertension and increases uterine blood flow by 15 per cent.[181] In comparison with sodium nitroprusside, hydralazine is slower in onset but produces a greater increase in cardiac output and heart rate and a greater decrease in systemic vascular resistance at the same systemic pressure.[181]

Direct Current Cardioversion

Use of direct current cardioversion during pregnancy has been reported by Vogel et al.,[31] Sussman et al.[153] and Schroeder and Harrison.[32] Energies as high as 100 watt-seconds were used. Gestation and delivery were normal in all cases. Monitoring of fetal heart rate revealed no apparent effect on the fetus.

References

1. Mendelson CL: *Cardiac Disease in Pregnancy.* F. A. Davis, Philadelphia, 1960.
2. Mendelson CL: Heart disease and pregnancy. Clin Obstet Gynecol 42:603, 1968.
3. Barnes CG: *Medical Disorders in Obstetrics Practice,* ed 3. Blackwell, Oxford, 1970.
4. Szekely P, Snaith L: *Heart Disease and Pregnancy.* Churchill Livingstone, London, 1974.
5. Ueland K: Cardiovascular diseases complicating pregnancy. Clin Obstet Gynecol 21:429, 1978.

6. Niswander K, Berendes H, Deutschberger J, et al.: Fetal mortality following potentially anoxigenic conditions. Am J Obstet Gynecol 98:871, 1967.
7. Burwell CS, Metcalfe J: Heart Disease and Pregnancy. Little, Brown, and Co., Boston, 1958, pp 210, 217, 220.
8. Szekely P, Snaith L: Atrial fibrillation and pregnancy. Br Med J 1:1407, 1961.
9. Cannell DE, Vernon CP: Congenital heart disease and pregnancy. Am J Obstet Gynecol 85:744, 1961.
10. Kerr M: Cardiovascular dynamics in pregnancy and labor. Br Med Bull 24:19, 1968.
11. Liley AW: Clinical and laboratory significance of variations in maternal and plasma volume in pregnancy. Int J Gynecol Obstet 8:358, 1970.
12. Metcalfe J, Ueland K: Maternal cardiovascular adjustments to pregnancy. Prog Cardiovasc Dis 16:363, 1974.
13. Ueland K, Novy M, Peterson E, et al.: Maternal cardiovascular dynamics. IV. The influence of gestational age on the maternal cardiovascular response to posture and exercise. Am J Obstet Gynecol 104:156, 1969.
14. Ueland K, Hansen J: Maternal cardiovascular dynamics. III. Labor and delivery under local and caudal analgesia. Am J Obstet Gynecol 103:8, 1969.
15. Ueland K, Hansen J: Maternal cardiovascular dynamics. II. Posture and uterine contractions. Am J Obstet Gynecol 103:1, 1969.
16. Braunwald E, Ross J, Sonnenblick E: Mechanisms of contraction of the normal and failing heart. Little, Brown, and Co., Boston, 1976.
17. Hurst JW: The Heart. McGraw-Hill, New York, 1978.
18. Fowler NO: Cardiac Diagnosis and Treatment. Harper & Row, New York, 1976.
19. Sonnenblick E, Lesch M: Valvular Heart Disease Grune & Stratton, New York, 1974.
20. Spagnuolo M, Pasternack B, Taranta A: Risk of rheumatic fever recurrences after streptococcal infections. N Engl J Med 285:641, 1971.
21. Jones TD: The diagnosis of rheumatic fever. JAMA 126:481, 1944.
22. Rapaport E: Natural history of aortic and mitral valve disease. Am J Cardiol 35:221, 1975.
23. Selzer A, Cohn E: Natural history of mitral stenosis: A review. Circulation 45:878, 1972.
24. Wood P: An appreciation of mitral stenosis. Br Med J 1:1051, 1954.
25. Keith TA, Fowler NO, Helmsworth JA, et al.: The course of surgically modified mitral stenosis. Am J Med 34:308, 1963.
26. Hultgren H, Hubis H, Shumway N: Cardiac function following mitral valve replacement. Am Heart J 75:302, 1968.
27. Braunwald E, Braunwald NS, Ross J Jr: Effects of mitral valve replacement on the pulmonary vascular dynamics of patients with pulmonary hypertension. N Engl J Med 273:509, 1965.
28. Stott DK, Marpole DGF, Bristow JD, et al: The role of left atrial transport in aortic and mitral stenosis. Circulation 41:1031, 1970.
29. Hildner FJ: Myocardial dysfunction associated with valvular heart disease. Am J Cardiol 30:310, 1972.
30. Arani DT, Carleton RA: The deleterious role of tachycardia in mitral stenosis. Circulation 36:511, 1967.
31. Vogel JHK, Pryor R, Blount SG Jr: Direct-current defibrillation during pregnancy. JAMA 193:970, 1965.
32. Schroeder JS, Harrison DC: Repeated cardioversion during pregnancy: Treatment of refractory paroxysmal atrial tachycardia during three successive pregnancies. Am J Cardiol 27:445, 1971.
33. Perloff JK, Roberts WC: The mitral apparatus: Functional anatomy of mitral regurgitation. Circulation 46:227, 1972.
34. Braunwald E: Mitral regurgitation, physiological, clinical and surgical considerations. N Engl J Med 281:425, 1969.
35. Baxley WA, Kennedy JW, Feild B, et al.: Hemodynamics in ruptured chordae tendinae and chronic rheumatic mitral regurgitation. Circulation 48:1288, 1973.
36. Goodman DJ: Effect of nitroprusside on left ventricular dynamics in mitral regurgitation. Circulation 50:1025, 1974.
37. Marcus FI, Ewy GA, O'Rourke RA, et al.: The effect of pregnancy on the murmurs of mitral and aortic regurgitation. Circulation 41:795, 1970.
38. Dack S, Bader ME, Bader RA, et al.: Heart Disease. Medical, Surgical and Gynecologic Complications of Pregnancy, JJ Rovinsky and AF Guttmacher, eds, ed 2. Williams & Wilkins, Baltimore, 1965. p. 1.
39. Brawley RK, Morrow AG: Direct determinations of aortic blood flow in patients with aortic regurgitation. Circulation 35:32, 1967.
40. Schlant RC, Nutter DO: Heart failure in valvular heart disease. Medicine 50:421, 1971.
41. Judge TP, Kennedy JW, Bennett LJ, et al.: Quantitative hemodynamic effects of heart rate in aortic regurgitation. Circulation 44:355, 1971.
42. Finegan RE, Gianelly RE, Harrison DC: Aortic stenosis in the elderly. N Engl J Med 281:1261, 1969.
43. Frank S, Johnson A, Ross J Jr: Natural history of aortic valvular stenosis. Br Heart J 35:41, 1973.
44. Ueland K, Novy MJ, Peterson EN, et al.: Hemodynamic responses of patients with heart disease to pregnancy and exercise. Am J Obstet Gynecol 113:47, 1972.
45. Frank S, Ross J Jr: The natural history of severe acquired valvular aortic stenosis. Am J Cardiol 19:128, 1967.
46. Liedtke AJ, Gentzler RD II, Babb JD, et al.: Determinants of cardiac performance in severe aortic stenosis. Chest 69:192, 1976.
47. Lee SJK, Jonsson B, Bevegard S, et al.: Hemodynamic changes at rest and during exercise in patients with aortic stenosis of varying severity. Am Heart J 79:318, 1970.

48. Bloomfield DK: The natural history of ventricular septal defect in patients surviving infancy. Circulation 29:914, 1964.
49. Snaith L, Szekely P: Cardiovascular surgery in relation to pregnancy. In *Advances in Obstetrics and Gynecology*, SL Marcus and CC Marcus, eds. Williams & Wilkins, Baltimore, 1967 p 220.
50. Rudolph AM: *Congenital Diseases of the Heart*. Year Book Medical Publishers, Chicago, 1974.
51. Ullery JC: The management of pregnancy complicated by heart disease. Am J Obstet Gynecol 67:834, 1954.
52. Jones AM, Howitt G: Eisenmenger syndrome in pregnancy. Br Med J 1:1627, 1965.
53. Neilson G, Galea EG, Blunt A: Eisenmenger's syndrome and pregnancy. Med J Aust 1:431, 1971.
54. Ueland K: Cardiac surgery and pregnancy. Am J Obstet Gynecol 92:148, 1965.
55. Campbell M: The incidence and later distribution of malformations of the heart. In *Paediatric Cardiology*, H Watson, ed. Lloyd-Luke, London, 1968, p 71.
56. Jewett JF, Ober WB: Primary pulmonary hypertension as a cause of maternal death. Am J Obstet Gynecol 71:1335, 1956.
57. Copeland WE, Wooley CF, Ryan JM, et al.: Pregnancy and congenital heart disease. Am J Obstet Gynecol 86:107, 1963.
58. Meyer EC, Tulsky AS, Sigmann P, et al.: Pregnancy in the presence of tetralogy of Fallot. Am J Cardiol 14:874, 1964.
59. Jacoby WJ: Pregnancy with tetralogy and pentalogy of Fallot. Am J Cardiol 14:866, 1964.
60. Kirklin JW, Karp RB: *The Tetralogy of Fallot*. W. B. Saunders, Philadelphia, 1970.
61. Duborg G, Broustet P, Bricaud H, et al.: Correction complete d'une triade de Fallott en circulation extracorporelle chez une femme enceinte. Arch Mal Coeur 52:1389, 1959.
62. Baker JL, Russell CS, Grainger RG, et al.: Closed pulmonary valvotomy in the management of Fallot's tetralogy complicated by pregnancy. J Obstet Gynaecol Br Commonw 70:154, 1963.
63. Cutforth R, Catchlove B, Knight LW, et al.: The Eisenmenger syndrome and pregnancy. Aust N Z J Obstet Gynaecol 8:202, 1968.
64. Goodwin JF: Pregnancy and coarctation of the aorta. Clin Obstet Gynecol 4:645, 1961.
65. Deal K, Wooley CF: Coarctation of the aorta and pregnancy. Ann Intern Med 73:706, 1973.
66. Cohen LS, Friedman WF, Braunwald E: Natural history of mild congenital aortic stenosis elucidated by serial hemodynamic studies. Am J Cardiol 30:1, 1972.
67. Pansegrau DG, Kilschos JM, Durnin RE, et al.: Supravalvular aortic stenosis in adults. Am J Cardiol 31:635, 1973.
68. Parker B: The course in idiopathic hypertrophic muscular subaortic stenosis. Ann Intern Med 70:903, 1969.
69. Varghese PH, Izukawa T, Rowe RD: Supravalvular aortic stenosis as part of rubella syndrome with discussion of pathogenesis. Br Heart J 31:59, 1969.
70. Roberts WC: The congenitally bicuspid aortic valve: A study of 85 autopsy cases. Am J Cardiol 26:72, 1970.
71. Bacon APC, Matthews MB: Congenital bicuspid aortic valves and the etiology of isolated aortic valvular stenosis. Q J Med 28:545, 1959.
72. Kirklin JW, Connolly DC, Ellis FH Jr, et al.: Problems in the diagnosis and surgical treatment of pulmonic stenosis with intact ventricular septum. Circulation 8:849, 1953.
73. Bentivoglio LG, Maranhao V, Downing DF: Electrocardiogram in pulmonary stenosis with intact septa. Am Heart J 59:347, 1960.
74. Cayler GG, Ongley P, Nadas AS: Relation of systolic pressure in the right ventricle to the electrocardiogram: A study of patients with pulmonary stenosis and intact ventricular septum. N Engl J Med 258:979, 1958.
75. Moller I, Wennevold A, Lyngborg KE: The natural history of pulmonary stenosis: Long-term follow-up with serial heart catheterizations. Cardiol 58:193, 1973.
76. Kaufman JM, Ruble PE: The current status of the pregnant cardiac. Ann Intern Med 48:1157, 1958.
77. Avido DM: *The Lung Circulation*. Pergamon Press, Oxford, 1965.
78. Wagenvoort CA, Wagenvoort N: *Pathology of Pulmonary Hypertension*. John Wiley & Sons, New York, 1977.
79. Coleman PN, Edmunds AWB, Tregillus J: Primary pulmonary hypertension in three sibs. Br Heart J 1:81, 1959.
80. Stoelting RK, Reis RR, Longnecker DE: Hemodynamic responses to nitrous oxide-halothane and halothane in patients with valvular heart disease. Anesthesiology 37:430, 1972.
81. Sullivan JM: Blood pressure elevation in pregnancy. Prog Cardiovasc Dis 16 (4):375, 1974.
82. Barnes CG: *Medical Disorders in Obstetric Practice*, ed. 34. Blackwell, Oxford, 1970, pp 50–52, 54–56, 58, 60.
83. Browne FJ: Chronic hypertension and pregnancy. Br Med J 2:283, 1947.
84. Wallen I: The infant mortality in specific hypertensive disease of pregnancy and in essential hypertension. Am J Obstet Gynecol 66:36, 1953.
85. Greenhill JP, Friedman EA: *Biological Principles and Modern Practice of Obstetrics*. W. B. Saunders, Philadelphia, 1974, p 394.
86. Kincaid-Smith P, Bullen M, Mills J: Prolonged use of methyldopa in severe hypertension in pregnancy. Br Med J I:274, 1966.
87. Leather HM, Humphreys DM, Baker P, et al: A controlled trial of hypotensive agents in hypertension in pregnancy. Lancet II:488, 1968.
88. Ross JH, Wright JA: Successful twin pregnancy after treatment of malignant essential hypertension. Br Med J II:545, 1958.
89. Hamilton M: Presymptomatic diagnosis of hypertension. In *Proceedings of the 5th Interna-*

tional Congress of Hygiene and Preventive Medicine, vol 1. Rome, 1968, p 132.
90. Smith SL, Douglas BH, Langford HG: A model of preeclampsia. Johns Hopkins Med J 120:220, 1967.
91. Chesley LC, Talledo E, Bohler CS, et al.: Vascular reactivity to angiotensin II and norepinephrine in pregnant and nonpregnant women. Am J Obstet Gynecol 91:837, 1965.
92. Dieckmann WJ, Michel HL: Vascular effects of posterior pituitary extracts in pregnant women. Am J Obstet Gynecol 33:131, 1937.
93. Talledo OE, Chesley LC, Zuspan FP: Renin-angiotensin system in normal and toxemic pregnancies. Am J Obstet Gynecol 100:218, 1968.
94. Brust AA, Assali NS, Ferris EB: Evaluation of neurogenic and humoral factors in blood pressure maintenance in normal and toxemic pregnancy using tetraethylatamonium chloride. J Clin Invest 27:717, 1948.
95. Assali NS, Prystowsky H: Studies on autonomic blockade. J Clin Invest 29:1354, 1950.
96. Koch-Weser J: Correlation of pathophysiology and pharmacotherapy in primary hypertension. Am J Cardiol 32:499, 1973.
97. Walsh JJ, Burch GE: Postpartal heart disease. Arch Intern Med 108:817, 1961.
98. Goodwin JF, Oakley CM: The cardiomyopathies. Br Heart J 34:545, 1972.
99. Demakis JG, Rahimtoola SH: Peripartum cardiomyopathy. Circulation 44:964, 1971.
100. Stuart KL: Cardiomyopathy of pregnancy and the puerperium. Q J Med 34:463, 1968.
101. Kitchen DH: Dissecting aneurysm of the aorta in pregnancy. J Obstet Gynaecol Br Commonw 81:410, 1974.
102. Schnitker MA, Bayer CA: Dissecting aneurysm of the aorta in young individuals, particularly in association with pregnancy: With report of a case. Ann Intern Med 20:486, 1944.
103. McGeachy TE, Paullin JE: Dissecting aneurysm of the aorta. JAMA 108:1690, 1937.
104. Frank S, Braunwald E: Idiopathic hypertrophic subaortic stenosis: Clinical analysis of 126 patients with emphasis on the natural history. Circulation 37:759, 1968.
105. Powell JW Jr, Whiting RB, Dinsmore RE, et al.: Symptomatic prognosis in patients with idiopathic hypertrophic subaortic stenosis (IHSS). Am J Med 55:15, 1973.
106. Reis RL, Peterson LM, Mason DT, et al.: Congenital fixed subvalvular aortic stenosis: An anatomical classification and correlations with operative results. Circulation 43:11, 1971.
107. Swan DA, Bell B, Oakley CM, et al.: Analysis of symptomatic course and prognosis and treatment of hypertrophic obstructive cardiomyopathy. Br Heart J 33:671, 1971.
108. Brown AK, Doukas N, Riding WD, et al.: Cardiomyopathy and pregnancy. Br Heart J 29:387, 1967.
109. Turner GM, Oakley CM, Dixon HG: Management of pregnancy complicated by hypertrophic obstructive cardiomyopathy. Br Med J II:281, 1968.
110. Braunwald E, Lambrew CT, Rockoff SD, et al.: Idiopathic hypertrophic subaortic stenosis. I. A description of the disease based upon an analysis of 64 patients. Circulation 30:3, 1964.
111. Mason DT, Braunwald E, Ross J Jr: Effects of changes in body position on the severity of obstruction to left ventricular outflow in idiopathic hypertrophic subaortic stenosis. Circulation 33:374, 1966.
112. Glancy DL, Shepherd RL, Beiser GD, et al.: The dynamic nature of left ventricular outflow obstruction in idiopathic hypertrophic subaortic stenosis. Ann Intern Med 75:589, 1971.
113. Watson H, Emslie-Smith D, Herring J, et al.: Myocardial infarction during pregnancy and the puerperium. Lancet II:523, 1960.
114. Fletcher E, Knox EW, Morton P: Acute myocardial infarction in pregnancy. Br Med J III:586, 1967.
115. Ginz B: Myocardial infarction in pregnancy. J Obstet Gynaecol Br Commonw 77:610, 1970.
116. Husaini MH: Myocardial infarction during pregnancy: Report of two cases with a review of the literature. Postgrad Med J 47:660, 1971.
117. Curry JJ, Quintana FJ: Myocardial infarction with ventricular fibrillation during pregnancy treated by direct current defibrillation with fetal survival. Chest 58:82, 1970.
118. Canning B St J, Green AT, Mulcahy R: Coronary heart disease in the puerperium. J Obstet Gynaecol Br Commonw 76:1018, 1969.
119. Schenker JG, Polishuk WZ: Pregnancy following mitral valvotomy: A survey of 182 patients. Obstet Gynecol 32:214, 1968.
120. Wallace WA, Ellis LB: Pregnancy following closed mitral valvuloplasty: Long-term follow-up. Circulation 40:211, 1969.
121. Wallace WA, Harken DE, Ellis LB: Pregnancy following closed mitral valvuloplasty: Long-term study with remarks concerning necessity for cardiac management. JAMA 217:297, 1971.
122. Harrison RC, Roschke EJ: Pregnancy in patients with cardiac valve prostheses. Clin Obstet Gynecol 18:107, 1975.
123. Villoria FE, Montoya L, Recasens E: Protesis valvulares y'embarazo. Rev Clin Esp 140:537, 1976.
124. Lutz DJ, Noller KL, Spittell J Jr, et al.: Pregnancy and its complications following cardiac valve prosthesis. Am J Obstet Gynecol 131:460, 1978.
125. Iberra-Perez C, Arevalo-Toledo N, Alvarez-De la Cadena, O, et al.: The course of pregnancy in patients with artificial heart valves. Am J Med 61:504, 1976.
126. Buxbaum A, Aygen MM, Shahin W, et al.: Pregnancy in patients with prosthetic heart valves. Chest 59:639, 1971.
127. Braunwald E, Braunwald N, Ross J: Effects of mitral valve replacement on the pulmonary vascular dynamics of patients with pulmonary hypertension. N Engl J Med 273:509, 1965.

128. Kloster F, Bristow D, Starr A, et al.: Serial cardiac output and blood volume studies following cardiac valve replacement. Circulation 33:528, 1966.
129. Austen W, Corning H, Moran J, et al.: Cardiac hemodynamics immediately following mitral valve surgery. J Thorac Cardiovasc Surg 51:468, 1966.
130. Hultgren H, Hubis H, Shumway N: Cardiac function following mitral valve replacement. Am Heart J 75:302, 1968.
131. Gilbert CS, Sullivan GJ, McLaughlin JJ: Heart disease in pregnancy: Ten year report from the Lewis Memorial Maternity Hospital. Obstet Gynecol 9:58, 1957.
132. Tejani N: Anticoagulant therapy with cardiac valve prosthesis during pregnancy. Obstet Gynecol 42:785, 1973.
133. Varkey GP, Brindle GF: Peripheral anesthesia and anticoagulant therapy. Can Anaesth Soc J 21:106, 1974.
134. Shaul WL, Hall JG: Multiple congenital anomalies associated with oral anticoagulants. Am J Obstet Gynecol 125:191, 1977.
135. Bloomfield DK: Fetal deaths and malformations associated with the use of coumarin derivatives in pregnancy. Am J Obstet Gynecol 118:883, 1970.
136. Saka DM, Marx GF: Management of a parturient with cardiac valve prosthesis. Anesth Analg 55:214, 1976.
137. Bristow JD, McCord CW, Starr A, et al.: Clinical and hemodynamic results of aortic valvular replacement with a ball-valve prosthesis. Circulation 29:36, 1964.
138. McHendry MM, Smeloff EA, Davey TB, et al.: Hemodynamic results with full-flow orifice prosthetic valves. Circulation 35:24, 1967.
139. Ross J Jr, Morrow AG, Mason DT, et al.: Left ventricular function following replacement of the aortic valve: Hemodynamic response to muscular exercise. Circulation 33:507, 1966.
140. Kay C, Smith K: Surgery of the pregnant cardiac patient. Am J Cardiol 12:293, 1963.
141. Zuhdi N, Carey JL, Schmidt A, et al.: Total body perfusion and pregnancy. J Int Coll Surg 43:43, 1965.
142. Lee WH Jr, Pate JW: Surgical aspects of heart disease in pregnancy. GP 28:78, 1963.
143. Jacobs WM, Cooley D, Goen GP: Cardiac surgery with extracorporeal circulation during pregnancy. Obstet Gynecol 25:167, 1965.
144. Harthorne JW, Buckley MJ, Grover JW, et al.: Valve replacement during pregnancy. Ann Intern Med 67:1032, 1967.
145. Zitnik RS, Brandenburg RO, Sheldon R, et al.: Pregnancy and open-heart surgery. Circulation (Suppl I) 39 and 40:I-257, 1969.
146. Upshaw CB: A study of maternal electrocardiograms recorded during labor and delivery. Am J Obstet Gynecol 107:17, 1970.
147. Spritzer RC, Seldon M, Mattes LM, et al.: Serious arrhythmias during labor and delivery in women with heart disease. JAMA 211:1005, 1970.
148. Szekely P, Snaith L: Atrial fibrillation and pregnancy. Br Med J I:1407, 1961.
149. Pine HL, Fox L, Shook D McK: Paroxysmal ventricular tachycardia complicating pregnancy. Am J Cardiol 15:732, 1965.
150. Szekely P, Snaith L: Paroxysmal tachycardia in pregnancy. Br Heart J 15:195, 1953.
151. Mendelson CL: Disorders of the heart beat in pregnancy. Am J Obstet Gynecol 72:1268, 1956.
152. Mowbray R: Heart block and pregnancy: A review. J Obstet Gynaecol Br Emp 55:432, 1948.
153. Sussman HF, Duque D, Lesser ME: Atrial flutter with 1:1 A-V conduction. Dis Chest 49:99, 1966.
154. Greiss FC, Still JG, Anderson S: Effects of local anesthetic agents on the uterine vasculatures and myometrium. Am J Obstet Gynecol 124:889, 1976.
155. Biehl D, Shnider SM, Levinson G, et al.: The direct effects of circulating lidocaine on uterine blood flow and foetal well being in the pregnant ewe. Can Anaesth Soc J 24:445, 1977.
156. Biehl D, Shnider SM, Levinson G, et al.: Placental transfer of lidocaine. Anesthesiology 48:409, 1978.
157. Joelsson I, Barton MD, Daniel S, et al.: The response of the unanesthetized sheep fetus to sympathomimetic amines and adrenergic agents. Am J Obstet Gynecol 114:43, 1972.
158. Joelsson I, Barton MD: The effect of blockade of the receptors of the sympathetic nervous system of the fetus. Acta Obstet Gynecol Scand (Suppl 3) 48:75, 1969.
159. Barnes AG: Chronic propranolol administration during pregnancy. J Reprod Med 5:79, 1970.
160. Renou P, Newman W, Wood C: Autonomic control of fetal heart rate. Am J Obstet Gynecol 105:949, 1969.
161. Tunstall ME: The effect of propranolol on the onset of breathing at birth. Br J Anaesth 41:792, 1969.
162. Reed RL, Cheney CB, Fearon RE, et al.: Propranolol therapy throughout pregnancy: A case report. Anaesth Analg 53:214, 1974.
163. Greiss FC, Crandell DL: Therapy for hypotension induced by spinal anesthesia during pregnancy. JAMA 191:793, 1965.
164. Greiss FC, Pick, JR: The uterine vascular bed: Adrenergic receptors. Obstet Gynecol 23:209, 1964.
165. Cibils LA, Pose SV, Zuspan FP: Effect of l-norepinephrine infusion on uterine contractility and the cardiovascular system. Am J Obstet Gynecol 84:307, 1962.
166. James FM III, Greiss FC, Kemp RA: An evaluation of vasopressor therapy for maternal hypotension during spinal anesthesia. Anesthesiology 33:25, 1970.
167. Lucas W, Kirschbaum T, Assali NS: Spinal shock and fetal oxygenation. Am J Obstet Gynecol 93:583, 1965.
168. Levinson G, Shnider SM: Vasopressors in obstetrics. In Clinical Anesthesia. HL Zauder, ed

F. A. Davis, Philadelphia, 1973. p. 77.
169. Shnider SM, deLorimier AA, Holl JW, et al.: Vasopressors in obstetrics. I. Correction of fetal acidosis with ephedrine during spinal hypotension. Am J Obstet Gynecol 102:911, 1968.
170. Kaiser IH, Harris JS: The effect of adrenalin on the pregnant human uterus. Am J Obstet Gynecol 59:775, 1950.
171. Kresnow N, Rolett EL, Yurchak PM, et al.: Isoproterenol and cardiovascular performance. Am J Med 37:514, 1964.
172. Mahon WA, Reid DWJ, Day RA: The in vivo effects of beta adrenergic stimulation and blockade on the human uterus at term. J Pharmacol Exp Ther 156:178, 1967.
173. Blanchard K, Dandavino A, Nuwayhid B, et al.: Systemic and uterine hemodynamic responses to dopamine in pregnant and non-pregnant sheep. Am J Obstet Gynecol 130:669, 1978.
174. Callender K, Levinson G, Shnider SM, et al.: Dopamine administration in the normotensive pregnant ewe. Obstet Gynecol 51:586, 1978.
175. Rolbin SH, Levinson G, Shnider SM, et al.: Dopamine treatment of spinal hypotension decreases uterine blood flow in the pregnant ewe. Anesthesiology 51:22, 1979.
176. Clark RB, Brunner JA: Dopamine as a vasopressor for the treatment of spinal hypotension during cesarean section. In press.
177. Hernandez A, Burton RM, Goldring D, et al.: The effects of maternally administered digoxin upon the cardiovascular hemodynamics of the fetal lamb. Am Heart J 85:511, 1973.
178. Berman W, Ravenscroft PJ, Sheiner LB, et al.: Differential effects of digoxin at comparable concentrations in tissues of fetal and adult sheep. Circ Res 41:635, 1977.
179. Okita GT, Plotz EJ, Davis ME: Placental transfer of radioactive digitoxin in pregnant women and its fetal distribution. Circ Res 4:376, 1956.
180. Sherman JL, Locke RV: Transplacental neonatal digitalis intoxication. Am J Cardiol 6:834, 1960.
181. Ring G, Krames E, Shnider SM, et al.: Comparison of nitroprusside and hydralazine in hypertensive pregnant ewes. Obstet Gynecol 51:598, 1977.
182. Naulty JS, Cefalo R, Rodkey FL: Placental transfer and fetal toxicity of sodium nitroprusside. In Abstracts of Scientific Papers, Annual Meeting, American Society of Anesthesiologists, San Francisco, 1976, p 543.

CHAPTER 14

Anesthetic Considerations for Preeclampsia-Eclampsia

Brett B. Gutsche, M.D.

Each year approximately 250,000 American women develop hypertension during pregnancy. These women have a significantly higher incidence of maternal, fetal and neonatal morbidity and mortality. The current classification of hypertensive disorders of pregnancy, as recommended by the American College of Obstetricians and Gynecologists, is:

I. Preeclampsia—eclampsia
II. Chronic hypertension
III. Chronic hypertension with superimposed preeclampsia (or eclampsia)
IV. Gestational hypertension (also called late or transient hypertension of the third trimester)

Preeclampsia is a syndrome of hypertension, proteinuria and generalized edema occurring after the twentieth week of gestation and usually abating within 48 hours of delivery. **Eclampsia** is the occurrence of convulsions superimposed on preeclampsia. The term **toxemia of pregnancy** refers specifically to preeclampsia and eclampsia. It is most commonly seen in young and elderly primagravidas, particularly those who have received inadequate prenatal care. It has a higher occurrence in conditions causing rapid uterine enlargement such as multiple gestations, diabetes mellitus, polyhydramnios and hydatidiform mole.

Chronic hypertension is the presence of persistent hypertension, regardless of etiology, before the twentieth week of gestation or beyond 6 weeks postpartum. **Gestational hypertension** is characterized by the development of hypertension without proteinuria or generalized edema during the last weeks of pregnancy or immediate postpartum period.

PATHOPHYSIOLOGY OF PREECLAMPSIA-ECLAMPSIA

The etiology of preeclampsia is unknown, but three factors which may be involved are immunologic injury of the placenta, uterine ischemia and the development of intravascular coagulopathy.[1-4] Recent evidence would indicate that vascular changes of the placenta developing in the first trimester of pregnancy are the cause of preeclampsia. An antigen-antibody reaction between maternal and fetal tissue activates a placental vasculitis. Later in pregnancy, this leads to tissue anoxia and the release of a thromboplastin-like substance into the general circulation of the mother, causing the signs and symptoms of preeclampsia (Figure 14.1). Uteroplacental ischemia results in the excretion of a renin-like substance, causing the increased production of angiotensin and aldosterone. It is also postulated that the synthesis of vasodepressor substances, particularly the prostaglandins, may be inhibited.[3,4] As previously stated, the triad

ANESTHETIC CONSIDERATIONS FOR ECLAMPSIA-PREECLAMPSIA

```
                    Decreased
                   Uteroplacental
                    Blood Flow
                         ↓ ↑
                  Decreased Placental
                    Prostaglandin
                         ↓ ↑
  Release of  ←──  "UTERINE ISCHEMIA"  ──→  Release of
  Trophoblastic                              Uterine Renin
  Material
      ↓                                          ↓
                        Angiotensinogen ──→ Angiotensin I
  Liberation of                                  ↓
  Thromboplastin      VASOCONSTRICTION  ←── Angiotensin II
      ↓                                          ↓
  Fibrin deposition                         Adrenal ──→ Aldosterone
      ↓
  Renal Glomerular
  Lesion
                                          Decreased Glomerular
                                          Filtration Rate
                                                 ↓
                                          Increased Sodium ←
                                          Reabsorption
      ↓                 ↓                        ↓
  ┌───────────┐  ┌──────────────┐         ┌──────────┐
  │PROTEINURIA│  │ HYPERTENSION │         │  EDEMA   │
  └───────────┘  └──────────────┘         └──────────┘
```

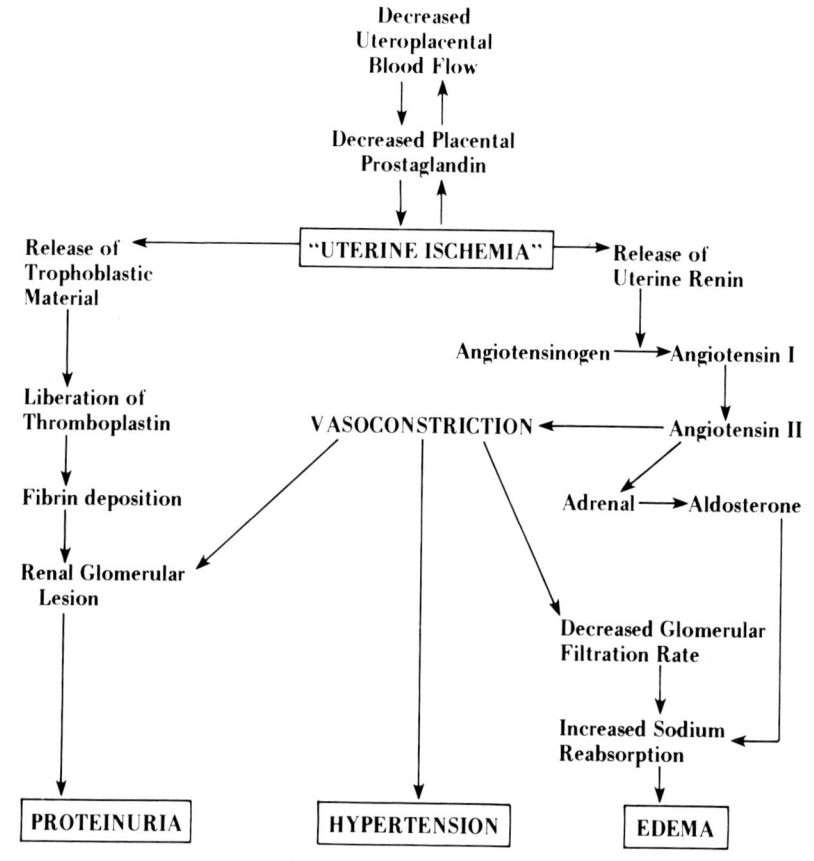

Figure 14.1. Proposed scheme of pathophysiologic changes in toxemia of pregnancy. (Modified by permission from Speroff L: Toxemia of pregnancy: Mechanism and therapeutic management. Am J Cardiol 32:582, 1973.)

of hypertension, proteinuria and generalized edema characterize preeclampsia, but occasionally generalized edema is not readily obvious. A blood pressure above 140/90, or a rise above normal in systolic pressure of 30 torr or diastolic pressure of 15 torr with a urine protein loss in excess of 2 gm a day are usually sufficient evidence for the diagnosis. A blood pressure exceeding 160/110, a proteinuria greater than 5 gm a day, headache, visual disturbances or epigastric pain indicate severe preeclampsia and impending eclampsia. If one or more grand mal convulsions occur in the presence of preeclampsia, a diagnosis of eclampsia is made, which significantly worsens the prognosis of both mother and fetus.

Maternal pathophysiology involves nearly every organ system.[3, 5-9] There is generalized vasoconstriction with a marked increased sensitivity to vasopressors. Therefore, ergots and their derivatives are best avoided or used with great caution in the toxemic patient because of their marked vasopressor and hypertensive activity. While sodium and water are retained, causing generalized edema, the intravascular volume is markedly decreased, often below non-pregnant levels, causing an increased hematocrit but representing a relative anemia (Table 14.1).

Table 14.1
Mean Plasma Volume, Albumin and Hematocrit in Non-pregnancy, Normal Pregnancy and Preeclampsia*

	Non-pregnancy	Normal Pregnancy	Preeclampsia
Number	22	55	14
Plasma volume (ml)	2242 ± 271	3133 ± 97	2590 ± 108
Albumin (gm %)	5.45 ± 0.01	3.92 ± 0.08	3.48 ± 0.08
Hematocrit (%)	39.0 ± 0.04	34.2 ± 0.54	39.3 ± 0.70

* Reprinted by permission from Bletka M, Hlavatj V, Trnkova M, et al.: Volume of whole blood and absolute amount of serum proteins in the early stages of late toxemia of pregnancy. Am J Obstet Gynecol 106:10, 1970.

There is a hyper-reflexia and often increased central nervous system irritability. Toxemic coma may develop in the absence of convulsions. The glomerular filtration rate is decreased with characteristic renal lesions showing swelling of capillary endothelial cells with a narrowing of glomerular capillaries and, frequently, fibrin deposits within the glomeruli. Blood uric acid levels are increased in toxemia and, in the patient not receiving thiazides, may be indicative of the severity of the process. In severe preeclampsia or eclampsia, periportal hemorrhage and ischemic lesions of the liver have been seen at autopsy. Edema of the upper airway and larynx seen in normal pregnancy may be exaggerated. Abnormalities in the coagulation system can occur (Figure 14.2) and, at times, progress to frank disseminated intravascular coagulation. The uterus becomes hyperactive, with an increased sensitivity to oxytocin. Rapid and premature labor is common. The placenta often shows infarcts, fibrin deposition or frank abruption.

With eclampsia and convulsions, frank pulmonary edema with congestive heart failure is common, often leading to demise. Maternal asphyxiation may result from inadequate respirations or pulmonary aspiration of stomach contents, which may occur during convulsions. Coma with cerebral edema may follow convulsions. Causes of maternal death include sequelae of hypertensive cerebral encephalopathy, cerebral hemorrhage, placental abruption, renal failure and pituitary necrosis.

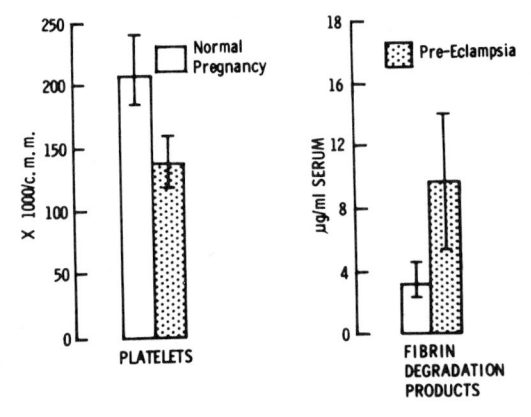

Figure 14.2. Comparison of platelet counts and serum fibrin/fibrinogen degradation products in 10 patients with severe preeclampsia and matched control pregnancies (mean ± SD). (Reprinted by permission from Lindheimer MD, et al.: *Hypertension in Pregnancy.* John Wiley & Sons, New York, 1976, p 87.)

The fetus is at great risk in preeclampsia due to marginal placental function, which may become inadequate, particularly in the presence of increased uterine activity. Aortocaval compression, induced hypotension from maternal therapy or anesthesia and the use of depressant drugs greatly enhance the danger to the fetus. Both premature as well as small-for-gestational-age neonates, frequently born through thick meconium, are common.

THERAPY OF THE TOXEMIC PATIENT

Therapy for preeclampsia varies greatly. In general its aims are to minimize vasospasm; improve circulation, particularly to the uterus, placenta and kidneys; improve intravascular volume; correct acid-base and electrolyte imbalances; and decrease both central nervous system and reflex hyperactivity. Frequently, with early detection and proper therapy, the process may be minimized and the pregnancy carried to term. Therapy as a rule is symptomatic, definitive treatment being delivery of the fetus and, most important, the placenta.

Hospitalization and bed rest in the lateral decubitus position to prevent aortocaval compression and improve uterine blood flow are often most effective.[4, 8] The upright and supine positions, which favor aortocaval compression, seem to aggravate the condition.[6] Although preeclampsia is associated with water and salt retention, fluids should not be restricted.[10] In the past, severe sodium restriction was recommended, which frequently led to sodium depletion and possible further production of renin, angiotensin and aldosterone.[6, 7]

Evidence now favors adequate sodium intake with minimal, if any, sodium restriction.[4, 7] Intravenous fluids should contain sodium, particularly if oxytocin is used, or water intoxication with convulsions can occur. The diet should be adequate, with no attempt at weight reduction as was taught in the past. Often just bed rest in the lateral decubitus position with adequate fluid and dietary intake will promote a diuresis and fall in blood pressure.

Until recently, much reliance was placed on diuretics, particularly the thiazides. These produced a diuresis at the expense of the already depleted intravascular volume. They also lead to electrolyte depletion, increased blood uric acid levels (which are already elevated in toxemia) and glucose intolerance in both mother and fetus. The routine use of diuretics should be discouraged,[8, 10, 11] except in cases of severe hypertension, congestive heart failure, severe fluid retention or when required to potentiate the action of antihypertensive drugs.

In the United States, parenterally administered magnesium is widely used in the treatment of toxemia of pregnancy. Magnesium is a central nervous system depressant. It also effectively reduces hyper-reflexia by depression at the neuromuscular junction.[12] Magnesium decreases the amount of acetylcholine liberated at the neuromuscular junction, diminishes the sensitivity of the endplate to acetylcholine and depresses the excitability of the muscle membrane.[13] Magnesium is a mild vasodilator and, in addition, depresses uterine hyperactivity, thus improving uterine blood flow. Therapeutic maternal blood levels are in the vicinity of 4 to 6 mEq/L (Table 14.2).

Magnesium therapy is associated with both maternal and neonatal side effects. Overdose can lead to maternal muscle

Table 14.2
Effects of Increasing Plasma Magnesium Levels

Observed Condition	mEq/L
Normal plasma level	1.5–2.0
Therapeutic range	4.0–6.0
ECG changes (P-Q interval prolonged, QRS complex widens)	5.0–10
Loss of deep tendon reflexes	10
Sinoatrial and atrioventricular block	15
Respiratory paralysis	15
Cardiac arrest	25

weakness, respiratory insufficiency and even cardiac failure.[12] Fortunately, these complications do not usually arise until after the deep tendon reflexes are depressed. Marked depression of deep tendon reflexes is an indication to decrease or omit the dose of magnesium. Magnesium will also increase the sensitivity of the mother to both the depolarizing and nondepolarizing skeletal muscle relaxants[14, 15] (Figure 14.3). Because magnesium crosses the placenta, its effects on the fetus often result in a newborn that has markedly decreased muscle tone at birth. With high magnesium levels the newborn may show respiratory depression and apnea. Intravenous calcium may partially overcome the neuromuscular blocking properties of magnesium in both mother and newborn. As magnesium is excreted by the kidneys, it must be given with care and in reduced doses in the presence of a decreased urine output or impaired renal function.

If the diastolic blood pressure remains

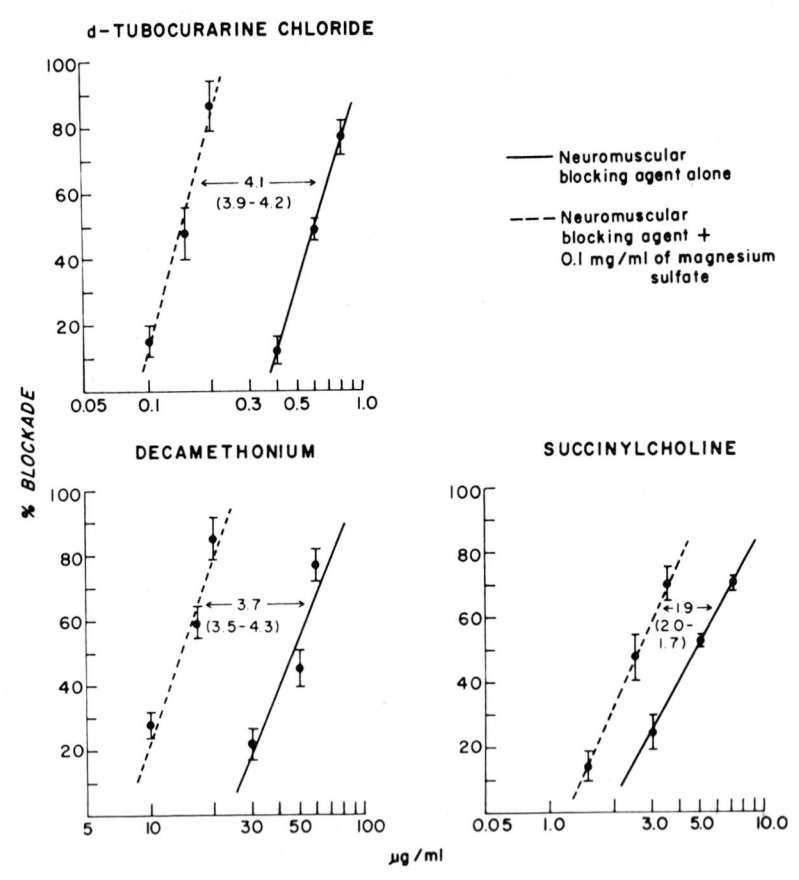

Figure 14.3. Dose response curves of *d*-tubocurarine, decamethonium and succinylcholine, using the rat phrenic nerve-diaphragm preparation. Each *point* represents the mean of five observations. *Vertical bars* indicate standard error. 0.1 mg/ml of magnesium sulfate is a subliminal dose. The magnitude of potentiation is shown in between the curves with their fiducial limits. (Reprinted by permission from Ghoneim MM, Long JP: Interaction between magnesium and other neuromuscular blocking agents. Anesthesiology 32:23, 1970.)

over 110 torr despite magnesium therapy, antihypertensives are usually required. In the past, large intravenous doses of veratrum alkaloids or reserpine were used effectively. However, they were frequently associated with neonatal respiratory obstruction due to nasal congestion of the newborn, who is an obligate nose breather. Nasal decongestants, such as Neosynephrine, usually alleviated the condition. Hydralazine (Apresoline) is frequently used today because of the following desirable properties: (1) rapid action when given intravenously, (2) it increases renal blood flow; and (3) if the blood pressure fall is more than desired, it is of short duration and easily treated by increasing venous return to the heart.[16, 17] It is also associated with tachycardia and increased cardiac output. Some of the newer antihypertensives have been recommended. Methyldopa has the disadvantage of a long latency period (6 to 8 hours) and may add to liver dysfunction. It may be useful after initial control of hypertension is accomplished with hydralazine or for use in the chronic hypertensive.[17] Diazoxide, (Hyperstat) a thiazide derivative without a diuretic activity, has its proponents.[17, 18] However, diazoxide has the disadvantage of interfering with glucose metabolism and uric acid excretion. Diazoxide is also a potent inhibitor of uterine activity. In a hypertensive crisis a continuous 0.1 per cent infusion of trimethaphan (Arfonad) can be lifesaving. For reasons discussed fully in chapter 3, nitroprusside is not used antepartum. When using antihypertensives, fetal heart rate should be carefully and continuously monitored. Sudden falls in maternal blood pressure can rapidly produce fetal distress and demise as the utero-placental circulation becomes further compromised. One usually aims only to produce a partial return of maternal blood pressure toward normal levels with a diastolic pressure of about 100 torr until after delivery.

Anticonvulsives and sedation may be required in severe preeclampsia or eclampsia. In the past, heavy sedation with barbiturates and narcotics was recommended, but this frequently resulted in severe neonatal depression. More recently, diazepam has been used with success.[16-18] However, diazepam may cause neonatal hypotonia, respiratory depression and loss of body heat regulation (chapter 7). More recently the British have been using chlormethiazole, a hypnotic and anticonvulsant, in a continuous infusion.[16, 19] During labor, perhaps the best means of sedation is expertly managed regional analgesia, which will be discussed later.[19]

With the development of eclampsia, the first priority is the control of grand mal convulsions and maintenance of adequate ventilation. Initially, a small intravenous dose of a rapidly acting barbiturate, such as thiopental 50 to 100 mg or diazepam 5 mg, is used. One should administer high concentrations of oxygen to the mother during the convulsion. It may be necessary initially to use a rapidly acting muscle relaxant and to intubate the mother, protecting her from pulmonary aspiration and ensuring adequate ventilation. Postictal depression may require support of ventilation to assure adequate oxygenation and to prevent hypercapnea and respiratory acidosis. Because convulsions are often associated with the development of a metabolic acidosis, correction with bicarbonate is indicated after determination of arterial blood gases and pH. In severe preeclampsia or eclampsia, frank congestive cardiac failure with pulmonary edema may occur. In these cases, a rapidly acting intravenous diuretic such as furosemide is useful. Digitalization may be indicated. If cerebral edema is suspected, an osmotic diuretic such as mannitol is used, but only in the presence of good urinary output. Dexamethasone may also be of use in this condition.[16] Further therapy is aimed at preventing additional convulsions and controlling blood pressure. In severe preeclampsia or eclampsia frank disseminated intravascular coagulation may develop.[9, 20] Therapy frequently includes administration of platelets, fresh frozen plasma, fresh whole blood and, occasionally, heparin.

Delivery of the fetus and placenta is the definitive therapy of toxemia of pregnancy. The timing and the method of delivery obviously remain in the domain of the obstetrician. However, before anesthesia for cesarean section is administered convulsions must be controlled, hypertension treated and blood volume restored toward normal. Continuous electronic monitoring of maternal arterial pressure through an arterial cannula and monitoring of central venous pressure to aid in fluid replacement are usually indicated. The delivery of a premature neonate may be indicated by the deterioration of the mother, although this situation is avoided in many cases by early hospitalization and proper obstetric care. As the uterus is sensitive to oxytocin, vaginal delivery before term is often possible by induction of labor, especially because the fetus is usually small. Emergency cesarean section is frequently necessary, usually because of fetal distress developing during the stress of labor superimposed on an already compromised utero-placental vascular insufficiency or due to the development of placental abruption.

ANESTHESIA FOR THE TOXEMIC PATIENT

The anesthesiologist should play a major role in the delivery of the toxemic patient. Because of his expertise in pain control, airway management, ventilatory care and monitoring and the significant effects that both toxemia and its management may have on anesthesia, the anesthesiologist should be consulted early and assume a major role in the care of these patients.

Calling the anesthesiologist just before delivery and instructing him to "take her down now" is unacceptable medical practice.

The toxemic patient requires a reliable means of intravenous administration with a minimum of an 18-guage indwelling catheter. Intravenous fluids should not consist of dextrose in water alone, especially if oxytocin is used, due to the danger of water intoxication. Urinary output should be monitored to help guide fluid replacement. In the severe preeclamptic or eclamptic, a functioning central venous pressure line will be of great value for fluid and blood replacement. Recently it has been suggested that 20 per cent serum albumin or other plasma expanders be given while monitoring the central venous pressure to replenish the diminished intravascular volume.[21] Whole blood should be typed, cross-matched and available. The patient should be encouraged to remain on her left side, avoiding aortocaval compression. Supplemental oxygen during labor and delivery is indicated. Continuous electronic monitoring of fetal heart rate and uterine contractions during labor may detect early fetal distress. Its use is mandatory with oxytocin-induced or -augmented labor or during major conduction anesthesia (subarachnoid, lumbar epidural or caudal epidural block) to detect fetal heart rate patterns indicative of utero-placental insufficiency.[22, 23]

The choice of analgesia depends on the obstetric situation. For vaginal delivery narcotics, if used, should be given in minimal dosage early in labor to minimize newborn depression. Although providing analgesia, narcotics have no anticonvulsant activity. Tranquilizers and other adjuncts often used with narcotics should also be given in small doses, particularly because there is no effective antagonist for these drugs as there is for narcotics namely naloxone. For the later first stage of labor and delivery continuous adminis tration of 30 to 40 per cent nitrous oxide in oxygen will provide good analgesia, increased oxygenation, minimal cardiovascular depression and negligible neonatal depression. At delivery, augmentation with pudendal block or local infiltration of the perineum will allow most forceps deliveries. Small amounts of methoxyflurane (0.2 to 0.4 per cent) may be added to 30 to 40 per cent nitrous oxide at the time of delivery to increase analgesia, but many believe it should be avoided because of its potentially deleterious effects on the kidneys. In the unlikely event general anesthesia is required for vaginal delivery, the technique described in chapter 10 should be used. Although some maintain that paracervical block is safe to provide analgesia for the first stage of labor,[24] the possibility of its causing fetal distress in the already compromised fetus leaves this open to question.

The use of major conduction analgesia in the severe preeclamptic or eclamptic has long been debated. Pritchard and Pritchard,[25] who successfully treated 154 consecutive eclamptic patients, avoided its use because of the fear of further compromising utero-placental circulation secondary to sympathetic block and maternal hypotension. On the other hand, various other investigators[16, 19, 26, 27] have recommended continuous epidural anesthesia in severe preeclampsia and eclampsia to (1) help control blood pressure, (2) increase renal and uterine perfusion and (3) control pain. However, sudden falls in maternal blood pressure in toxemic patients, regardless of how induced, can be associated with decreased uterine blood flow and fetal asphyxia.[23, 28] Although epidural or caudal anesthesia is useful in preventing the rise of blood pressure during a painful labor, regional anesthesia should not be used for antihypertensive therapy. Similarly, regional anesthesia per se does not increase renal or uterine blood flow. It may prevent endogenous catecholamine secretion associated with anxiety and pain and thereby prevent further reductions in renal and uterine perfusion. Smith et al.[29] showed that both mother and newborn had fewer complications when vaginal delivery was accomplished under low subarachnoid block than when cyclopropane anesthesia was used. **The consensus of opinion today is that properly administered continuous lumbar epidural analgesia is in most instances the preferred method of analgesia for labor and vaginal delivery for preeclamptic patients under good medical control.** Its primary advantages are (1) complete maternal pain relief, (2) that it provides excellent conditions for the obstetrician and (3) that it can be rapidly extended to allow abdominal delivery. When properly administered, epidural analgesia is associated with minimal newborn depression. The use of local anesthetics in proper dosage in convulsive disorders is not contraindicated.[30]

Before instituting continuous lumbar epidural analgesia the patient ideally should have a central venous pressure (CVP) monitor placed and receive hydration infusion of a balanced salt solution and/or plasmanate until CVP is 6 to 8 cm of H_2O. Usually this can be accomplished by 250 ml of plasmanate and 250 ml of lactated Ringers solution. Because labor tends to be rapid in the toxemic patient, placement of the epidural catheter is indicated early in established labor. This will frequently avoid the necessity of the use of narcotics with their depressant effect on the fetus. Coagulation studies in **severe** preeclamptics are indicated before performing epidural analgesia to avoid the danger of epidural hematoma with neurologic sequelae should severe coagulation abnormalities exist. Initially, by using a small dose of a low concentration of local anesthetic (chapter 8) a segmental block that includes T10 to L1 will provide complete relief associated with uterine contractions. This is repeated as necessary. As the fetus descends in the pelvis and the second stage of labor is entered, the dose and the concentration of the local anesthetic are increased to provide perineal analgesia. Placing the patient in the semi-sitting position will help obtain adequate perineal analgesia. Because of the hypersensitivity of maternal vasculature to vasopressors, the author prefers to omit epinephrine in the local anesthetic for the toxic patient, especially because it may decrease uterine blood flow (chapter 3).

In the past, continuous caudal epidural analgesia was widely used and recommended for preeclampsia.[31] Its disadvantages include (1) early anesthesia of the perineum, (2) the need for larger doses of local anesthetics, (3) the greater difficulty of placing the catheter and (4) the inability to extend the block to an adequate level to allow for cesarean section without the use of potentially toxic doses of local anesthetics.

If vaginal delivery is imminent, a low spinal anesthetic with a T10 sensory level will provide rapid and complete analgesia. Its major disadvantage is the possible rapid onset of severe hypotension. Hypotension can usually be prevented with acute intravenous hydration as outlined above, a slight head-down position to increase venous return to the heart and sustained left uterine displacement.

Because of an already compromised utero-placental perfusion, a sudden fall in blood pressure may result in severe fetal distress and rapid deterioration. Normally, maternal hypotension is considered to have occurred when there is a fall greater than 25 per cent of the pre-block systolic pressure or a systolic pressure less than 100 torr, whichever occurs first. Such a fall in maternal blood pressure may not be tolerated by the fetus, as evidenced by the development of late decelerations of the fetal heart rate (chapter 24). For this reason, all toxic patients should have continuous electronic fetal heart rate monitoring when major conduction anesthesia is used. Should hypotension with late decelerations develop, treatment consists of high inspired oxygen, further left uterine displacement and increased hydration with a balanced salt solution. If this is not effective, small (2.5 mg) intravenous doses of ephedrine are given until the blood pressure is corrected and remains stable. Every effort is made to avoid sudden rises and falls in maternal blood pressure.

Emergency cesarean section in an unanesthetized parturient may be required for fetal distress. In such situations, a balanced general anesthetic is indicated, both because of its rapidity and because it avoids the problem of maternal hypotension. The technique for general anesthesia is described in chapter 17. This standard technique is modified to (1) avoid prolonged paralysis due to the interaction of magnesium with muscle relaxants, (2) permit the easier control of hypertension and (3) avoid potentially nephrotoxic or hypertensive agents. The use of curare or pancuronium to prevent fasciculations is probably unnecessary because magnesium will accomplish this. When these non-depolarizing drugs are used for muscle relaxation, only half the usual dose will be necessary. Similarly, succinylcholine will also be potentiated by magnesium, and, if an infusion is administered, smaller doses are effective. Whenever muscle relaxants are used in a patient who is receiving magnesium, monitoring with a nerve-muscle stimulator is very useful.

Cesarean section with unsupplemented nitrous oxide and oxygen anesthesia is often associated with maternal hypertension. The addition of 0.5 per cent halothane will frequently avoid this problem. Methoxyflurane and enflurane are potentially nephrotoxic and should be avoided. Ketamine, sometimes used for induction of general anesthesia in bleeding parturients, should be avoided because of its tendency to produce hypertension.

Table 14.3
Effect of Preeclampsia on Fetal and Neonatal Parameters*

Severity of Pre-eclampsia	Number of Cases	Prematurity %	Small for Gestational Age	Apgar Score <6 %	Meconium-stained Amniotic Fluid %	Perinatal Death %
Mild	63	13	23	24	29	9
Moderate	67	16	39	39	38	16
Severe	38	45	48	48	29	37

* Reprinted by permission from Muller G, Philippe E, Lefakis P, et al.: Les lésions placentaires de la gestose; étude anatomo-clinique. Gynecol Obstet (Paris) 70:309, 1971.

If cesarean section is required in a toxemic patient with a functioning epidural catheter in place, the level of anesthesia can be extended and used for abdominal delivery, particularly if there is no fetal distress. However, in an emergency, surgery should not be delayed in order to establish an adequate sensory block. The author would be reluctant to use a spinal anesthetic in a severe preeclamptic for cesarean section, because of the danger of sudden maternal hypotension common after the use of high subarachnoid block.

As indicated previously, the neonate born of the toxemic mother is at high risk (Table 14.3). He may be suffering from any of the following problems: (1) prematurity, (2) small for gestational age, (3) asphyxia, (4) drug depression and (5) meconium aspiration. If he is to survive intact, prompt and proper resuscitation will be required. In his first days of life, he may require intensive therapy. It is our policy to have both a pediatrician and a second anesthesiologist present at the time of delivery of a toxemic patient to work as a team to resuscitate this neonate. If the neonate is depressed or if there is any question as to his ability to adjust to neonatal life, he is taken from the delivery room directly to the neonatal intensive care unit for further observation and treatment.

With the birth of the newborn, not infrequently the physicians involved give a sigh of relief and let down their guard. The toxemic patient may require several days postpartum to stabilize. It is not uncommon to see the severely preeclamptic patient convulse and become eclamptic within the first 24 hours postpartum. In a large series of severe preeclamptic patients, all managed with epidural analgesia, four patients convulsed all in the postpartum period after the epidural had been allowed to dissipate.[19] The toxemic patient requires her therapy to be continued. She deserves appropriate close supervision, often in an intensive care unit. The first 48 hours postpartum for this patient may be as critical as any part of her antenatal management.

References

1. Marx GF: Obstetric anesthesia in the presence of medical complications. Clin Obstet Gynecol 172:165, 1974.
2. Nadji P, Sommers SC: Lesions of toxemia in first trimester pregnancies. Am J Clin Path 58:344, 1973.
3. Simmon NM, Krumlovsky FA: The pathophysiology of hypertension in pregnancy. J Reprod Med 8:102, 1972.
4. Speroff L: Toxemia of pregnancy: Mechanism and therapeutic management. Am J Cardiol 32:582, 1973.
5. Craig CJT: Eclampsia and the anaesthetist. S Afr Med J 46:348, 1972.
6. Page EW: On the pathogenesis of preeclampsia and eclampsia. J Obstet Gynaecol Br Commonw 79:883, 1972.
7. Sims EAH: Preeclampsia and related complication of pregnancy. Am J Obstet Gynecol 107:154, 1970.
8. Sullivan JM: Blood pressure elevation in pregnancy. Prog Cardiovasc Dis 16:375, 1974.
9. Pritchard JA, Cunningham FG, Mason RA: Coagulation changes in eclampsia: Their frequency

and pathogenesis. Am J Obstet Gynecol 124:855, 1976.
10. Atkinson SM Jr: Salt, water and rest as a preventative for toxemia of pregnancy. J Reprod Med 9:223, 1972.
11. Kraus GW: Prophylactic use of hydrochlorothiazide in pregnancy. JAMA 198:1150, 1966.
12. Aldrete JA: Clinical implications of magnesium therapy. In *The Anesthesiologist, Mother and Newborn*, SM Shnider and F Moya, eds. Williams & Wilkins, Baltimore, 1974, pp 128–135.
13. Foldes FF: Factors which alter the effects of muscle relaxants. Anesthesiology 20:464, 1959.
14. Giesecke AG, Morris RE, Dalton MD, et al.: On magnesium, muscle relaxants, toxemic patients and cats. Anesth Analg 47:689, 1968.
15. Ghoneim MM, Long JP: Interaction between magnesium and other neuromuscular blocking agents. Anesthesiology 32:23, 1970.
16. Hibbard BM, Rosen M: The management of severe preeclampsia and eclampsia. Br J Anaesth 49:3, 1977.
17. Ferris TF: In *Toxemia and Hypertension from Medical Complications during Pregnancy*, GN Burrow and TF Ferris, eds. W. B. Saunders, Philadelphia, 1975, pp 53–104.
18. Martin JD: A critical survey of drugs used in the treatment of hypertensive crisis of pregnancy. Med J Aust 2:252, 1974.
19. Moir DD, Victor-Rodrigues L, Willocks J: Extradural analgesia during labour in patients with preeclampsia. J Obstet Gynaecol Br Commonw 79:465, 1972.
20. Beecham JB, Watson WJ, Clapp FF: Eclampsia, preeclampsia and disseminated intravascular coagulation. Obstet Gynecol 43:576, 1974.
21. Cloeren SE, Lippert TH, Hinselmann M: Hypovolemia in toxemia of pregnancy: Plasma expander therapy with surveillance of central venous pressure. Arch Gynaekol 215:123, 1973.
22. Schifrin BS: Fetal heart rate patterns following epidural anaesthesia and oxytocin infusion during labour. J Obstet Gynaecol Br Commonw 79:332, 1972.
23. Gibbs CP: Anesthetic management of the high-risk gravida. In *Management of the High-risk Pregnancy*, WN Spellacy, ed. University Park Press, Baltimore, 1976, pp 209–226.
24. McDonald JS: Considerations in anesthesia for obstetric complications. Int Anesthesiol Clin 11:93, 1973.
25. Pritchard JA, Pritchard SA: Standardized treatment of 154 consecutive cases of eclampsia. Am J Obstet Gynecol 123:543, 1975.
26. Bigler von R, Stamm O: Die periduralanasthesis zur verhinderung des eklamptischen anfalls und als therapie des eklamptischew comas. Gynaecologia 158:228, 1964.
27. Alper MH, Roaf ER: Anesthetic management of the high risk pregnancy. Clin Obstet Gynecol 16:347, 1973.
28. Lander CN: Dynamics of uterine circulation in pregnant and non-pregnant sheep. Am J Physiol 218:257, 1970.
29. Smith BE, Cavanagh D, Moya F: Anesthesia for vaginal delivery of the patient with toxemia of pregnancy. Anesth Analg 45:853, 1966.
30. deJong RH: *Physiology and Pharmacology of Local Anesthesia*. Charles C Thomas, Springfield, Ill, 1970, p 211.
31. Hingson RA, Edwards WB: Continuous caudal anesthesia. JAMA 123:538, 1943.
32. Hon EH, Reid BL, Hehre FW: The electronic evaluation of fetal heart rate. II. Changes with maternal hypotension. Am J Obstet Gynecol 79:209, 1960.
33. Munson EF, Embro WJ: Enflurane, isoflurane and halothane and isolated human uterine muscle. Anesthesiology 46:11, 1977.
34. Naftalin NJ, McKay DM, Phear WPC, et al.: Effects of halothane on pregnant and non-pregnant human myometrium. Anesthesiology 46:15, 1977.
35. Marx GF, Kim YI, Lin CC, et al.: Postpartum uterine pressures under halothane or enflurane anesthesia. Obstet Gynecol 51:695, 1978.
36. Moir DD: Anesthesia for caesarean section. An evaluation of a method using low concentrations of halothane and 50 per cent of oxygen. Br J Anaesth 42:136, 1970.
37. Baraka A: Correlation between maternal and foetal P_{o2} and P_{co2} during caesarean section. Br J Anaesth 42:432, 1970.
38. Marx GF, Mateo CV: Effects of different oxygen concentrations during general anesthesia for elective cesarean section. Can Anaesth Soc J 18:587, 1971.

CHAPTER 15

Coagulation Disorders in the Obstetric and Surgical Patient

Russell K. Laros, Jr., M.D.

On occasion the obstetrician-gynecologist and anesthesiologist are confronted by the need to anesthetize and deliver or operate on a patient with a congenital or acquired coagulation disorder. When the history suggests an undiagnosed abnormality of coagulation, a pre-operative laboratory screen (bleeding times, platelet count, prothrombin time, partial thromboplastin time, and thrombin time) will usually indicate either normalcy or the need for further studies to specifically identify the abnormality. Although most bleeding disorders can be anticipated and diagnosed pre-operatively by history and laboratory evaluation, on occasion they may present themselves for the first time dramatically during surgery. In either instance, a clear understanding of the coagulation mechanism, the laboratory evaluation of coagulation and therapy of the common disorders of hemostasis is essential.

THE COAGULATION MECHANISM

The initial coagulation mechanism for thrombus formation *in vivo* is adhesion of platelets to the injured vessel walls. Collagen fibrils in the injured tissue initiate adhesion, which is promptly followed by a change in shape of the platelet.

$$\text{Injury + platelets} \xrightarrow[\text{aggregation}]{\text{adhesion}} \text{platelet factor 3 + ADP}$$

During this change in shape, degranulation occurs and an adenosine diphosphate (ADP) and other constituents are released.[1] Additionally, platelet factor 3 (PF3), a lipoprotein surface component of the platelet membrane, becomes available. The ADP released from platelets attracts more platelets to the area, resulting in **platelet aggregation.** The aggregation phenomenon tends to perpetuate itself, because newly attracted platelets in turn release ADP and attract additional platelets. Increasingly large amounts of platelet factor 3 become available for initiation of the plasma phase of coagulation.

Table 15.1 details some of the properties of the coagulation factors.[2] With the exception of fibrinogen, prothrombin and calcium, the coagulation factors are trace proteins. Factor III is not listed in the table and is, in fact, the tissue factor thromboplastin. The preferred descriptive name and several common synonyms for the coagulation factors are as follows: V, proaccelerin or labile factor; VII, proconvertin or serum prothrombin conversion accelerator; VIII, antihemophilic factor or antihemophilic globulin; IX, plasma

Table 15.1
Some Properties of Coagulant Factors

Factor	Biochemistry	Biosynthesis	Biologic half-life	Function
			hrs	
Fibrinogen (I)	Glycoprotein; MW 340,000; 3 globular subunits	Liver	72–120	Common pathway; fibrin precursor
Prothrombin (II)	Glycoprotein, MW 69,000; α-2 or β-globulin	Liver; vitamin K*	72	Common pathway; proenzyme precursor of thrombin
Calcium (IV)	Ionic calcium			Extrinsic, intrinsic and common pathways
Factor V	? lipoprotein; MW > 200,000	Liver	12–36	Common pathway
Factor VII	Glycoprotein; MW 48,000–100,000; α- or β-globulin	Liver; vitamin K	4–6	Extrinsic pathway; proenzyme
Factor VIII	Lipoglycoprotein; MW > 2,000,000; α- or β-globulin	? liver, ? reticuloendothelial system	10–14	Intrinsic pathway
Factor IX	Glycoprotein; MW 50,000–200,000; α- or β-globulin	Liver; vitamin K	24	Intrinsic pathway; proenzyme
Factor X	Glycoprotein; MW 50,000–100,000; α-globulin or prealbumin	Liver; vitamin K	24–60	Common pathway; proenzyme
Factor XI	β- or γ-globulin; MW 50,000–200,000	Liver	48–84	Intrinsic pathway; proenzyme
Factor XII	β- or γ-globulin; MW $\approx$80,000	Unknown	52–60	Intrinsic pathway; proenzyme
Factor XIII	α-2-globulin; MW 320,000 4 subunits	Liver	72–120	Common pathway; proenzyme; transglutaminase

* "Vitamin K" indicates that synthesis is dependent on vitamin K.

thromboplastin component or Christmas factor; X, Stuart factor or Prower factor; XI, plasma thromboplastin antecedent; XII, Hageman factor or glass or contact factor; XIII, fibrin stabilizing factor.

The third column in the table indicates the site of biosynthesis for each factor. It is noteworthy that prothrombin, Factor VII, Factor IX and Factor X are dependent on vitamin K for their synthesis and, thus, are the factors depleted when a patient is receiving a vitamin K antagonist such as sodium warfarin. The biologic half-life is also listed for each factor and can be used to estimate roughly the frequency of replacement therapy needed during an acute bleeding problem.

The remainder of the coagulation process can be broadly divided into three phases: the extrinsic pathway, intrinsic pathway and common pathway. The pathway of function for each of the plasma factors is also noted in Table 15.1.

The total coagulation scheme can be summarized by the following schematized seven formulas:

COAGULATION DISORDERS IN THE OBSTETRIC AND SURGICAL PATIENT

1. Injury + platelets $\xrightarrow[\text{aggregation}]{\text{adhesion}}$ platelet factor 3 + ADP

2. Tissue thromboplastin + VII $\xrightarrow{Ca^{++}}$ extrinsic activator

3. XII + XI + IX + PF3 + VIII $\xrightarrow{Ca^{++}}$ intrinsic activator

4. X + V + PF3 + Ca^{++} $\xrightarrow[\text{intrinsic activator}]{\text{extrinsic activator}}$ common activator

5. Prothrombin $\xrightarrow[Ca^{++}]{\text{common activator}}$ thrombin

6. Fibrinogen $\xrightarrow{\text{thrombin}}$ fibrin polymer

7. Fibrin polymer + VIII $\xrightarrow{Ca^{++}}$ stabilized fibrin

The basic feature of coagulation is the conversion of circulating fibrinogen into a stabilized fibrin clot; it occurs in two steps. First, fibrinogen is enzymatically converted to fibrin monomer by the action of thrombin, and the fibrin monomeric units polymerize (formula 6). Next, the resulting fibrin clot is strengthened and further rendered insoluble by the action of Factor XIII (formula 7).

In order for fibrinogen to be converted to fibrin, thrombin must be generated from its precursor prothrombin. This reaction is catalyzed by a complex, common activator which consists of the activated form of Factor X, Factor V, calcium and PF3 (formula 5). The production of the common activator can occur as a result of two different pathways, the intrinsic and extrinsic. The intrinsic is so named because all its components are present in the circulating plasma (formula 3). This pathway is probably triggered by both endothelial damage and PF3. The extrinsic pathway is so named because it is triggered by tissue thromboplastin (formula 2).

Finally, the fibrinolytic system must be briefly considered. Fibrinolysis is the major physiologic means by which fibrin is disposed of after its hemostatic function has been fulfilled. The mechanism of fibrinolysis is schematically summarized by formulas 8 and 9:

8. Plasminogen $\xrightarrow{\text{activators}}$ plasmin

9. $\left.\begin{array}{l}\text{Fibrin}\\\text{Fibrinogen}\\\text{Complement}\\\text{Factor VIII}\end{array}\right\} \xrightarrow{\text{plasmin}}$ degradation products

Plasminogen is a β-globulin with a molecular weight of 81,000 daltons. It circulates in the plasma in concentrations of 10 to 20 mg/dalton. It is activated by a heterogeneous group of substances termed "plasminogen activators" (formula 8). Activators reside within the lysozyme of most cells, and urokinase and streptokinase are examples of specifically identified activators. The activated form of plasminogen, plasmin, is a proteolytic enzyme with a rather wide spectrum of activity. It cleaves arginyl-lysine bonds in a large variety of substrates, including fibrinogen, fibrin, Factor VIII and various components of complement (formula 9). It has a very short life in plasma, owing to its inactivation by humoral antiplasmins.

LABORATORY METHODS FOR STUDY OF BLOOD COAGULATION

There is no single test that is suitable as an over-all laboratory screening study of hemostasis and blood coagulation. Commonly, the combination of bleeding time, platelet count, partial thromboplastin time (PTT), prothrombin time (PT) and thrombin time are used as a screening battery.

Table 15.2 indicates which factors are measured by each study and indicates the normal value for the study in question. There are a large number of additional studies which define specific abnormalities of platelet function or allow measurements of a specific plasma clotting factor. The Rumpel-Leede test, platelet adhesiveness, platelet aggregation, whole blood prothrombin activation rate and clot retraction are all examples of studies which further define abnormalities of platelet function.

Precise levels of each circulating plasma factor can be defined by either the thromboplastin generation test or cross-correction studies with normal plasma and plasma known to be deficient in the factor being assayed. A specific assay for Factor XIII is also available.[3,4] Several accurate methods are now available for the quantitative assay of plasma fibrinogen.[5] Normal values range from 160 to 415 mg/per cent and are abnormal in acquired hypofibrinogenemia secondary to disseminated intravascular coagulation and in the hereditary afibrinogenemias and dysfibrinogenemias.[5]

Studies used in the evaluation of fibrinolysis include the euglobulin clot lysis time and the demonstration of fibrin-fibrinogen degradation products by a variety of techniques.

Table 15.3 correlates the results of several coagulation studies with hemostasis during major and minor surgery. It is important to remember that the screening coagulation studies do not provide one with a specific etiologic diagnosis. Such a diagnosis is important because only then is it possible to optimally treat excessive bleeding should it occur during surgery. Furthermore, the presence of an adequate coagulation screen in a patient suspected of having a coagulation abnormality does not diminish the necessity of pursuing a specific diagnosis and making available specific therapy should it be needed.

TREATMENT OF COAGULATION ABNORMALITIES

The author will not attempt to discuss all possible congenital and acquired coagulation disorders but will only consider those most commonly seen by the obstetrician-gynecologist and anesthesiologist dealing with obstetric patients. Acquired disorders are far more common than congenital, and those seen most frequently include idiopathic thrombocytopenic purpura, disseminated intravascular coagulation, liver disease and anticoagulant therapy. The congenital disorders seen most frequently are von Willebrand's disease and Factor XI deficiency.

Platelet Disorders

Thrombocytopenia is the most common platelet disorder and is due to either a diminished production or an increased destruction of platelets. The severity of bleeding in thrombocytopenia is roughly

Table 15.2
Screening Coagulation Tests

Study	Measures	Normal Values
Bleeding time	Platelets and vascular integrity	1–5 min (Ivy)
Platelet count	Number of platelets	140–440 × 10^3/mm^3
Partial thromboplastin time	II, V, VIII, IX, X, XI	24–36 sec
Prothrombin time	II, V, VII, X	11–12 sec
Thrombin time	I, II, circulating split products, heparin	16–20 sec

Table 15.3
Abnormal Coagulation Studies and Surgery

Normal	Inadequate for Surgery	Adequate for Minor Surgery	Adequate for Major Surgery
Bleeding time (min)	>15	<10	<8
Platelets (per mm³)	<10,000	>50,000	>100,000
Prothrombin time (sec)	>40	<35	<13
Partial thromboplastin time (sec)	>60	<45	<38
Thrombin time (sec)	>60	<32	<24

proportional to the degree to which the platelet count has been lowered.

A specific diagnosis is obviously essential for the proper total management of a patient with thrombocytopenia. However, when hemorrhage is due to thrombocytopenia, platelet transfusions are frequently of value.[6] The success of platelet transfusion therapy is dependent on the functional integrity of the transfused platelets, the underlying cause of the platelet defect in the recipient and the presence and level of antiplatelet antibodies. Platelet transfusions are available both as platelet-rich plasma and platelet concentrates. When platelet concentrates are used, a relatively large number of platelets remain in the bag and can be harvested by adding a small amount of normal saline solution after evacuation of each bag to resuspend platelets remaining in the bag. One can expect an increase in platelet count of 5,000 to 10,000/μ^3/unit of platelets transfused. The exact incremental rise and the length of platelet survival are dependent both on the underlying disease process and the freshness of the platelets.

The complications of platelet transfusion are less common and less serious than those accompanying transfusion of whole blood. They include bacterial contamination, infectious hepatitis, febrile transfusion reaction and post-transfusion purpura.

Management of idiopathic thrombocytopenic purpura during pregnancy requires concern for both fetus and mother. A review of 14 pregnancies complicated by idiopathic thrombocytopenic purpura revealed significant maternal morbidity but no maternal deaths.[7] The perinatal mortality was 21 per cent. Current recommendations for management include: (1) corticosteroids, (2) splenectomy if response is unsatisfactory with corticosteroids alone, (3) liberal use of platelet transfusion if surgical intervention is required in the face of significant thrombocytopenia and (4) careful observation of the newborn infant and treatment with corticosteroids and/or platelets if thrombocytopenia is severe.

Acquired and Congenital Plasma Factor Disorders

Von Willebrand's disease is inherited as an autosomal dominant trait and is characterized by abnormal bleeding of varying severity. The pathophysiologic basis for the disease is a marked decrease or absence of both clottable and antigenic Factor VIII. Criteria for laboratory diagnosis are as yet not completely satisfactory but include slight to moderate reduction in the PTT, a clottable Factor VIII level 15 to 30 per cent of normal, a prolonged bleeding time, abnormal platelet adhesiveness and a lack of ristocetin-induced platelet aggregation.[8, 9]

Patients undergoing surgical procedures where difficulty is anticipated in securing adequate surgical hemostasis (such as a retropubic urethropexy) should be treated prior to surgery. The therapeutic material should be either cryoprecipitate, in a dose of one bag per 10 kg of body weight per day or fresh frozen plasma in a dose of 10 ml/kg of body weight per day. Treatment should begin 24 hours pre-operatively to allow new Factor VIII synthesis in addition to the elevation obtained from the therapeutic material. When unanticipated acute bleeding is encountered, the initial therapeutic dose should be increased by approximately 50 per cent and a second dose should be given approximately 12 hours later.[10] Because Factor VIII levels are usually improved during pregnancy, most parturients will deliver without hemorrhage. The Factor VIII level should be checked periodically during the antenatal course, and pre-treatment should be reserved for patients with levels less than 25 per cent of normal. Levels should be checked daily after vaginal delivery or cesarean section and therapy given if the level falls below 25 per cent or bleeding occurs.[11, 12]

In **liver disease** virtually every hemostatic function may be impaired. Deficiencies of prothrombin and of Factors VII, IX and X generally result from decreased synthesis by the damaged liver. Factor V and fibrinogen are also synthesized by the liver; however, their levels are usually not so severely depressed. The diversity of the coagulation abnormality will be reflected in the laboratory studies by abnormalities in the PTT, PT and fibrinogen level and by abnormal fibrinolysis.

Treatment consists of both vitamin K administration and procoagulant replacement therapy. Vitamin K can be administered as vitamin K_1 in a dose of 50 mg intramuscularly; it will produce improvement in approximately 30 per cent of patients with liver disease. Replacement therapy is accomplished with fresh frozen plasma in a dose of 10 to 20 ml/kg.[13]

Factor XI deficiency (plasma thromboplastin antecedent deficiency) is a hereditary disorder transmitted as an incompletely recessive autosomal trait manifested either as a major defect in homozygous individuals with Factor XI levels below 20 per cent or as a minor defect in heterozygous individuals with levels ranging from 30 to 65 per cent of normal.[14] Severity of bleeding, however, does not always correlate with the level of Factor XI.[15, 16] The PTT is usually prolonged in individuals with Factor XI deficiency, and the specific diagnosis is confirmed by demonstrating a Factor XI level that is below 65 per cent of normal.

Despite the fact that Factor XI normally decreases during pregnancy,[17] most gravidas do not encounter bleeding problems. In one series nine women went through 17 pregnancies without a major hemorrhage.[18] Therapy is based on maintaining the Factor XI level above 40 per cent for minor procedures (including delivery) and above 50 per cent for major procedures. Treatment consists of a loading dose of fresh frozen plasma of 10 ml/kg followed by a maintenance dose of 5 ml/kg per day.

Disseminated intravascular coagulation is really a syndrome produced as part of an underlying disease which in some way leads to initiation of the clotting mechanism.[19] In the area of obstetrics and gynecology, disseminated intravascular coagulation is seen in association with placental abruption,[20] the dead fetus syndrome,[21] amniotic fluid embolism,[22] gram-negative sepsis,[23] saline abortions,[24] and severe pre-eclampsia-eclampsia.[25]

Laboratory diagnosis is based on demonstrating consumption of procoagulants: (1) a decrease in fibrinogen, a decrease in platelet count and variable prolongation of the PT and PTT; (2) demonstration of circulating fibrin-fibrinogen degradation products (prolongation of the TCT and a positive study for fibrin degradation products); and (3) indirect evidence of obstruction of the microcirculation such as abnormal red cell morphology (increased red cell fragmentation).

Treatment consists of: (1) treatment of the underlying disease, that is, removal of the source of thromboplastin whenever possible; (2) anticoagulant therapy with heparin to stop consumption and generation of split products; and (3) administration of procoagulants to replace factors that have been consumed.[19] Heparin is administered in a dose of 500 to 1000 units per hour intravenously after a loading dose of 5000 units. Laboratory control of heparin therapy may be difficult. However, unless the fibrinogen level is very low, an adequate end point can usually be obtained and consists of an increased TCT or activated clotting time to approximately one and one-half times the control value. Procoagulants can be administered in the form of fresh platelet-rich plasma following the guidelines above for platelet transfusions. Platelet transfusions are particularly indicated if heparin is to be administered in the face of significant thrombocytopenia ($<30,000/\mu^3$).

Finally, surgery or delivery in the **anticoagulated patient** must be considered. Patients receiving coumarin anticoagulants will generally withstand minor surgery if the PT is less than 35 seconds and major surgery if the PT is less than 13 seconds. Correction of a bleeding disorder secondary to coumarin therapy is accomplished by withholding the drug and administering vitamin K_1 in a dose of 5 to 50 mg intravenously. Although the larger doses of vitamin K_1 will speed the rate of return to normal, this is accomplished at the cost of making reanticoagulation with coumarin difficult for a week or more. When prompt correction is required, it can also be accomplished by administering fresh frozen plasma as outlined above.

In a number of situations it is desirable to have a patient fully anticoagulated with heparin during delivery or a surgical procedure. If adequate hemostasis becomes a problem, heparin can be discontinued and instantly counteracted by the administration of protamine sulfate in a dose of 50 mg intravenously. If bleeding continues following this dose and the thrombin time or activated clotting time is still prolonged, a second dose of 50 mg should be given and this regimen repeated as needed until correction is obtained.

References

1. Deykin D: Emerging concepts of platelet function. N Engl J Med 290:144, 1974.
2. Wintrobe MW: *Clinical Hematology*. Lea and Febiger, Philadelphia, 1974, p 409.
3. Tocantins LM, Kazal LA: *Blood Coagulation, Hemorrhage and Thrombosis*, Grune & Stratton, New York, 1965.
4. Penner JA: *Blood Coagulation Laboratory Manual*. Department of Postgraduate Medicine, University of Michigan, Ann Arbor, 1972.
5. Grannis GF: Plasma fibrinogen: Determination, normal values, physiologic shifts and fluctuations. Clin Chem 16:486, 1970.
6. Freireich EJ: Platelet transfusion procedures. Cancer Chemother Rep 1:1, 1968.
7. Laros RK, Sweet RL: Management of idiopathic thrombocytopenic purpura during pregnancy. Am J Obstet Gynecol 122:182, 1975.
8. Veltkamp JJ, van Tilburg NH: Autosomal haemophilia. Br J Haematol 26:141, 1974.
9. Weiss HJ, Hoyer LW, Rickles FR, et al.: Quantitative assay of a plasma factor deficiency in von Willebrand's disease that is necessary for platelet aggregation. J Clin Invest 52:2708, 1973.
10. Shulman, NR: The physiological basis for therapy of classical hemophilia and related disorders. Ann Intern Med 67:856, 1967.
11. Noller KL, Bowie EJW, Kempers RD, et al.: Von Willebrand's disease in pregnancy. Obstet Gynecol 41:865, 1973.
12. Krishnamurth M, Miotti AB: Von Willebrand's disease and pregnancy. Obstet Gynecol 49:244, 1977.
13. Slocter I, Corn M: Laboratory tests of hemostasis: The relation to hemorrhage in liver disease. Arch Intern Med 119:577, 1967.
14. Leiba H, Ramot B, Many A: Heredity and coagulation studies in ten families with Factor XI deficiency. Br J Haematol 11:654, 1965.
15. Rimon A, Schiffman S, Feinstein D, et al.: Factor XI activity and Factor XI antigen in homozygous and heterozygous Factor XI deficiency. Blood 48:165, 1976.
16. Purcell G, Nossel HL: Factor XI (PTA) deficiency. Obstet Gynecol 35:69, 1970.

17. Phillips LL, Rosano L, Skrodelis V: Changes in Factor XI levels during pregnancy. Am J Obstet Gynecol 116:1114, 1973.
18. Rapaport SI, Proctor RR, Patch MJ, et al.: The mode of inheritance of PTA deficiency. Blood 18:149, 1961.
19. Deykin D: The clinical challenge of disseminated intravascular coagulation. N Engl J Med 283:636, 1970.
20. Sutton DMC, Hauser R, Kulaping S, et al.: Intravascular coagulation in abruptio placentae. Am J Obstet Gynecol 109:604, 1971.
21. Phillips LL, Skrodelis V, Kers TA: Hypofibrinogenemia and intrauterine fetal death. Am J Obstet Gynecol 89:907, 1964.
22. Phillips LL, Davidson EC: Procoagulant properties of amniotic fluid. Am J Obstet Gynecol 113:911, 1972.
23. Phillips LL, Skrodelis V, Quigley HJ: Intravascular coagulation in septic abortion. Obstet Gynecol 30:350, 1967.
24. Laros RK, Penner JA, Collins J, et al.: Coagulation changes in saline-induced abortion. Am J Obstet Gynecol 116:277, 1973.
25. Davidson EC, Phillips LL: Coagulation studies in the hypertensive toxemias of pregnancy. Am J Obstet Gynecol 113:905, 1972.

CHAPTER 16

Antepartum and Postpartum Hemorrhage

Diane R. Biehl, M.D.

Hemorrhage in the obstetric patient is the leading cause of maternal mortality.[1] Reduction in morbidity and mortality depends on accurate, early diagnosis and prompt, skillful treatment by both the obstetrician and the anesthesiologist.

ANTEPARTUM HEMORRHAGE

A patient may bleed at any time during her pregnancy, but the most severe bleeding usually occurs in the third trimester. The major causes are placenta praevia and abruptio placenta.

Placenta Praevia

The incidence of placenta praevia varies from 0.1 to 1.0 per cent.[2] It is highest in the multigravida, although the association is actually with age rather than parity. If a patient has a placenta praevia in one pregnancy, the chance of recurrence is 12 times that for the normal parturient.[3]

Placenta praevia varies in degree and may be complete (37 per cent), partial (27 per cent) or marginal (low implantation) (46 per cent) (Figure 16.1). The main symptom is painless vaginal bleeding. The patient may bleed and then stop spontaneously (the usual situation), but sudden severe hemorrhage may recur at any time.

Although placenta praevia is the cause of vaginal bleeding in only about one-third of antepartum hemorrhages,[4] all patients who present with vaginal bleeding in the third trimester should be considered to have placenta praevia until disproved. If the diagnosis of placenta praevia is suspected, the placenta may be located by means of B-scan ultrasonography (Figures 16.2 and 16.3). The recent development of gray imaging has provided even more accurate localization of placental position in low-lying and placental praevia implantation. If ultrasound is unavailable, radioisotope scanning using radioiodinated serum albumin or 99 TE-labeled albumin (technetium scan) may be used to locate the placenta. If ultrasound or radioisotope scan is not conclusive, definitive diagnosis is made by direct examination of the cervical os. This procedure should be done in the delivery room only after all preparations have been made to do a cesarean section, i.e. "the double set-up" (Table 16.1). A vaginal examination is carried out to determine whether the placenta is covering or encroaching on the lower segment of the uterus.

Prior to term the patient is usually managed with bed rest in the hope that the bleeding will cease spontaneously. Once the patient is near term, fetal maturity is assessed by amniocentesis (chapter 23), and the mother is delivered by cesarean section. In most instances a vaginal examination is still done immediately prior to cesarean section to confirm the diagnosis. If, during pregnancy, the patient begins

244   ANESTHESIA FOR OBSTETRICS

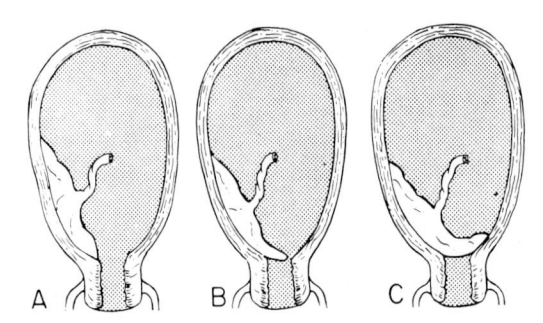

Figure 16.1. Types of placenta praevia. A, low implantation of placenta; B, partial placenta praevia; C, total placenta praevia. (Reprinted by permission from Bonica JJ, Johnson WL: Placenta praevia, abruptio placentae or rupture of the uterus. In *Principles and Practice of Obstetric Analgesia and Anesthesia,* vol 2. F. A. Davis, Philadelphia, 1969, p 1164.)

to bleed and does not stop spontaneously, emergency cesarean section must be carried out despite the gestational age of the fetus. If cesarean section is performed prior to 30 weeks' gestation, fetal and neonatal mortality is in the range of 60 to 70 per cent.[5] The fetus becomes compromised quickly if maternal hypotension occurs (Figure 16.4). It is also possible for the placental bleeding to cause fetal exsanguination. The fetus becomes asphyxiated and, if delivered prematurely, usually succumbs to a combination of asphyxia and hyaline membrane disease.

ANESTHETIC MANAGEMENT

"Double set-up." Prior to the double set-up, if the patient has bled profusely as

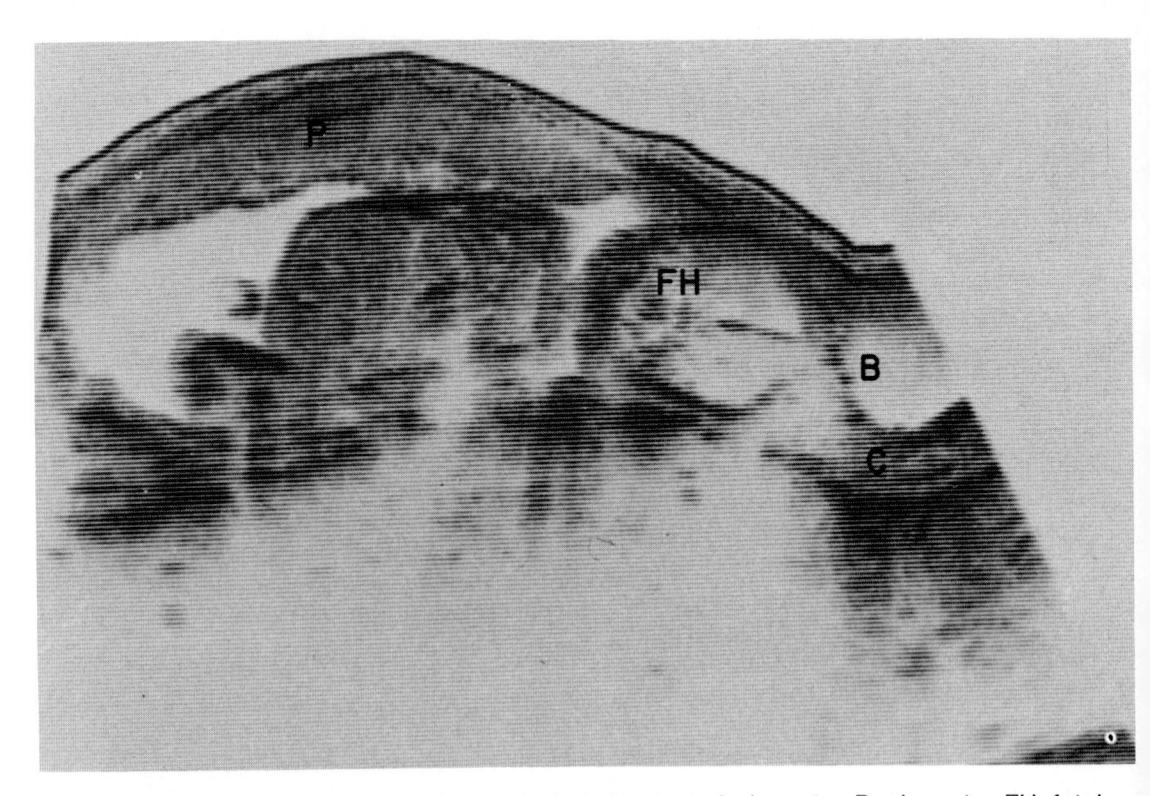

Figure 16.2. Ultrasonogram of an anteriorly implanted placenta. *P,* placenta; *FH,* fetal head; *B,* maternal bladder; *C,* cervix. (Courtesy of Dr. R. Filly, University of California, San Francisco.)

ANTEPARTUM AND POSTPARTUM HEMORRHAGE

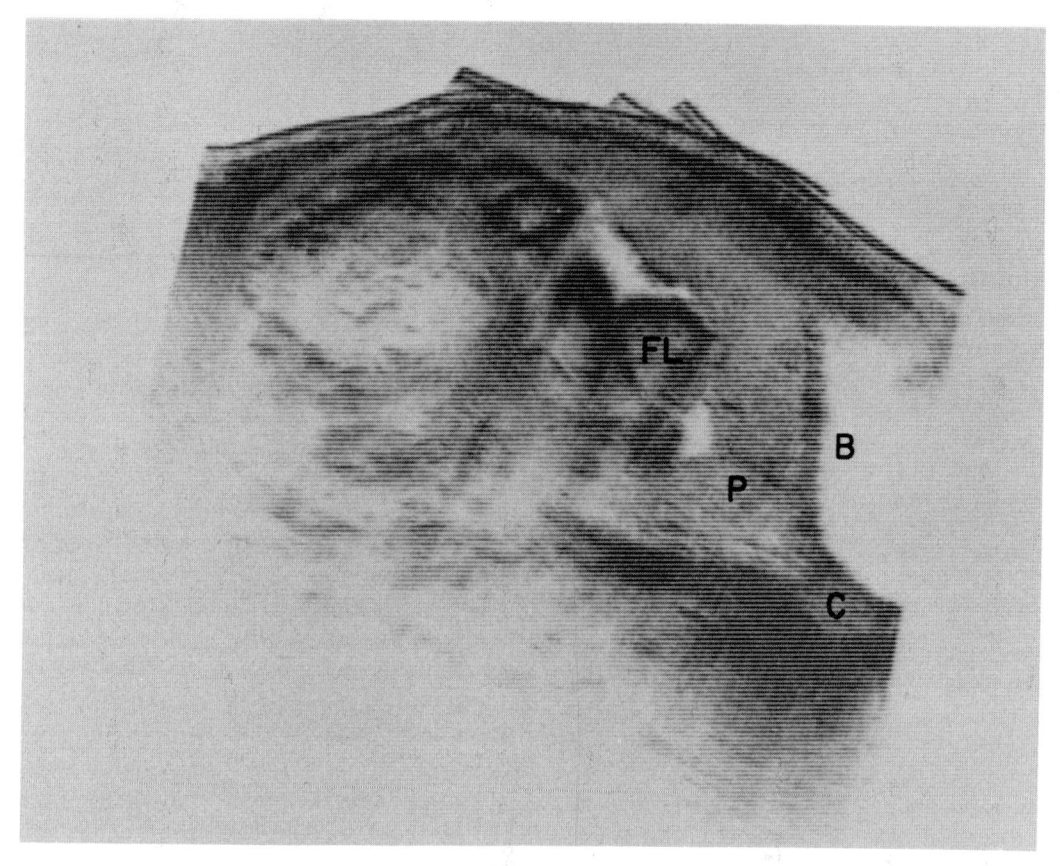

Figure 16.3. Ultrasonogram of a complete placenta praevia. *P*, placenta; *FL*, fetal limb; *B*, maternal bladder; *C*, cervix. (Courtesy of Dr. R. Filly, University of California, San Francisco.)

manifested by postural or obvious hypotension, blood volume should be restored. A central venous pressure line is especially useful in evaluating and treating hypovolemia.

During the vaginal examination for the diagnosis of placenta praevia, sudden severe maternal hemorrhage may occur, necessitating immediate emergency cesarean section. Therefore, with the patient in the lithotomy position, the abdomen is prepped and draped and all preparations for cesarean section are completed. It is mandatory that at least one and preferably two intravenous lines be established with either 16- or 18-gauge catheters. The patient must be cross-matched, and at least 2 units of blood must be present in the operating room prior to examination of the patient.

Preparation for general anesthesia should include administration of oral antacid within 15 to 30 minutes of the examination and a non-depolarizing muscle relaxant (e.g. curare 3 mg) and pre-oxygenation within 3 to 5 minutes of the examination. An assistant should be present to provide cricoid pressure if necessary. The examination of the cervical os is then performed, and the diagnosis is made.

Placenta praevia—actively bleeding. If the diagnosis of placenta praevia is con-

Table 16.1
Antepartum Hemorrhage: "The Double Set-up"

Preparation
   2 I.V.'S – 16- or 18-gauge plastic catheters
   Blood pump I.V. set
   Blood in room
   Oral antacid
   Oxygen
   i.v. – atropine 0.6 mg
   i.v. – curare 3 mg
   Assistant near by
Bleeding and cesarean section
   Treat hypovolemia
   Induce ketamine 1 mg/kg plus succinylcholine 1.5 mg/kg
   Intubate – provide cricoid pressure
   O_2 or 50% N_2O and O_2 until baby delivered
   Awake extubation

firmed and the patient is actively bleeding, then an emergency cesarean section under general anesthesia is performed immediately.

Where the mother is bleeding copiously and may be in hemorrhagic shock, resuscitation of the mother may be extremely difficult. Unlike some anesthetic emergencies, it may not be possible to correct the blood loss completely prior to surgery, because the hemorrhaging will continue until the placenta is removed. Blood, plasmanate or crystalloid should, nevertheless, be infused as rapidly as possible.

Induction of anesthesia is accomplished with either an appropriate dose of thiopental (usually less than 100 mg) or ketamine (0.5 to 1.0 mg/kg) plus succinylcholine 1.5 mg/kg and endotracheal intubation. Ketamine, in contrast to thiopental, has the advantage of not causing cardiovascular depression. In a dose of 1 mg/kg, it stimulates heart rate and may actually increase blood pressure in the patient who is not severely hypovolemic. In the hypotensive moribund patient neither ketamine nor thiopental should be used. Succinylcholine may be used to facilitate intubation. In this severe situation the possibility of maternal recall should be disregarded in order to provide maximum maternal safety.

Maintenance of anesthesia prior to delivery depends on the clinical condition of the mother. Pancuronium (2 to 4 mg) or succinylcholine (0.1 to 0.2 per cent) infusion will provide optimum operating conditions. Initially, 100 per cent oxygen is administered. Nitrous oxide, up to 70 per cent, may be added as tolerated by the patient. Alternatively, nitrous oxide 50 per cent and halothane 0.5 per cent may be used.

Once the uterus has been opened and the infant and placenta removed, the threat to the mother is much less. Blood volume, as assessed by blood pressure, central venous pressure and urine output, is restored to normal, and anesthesia is maintained with either the inhalational agent or narcotics and muscle relaxants.

The neonate may require intensive resuscitation at birth. These infants may be asphyxiated, acidotic and hypovolemic. Immediate intubation and ventilation with 100 per cent oxygen should be instituted, and an umbilical arterial catheter should be placed for monitoring blood pressure and blood gases and for giving infusions of plasma, albumin and crystalloid (chapter 26). Ideally, another anesthetist or a neonatologist should be present to attend to the neonate. Transfer to an intensive care nursery for further close observation and treatment should be accomplished as soon as possible.

Placenta praevia—not bleeding. If the diagnosis of placenta praevia is confirmed and the patient is not bleeding, cesarean section is still usually performed at this time. Despite the fact that the patient has been prepared for a general anesthetic as part of the double set-up, spinal or epidural anesthesia may be used if the patient requests it and if no evidence of hypovolemia is present. The technique for regional or general anesthesia in these patients is

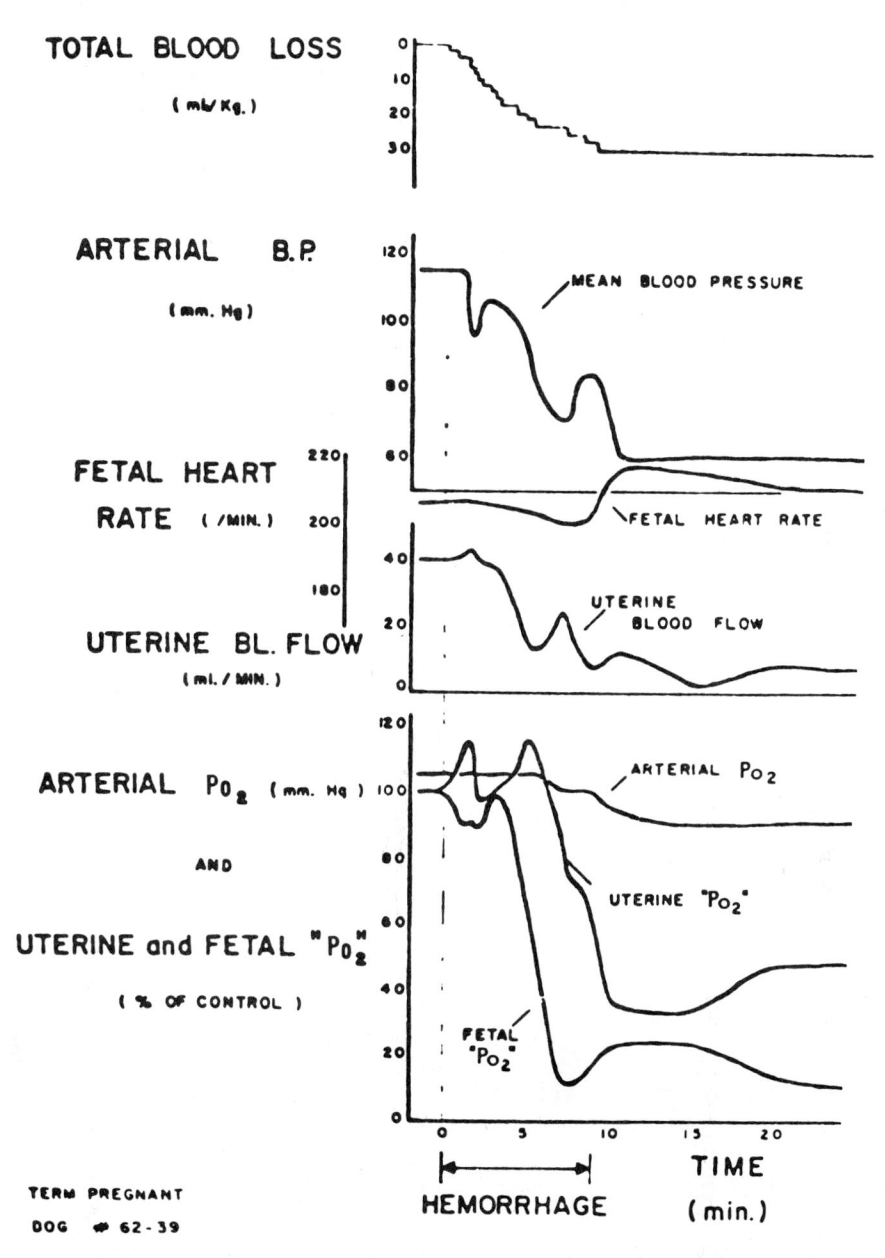

Figure 16.4. Effects of acute hemorrhage in pregnant dogs. Rapid bleeding produced a prompt fall in mean maternal arterial blood pressure, a comparable fall in uterine blood flow, decreased fetal tissue PO$_2$ and fetal bradycardia. (Modified by permission from Romney SL, Gabel PV, Takeda Y: Experimental hemorrhage in late pregnancy. Am J Obstet Gynecol 87:636, 1963.)

Abruptio Placentae

The term abruptio placentae refers to the separation of a normally implanted placenta after 20 weeks' gestation and before the birth of the fetus. The term "marginal separation of the placenta" refers to a mild form of abruptio placentae. The incidence of abruptio placentae varies from 0.2 to 2.4 per cent.[6] Maternal mortality is significant, probably 1.8 to 2.8 per cent.[7] Perinatal mortality may be as high as 50 per cent of cases.[8]

The etiology of abruptio placentae is not well defined but is associated with hypertensive disorders of pregnancy, high parity, uterine abnormalities (tumors, etc.) and previous placental abruption. Dietary deficiencies, particularly of folate, are thought by some investigators also to contribute to this disease entity.[9]

The clinical manifestations of this disease depend primarily on the site and degree of placental separation (Figure 16.5) and the amount of blood loss. Bleeding from the abruptio may appear through the vagina (external or revealed hemorrhage) or remain concealed in the utero-placental unit (internal or concealed hemorrhage). The degree of revealed vaginal bleeding is often misleading, and concealed hemorrhage (retroplacental clot) provides one of the main problems for the anesthetist in coping with these patients on an emergency basis. The amount of blood loss is commonly underestimated, and as much as 4,000 ml of blood may be sequestered in the uterus. Abruptio placentae has been classified as mild, moderate or severe. In mild or moderate abruption there is usually no maternal hypotension or coagulopathies and no fetal distress. Severe abruption is characterized by maternal hypotension, uterine irritability, hypertonus and pain, fetal distress or death and clotting abnormalities. Of all abruptions, mild to moderate account for 85 to 90 per cent and severe account for 10 to 15 per cent.

CLOTTING ABNORMALITIES ASSOCIATED WITH ABRUPTIO PLACENTAE

Besides the problem of hemorrhage in the mother, severe abruptio placentae may result in blood coagulation defects.[10] Two theories have evolved to explain the observed clotting defects: (1) Placental abruption causes circulating plasminogen to be activated, which enzymatically destroys circulating fibrinogen (fibrinolysis). (2) Thromboplastin from placenta and decidua triggers the activation of the extrinsic clotting pathway, causing thrombin to convert fibrinogen to fibrin (disseminated intravascular coagulation).

It is unlikely that either mechanism operates exclusively. In the clinical situation, the end result is hypofibrinogenemia, platelet deficiency and decreased Factor V and VIII. Once the clotting mechanism has been activated, degeneration products of the fibrin-fibrinogen system also appear in the circulation. The patient then manifests widespread bleeding from the intravenous

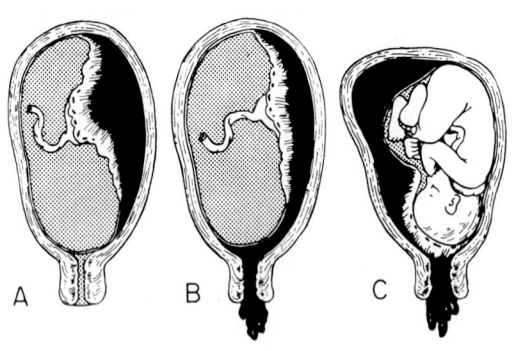

Figure 16.5. Abruptio placentae. *A*, internal or concealed hemorrhage; *B*, external hemorrhage; *C*, prolapse of the placenta. (Reprinted by permission from Bonica JJ, Johnson WL: Placenta praevia, abruptio placentae or rupture of the uterus. In *Principles and Practice of Obstetric Analgesia and Anesthesia*, vol 2. F. A. Davis, Philadelphia, 1969, p 1166.)

sites, gastrointestinal tract and subcutaneous tissues, as well as the uterus.

In all patients suspected of having abruptio placentae, clotting parameters should be measured. With sophisticated laboratory equipment actual amounts of the clotting factors present in the blood, as well as degradation products, can be measured. However, the clinical situation is often acute, and treatment must be instituted before test results are known. For this reason, a simple clot observation test which can be performed in the delivery suite is often preferred. In this test, 5 ml of maternal venous blood are drawn into a clean glass test tube, shaken gently and allowed to stand. If a clot does not form within 6 minutes or the clot is lysed within 1 hour, a clotting defect is present. If the clot fails to form within 30 minutes, the fibrinogen level is probably less than 100 mg/100 ml.

When the blood sample is drawn for the clot observation test, a sample should also be sent to the laboratory for complete analysis, including hemoglobin, hematocrit, platelet count, prothrombin time, partial thromboplastin time, fibrinogen level and fibrin degradation products. The complete results will then be useful for the management of these patients both intrapartum and postpartum. Analyses should be repeated frequently to monitor treatment, because the clotting parameters may take several days to return to normal.

MANAGEMENT OF ABRUPTIO PLACENTAE

The definitive management of abruptio placentae is to empty the uterus. The method by which this is done depends on: (1) the degree of abruption; (2) the time in gestation at which abruption occurs; (3) the stability of the maternal cardiovascular and hematologic systems; and (4) the status of the fetus.

The diagnosis of mild or moderate abruption is usually made by excluding placenta praevia at a double set-up. After the diagnosis, if the fetus is mature, an amniotomy is performed, labor is induced or augmented with oxytocin if necessary and the fetus is monitored continuously by electronic means. Baseline clotting studies are obtained. If there are no signs of maternal hypovolemia, clotting studies are normal and there is no evidence of uteroplacental insufficiency, continuous lumbar epidural, caudal or subarachnoid block may be used for labor and vaginal delivery.

In severe abruption, if emergency cesarean section is performed to save the life of the fetus or the mother, general anesthesia should be used. Regional anesthesia is contraindicated in patients with hypovolemic shock and/or severe coagulation abnormalities. The induction and maintenance of general anesthesia are similar to the procedures used for "Placenta Praevia—Actively Bleeding" as outlined above.

If the infant is alive at delivery, intensive resuscitation is usually required. These infants are usually severely asphyxiated and severely hypovolemic. In addition, they may also be premature.

After delivery of the infant and removal of the placenta, subsequent management of the mother may continue to be difficult. If blood has extravasated into the myometrium, the uterus may not contract, and bleeding may continue. Oxytocin by infusion (20 to 40 units in 500 ml of normal saline) should be started as soon as the infant is delivered. If this is not effective, then intravenous ergot preparations may be tried. As a last resort internal iliac artery ligation or hysterectomy may be required as a lifesaving procedure for the mother.

Massive and rapid blood transfusion restores the depleted blood volume, maintains tissue perfusion and prevents renal damage. If blood is not immediately available, crystalloid, albumin or plasmanate should be used to maintain the circulating blood volume. When necessary, fresh frozen plasma will restore the Factor V and VIII components, and, in severe situations, platelet concentrate may also be required (6 to 12 units). Cryoprecipitate contains 23 per cent of the fibrinogen in a unit of plasma and, thus, provides concentrated fibrinogen and Factor VIII in a small volume. Infusion of fibrinogen is no longer recommended because: (1) it may only aggravate the disseminated intravascular coagulation and (2) it carries a high risk of serum hepatitis.

The use of heparin in these patients remains controversial but for the most part has been abandoned. Pritchard maintains that if the uterus is well contracted and blood loss is replaced, heparin is not required.[10] The clotting parameters will return to normal within several hours after the uterus is empty.

During an apparently normal vaginal delivery, abruptio placentae may occur just prior to birth of the infant. In this situation, the problems are maternal hemorrhage and fetal asphyxia. Clotting deficits do not usually become manifest. The anesthesiologist should resuscitate the mother by establishing intravenous lines, monitoring vital signs and supporting the circulation with crystalloid solution and blood when available. Intravenous infusion of oxytocin should be begun as soon as the infant and placenta are delivered. General anesthesia may be required if extraction of the infant is necessary. The technique of rapid induction, previously described, should be used.

These patients, regardless of the mode of delivery, are extremely susceptible to postpartum hemorrhage due to uterine atony. Frequent monitoring of maternal vital signs, urine output and fundal firmness is necessary.

Other Causes of Antepartum Hemorrhage

Placenta praevia and abruptio placentae account for one-half to two-thirds of all cases of antepartum hemorrhage. The remainder are due to cervical pathology, e.g. polyps, carcinoma, vaginal and vulvar varicosities, circumvallate placenta and vasopraevia. The latter two causes do not present a threat to the mother as much as to the fetus, because the bleeding is primarily from fetal vessels. Other obstetric problems may give rise secondarily to hemorrhage as a result of derangement of the clotting mechanisms (chapter 15). Severe preeclampsia, maternal infection, amniotic fluid embolism and intrauterine death may all result in disseminated intravascular coagulation and hemorrhage if the diagnosis is not established quickly and treatment instituted.

UTERINE RUPTURE

Uterine rupture is an uncommon but potentially catastrophic obstetric complication which may occur antepartum, intrapartum or postpartum. It occurs in about 1 in 1,250 births and causes approximately 5 per cent of all maternal deaths.[11] Causes include: (1) separation of uterine scar; (2) rupture of myomectomy scar; (3) previous difficult deliveries; (4) rapid, spontaneous, tumultuous labor; (5) prolonged labor in association with excessive oxytocin stimulation or cephalo-pelvic disproportion; (6) weak or stretched uterine muscles as might be found in the grand multipara, multiple gestation, polyhydramnios; and (7) traumatic rupture (iatrogenic) occurring from intrauterine manipulations, difficult forceps applications and excessive suprafundal pressure.

Although the uterine rupture is usually found at the site of a previous operation or injury, several recent reviews[12, 13] have indicated that maternal mortality is low in these circumstances because rupture is recognized and promptly treated. With traumatic rupture or spontaneous rupture and no uterine scar, maternal mortality from obstetric hemorrhage was 26 and 66 per cent respectively.[14] Maternal death from rupture apparently occurs because the possibility is not considered, and blood transfusions are inadequate and laparotomy is delayed or not done.

Signs and symptoms depend on the extent of the rupture and include vaginal bleeding, severe uterine or lower abdominal pain, shoulder pain from subdiaphragmatic irritation by blood, disappearance of fetal heart tones and severe maternal hypotension and shock. Anesthetic management for the laparotomy, uterine repair, hysterectomy or hypogastric ligation is similar to that outlined above for the actively bleeding, acutely hypovolemic patient.

Many women with previous cesarean sections are now being allowed to deliver vaginally. The incidence of uterine rupture from a low transverse segment scar is less than 0.5 per cent and with a classical cesarean section scar 2 per cent.[11] This risk, therefore, demands continuous observation of these patients throughout labor and ability to treat a uterine rupture promptly. Because abdominal pain is one of the cardinal symptoms and often the first indication of impending or actual rupture, the author believes major conduction anesthesia is contraindicated in these patients. On the other hand, Crawford has stated that segmental epidural anesthesia will not mask the pain of uterine rupture and may be used, providing the patient is monitored closely.[15]

POSTPARTUM HEMORRHAGE

The postpartum period is defined as the 6-week period after delivery of the infant. The main causes of hemorrhage in this group of women (3 to 5 per cent of all deliveries) occur within minutes of birth and are due to retained products of conception; uterine atony; cervical, vaginal or, in some cases, uterine lacerations; or bleeding from the episiotomy site. Twenty per cent of all patients who have antepartum hemorrhage will also bleed postpartum. Severe postpartum hemorrhage often occurs with little or no warning. For this reason immediately after delivery the anesthesiologist must observe the patient closely and be prepared to institute resuscitation of the mother and/or give an anesthetic at a few seconds notice.

Retained Placenta

The incidence of retained placenta is approximately 1 per cent of all vaginal deliveries, and retained products of conception usually require a manual exploration of the uterus. In the multiparous patient, this can sometimes be done without an anesthetic, but usually the mother is severely distressed and the obstetrician may encounter difficulty in exploring a uterus that is partially contracted. For these reasons, analgesia is usually necessary. If the mother has an epidural or spinal block encompassing T10 to S4, manual removal of the placenta can be accomplished. The anesthesiologist must remember, however, that, should severe bleeding occur, the sympathectomy imposed by the block may make resuscitation more difficult and may result in severe maternal hypotension.

If the parturient does not have a regional block prior to delivery, manual removal of the placenta should first be attempted under continuous inhalation analgesia (Table 10.2). After 10 minutes of continuous administration of 30 to 40 per cent nitrous oxide and 0.2 to 0.3 per cent methoxyflurane the awake patient will usually tolerate manual removal of the placenta. If the uterus remains firmly contracted around the placenta and uterine relaxation is required, this is best accomplished under general endotracheal anesthesia. Following the usual technique for rapid induction and intubation, the patient is given sufficient halothane and oxygen, with or without nitrous oxide, to provide adequate uterine relaxation (Table 10.3). The halothane should be discontinued as soon as the uterus has relaxed enough to allow manual removal. An oxytocin infusion should be initiated immediately after removal of the placenta. Because ketamine anesthesia increases uterine tone, it should be avoided when uterine relaxation is needed.

Uterine Atony

Uterine atony, in varying degrees, occurs in approximately 2 to 5 per cent of all vaginal deliveries.[16] A completely atonic uterus may result in a loss of 2 liters of blood in less than 5 minutes. In a recent report of 501 consecutive maternal deaths, postpartum uterine atony was the leading cause of death in the parturient.[13]

Uterine atony is increased with high parity, multiple births, polyhydramnios, large infants, retained placenta or operative intervention, such as internal version and extraction. It may occur immediately or several hours after delivery of the infant.

Resuscitation of the mother necessitates: (1) replacement of blood loss initially with crystalloid and colloid solution and then whole blood as soon as it can be obtained; (2) intravenous infusion of oxytocin to cause contraction of the uterus; (3) general supportive measures, i.e. oxygen by face mask, with the patient in the Trendelenburg position; (4) close monitoring of vital signs, including central venous pressure and urine output.

In situations in which the above measures do not correct the problem, emergency hysterectomy or internal iliac artery ligation may be required. The considerations here are very similar to those for placenta praevia or abruptio placenta, except that there is no infant to influence management. The patient in an unstable condition prior to operation can be expected to lose anywhere from 2 to 18 liters of blood before completion of the hysterectomy.[17]

Cervical and Vaginal Lacerations

Both of these conditions may result in hemorrhagic shock. One of the main problems with lacerations is that they may be undiagnosed due to other complications. Blood loss may also go undetected if it occurs after the patient has been removed from the delivery room. In these situations, resuscitation should be started and the patient should be transferred back to the delivery room. A careful search for the source of bleeding may require a general anesthetic to allow the obstetrician to explore the uterus and examine the cervix and vaginal vault. If the bleeding source is not found, in rare cases laparotomy may be required.

Blood Loss at Cesarean Section

In most high-risk obstetric units, the incidence of cesarean sections has doubled in the last 10 years. Regardless of the indication for cesarean section, the obstetric anesthetist must remember that sudden hemorrhage may occur with any manipulation of the highly vascular term uterus. Blood loss at "elective" cesarean sections is estimated at between 800 and 1,200 ml, which is 10 to 15 per cent of the circulating blood volume of the normal pregnant women at term. Any further bleeding may result in a compromised patient. With repeat cesarean sections, adhesions, varicosities in the uterus or rupture of the previous scar may give rise to sudden, severe hemorrhage. The anesthetist in any obstetric unit must be prepared to institute suddenly any of the measures previously discussed to resuscitate a parturient in hemorrhagic shock.

CONCLUSION

Hemorrhage in the obstetric patient is still a leading cause of maternal deaths in modern obstetrics and contributes heavily to perinatal mortality as well. The pregnant patient often bleeds unexpectedly and may exsanguinate in a matter of minutes. Because of this, no obstetric patient should be treated "routinely," and every obstetric anesthetist should be prepared to diagnose and treat hemorrhagic shock immediately.

References

1. Pritchard JA: Obstetrics in broad perspective. In *Williams Obstetrics,* JA Pritchard and PC McDonald, eds, ed 15. Appleton-Century-Crofts, New York, 1976, p 3.
2. Greenshaw JRC, Jones DED, Parker RT: Placenta previa: A survey of twenty years' experience with improved perinatal survival by expectant therapy and cesarean section delivery. Obstet Gynecol Surv 28:461, 1973.
3. Hellman LM, Pritchard JA, Wynn RM: Placenta previa and abruptio placenta. In *Williams Obstetrics,* NJ Newman and LM Hellman, eds, ed 14. Appleton-Century-Crofts, New York, 1971.
4. Greenhill JP, Friedman EA: *Biological Principles and Modern Practice of Obstetrics.* W. B. Saunders, Philadelphia, 1974, p 418.
5. Hibbard LT: Fetal mortality in placenta previa. Obstet Gynecol 8:613, 1956.
6. Leenan CB: The management of abruptio placenta. J Obstet Gynaecol Br Emp 80:120, 1973.
7. Porter J: Conservative treatment of abruptio placenta. Obstet Gynecol 15:690, 1960.
8. Hibbard BM, Jeffloate TNA: Abruptio placenta. Obstet Gynecol 27:1955, 1966.
9. Pritchard JA, Mason R, Conley M, et al.: Genesis of severe placental abruption. Am J Obstet Gynecol 108:22, 1970.
10. Pritchard JA: Hematological problems associated with delivery, placental abruption, retained dead fetus and amniotic fluid embolism. Clin Haematol 2:563, 1973.
11. Eastman NJ, Hellman LM, eds: Rupture of the Uterus. In *Williams Obstetrics,* ed 13. Appleton-Century-Crofts, New York, 1966, pp 924–925.
12. Hughes EC, Cochrane NE, Czyz PL: Maternal mortality study—1970–1975. N Y State J Med 76:2206, 1976.
13. Gibbs CE, Locke WE: Maternal deaths in Texas, 1969 to 1973. Am J Obstet Gynecol 126:687, 1976.
14. Ware HH Jr: Rupture of the uterus. Clin Obstet Gynecol 3:637, 1960.
15. Crawford JS: Epidural analgesia and uterine rupture (Letter to the Editor). Lancet 1:361, 1974.
16. Newton M: Postpartum hemorrhage. Am J Obstet Gynecol 54:51, 1967.
17. Pritchard JA: Obstetric hemorrhage. In *Williams Obstetrics,* JA Pritchard and PC McDonald, eds, ed 15. Appleton-Century-Crofts, New York, 1976, p 398.

CHAPTER 17

Anesthesia for Cesarean Section

Sol M. Shnider, M.D.
Gershon Levinson, M.D.

Delivery of a baby by cesarean section has become increasingly common. In the past, 4 to 6 per cent of deliveries were via the abdominal route. The most common indications were cephalo-pelvic disproportion, uterine dystocia, hemorrhage, and acute fetal distress. Currently cesarean section rates of 10 to 15 per cent are common; in high-risk centers with disproportionately increased incidences of pre-eclampsia-eclampsia, diabetes, Rh isoimmunization, prematurity, and other high-risk problems, rates as high as 25 per cent are not unusual.[1] Likely there are two major factors accounting for the increased section rate. First, the widespread use of electronic and biochemical fetal monitoring prior to and during labor (chapters 23 and 24) has made it easier to identify the fetus in jeopardy. Second, it has become commonly accepted that serious trauma to the baby can be eliminated by avoiding potentially difficult mid-forceps or vaginal breech deliveries. Furthermore, in many obstetric units maternal mortality rates are the same for vaginal or cesarean deliveries, thus swaying obstetricians toward cesarean section in borderline cases. Because the most common indication for a cesarean section is a previous cesarean section, the increased rate of primary or emergency section will further increase the over-all rate. Indications for cesarean section are listed in Table 17.1.

CHOICE OF ANESTHESIA

The choice of anesthesia for cesarean section depends on the reason for the operation, the degree of urgency, the desires of the patient and the skills of the anesthesiologist. There is no one ideal method of anesthesia for cesarean section; the advantages and disadvantages of spinal, epidural and general anesthesia will be discussed in this chapter and suggested methods for these techniques will be outlined. The anesthesiologist must choose the method that he believes is (1) safest and most comfortable for the mother, (2) least depressant to the newborn and (3) provides the optimal working conditions for the obstetrician.

Two recent surveys indicate that conduction anesthesia is the most commonly used anesthetic for cesarean section[2] (Table 17.2). Spinal anesthesia appears to be the preferred technique nationwide. However, in residency training programs spinal anesthesia is less popular. Whereas the American College of Obstetricians and Gynecologists survey of all maternity units

ANESTHESIA FOR CESAREAN SECTION

Table 17.1
Common Indications for Cesarean Section

Previous section
Cephalo-pelvic disproportion
Failure to progress
Failure of induction
Malpresentation
Breech
Failed forceps
Hemorrhage
Placenta praevia
Toxemia
Chorioamnionitis
Herpes genitalia
Fetal distress
Chronic utero-placental insufficiency
Rh isoimmunization
Prolapsed cord
Hypertonic uterus

Table 17.2
Cesarean Sections Classified by Type of Anesthesia Used

| | Percent Cent of Cesarean Sections ||
	All Maternity Units*	Obstetric Anesthesia Centers†
Spinal	53	24
Inhalation	32	43
Combination	9	
Epidural	3	32
Local	1	1
Other	1	

* Data from American College of Obstetricians and Gynecologists: *A Report of the Committee on Maternal Health: National Study of Maternity Care. Survey of Obstetric Practice and Associated Services in the Hospitals in the United States.* American College of Obstetricians and Gynecologists, Chicago, 1970.
† Data from Hicks JS, Levinson G, Shnider SM: Obstetric anesthesia training centers in the U.S.A.–1975. Anesth Analg 55:839, 1976.

showed that epidural anesthesia was used in only 3 per cent of cesarean sections, in the training programs it is used in 32 per cent. Likely the preference for epidural over spinal anesthesia will be reflected nationwide in years to come.

Regional Anesthesia

Epidural or spinal anesthesia for cesarean section allows the mother to be awake, minimizes or completely avoids the problems of maternal aspiration and avoids neonatal drug depression from general anesthetics.

CHOICE OF REGIONAL TECHNIQUE

A subarachnoid block is easily administered and rapidly and reliably produces profound analgesia. Nevertheless, many anesthesiologists prefer the continuous epidural technique. It is their belief that, with epidural anesthesia, hypotension occurs less precipitously and, consequently, is easier to prevent or treat. The anesthetic level is also more controllable with epidural anesthesia, because if the initial dose does not produce a satisfactory sensory block, more drug can be injected through the epidural catheter. A suggested technique for regional anesthesia for cesarean section is outlined in Tables 17.3, 17.4 and 17.5. The rationale for these recommendations is discussed below.

Table 17.3
Preparation for Regional Anesthesia for Cesarean Section

1. Give 30 to 60 ml of oral antacid within 4 hours of induction of anesthesia.
2. Transport the patient to the operating room in the lateral position.
3. Measure vital signs. Supine hypotension unresponsive to left uterine displacement may make regional anesthesia inadvisable; if blood pressure is normal, administer 25 mg of ephedrine I.M. Avoid in hypertensive or preeclamptic patients.
4. Administer intravenously 1,000 ml of balanced salt solution rapidly.
5. Before starting block check (1) oxygen delivery system in the anesthesia machine, (2) airways, (3) laryngoscope, (4) endotracheal tubes, (5) thiopental or diazepam for possible convulsion, (6) ephedrine for hypotension and (7) suction apparatus.

Table 17.4
Regional Anesthesia for Cesarean Section: A Suggested Technique

1. *Spinal Anesthesia*: Use smallest needle possible (25-gauge preferred). Give 7 to 9 mg of tetracaine or 50 to 75 mg of lidocaine made hyperbaric with dextrose.
2. *Epidural Anesthesia*: 0.5 or 0.75 per cent bupivacaine without epinephrine or 3 per cent chloroprocaine. Use 2-ml test dose. Wait 2 minutes and if there are no signs of spinal anesthesia administer another 5 ml of drug. Wait 30 seconds and if there are no signs of a systemic reaction due to inadvertent intravenous injection then administer up to a total of 20 ml of local anesthetic. Insert epidural catheter. Inject additional drug as required through catheter (after test dose) to obtain sensory blockade up to fourth thoracic dermatome.
3. Position patient with left uterine displacement and slight (10°) Trendelenburg tilt.
4. Administer oxygen by plastic face mask.
5. Monitor arterial blood pressure every minute for 20 minutes, then every 5 minutes for duration of block.

Table 17.5
Management of Complications

1. If systolic blood pressure falls by 30 per cent or below 100 torr, assure left uterine displacement, increase I.V. infusion rate. If blood pressure is still not restored, administer 5 to 10 mg of ephedrine I.V.; repeat if necessary.
2. Treat anxiety and incomplete or "spotty" anesthesia with one or more of the following agents prior to delivery of the infant: (1) 2.5 mg of diazepam in increments up to 10 mg I.V.; (2) 40 per cent nitrous oxide and/or 0.25 per cent methoxyflurane; (3) 0.25 mg/kg of ketamine I.V.
3. If analgesia is inadequate, proceed to general anesthesia with endotracheal intubation.
4. If supplementation to spinal or epidural blockade is necessary after delivery, administer small doses of narcotic.

ANTACID ADMINISTRATION

The hazards of aspiration pneumonitis and the use of oral antacids are discussed fully in chapter 19. Approximately 30 per cent of women undergoing elective scheduled cesarean section will have significant amounts of acidic contents in their stomach unless they have received antacid within 4 hours before surgery.[3] Because a small proportion of patients receiving a block will require a general anesthetic, it is prudent to give all patients an oral antacid prior to cesarean section.

MATERNAL HYPOTENSION: PREVENTION AND THERAPY

Pregnant women are particularly prone to arterial hypotension following sympathetic blockade. When the parturient lies in the supine position, her gravid uterus compresses the inferior vena cava and decreases venous return to the heart. With sympathetic blockade she may not be able to compensate adequately for the venous obstruction. A fall in blood pressure is associated with a comparable fall in uterine blood flow and placental perfusion and may lead to fetal hypoxia and acidosis. Therefore, the patient should not be permitted to lie in the supine position either in transit to the operating room or after the block is performed. After regional blockade the patient should be positioned with left uterine displacement to prevent aortocaval compression and with slight Trendelenburg position to increase venous return. The authors have found that the incidence of hypotension can be decreased from more than 80 per cent if no prophylactic measures are instituted to 17 per cent with prophylaxis. The recommended prophylaxis is (1) intravenous hydration with 1 liter of balanced salt solution, (2) ephedrine 25 mg given intramuscularly—both administered within 15 minutes of the block—and (3) left uterine displacement with either a mechanical device* or

---

* Kennedy device manufactured by H. E. Richards Company, Box 345, Toledo, Ohio 43601. Colon-Morales device manufactured by Resuscitation Laboratories, P. O. Box 3051, Bridgeport, Connecticut 06605.

ANESTHESIA FOR CESAREAN SECTION

a pillow placed under the patient's right hip immediately after the block (Table 17.6).† The blood pressure should be monitored every minute for the first 20 minutes and then every 5 minutes for the duration of surgery. If hypotension occurs (either a systolic pressure of less than 100 torr or a fall of 30 per cent from pre-anesthetic levels) left uterine displacement should be increased and fluids rapidly infused. If hypotension is not corrected within 30 to 60 seconds an additional dose of ephedrine (5 to 10 mg intravenously) should be administered.

In the past, the use of vasopressors in the pregnant patient has been criticized on the basis of uterine vasoconstriction that could lead to fetal hypoxia and acidosis.[4] This problem can be avoided by using vasopressors such as ephedrine and mephentermine (Wyamine). These drugs, in contrast to methoxamine (Vasoxyl) and phenylephrine (Neosynephrine), have little α-adrenergic activity and do not cause uterine vasoconstriction[5,6] (Figure 3.7). In the experimental animal, ephedrine restores uterine blood flow toward normal when used to treat spinal hypotension. A prophylactic dose of the vasopressor similarly has no adverse effect on uterine blood flow[7] (Figure 3.8).

TOXIC REACTIONS AND TOTAL SPINALS

With administration of a spinal or epidural block, a total spinal with hypotension and respiratory insufficiency or a toxic reaction with convulsions, hypoxia and cardiovascular collapse may occur. Therefore, before starting any block the anesthesia machine, laryngoscope, airways, endotracheal tubes, suction apparatus and monitoring equipment should be checked, and thiopental and ephedrine should be immediately available. Treatment of these complications is outlined in chapter 8.

† Data presented in Tables 17.6, 17.8, 17.14, 17.18, 17.19, 17.20, 17.21 and 17.22 are in part based on a review of each cesarean section performed at the University of California, San Francisco over 10 consecutive years.

Table 17.6
Prevention of Hypotension*: Epidural Anesthesia for Cesarean Section

Prophylaxis	Hypotension before Birth
	%
None	80
Fluids alone	53
Fluids and ephedrine I.M.	41
Fluids and mechanical uterine displacer	34
Fluids, ephedrine I.M. and mechanical uterine displacer	17

* Systolic pressure less than 100 torr or 30 per cent fall from control.

CHOICE OF LOCAL ANESTHETICS

Subarachnoid block. The most popular drug for spinal anesthesia for cesarean section is tetracaine (Pontocaine), although some prefer lidocaine (Xylocaine) because of its short action. Because the dose of either drug administered for subarachnoid block is low, toxic maternal reactions and placental transfer are not clinical problems.

Engorgement of the epidural veins during late pregnancy results in a smaller subarachnoid and epidural space. The dose required to achieve a given level with spinal anesthesia is approximately 50 to 70 per cent of the dose required for non-pregnant women.[8] With epidural anesthesia, some have reported that dose requirements are also reduced[9] (Figure 17.1). On the other hand, recent work suggests that with equal amounts of local anesthetic there is no significant difference in sensory levels in pregnant and non-pregnant patients[10] (Table 17.7).

Epidural anesthesia. With epidural in contrast to spinal anesthesia, large amounts of local anesthetic are required, and the fetus and neonate may be affected adversely by placental transfer of these drugs. The ester-type local anesthetics such as chloroprocaine (Nesacaine) have low maternal and fetal toxicity because of rapid hydrolysis by maternal plasma cholinesterase. The half-life of chloroprocaine in maternal blood is 21 seconds,[11] and very little agent crosses the placenta. Fetal blood levels of amide-type local anesthetics are primarily influenced by maternal and fetal protein binding. Bupivacaine (Marcaine) and etidocaine (Duranest), which are bound to protein to the greatest degree, have the lowest fetal blood levels.[12,13]

Neurobehavioral assessment as described by Scanlon and co-workers[14] is a sensitive method for detecting subtle changes in the newborn due to maternally administered drugs. Multiple tests are performed to assess muscle strength and tone as well as ability of the infant to adapt to his environment. Infants whose mothers receive epidural anesthesia for cesarean section with bupivacaine do not demonstrate any measurable difference from infants born after spinal anesthesia,[15] nor do they exhibit the decrease in muscle tone seen in infants whose mothers receive epidural anesthesia with lidocaine or mepivacaine (Carbocaine).[16]

Many recommend that epinephrine be added to local anesthetics in order to decrease systemic absorption, provide a longer duration of action and intensify the motor block. In obstetric anesthesia the authors believe that the addition of epinephrine to chloroprocaine or bupivacaine is unnecessary because of (1) the low toxicity of these agents combined with the reduced anesthetic requirement in the parturient, (2) the long duration of bupivacaine if this characteristic is required and (3) the lack of need for profound motor block.

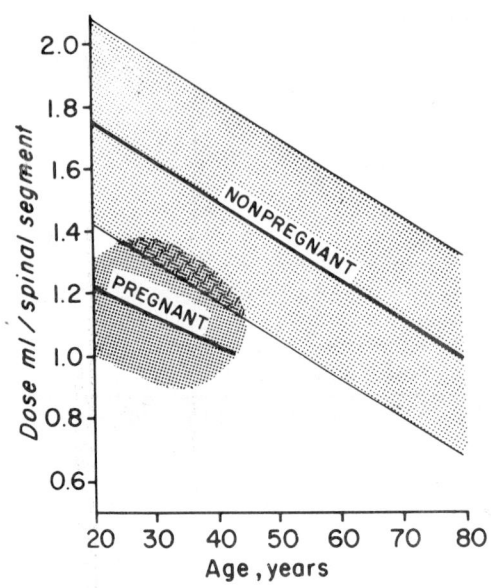

Figure 17.1. Regression lines for dose of epidural solution and age in non-pregnant women and in pregnant women at term. The gravida obviously requires much less drug. (Reprinted by permission from modification by Bonica JJ: *Principles and Practice of Obstetric Analgesia and Anesthesia*, vol 1. F. A. Davis, Philadelphia, 1967, p 624, of Bromage PR: Continuous lumbar epidural analgesia for obstetrics. Can Med Assoc J 85:1136, 1961.)

Table 17.7
Comparison of Spread of Epidural Anesthesia in Pregnant and Non-pregnant Women*

Volume of Bupivacaine 0.75 Per Cent		Most Cephalad Thoracic Dermatome Anesthetized to Pinprick
	ml	
Non-pregnant (n = 32)	15	5.7 ± 1.7
Pregnant (n = 60)	15	5.5 ± 1.2
Non-pregnant (n = 29)	20	4.7 ± 1.7
Pregnant (n = 29)	20	4.2 ± 1.5

* Adapted from Grundy EM, Zamora AM, Winnie AP: Comparison of Spread of epidural anesthesia in pregnant and nonpregnant women. Anesth Analg 57:544, 1978.

SUPPLEMENTARY OXYGEN

Immediately after administering a spinal or epidural block the mother should be given supplementary oxygen. The use of nasal prongs or a clear plastic face mask is more acceptable to most parturients than an anesthesia face mask. The added maternal oxygen may increase fetal oxygenation and provide additional maternal safety should maternal hypoventilation or hypotension not be recognized immediately.

SUPPLEMENTARY DRUGS FOR ANXIETY AND ANALGESIA

Treatment of maternal anxiety may often facilitate performance of the regional block and, with attainment of an adequate sensory level, provide the mother with a more pleasant delivery. Low doses of intravenous diazepam (2.5-mg increments up to 10 mg) may be used with minimal neonatal effects.[17] If the sensory block is not completely satisfactory, then 30 to 40 per cent nitrous oxide with or without 0.25 to 0.3 per cent methoxyflurane and oxygen or a low dose of ketamine (0.25 mg per kg) intravenously[18] may be used safely as long as the mother remains awake and maintains her laryngeal reflexes. If the sensory level is clearly inadequate, then general anesthesia with endotracheal intubation should be performed.

In the authors' experience (Table 17.8) between 12 and 14 per cent of patients will require supplementary analgesia before birth of the baby.

POST-DURAL PUNCTURE HEADACHE

One of the most troublesome and annoying complications of spinal anesthesia is post-dural puncture headache. The incidence can be minimized by using the smallest needle possible (Table 17.9).

The occurrence of inadvertent dural puncture associated with epidural anesthesia will, of course, vary with the experience of the anesthesiologist. In training centers the incidence reported is usually between 2 and 3 per cent.[28] If a dural puncture occurs after the use of a 16-gauge

Table 17.8
Maternal Analgesia: Cesarean Section Conduction Anesthesia

	Spinal	Epidural
Number of patients	343	1210
Analgesia		
Good to excellent	86%	84%
Fair	3%	2%
Insufficient		
Regional anesthesia supplemented with nitrous oxide, methoxyflurane or low-dose ketamine	6%	4%
General anesthesia required before birth	6%	10%

Table 17.9
Influence of Size and Bevel of Needle on Incidence of Post-puncture Headache*

Author	Gauge and Bevel of Needle	Incidence of Headache
		% of cases
Arner[19]	24	3.2
	22	5.4
Greene[20]	20	41
	22	26
	24	8
	26	0.4
Harris and Harmel[21]	18 and larger	24
	20	8
	24	3.5
Krueger[22]	20; regular	22
	20; pencil point	7
Hart and Whitacre[23]	20; regular	5
	20; pencil point	2
Ebner[24]	25	1.0
Phillips et al.[25]	25	0.9
Myers and Rosenberg[26]	26	0.33
Tarrow[27]	25 or 26	0.2

*Reprinted by permission from Bonica JJ: Postspinal complications. In *Obstetrical Anesthesia: Current Concepts and Practice,* SM Shnider, ed. Williams & Wilkins, Baltimore, 1970, p 175.

needle and the epidural technique is abandoned, almost 80 per cent of patients develop a headache. If, however, an epidural anesthetic is administered using another interspace (directing the catheter away from the dural hole) approximately 55 per cent of patients develop a headache. This headache can be severely incapacitating. Conservative therapy consists of bed rest in the prone or supine position, analgesics, hydration and a tight abdominal binder to increase epidural pressure and decrease the leak of cerebrospinal fluid.

BLOOD PATCH EPIDURAL

A blood patch epidural using autologous blood may be performed in patients suffering from severe refractory post-dural puncture headaches. Under a rigidly aseptic technique, 10 ml of blood are withdrawn via a venipuncture and immediately placed into the epidural space at the site of the dural rent. The success rate reported has ranged between 94 and 100 per cent (Table 17.10). A long-term follow-up of 118 patients for 2 years has indicated that epidural blood patch is without serious complication. No cases of infection, adhesive arachnoiditis or cauda-equina syndrome have been reported.[38] Backache is the most common complication. It is seldom severe or incapacitating and usually disappears within 48 hours, although it may occasionally last up to 3 months.

General Anesthesia

In contrast to regional anesthesia, general anesthesia has the advantages of a more rapid induction, less hypotension and cardiovascular instability and better control of the airway and ventilation. Some patients are terrified of "needles in the back" or the prospect of being awake during major abdominal surgery. In addition, general anesthesia may be preferable in patients with pre-existing neurologic or lumbar disc disease, coagulopathies or infections.

Management of general anesthesia for cesarean section, as outlined in Table 17.11, is based on the following considerations.

PREVENTION OF ASPIRATION

Aspiration of gastric contents during general anesthesia is a major cause of ma-

Table 17.10
Blood Patch Epidural for Dural Puncture Headache

Investigator	Number of Patients	Success Rate
		%
Gormley[29]	7	100
DiGiovanni and Dunbar[30]	45	91.1
DiGiovanni et al.[31]	63	96.8
Glass and Dupont[98]	43	93
Glass and Kennedy[32]	50	94
Dupont and Shire[33]	41	97.5
Vondrell and Bernards[34]	60	96.5
Blok[35]	22	91
Balagot et al.[36]	7	100
Ostheimer et al.[37]	185	98.5
Abouleish et al.[38]	118	97.5
Loeser et al.[39]	31	96
Abouleish[40]	3	100
Total:	675	Average: 96

Table 17.11
General Anesthesia for Cesarean Section: A Suggested Technique

1. Give 30 to 60 ml of oral antacid 1 hour before induction.
2. Utilize left uterine displacement.
3. Start I.V. infusion with a large-bore plastic cannula.
4. Pre-oxygenate 3 minutes at high flow rates (greater than 6 L/min).
5. Administer 0.4 mg of atropine or 0.2 mg of glycopyrrolate and 3 mg of curare or 0.5 mg of pancuronium I.V. within 5 minutes of induction.
6. When the surgeon is ready to begin, administer 4 mg/kg of thiopental and 1.5 mg/kg of succinylcholine.
7. An assistant should apply cricoid pressure until the trachea is sealed by the cuff of the endotracheal tube.
8. Administer N_2O (6 L/min) + O_2 (3 L/min) or N_2O (5 L/min) + O_2 (5 L/min) + either halothane 0.5 per cent, enflurane 0.5 to 0.75 per cent or methoxyflurane 0.1 to 0.2 per cent. Use muscle relaxant as necessary.
9. Avoid maternal hyperventilation.
10. Five minutes before delivery increase oxygen concentration to 50 per cent.
11. After umbilical cord is clamped, deepen anesthesia with nitrous oxide, narcotic or barbiturate; the halothane may be discontinued.
12. Extubate when the patient is awake.

---

ternal morbidity and mortality. Routine administration of antacid prior to induction significantly raises gastric pH.[41] However, use of antacids will not diminish the risk of aspiration of particulate matter.

The risk of regurgitation and aspiration is decreased by (1) rapid endotracheal intubation, (2) use of 0.4 mg of atropine or 0.2 mg of glycopyrrolate intravenously to possibly increase the tone of the cardio-esophageal sphincter, (3) pre-treatment with 3 mg of curare or 0.5 mg of pancuronium to prevent fasciculations and the associated rise in intragastric pressure secondary to succinylcholine administration,[42] (4) avoiding positive-pressure ventilation prior to intubation which could inflate the stomach and make the patient more prone to regurgitate, (5) use of cricoid pressure (Sellick maneuver) to occlude the esophagus and prevent passive regurgitation during endotracheal intubation[43] and (6) extubating the patient only after she is fully awake and able to protect her airway.

PRE-OXYGENATION

Oxygen consumption at term is 20 per cent higher than in the non-pregnant state.[44] Furthermore, in pregnant women, functional residual capacity is reduced 20 per cent because of upward displacement of the diaphragm.[45] Because of the reduced functional residual capacity the mother is more likely to become hypoxic during induction of anesthesia than is the non-pregnant patient. During a 1-minute period of apnea (due to paralysis after pre-oxygenation) a parturient will sustain a 150-torr reduction in PaO_2, in contrast to a 50-torr reduction in a non-pregnant woman.[46] Occasionally, difficult laryngoscopy and several attempts at intubation are encountered. Thus, maternal hypoxia is less likely with pre-oxygenation before induction.

REDUCED ANESTHETIC REQUIREMENTS

Anesthetic requirements are decreased during pregnancy. In the experimental animal, MAC for halothane, isoflurane or methoxyflurane is 25 to 40 per cent less in pregnant animals than in non-pregnant animals[47] (Table 17.12). Also, the reduced maternal functional residual capacity results in a faster rate of equilibration between inspired and alveolar (brain) gas tension. Therefore, the rate of induction of anesthesia is much more rapid in the pregnant patient, and overdose may easily occur.

MATERNAL VENTILATION

Under anesthesia, excessive positive-pressure ventilation (maternal $PaCO_2$ less than 20 torr) may result in fetal hypoxemia and acidosis.[48] The etiology includes reduced uterine and umbilical blood flow and increased affinity of maternal hemoglobin for oxygen (Bohr effect), resulting in less placental transfer of oxygen (Figures 17.2 and 17.3). The anesthesiologist should try to maintain a normal $PaCO_2$,

Table 17.12
MAC Presented as Per Cent End-tidal Anesthetic Concentration (Means ± SE)*

	Non-pregnant ewes (n = 6)	Pregnant ewes (n = 6)	Change
			%
Halothane	0.97 ± .04	0.73† ± .07	−25
Isoflurane	1.58 ± .07	1.01‡ ± .06	−40
Methoxyflurane	0.26 ± .02	0.18§ ± .01	−32

* Reprinted by permission from Palahniuk RJ, Shnider SM, Eger El II: Pregnancy decreases the requirements for inhaled anesthetic agents. Anesthesiology 41:82, 1974.
† $p < .001$.
‡ $p < .010$.
§ $p < .025$.

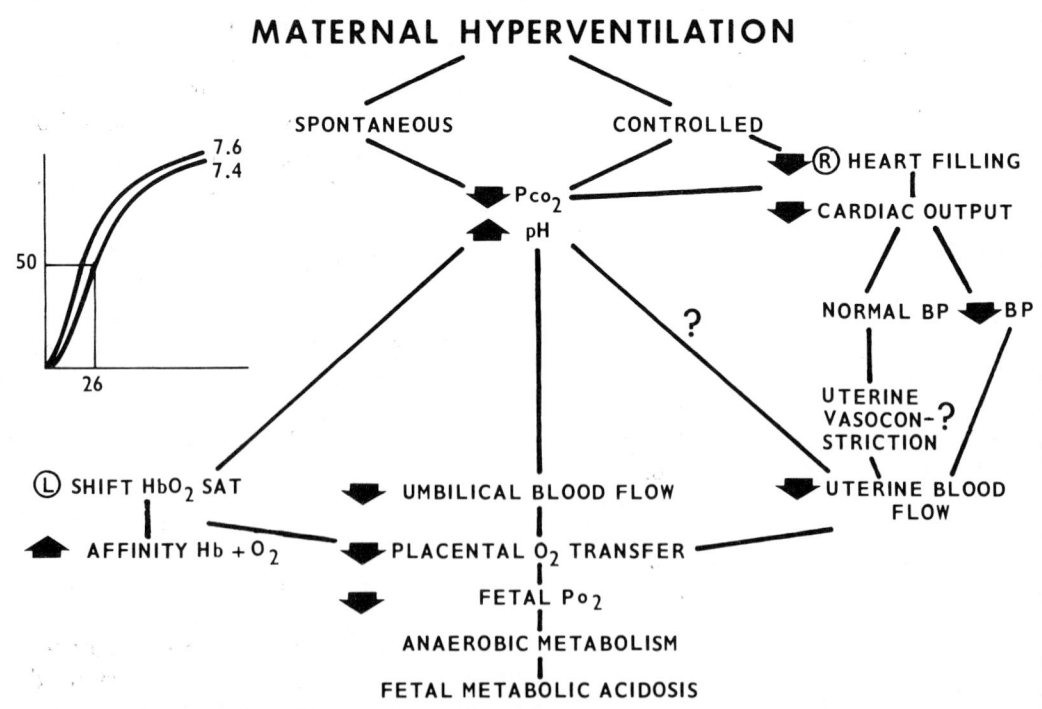

Figure 17.2. Pathophysiology of maternal hyperventilation. (Reprinted by permission from Shnider SM, Moya F: *The Anesthesiologist, Mother and Newborn.* Williams & Wilkins, Baltimore, 1973, p 98.)

ANESTHESIA FOR CESAREAN SECTION

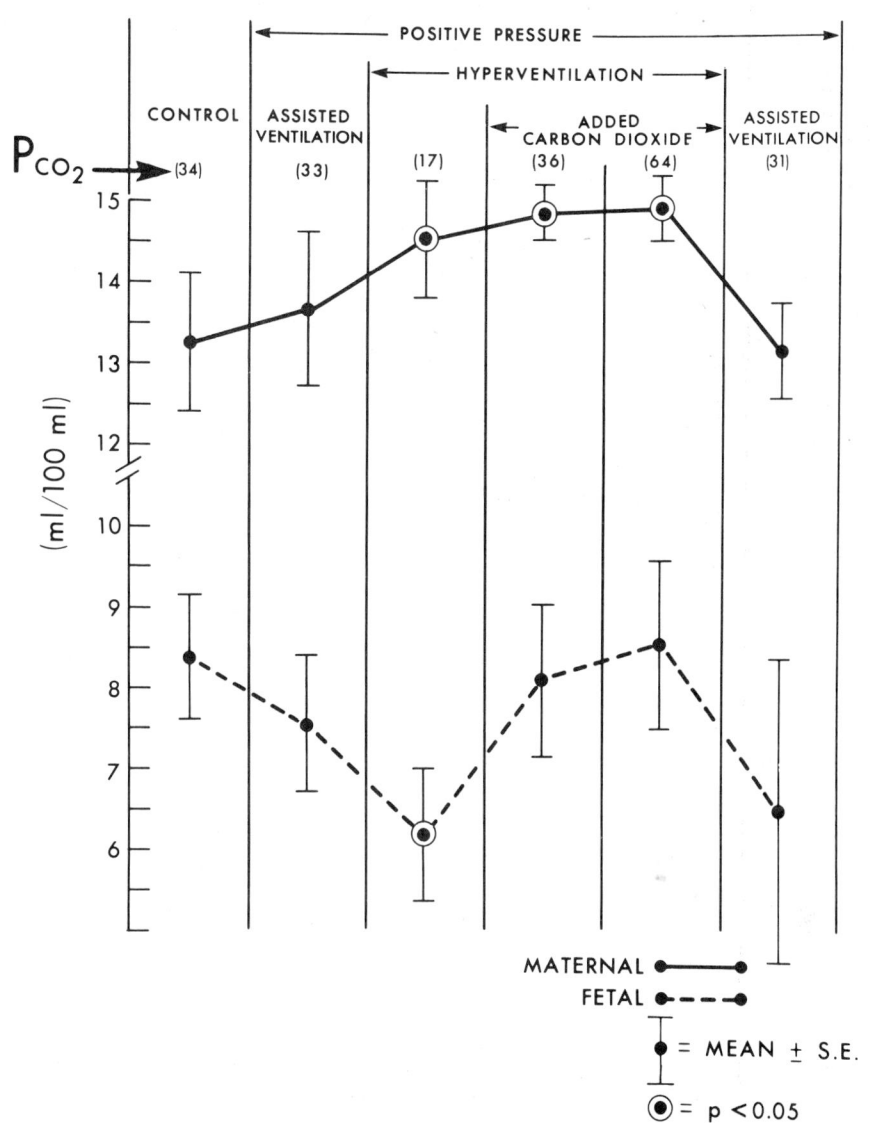

Figure 17.3. Changes from control values in mean maternal and fetal arterial oxygen content during five periods of positive-pressure ventilation. Mean maternal PaCO$_2$ during each period is indicated at the top of the figure. (Reprinted by permission from Levinson G, Shnider SM, deLorimier AA, et al.: Effects of maternal hyperventilation on uterine blood flow and fetal oxygenation and acid-base status. Anesthesiology 40:340, 1974.)

which at term ranges between 30 and 33 torr.

MATERNAL AND FETAL EFFECTS OF ANESTHETIC AGENTS

Thiopental. Thiopental rapidly crosses the placenta, and it is not possible to deliver the baby before the drug is transferred to the fetus. After a single maternal intravenous dose the drug can be detected in umbilical venous blood within 30 seconds[49] (Figure 17.4). Thiopental reaches its peak concentration in umbilical venous blood in 1 minute and in umbilical arterial

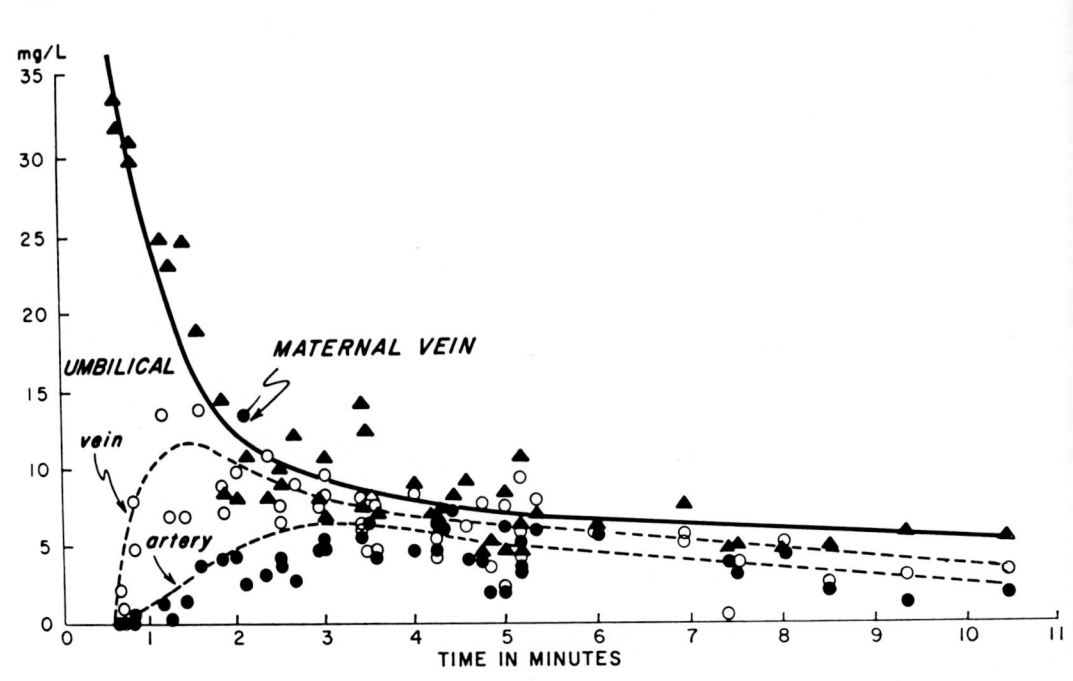

Figure 17.4. The level of thiopental in maternal vein, umbilical vein and umbilical artery after injection of a single dose of 4 mg/kg for induction of anesthesia. Note the rapid decay of the maternal venous blood level and the rapid transfer to the fetus. (Reprinted by permission from Kosaka Y, Takahashi T, Mark LC: Intravenous thiobarbiturate anesthesia for cesarean section. Anesthesiology 31:489, 1969.

blood in 2 to 3 minutes. Why, then, is the neonate not affected? The fetal brain will not be exposed to high concentrations of barbiturate if the induction dose is less than 4 mg/kg. With this dose umbilical arterial levels of thiopental are much lower than the umbilical venous levels[50] (Figure 17.5). Blood from the placenta first passes through the liver, so most of the thiopental is either cleared by the liver or diluted by blood from the lower extremities and viscera. Other reasons for lack of neonatal depression after a sleep dose of thiopental are swift decline of the drug concentration in maternal blood and non-homogeneity of blood in the intervillous space. There is no advantage to delaying delivery until the thiopental has redistributed in the mother or fetus. It should be stressed that after large doses of thiopental (8 mg/kg) babies are depressed.[50]

Muscle relaxants. Muscle relaxants are commonly used prior to delivery to facilitate rapid endotracheal intubation and provide optimum operating conditions in a lightly anesthetized patient. Muscle relaxants have low lipid solubility and are highly ionized at physiologic pH. When conventional doses are administered clinically, insignificant placental transfer occurs.[51, 52]

Succinylcholine administered to the mother in high doses (2 to 3 mg/kg) is detectable in fetal blood and may cause alterations in the electromyograph,[53] but it has no depressant effects on neonatal respiration. Only with maternal administration of massive doses (10 mg/kg) does enough placental transfer occur to cause neonatal depression.[54] Despite reduced plasma pseudocholinesterase in parturients,[55] metabolism of moderate doses of

ANESTHESIA FOR CESAREAN SECTION

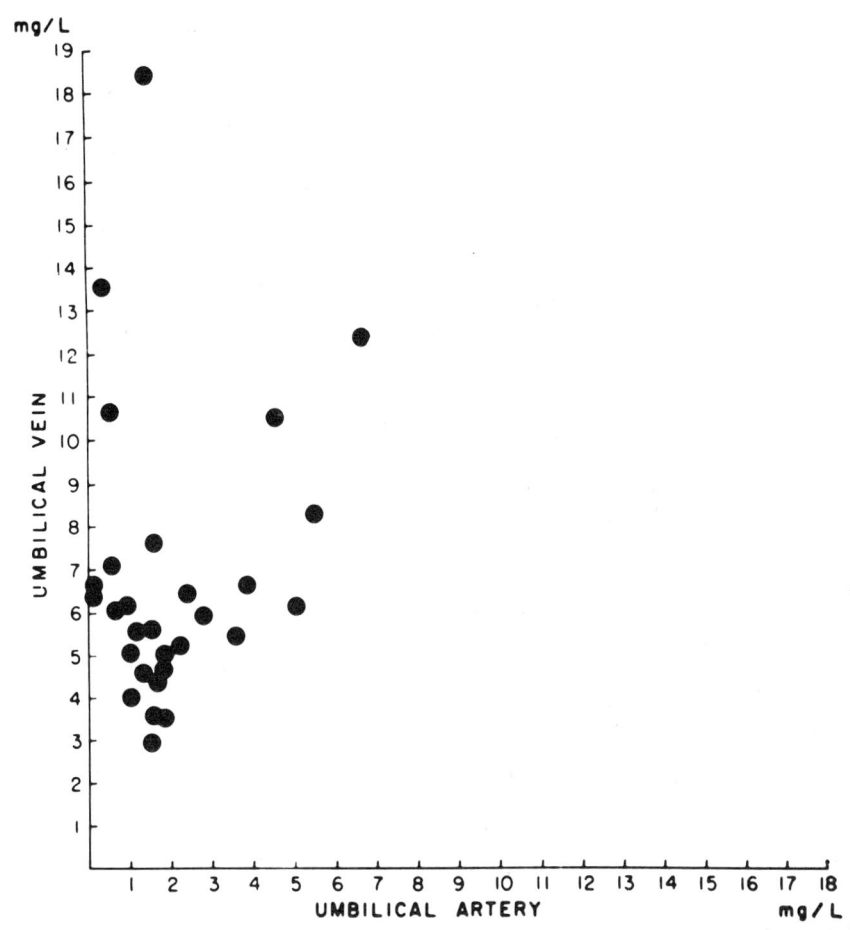

Figure 17.5. Relationship between the concentration of thiopental in umbilical artery and umbilical vein at birth. (Reprinted by permission from Finster M, Mark LC, Morishima HO, et al.: Plasma thiopental concentrations in the newborn following delivery under thiopental-nitrous oxide anesthesia. Am J Obstet Gynecol 95:621, 1966.)

succinylcholine is usually not prolonged[56] (Table 17.13). In some patients, however, pseudocholinesterase levels are so low as to result in a prolonged block.[55] Also, in patients with atypical cholinesterase, prolonged maternal and neonatal respiratory depression have been reported.[57] After injection of an intubating dose of succinylcholine, return of neuromuscular function should be assured before additional relaxant is administered.

Curare or pancuronium is administered in small doses to prevent fasciculations from succinylcholine and in larger doses to maintain muscle relaxation during surgery. Because these non-depolarizing relaxants are easily reversible, the authors prefer them to a continuous infusion of succinylcholine. Placental transfer of curare does occur, but fetal blood levels are only one-tenth of maternal blood levels,[58] and neonatal muscle weakness is not found. In clinical doses, pancuronium does not affect the neonate.[59]

Gallamine seems to be more easily transferred than the other relaxants, with relatively high fetal levels found after conventional maternal doses.[60] Even though

Table 17.13
Time to Twitch Recovery after Succinylcholine*

	Succinylcholine	Twitch Recovery 10%	50%	90%
	mg	minutes		
Non-pregnant women (n = 15)	144	10.2	11.9	13.3
Cesarean sections (n = 10)	148	9.9	11.5	12.9

* Adapted from Blitt CD, Petty WC, Alberternst EE, et al.: Correlation of plasma cholinesterase activity and duration of action of succinylcholine during pregnancy. Anesth Analg 56:78, 1977.

neonatal muscle weakness has not been reported, gallamine has not achieved popularity in obstetric anesthesia.

Nitrous oxide. Nitrous oxide is the most popular inhalation agent in obstetric anesthesia. It produces no significant uterine relaxation. It is rapidly transferred across the placenta, but fetal tissue uptake during the first 20 minutes reduces the fetal arterial concentration and subsequent neonatal depression[61, 62] (Figures 10.2 and 10.3). It is well documented that the longer the duration of anesthesia with nitrous oxide the more anesthetized the newborn may be.[63, 64] The authors' findings are shown in Table 17.14. Therefore, the duration of anesthesia prior to delivery should be as brief as possible. This can be accomplished by delaying induction of anesthesia until the patient is prepped and draped and the obstetrician is ready to begin the operation.

Halogenated agents. There has been much recent interest in the use of low-dose halothane (0.25 to 0.5 per cent), enflurane (0.5 to 0.75 per cent) or methoxyflurane (0.1 per cent) as supplements to nitrous oxide anesthesia. These agents (1) decrease the likelihood of maternal post-operative recall and awareness of intraoperative events, (2) permit higher maternal inspired oxygen tension, (3) may improve uterine blood flow, (4) do not result in increased uterine bleeding and (5) do not depress the newborn.

Maternal awareness. Several surveys

Table 17.14
Elective Cesarean Section: Duration of (General Anesthesia (N$_2$O-O$_2$) Antepartum and Apgar Scores

Minutes of Anesthesia	Apgar Score 7 to 10 Number	Per cent
<5	16	88
6–10	47	74
11–20	36	69
21–30	20	50
31–60	11	36

* Reprinted by permission from Rolbin SH, Levinson G, Shnider SM: Current status of anesthesia for cesarean section. Weekly Anesthesiology Update, Volume 1, Lesson 7. Weekly Anesthesiology Update, Inc. Princeton, N.J. 1977

have reported a high incidence of maternal awareness of surgery and birth with subsequent unpleasant experiences such as nightmares following nitrous oxide-oxygen-relaxant technique for vaginal delivery or cesarean section [65-73] (Table 17.15). The incidence of awareness appears to vary inversely with the concentration of nitrous oxide. For example, in one study approximately 9 per cent of parturients who received 67 per cent nitrous oxide in oxygen were aware of the delivery, whereas 26 per cent were aware if 50 per cent nitrous oxide was used.[65] No maternal awareness of pain has been reported if halothane 0.1 to 0.65 per cent or enflurane 0.5 to 1.5 per cent or methoxyflurane 0.1 per cent is added to 50 per cent nitrous

ANESTHESIA FOR CESAREAN SECTION

Table 17.15
Maternal Awareness of Surgery and Birth after Barbiturate-Relaxant Induction

Anesthetic	Incidence of Awareness
	%
Nitrous oxide 50 per cent	
Crawford[65]	26
Wilson and Turner[66]	19
Nitrous oxide 67 per cent to 75 per cent	
Crawford[65]	9
Wilson and Turner[66]	10
Moir[67]	4
Palahniuk[68]	5
Nitrous Oxide 25 per cent to 40 per cent + halothane 0.3 per cent to 0.5 per cent	
Galbert and Gardner[69]	0
Nitrous oxide 50 per cent + halothane 0.1 per cent to 0.65 per cent	
Wilson[70]	0
Latto and Waldron[71]	0
Moir[67]	0
Nitrous oxide 50 per cent + enflurane 0.5 per cent to 1.5 per cent	
Coleman and Downing[72]	0
Nitrous oxide 33 per cent + methoxyflurane 0.1 per cent	
Crawford et al.[73]	3.5
Nitrous oxide 50 per cent + methoxyflurane 0.1 per cent	
Palahniuk[68]	0

oxide before delivery.[67-71] Although methoxyflurane may cause dose-related nephrotoxicity, numerous studies in the obstetric patient have demonstrated no adverse renal effects.[74-78] The low doses necessary for cesarean section result in low non-toxic inorganic fluoride levels. Its use, however, is best avoided in patients with renal dysfunction such as preeclampsia or pyelonephritis.

Higher maternal oxygen. Maternal hyperoxia should improve fetal oxygenation and neonatal clinical condition at birth. In a study of 75 healthy women undergoing elective cesarean section under general anesthesia, oxygen tension, saturation and content of fetal blood increased significantly with increases in maternal inspired oxygen concentration to a maternal PaO_2 of 300 torr[79] (Table 17.16). The clinical condition of the newborn was also better in the higher oxygen groups. It was noted that there was no additional fetal or neonatal benefit if the maternal oxygen tension was above 300 torr.

Improved uterine blood flow. Anesthetic agents modify sympathetic activity. The authors have shown that in pregnant sheep noxious stimulation during nitrous oxide-oxygen anesthesia was associated with an increase in maternal blood pressure, a decrease in uterine blood flow and an increase in plasma norepinephrine compared to the awake control state.[80] By contrast noxious stimulation during nitrous oxide-oxygen anesthesia that was supplemented with either 0.5 per cent halothane or 1 per cent enflurane did not increase plasma catecholamines. Blood pressure remained unchanged in both groups, and uterine blood flow increased with halothane but did not change with enflurane (Figure 17.6).

Uterine bleeding. The main concern associated with the administration of halogenated agents is that they may decrease uterine muscle tone, and that postpartum blood loss will be increased. Halothane and enflurane produce a dose-related decrease in uterine contractility and tone.[81-85] However, several studies have failed to reveal any increased blood loss with low-dose halothane 0.1 to 0.8 per cent[67, 69-71] (Table 17.17) or enflurane 0.5 to 1.5 per cent[72] during cesarean section. At these low concentrations, the uterus in the immediate postpartum period is responsive to oxytocin stimulation.[85]

Neonatal depression. A potential hazard of the use of these potent inhalational agents is neonatal depression. Clinical experience, however, indicates that the slight increase in maternal anesthetic depth is not reflected in the neonate at birth.[67-73]

Table 17.16
Maternal Arterial, Umbilical Venous, and Umbilical Arterial Blood Oxygen Tensions and Neonatal Condition at Birth Improved with Increasing Maternal Oxygen Tension, but There Was No Further Change As Maternal Oxygen Tension Rose above 300 Torr*

Maternal arterial PO_2 (torr)	61–100	101–160	181–240	241–300	301–360	361–420	421–520
Number	13	12	3	10	19	11	7
Umbilical venous PO_2 (torr)	29	31	29	35	38	41	41
Umbilical artery PO_2 (torr)	16	20	21	23	25	26	25
Time necessary for infant to establish sustained respiration (seconds)	62	54	33	27	11	13	14
Number of infants with Apgar score of 6 or less	4	2	1	0	0	0	0

* Modified from: Marx GF, Mateo CV: Effects of different oxygen concentrations during general anaesthesia for elective caesarean section. Can Anaesth Soc J 18:587, 1971.

Table 17.17
Influence of Anesthesia on Blood Loss at 145 Cesarean Sections*

	Anesthetic			
	N_2O-O_2 (70:30) (50 Cases)	N_2O-O_2 (50:50) + 0.5% Halothane (50 Cases)	N_2O-O_2 (50:50) + 0.8% Halothane (25 Cases)	Epidural Analgesia (20 Cases)
		ml		
Loss (mean ± SD)	792 ± 388	688 ± 206	702 ± 294	378 ± 146

* Reprinted by permission from Moir DD: Anaesthesia for caesarean section: An evaluation of a method using low concentrations of halothane and 50 per cent of oxygen. Br J Anaesth 42:138, 1970.

Regional versus General Anesthesia: Condition of the Newborn

A neonate is conventionally evaluated by Apgar score, acid-base status and neurobehavioral examination. Although it is widely believed that regional anesthesia is safer for the newborn, recent studies suggest that either technique can result in vigorous, well oxygenated babies.

APGAR SCORE

Virginia Apgar was the first to point out that babies were more vigorous following cesarean section under conduction (spinal) than general (cyclopropane) anesthesia.[86] Since then numerous studies have confirmed these findings. For example the Collaborative Project (a research study involving 15 medical centers) found that in 405 normal gravidas undergoing elective repeat cesarean section more than five times as many neonates were depressed at 1 minute (Apgar 0 to 3) when delivery occurred under general anesthesia as compared to regional anesthesia.[87] Moreover, in this study, three times as many newborns had depressed Apgar scores at 5 minutes after general anesthesia in contrast to regional anesthesia. This prolonged depression, the authors believe, probably represents inadequate management of the newborn. The authors have found that, after general anesthesia—despite a high

ANESTHESIA FOR CESAREAN SECTION

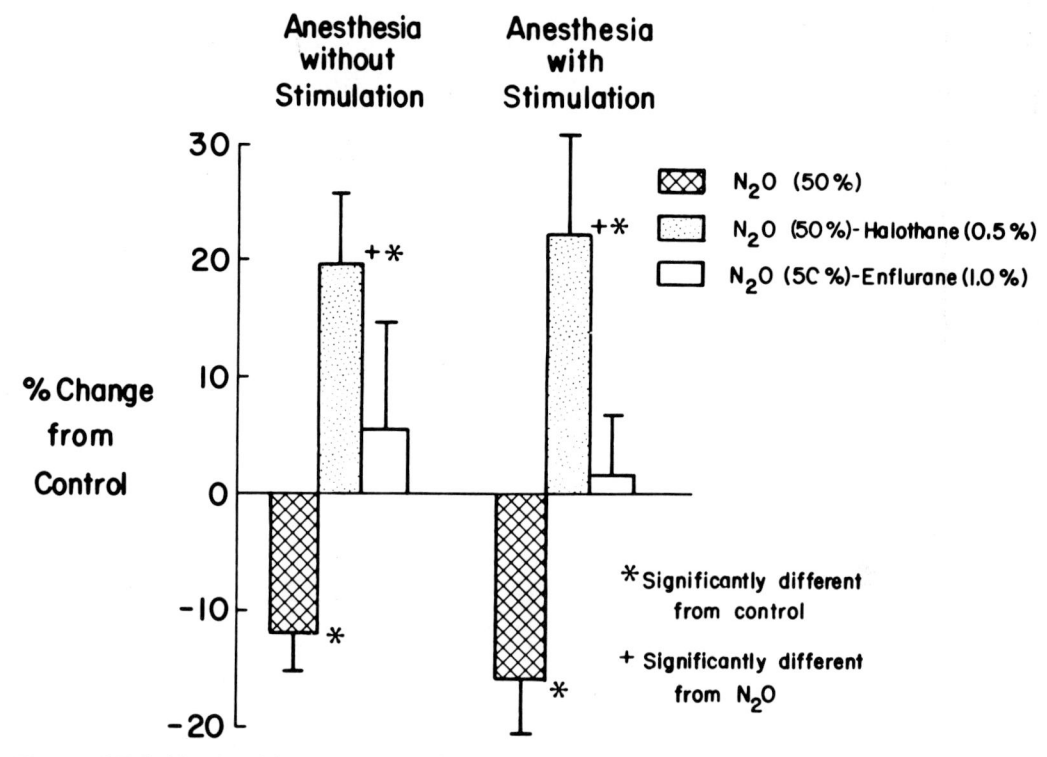

Figure 17.6. Uterine blood flow changes during anesthesia in the pregnant ewe with and without noxious stimulation. The three anesthetics administered for 1 hour each were nitrous oxide 50 per cent, nitrous oxide 50 per cent and halothane 0.5 per cent, and nitrous oxide 50 per cent and enflurane 1.0 per cent. (Reprinted by permission from Shnider SM, Wright RG, Levinson G, et al.: Plasma norepinephrine and uterine blood flow changes during endotracheal intubation and general anesthesia in the pregnant ewe. In *Abstracts of Scientific Papers*, Annual Meeting, American Society of Anesthesiologists, Chicago, 1978, p 115.)

incidence of depressed newborns at 1 minute—by 5 minutes of age—after stimulation and assisted ventilation—babies are as vigorous as those after regional anesthesia (Table 17.18). The low initial Apgar score in these babies is clearly due to transient sedation rather than asphyxia, as seen in Table 17.14.

Furthermore, babies delivered shortly after the induction of general anesthesia are as vigorous as those born with regional anesthesia (Tables 17.14 and 17.18). The authors' findings that neonatal depression after general anesthesia is related to the duration of anesthesia are in agreement with numerous other studies.[62, 63, 88, 89] For example, Stenger et al.[62] reported a 15 per cent incidence of depressed neonates when the mean duration of nitrous oxide

Table 17.18
Elective Cesarean Section: Clinical Condition of Newborn

	Apgar Score: 7 to 10	
	1 Minute	5 Minutes
	%	%
Spinal (n = 151)	92	97
Epidural (n = 327)	91	99
General (n = 163)	69	97

anesthesia was 15 minutes and a 54 per cent incidence when the duration was 36 minutes. Finster and Poppers[63] found that when duration of anesthesia was less than 10 minutes the mean Apgar score was 7.7; it decreased to 6.8 in the group delivered after 11 to 20 minutes and to 6.3 when the duration of anesthesia before delivery exceeded 21 minutes.

Thus, when general anesthesia is chosen, expeditious delivery of the newborn is necessary to minimize neonatal depression. If prolonged operating time is anticipated, regional anesthesia may be preferable. In contrast to general anesthesia, the authors have found that a prolonged duration of epidural anesthesia does not result in depressed neonates (Table 17.19). In addition, the hypotension so common with regional anesthesia, when properly and promptly treated, does not result in low Apgar scores (Table 17.20).

ACID-BASE STATUS

Numerous investigators have compared fetal acid-base status in umbilical cord blood sampled from a doubly clamped segment immediately after elective cesarean section delivery.[64, 90-93] Although results are conflicting, as seen in Tables 17.21 and 17.22, the differences between the techniques are minimal and probably not clinically significant. With any technique the acid-base status of the neonate should be in the normal range. Even with prolonged general anesthesia and depressed Apgar scores, i.e. sleeping babies, fetal acid-base status is normal. Patients with diabetes mellitus have been reported to be slightly more acidotic after spinal anesthesia than after general anesthesia. Acidosis was especially related to the occurrence of maternal hypotension.[91]

If fetal hypoxia and acidosis are found with elective cesarean section, then a number of etiologic factors may exist. With general anesthesia maternal hypoxia, excessive hyperventilation, aortocaval compression or anesthetic overdose may all cause fetal asphyxia. With regional anesthesia, unrecognized or improperly treated hypotension is the most likely cause of fetal acidosis.

With either technique a prolonged uterine incision to delivery time has been found to be directly related to fetal hypoxia and acidosis.

Crawford and Davies[94] found that with cesarean section under general anesthesia the condition of the infant, both clinical and biochemical, was directly related to the time which elapsed from the initial uterine incision to completion of delivery. This was confirmed by Datta et al.[95] who found that with both general and spinal

Table 17.19
Elective Cesarean Section: Duration of Epidural Anesthesia Antepartum and Apgar Scores

Minutes of Anesthesia	Apgar Score: 7 to 10	
	Numbers	Per Cent
<20	20	85
21–30	44	93
31–60	214	92
61–120	40	90
>120	5	100

Table 17.20
Elective Cesarean Section: Hypotension and Condition of Infant

		Number	Apgar Scores 7 to 10 (per cent)	
Spinal	Hypotension	104	91	ns*
	No hypotension	47	100	
Epidural	Hypotension	102	88	ns*
	No hypotension	227	93	

* No statistically significant difference between hypotension and no hypotension.

Table 17.21
General versus Spinal Anesthesia

		pH General	pH Spinal	Base Deficit General	Base Deficit Spinal
		units		(mEq/L)	
Marx et al.[90]	MA*	7.42	7.40	3.5	4.6
(14 general; 10 spinal)	UV	7.30	7.30	4.9	5.1
	UA	7.23	7.24	6.5	6.0
Datta and Brown[91]	MA	7.46	7.43	0.58	0.67
(15 general; 15 spinal)	UV	7.38	7.34		
	UA	7.30	7.28	1.87	1.40
Shnider[64]	MA	7.46	7.42	3.6	3.9
(26 spinal; 39 general)	UV	7.36	7.33	2.3	3.3
	UA	7.29	7.23	2.9	4.7

* MA, maternal artery; UV, umbilical vein; UA, umbilical artery.

Table 17.22
General versus Epidural Anesthesia

		pH General	pH Epidural	Base Deficit General	Base Deficit Epidural
		units		mEq/L	
Fox and Houle[92]	MA*	7.38	7.42	4.9	4.1
(13 general; 13 epidural)	UV	7.27	7.33	6.8	5.3
	UA	7.22	7.28	8.1	6.7
James et al.[93]	MA	7.47	7.44	3.0	3.0
(20 general; 15 epidural)	UV	7.38	7.35	1.9	1.6
	UA	7.32	7.30	1.8	1.3
Shnider	MA	7.46	7.45	3.6	3.8
(30 epidural; 41 general)	UV	7.36	7.32	2.3	5.1
	UA	7.29	7.23	2.9	5.7

* MA, maternal artery; UV, umbilical vein; UA, umbilical artery.

anesthesia uterine incision to delivery intervals exceeding 3 minutes were associated with a significantly lower pH in the baby and a higher incidence of depressed Apgar scores. Thus, it is apparent that prolonged uterine manipulation may adversely affect the placental blood flow.

NEUROBEHAVIORAL EXAMINATION

Even when neonates are not depressed at birth as ascertained by low Apgar scores, more subtle neurobehavioral changes in the subsequent neonatal period may occur. Using the early neonatal behavioral scale[14] on infants delivered by cesarean section, Scanlon et al.[96] reported that infants born after general anesthesia with nitrous oxide were more depressed 6 to 8 hours later than those born after spinal anesthesia. On the other hand, Palahniuk et al.[97] compared general anesthesia with nitrous oxide or methoxyflurane-oxygen and lumbar epidural. Methoxyflurane-oxygen anesthesia resulted in more alert normotonic newborns than the nitrous oxide (70 per cent)-oxygen group. Lumbar epidural anesthesia resulted in alert but hypotonic newborns. As far as the neurobehavioral status is concerned, the choice between regional and general anesthesia is still undecided.

Emergency Cesarean Section

Sudden unexpected complications during late pregnancy or labor which adversely affect the mother or fetus may necessitate an immediate emergency cesarean section. Examples include massive third trimester bleeding, prolapsed umbilical cord or severe fetal distress. When the mother or fetus is in immediate jeopardy cesarean section should not be delayed in order to establish an adequate sensory level with either a spinal or epidural block. For some emergency cesarean sections where neither the mother nor fetus is in immediate danger, immediate delivery is not crucial. Examples might include repeat section in early labor, failure of induction, failure to progress, failed forceps, chorioamnionitis and malpresentation. In these situations either regional or general anesthesia may be administered.

Anesthesia for cesarean section in the presence of some of the more common and significant obstetric and medical complications is discussed in previous chapters: preeclampsia-eclampsia, chapter 14; placenta praevia, abruptio placentae, ruptured uterus, chapter 16; and parturients with cardiac disease, chapter 13.

References

1. American College of Obstetricians and Gynecologists: Précis: An Update in Obstetrics and Gynecology. McGraw-Hill, New York, 1977, p 24.
2. Hicks JS, Levinson G, Shnider SM: Obstetric anesthesia training centers in the U.S.A.–1975. Anesth Analg 55:839, 1976.
3. Roberts RB, Shirley MA: The obstetrician's role in reducing the risk of aspiration pneumonitis with particular reference to the use of oral antacids. Am J Obstet Gynecol 124:611, 1976.
4. Greiss FC, Crandell DL: Therapy for hypotension induced by spinal anesthesia during pregnancy. JAMA 191:793, 1965.
5. James FM, Greiss FC, Kemp RA: An evaluation of vasopressor therapy for maternal hypotension during spinal anesthesia. Anesthesiology 33:25, 1970.
6. Shnider SM, deLorimier AA, Holl JW, et al.: Vasopressors in obstetrics. I. Correction of fetal acidosis with ephedrine during spinal anesthesia. Am J Obstet Gynecol 102:911, 1968.
7. Ralston DH, Shnider SM, deLorimier AA: Effects of equipotent ephedrine, metaraminol, mephentermine, and methoxamine on uterine blood flow in the pregnant ewe. Anesthesiology 40:354, 1974.
8. Assali NS, Prystowsky H: Studies on autonomic blockade. II. Observations on the nature of blood pressure fall with high selective spinal anesthesia in pregnant women. J Clin Invest 29:1367, 1950.
9. Bromage PR: Continuous lumbar epidural analgesia for obstetrics. Can Med Assoc J 85:1136, 1961.
10. Grundy EM, Zamora AM, Winnie AP: Comparison of spread of epidural anesthesia in pregnant and nonpregnant women. Anesth Analg 57:544, 1978.
11. O'Brien JE, Abbey V, Hinsvark O, et al.: Metabolism and measurement of 2-chloroprocaine, an ester-type local anesthetic. J Pharm Sci. 66:75, 1979.
12. Tucker GT, Boyes RN, Bridenbaugh PO, et al.: Binding of anilide-type local anesthetics in human plasma. II. Implications in vivo, with special reference to transplacental distribution. Anesthesiology 33:304, 1970.
13. Tucker GT: Plasma binding and disposition of local anesthetics. Int Anaesth Clin 13:33, 1975.
14. Scanlon JW, Brown WU, Weiss JB, et al.: Neurobehavioral responses of newborn infants after maternal epidural anesthesia. Anesthesiology 40: 121, 1974.
15. McGuinness GA, Merkow AJ, Kennedy RL, et al.: Epidural anesthesia with bupivacaine for cesarean section: Neonatal blood levels and neurobehavioral responses. Anesthesiology 49:270, 1978.
16. Scanlon JW, Ostheimer GW, Lurie AO, et al.: Neurobehavioral responses and drug concentrations in newborns after maternal epidural anesthesia with bupivacaine. Anesthesiology 45:400, 1976.
17. Rolbin SH, Wright RG, Shnider SM, et al.: Diazepam during cesarean section: Effects of neonatal Apgar scores, acid-base status, neurobehavioral assessment and maternal and fetal plasma norepinephrine levels. In Abstracts of Scientific Papers, Annual Meeting, American Society of Anesthesiologists, New Orleans, 1977, p 449.
18. Akamatsu TJ, Bonica JJ, Rehmet R, et al.: Experiences with the use of ketamine for parturition. I. Primary anesthetic for vaginal delivery. Anesth Analg 53:284, 1974.
19. Arner O: Complications following spinal anesthesia. Their significance and technic to reduce their incidence. Acta Chir Scand (Suppl) 167:7, 1952.
20. Greene BA: A 26-gauge lumbar puncture needle:

Its value in the prophylaxis of headache following spinal analgesia for vaginal delivery. Anesthesiology 11:464, 1950.
21. Harris LM, Harmel MH: The comparative incidence of postlumbar puncture headache following spinal anesthesia administered through 20 and 24 gauge needles. Anesthesiology 14:390, 1953.
22. Krueger JE: Etiology and treatment of postspinal headaches. Anesth Analg 32:190, 1953.
23. Hart JR, Whitacre RJ: Pencil-point needle in prevention of postspinal headache. JAMA 147:657, 1951.
24. Ebner H: An evaluation of spinal anesthesia in obstetrics. Anesth Analg 38:378, 1959.
25. Phillips OC, Lyons WB, Harris LC, et al.: Spinal anesthesia for vaginal delivery: A review of 2016 cases using Xylocaine. Obstet Gynecol 13:437, 1959.
26. Myers L, Rosenberg M: The use of the 26-gauge spinal needle: A survey. Anesth Analg 41:509, 1962.
27. Tarrow AB: Solution to spinal headaches. Int Anesth Clin 1:877, 1963.
28. Palahniuk RJ: Prophylactic blood patch does not prevent spinal headache. In *Abstracts of Scientific Papers*, Annual Meeting, Society for Obstetric Anesthesia and Perinatology, Seattle, 1977, p 21.
29. Gormley JB: Treatment of postspinal headache. Anesthesiology 21:565, 1960.
30. DiGiovanni AJ, Dunbar BS: Epidural injections of autologous blood for postlumbar-puncture headache. Anesth Analg 49:268, 1970.
31. DiGiovanni AJ, Galbert MW, Wahle WM: Epidural injection of autologous blood for postlumbar-puncture headache. II. Additional clinical experiences and laboratory investigation. Anesth Analg 51:226, 1972.
32. Glass PM, Kennedy WF Jr: Headache following subarachnoid puncture: Treatment with epidural blood patch. JAMA 219:203, 1972.
33. DuPont FS, Shire RD: Epidural blood patch: An unusual approach to the problem of post-spinal anesthetic headache. Mich Med 71:105, 1972.
34. Vondrell JJ, Bernards WC: Epidural "blood patch" for the treatment of postspinal puncture headaches. Wis Med J 72:132, 1973.
35. Blok RJ: Headache following spinal anesthesia: Treatment by epidural blood patch. J Am Osteopath Assoc 73:128, 1973.
36. Balagot RC, Lee T, Liu C, et al.: The prophylactic epidural blood patch (Letter). JAMA 228:1369, 1974.
37. Ostheimer GW, Palahniuk RJ, Shnider SM: Epidural blood patch for postlumbar-puncture headache (Letter). Anesthesiology 41:307, 1974.
38. Abouleish E, de la Vega S, Blendinger I, et al.: Long-term follow-up of epidural blood patch. Anesth Analg 54:459, 1975.
39. Loeser EA, Hill GE, Bennett GM, et al.: Time vs. success rate for epidural blood patch. Anesthesiology 49:147, 1978.
40. Abouleish E: Epidural blood patch for the treatment of chronic postlumbar-puncture cephalgia. Anesthesiology 49:291, 1978.
41. Roberts RB, Shirley MA: Reducing the risk of acid aspiration during cesarean section. Anesth Analg 53:859, 1974.
42. Miller RD, Way WL: Inhibition of succinylcholine-induced increased intragastric pressure by nondepolarizing muscle relaxants and lidocaine. Anesthesiology 34:185, 1971.
43. Sellick BA: Cricoid pressure to control regurgitation of stomach contents during induction of anaesthesia. Lancet 2:404, 1961.
44. Widlund G: Cardio-pulmonal function during pregnancy: A clinical-experimental study with particular respect to ventilation and oxygen consumption among normal cases in rest and after work tests. Acta Obstet Gynaecol Scand 25:1, 1945.
45. Cugell DW, Frank NR, Gaensler ER, et al.: Pulmonary function in pregnancy. I. Serial observations in normal women. Am Rev Tuberc 67:538, 1953.
46. Archer GW Jr, Marx GF: Arterial oxygen tension during apnoea in parturient women. Br J Anesth 46:358, 1974.
47. Palahniuk RJ, Shnider SM, Eger EI II: Pregnancy decreases the requirements for inhaled anesthetic agents. Anesthesiology 41:82, 1974.
48. Levinson G, Shnider SM, deLorimier AA, et al.: Effects of maternal hyperventilation on uterine blood flow and fetal oxygenation and acid-base status. Anesthesiology 40:340, 1974.
49. Kosaka Y, Takahashi T, Mark LC: Intravenous thiobarbiturate anesthesia for cesarean section. Anesthesiology 31:489, 1969.
50. Finster M, Mark LC, Morishima HO, et al.: Plasma thiopental concentrations in the newborn following delivery under thiopental-nitrous oxide anesthesia. Am J Obstet Gynecol 95:621, 1966.
51. Cohen EN, Paulson WJ, Wall J, et al.: Thiopental, curare, and nitrous oxide anaesthesia for cesarean section with studies on placental transmission. Surg Gynecol Obstet 97:456, 1953.
52. Moya F, Kvisselgaard N: The placental transmission of succinylcholine. Anesthesiology 22:1, 1961.
53. Drabkova J, Crul JF, Van Der Kleijn E: Placental transfer of ^{14}C-labelled succinylcholine in near-term Macaca mulatta monkeys. Br J Anaesth 45:1087, 1973.
54. Kvisselgaard N, Moya F: Investigation of placental thresholds to succinylcholine. Anesthesiology 22:7, 1961.
55. Shnider SM: Serum cholinesterase activity during pregnancy, labor and puerperium. Anesthesiology 26:355, 1965.
56. Blitt CD, Petty WC, Alberternst EE, et al.: Correlation of plasma cholinesterase activity and duration of action of succinylcholine during pregnancy. Anesth Analg 56:78, 1977.
57. Baraka A, Haroun S, Bassili M, et al.: Response of the newborn to succinylcholine injection in homozygote atypical mothers. Anesthesiology 43:115, 1975.
58. Kivalo I, Saarikoski S: Placental transmission and

59. Latto IP, Wainwright AC: Anaesthesia for caesarean section: Analysis of blood concentrations of methoxyflurane using 0.1 per cent methoxyflurane and 40 per cent oxygen. Br J Anaesth 44: 1050, 1972.
  foetal uptake of ^{14}C-dimethyltubocurarine. Br J Anaesth 44:557, 1972.
60. Crawford JS, Gardiner JE: Some aspects of obstetric anaesthesia. Part II. The use of relaxant drugs. Br J Anaesth 38:154, 1956.
61. Marx GF, Joshi CW, Orkin LR: Placental transmission of nitrous oxide. Anesthesiology 32:429, 1970.
62. Stenger VG, Blechner JN, Prystowsky H: A study of prolongation of obstetric anesthesia. Am J Obstet Gynecol 103:901, 1969.
63. Finster M, Poppers PJ: Safety of thiopental used for induction of general anesthesia in elective cesarean section. Anesthesiology 29:190, 1968.
64. Shnider SM: Anesthesia for elective cesarean section. In *Obstetrical Anesthesia: Current Concepts and Practice*, SM Shnider, ed. Williams & Wilkins, Baltimore, 1970, p 94.
65. Crawford JS: Awareness during operative obstetrics under general anesthesia. Br J Anaesth 43:179, 1971.
66. Wilson J, Turner DJ: Awareness during caesarean section under general anaesthesia. Br Med J 1:280, 1969.
67. Moir DD: Anaesthesia for caesarean section: An evaluation of a method using low concentrations of halothane and 50 per cent of oxygen. Br J Anaesth 42:136, 1970.
68. Palahniuk RJ: Personal Communication.
69. Galbert MW, Gardner AE: Use of halothane in a balanced technique for cesarean section. Anesth Analg 51:701, 1972.
70. Wilson J: Methoxyflurane in caesarean section. Br J Anaesth 45:233, 1973.
71. Latto IP, Waldron BA: Anaesthesia for caesarean section. Br J Anaesth 49:371, 1977.
72. Coleman AJ, Downing JW: Enflurane anesthesia for cesarean section. Anesthesiology 43:354, 1975.
73. Crawford JS, Burton OM, Davies P: Anaesthesia for section: Further refinements of a technique. Br J Anaesth 45:726, 1973.
74. Creasser CW, Stoelting RK, Krishna G, et al.: Methoxyflurane metabolism and renal function after methoxyflurane analgesia during labor and delivery. Anesthesiology 41:62, 1974.
75. Young SR, Stoelting RK, Bond VK, et al.: Methoxyflurane biotransformation and renal function following methoxyflurane administration for vaginal delivery or cesarean section. Anesth Analg 55:415, 1976.
76. Clark RB, Beard AG, Thompson DS, et al.: Maternal and neonatal plasma inorganic fluoride levels after methoxyflurane analgesia for labor and delivery. Anesthesiology 45:88, 1976.
77. Palahniuk RJ, Cumming M: Plasma fluoride levels following obstetrical use of methoxyflurane. Can Anaesth Soc J 22:291, 1975.
78. Clark RB, Beard AG, Thompson DS: Renal function in newborns and mothers exposed to methoxyflurane analgesia for labor and delivery. In *Abstracts of Scientific Papers*, Annual Meeting, American Society of Anesthesiologists, San Francisco, 1976, p 247.
79. Marx GF, Mateo CV: Effects of different oxygen concentrations during general anaesthesia for elective caesarean section. Can Anaesth Soc J 18:587, 1971.
80. Shnider SM, Wright RG, Levinson G, et al.: Plasma norepinephrine and uterine blood flow changes during endotracheal intubation and general anesthesia in the pregnant ewe. In *Abstracts of Scientific Papers*, Annual Meeting, American Society of Anesthesiologists, Chicago, 1978, p 115.
81. Naftalin NJ, Phear WPC, Goldberg AH: Halothane and isometric contractions of isolated pregnant rat myometrium. Anesthesiology 42:458, 1975.
82. Naftalin NJ, McKay DM, Phear WPC, et al.: The effects of halothane on pregnant and nonpregnant human myometrium. Anesthesiology 46:15, 1977.
83. Munson ES, Maier WR, Caton D: Effects of halothane, cyclopropane and nitrous oxide on isolated human uterine muscle. J Obstet Gynaecol Br Commonw 76:27, 1969.
84. Munson ES, Embro WJ: Enflurane, isoflurane, and halothane and isolated human uterine muscle. Anesthesiology 46:11, 1977.
85. Marx GF, Kim YI, Lin CC, et al.: Postpartum uterine pressures under halothane or enflurane anesthesia. Obstet Gynecol 51:695, 1978.
86. Apgar V, Holaday DA, James LS, et al.: Comparison of regional and general anesthesia in obstetrics. JAMA 165:2155, 1957.
87. Benson RC, Shubeck F, Clarke WM, et al.: Fetal compromise during elective cesarean section. Am J Obstet Gynecol 91:645, 1965.
88. Kalappa R, Ueland K, Hansen JM: Maternal acid-base status during cesarean section under thiopental, N$_2$O and succinylcholine anaesthesia. Am J Obstet Gynecol 109:411, 1971.
89. Hodges RJ, Tunstall ME: The choice of anaesthesia and its influence on perinatal mortality in caesarean section. Br J Anaesth 33:572, 1961.
90. Marx GF, Cosmi EV, Wollman SB: Biochemical status and clinical condition of mother and infant at cesarean section. Anesth Analg 48:986, 1969.
91. Datta S, Brown WU Jr: Acid-base status in diabetic mothers and their infants following general or spinal anesthesia for cesarean section. Anesthesiology 47:272, 1977.
92. Fox GS, Houle GL: Acid-base studies in elective caesarean sections during epidural and general anaesthesia. Can Anaesth Soc J 18:60, 1971.
93. James FM, Crawford JS, Hopkinson R, et al.: A comparison of general anesthesia and lumbar epidural analgesia for elective cesarean section. Anesth Analg 56:228, 1977.
94. Crawford JS, Davies P: A return to trichloroethylene for obstetric anesthesia. Br J Anaesth 47:482, 1975.

95. Datta S, Alper MH, Brown WU Jr, et al.: Anesthesia for cesarean section: Importance of induction-delivery and incision-delivery interval on neonatal outcome. In *Abstracts of Scientific Papers*, Annual Meeting, American Society of Anesthesiologists, Chicago, 1978, p 103.
96. Scanlon JW, Shea E, Alper MH: Neurobehavioral responses of newborn infants following general or spinal anesthesia for cesarean section. In *Abstracts of Scientific Papers*, Annual Meeting, American Society of Anesthesiologists, Chicago, 1975, p 91.
97. Palahniuk RJ, Scatliff J, Biehl D, et al.: Evaluation of methoxyflurane, nitrous oxide, and lumbar epidural anesthesia for elective cesarean section. In *Abstracts of Scientific Papers*, Annual Meeting, American Society of Anesthesiologists, San Francisco, 1976, p 249.
98. Glass PM, Dupont FS: Personal communication in DiGiovanni AJ, et al.[31]

SECTION FOUR

ANESTHETIC COMPLICATIONS

CHAPTER 18

Hypotension and Regional Anesthesia in Obstetrics

Richard G. Wright, M.D.
Sol M. Shnider, M.D.

Arterial hypotension is the most common complication of spinal or epidural anesthesia in the parturient. Mild to moderate reductions in maternal blood pressure which do not adversely affect the mother may have profound effects on uterine blood flow and fetal well-being.

ETIOLOGY

Despite an increase in blood volume of 40 per cent above pre-pregnant levels, the parturient at term is particularly susceptible to hypotension during major conduction anesthesia.[1,2] Partial or complete inferior vena cava and aortic occlusion from compression by the gravid uterus is present in the majority of parturients lying in the supine position. (Figures 18.1 and 18.2).[3-7] Vena caval obstruction not only impedes venous return to the heart, thereby causing hypotension (Figure 18.3), but also increases uterine venous pressure, further decreasing uterine blood flow. In most parturients, an increase in resting sympathetic tone compensates for the effects of caval compression, and blood pressure is maintained (Figure 18.4). However, when sympathetic tone is abolished, as with spinal or epidural anesthesia, marked falls in blood pressure may result. A diminished intravascular volume—as is frequently found with preeclampsia, antepartum bleeding or dehydration—may further promote maternal hypotension.

SIGNIFICANCE

Many healthy individuals, including most parturients, tolerate systolic blood pressures of 80 to 90 mm Hg without ill effects to their brain, heart and kidneys. The fetus, however, is highly sensitive to decreases in maternal arterial blood pressure. In contrast to other vital organs, there is no autoregulation of blood flow to the uterus. With spinal or epidural hypotension, uterine blood flow falls linearly with blood pressure.[8-10]

The fetal consequences of the reduced uterine blood flow are dependent on the degree and duration of the fall and the pre-existing status of the utero-placental circulation. When uterine blood flow is inadequate, fetal asphyxia will develop.[11-15] The precise degree and duration of hypotension necessary to cause fetal distress seems to be variable. Ebner et al.[16] reported that with conduction anesthesia a maternal systolic blood pressure of less than 70 mm Hg consistently produced sustained fetal bradycardia. When maternal systolic

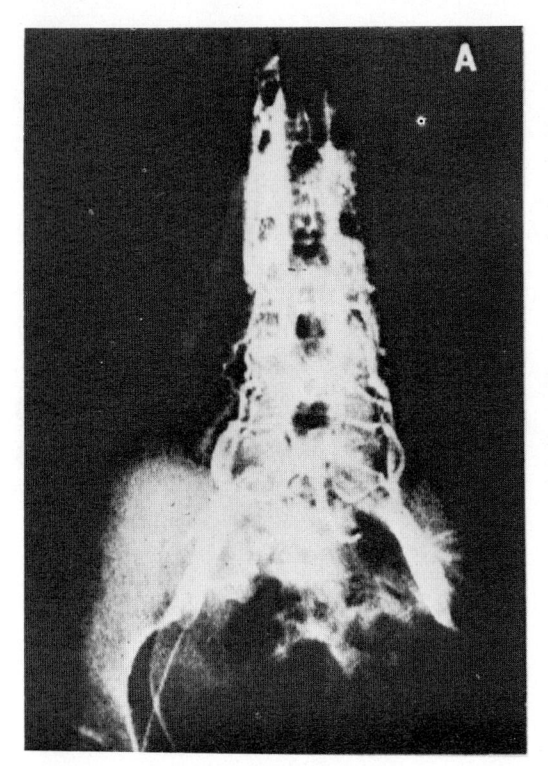

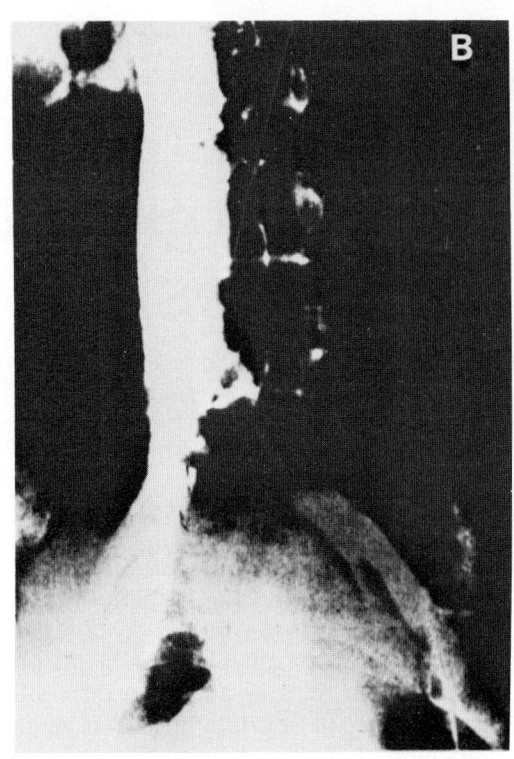

Figure 18.1. *A*, venogram in the supine position just before cesarean section. Dye has been injected into both femoral veins but does not reach the inferior vena cava, traversing instead the paravertebral veins. *B*, same patient just after cesarean section. The dye now easily reaches the inferior vena cava. (Reprinted by permission from Kerr MG, Scott DB, Samuel E: Studies of the inferior vena cava in late pregnancy. Br Med J 1:532, 1964.)

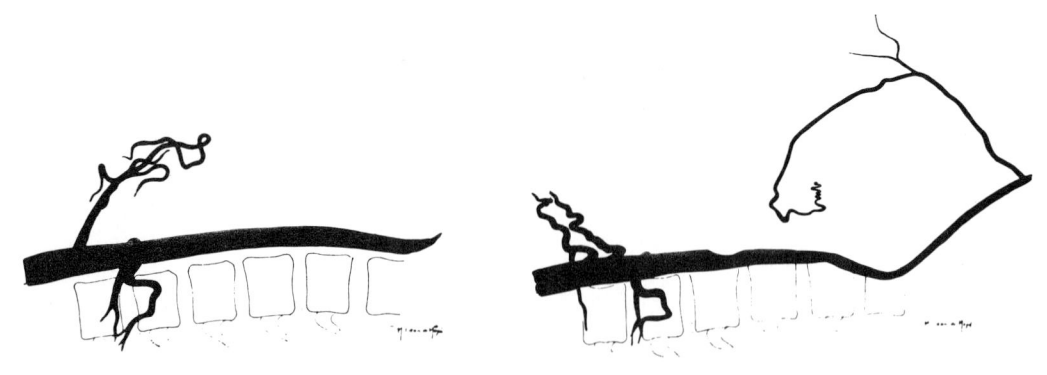

Figure 18.2. Schematic of lateral angiograms obtained from two women lying in the supine position. In the non-pregnant woman (*left*) there is a clear gap between the vertebral column and the aorta. Note the uniform width of the aorta. In the pregnant patient near term (*right*) the aorta is clearly displaced in the dorsal direction, encroaching on the shadow of the spine. The aorta is narrowed at the level of the lumbar lordosis. (Reprinted by permission from Bieniarz J. Crottogini JJ, Curuchet E, et al. : Aortocaval compression by the uterus in late human pregnancy. Am J Obstet Gynecol 100:203, 217, 1978.)

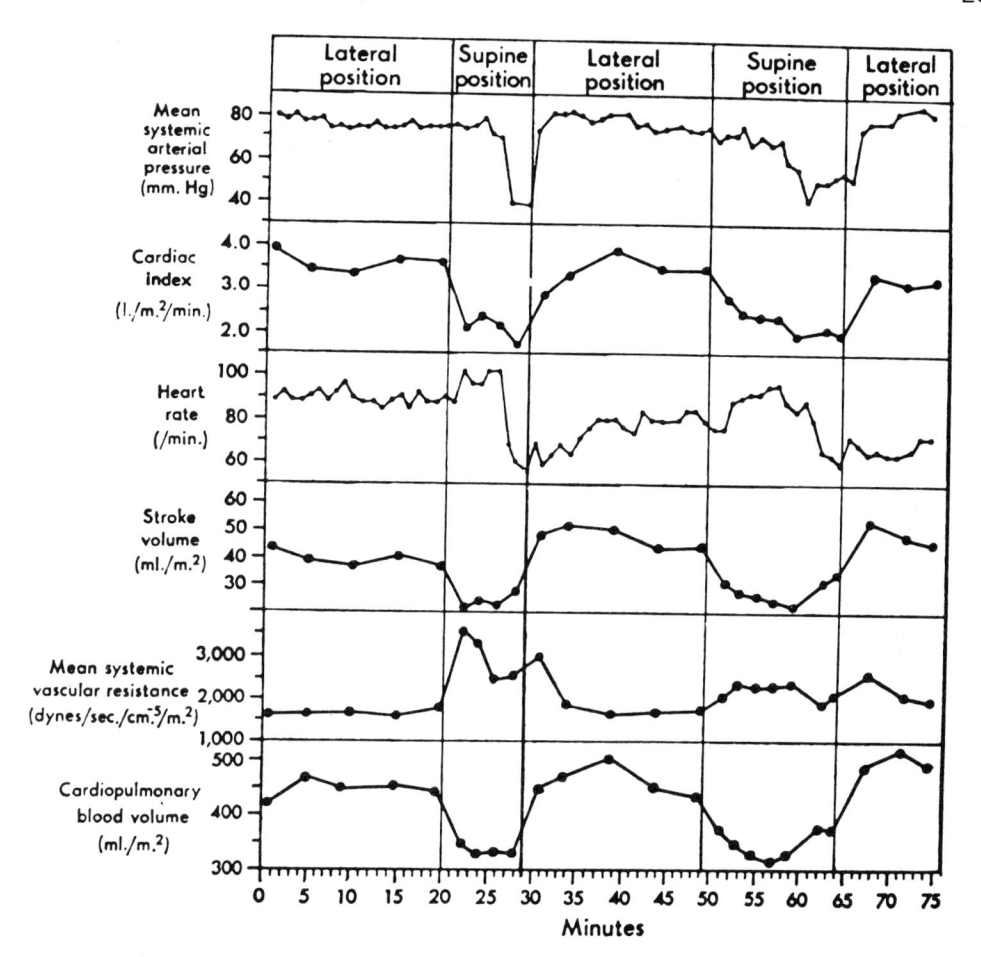

Figure 18.3. Serial hemodynamic studies in a patient who exhibited supine hypotension. After the patient was lying supine for 6 minutes, a profound fall in arterial pressure and pulse rate was seen. (Reprinted by permission from Kerr MG: Cardiovascular dynamics in pregnancy and labour. Br Med Bull 24:19, 1968.)

blood pressure was between 70 and 80 mm Hg for 4 minutes or longer, some fetuses developed sustained bradycardia. Hon et al.[17] and Bonica and Hon[18] found that with maternal systolic blood pressure less than 100 mm Hg for about 5 minutes abnormal fetal heart rate patterns developed. Zilianti[19] reported that a systolic pressure of less than 100 mm Hg for 10 to 15 minutes usually leads to fetal acidosis and bradycardia. In all these studies fetal heart rate returned to normal with correction of hypotension. Moya and Smith[20] reported an increased incidence of low Apgar scores when maternal systolic blood pressure fell to between 90 and 100 mm Hg for longer than 15 minutes (Figure 18.5). Women who had even greater falls in blood pressure but were promptly treated delivered vigorous neonates.

In summary, it seems that systolic blood pressures of less than 100 mm Hg in a previously normotensive parturient should be treated. In the hypertensive patient a fall of 20 to 30 per cent of pre-block pressure should probably be treated.

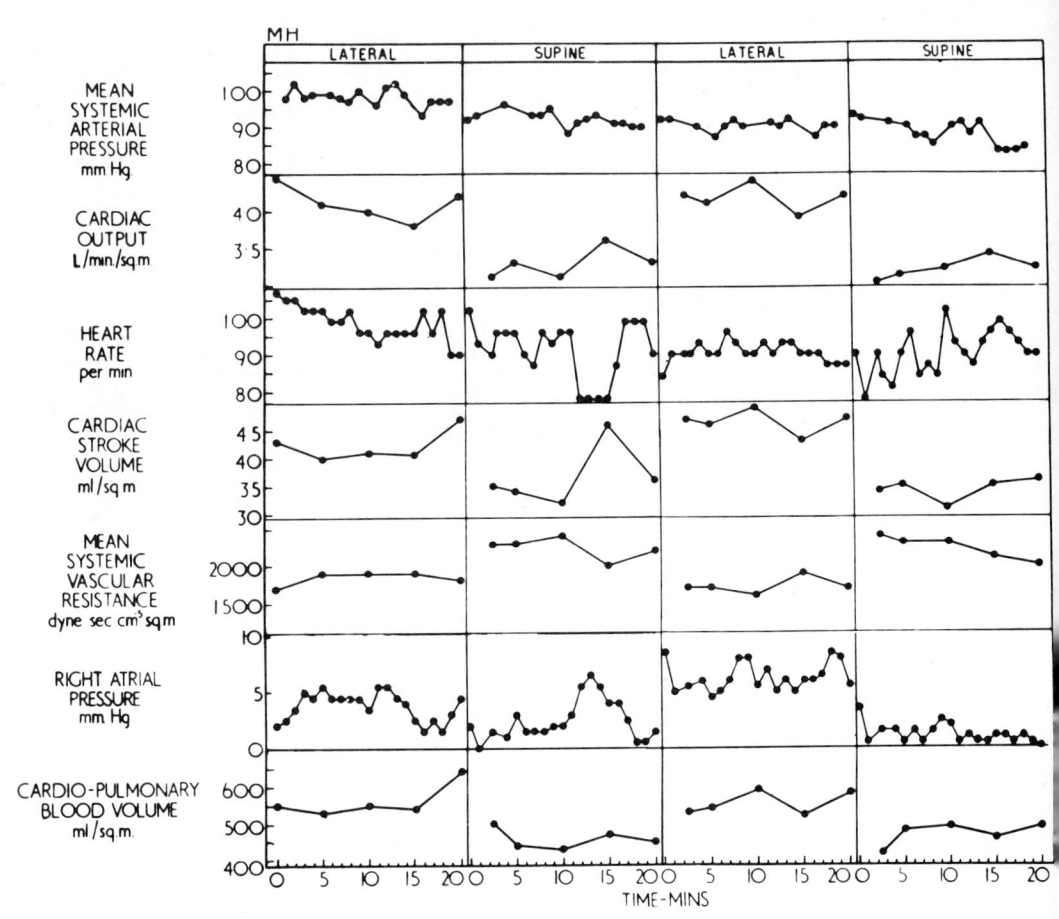

Figure 18.4. Hemodynamic parameters in a patient during late pregnancy who developed a reduced cardiac output in the supine position. The patient was asymptomatic. Note that the changes could be reproduced on turning the patient a second time. (Reprinted by permission from Scott DB: Inferior vena caval occlusion in late pregnancy. In *Parturition and Perinatology*, G F Marx, ed. F. A. Davis, Philadelphia, 1973, p 42.)

PREVENTION

Several preventive measures can be taken to minimize the incidence and severity of hypotension following conduction anesthesia in obstetrics. For routine spinal or epidural blocks the authors recommend the following:

1. Intravenous infusion of 1,000 ml of balanced electrolyte solution should be administered within 30 minutes of high spinal or epidural anesthesia (dermatome level of T4 for cesarean section) or 500 ml before a low epidural or saddle block (dermatome level of T10 for labor and delivery).

2. A predominantly centrally acting vasopressor, such as 25 to 50 mg of ephedrine, should be administered intramuscularly within 30 minutes of institution of high block.

3. Continuous left uterine displacement should be applied to minimize aortocaval compression. During labor fetal oxygenation can fall rapidly even with no concomitant fall in maternal oxygen after the mother is turned from the lateral to the supine position (Figure 18.6).[21] During the

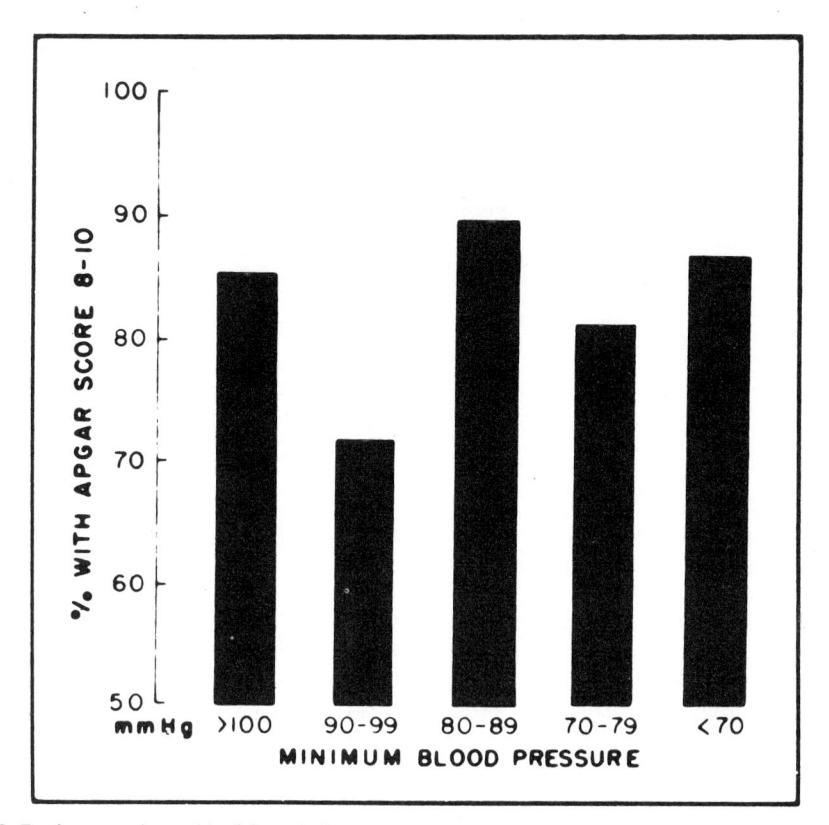

Figure 18.5. In a series of babies delivered by cesarean section under spinal anesthesia, maternal systolic blood pressures below 90 mm Hg were treated immediately. Mothers with blood pressures between 90 and 99 mm Hg were not considered to be hypotensive and were not treated. Note that even this mild degree of hypotension, when uncorrected, resulted in neonatal depression. (Reprinted by permission from Lichtiger M, Moya F: *Introduction to the Practice of Anesthesia.* Harper & Row, Hagerstown, Md., 1974, p 313.)

second stage of labor a time-related decrease in fetal pH has been reported when the mother was delivered in the supine lithotomy position. This fetal acidosis was not seen if the mother was tilted to the left.[22] With cesarean section, better fetal oxygenation, less fetal acidosis and higher Apgar scores have been reported when left uterine displacement was established as soon as the mother was placed on the operating room table.[23] During labor the patient should remain in the lateral or semilateral position. The semilateral position is best obtained by placing a wedge under the right hip. For cesarean section or vaginal delivery, uterine displacement may be accomplished either by tilting the delivery room table 15 to 30 degrees, placing a wedge under the right hip, manually displacing the uterus or using a mechanical uterine displacing device.[24,25]

4. Frequent monitoring of arterial blood pressure after institution of the block is mandatory. This will allow early recognition and prompt therapy of hypotension. Measurements should be made at 1- to 2-minute intervals for the first 20 minutes after the local anesthetic is injected and

then every 5 to 10 minutes until anesthesia is terminated.

In groups of parturients undergoing elective cesarean sections with epidural anesthesia, the authors have found that the incidence of hypotension can decrease from 82 per cent to 18 per cent by the prophylactic administration of ephedrine, lactated Ringer's solution and left uterine displacement (Table 17.6).

SAFETY OF PROPHYLAXIS

The safety of the above measures as prophylaxis for hypotension is well established. Acute hydration of the normal parturient with 1,000 ml of balanced salt solution has no significant effect on central venous pressure even in the absence of sympathetic blockade (Figure 18.7). In patients with cardiac disease, acute hydration should only be performed with monitoring of central venous or pulmonary arterial pressures.

In a study on the prophylactic administration of vasopressors in pregnant ewes, Ralston and co-workers[26] found that

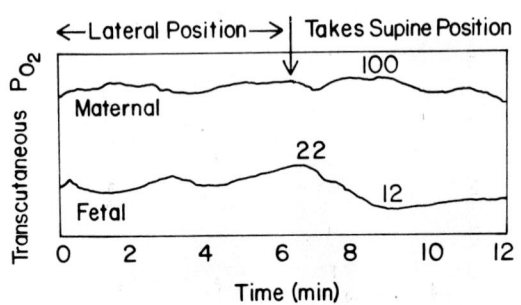

Figure 18.6. Continuous monitoring of maternal and fetal transcutaneous PO_2 during labor. Fetal PO_2 was monitored using a fetal scalp transcutaneous oxygen electrode. When mother turned from the lateral to the supine position, fetal PO_2 promptly fell. (Modified from Huch A, Huch R: Transcutaneous noninvasive monitoring of PO_2. Hosp Pract 11:43, 1976.)

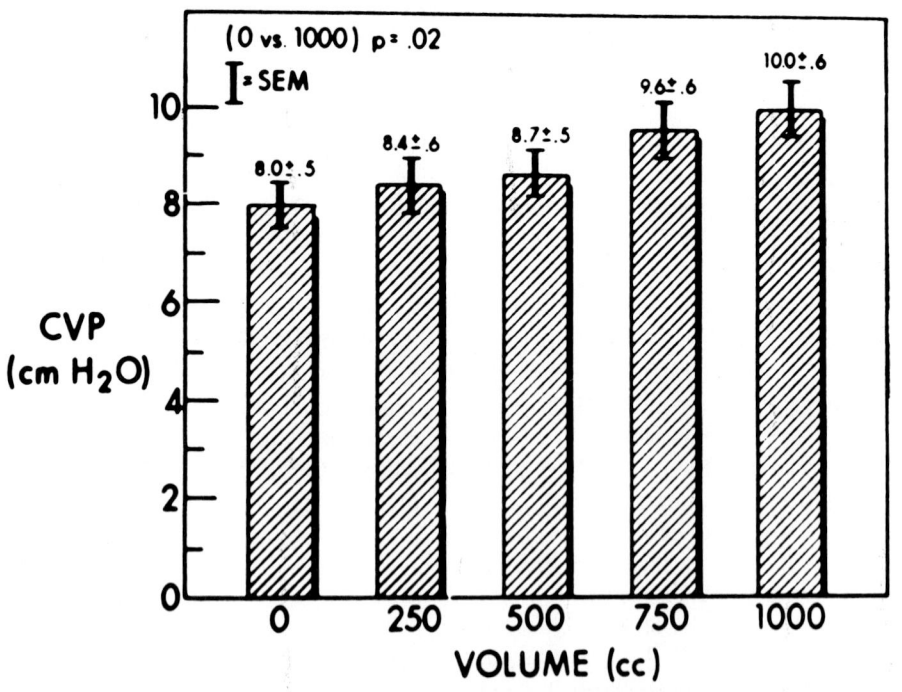

Figure 18.7. Response of central venous pressure (CVP) to rapid (14 to 20 minutes) infusion of 1,000 ml of 5 per cent dextrose in lactated Ringer's solution. (Reprinted by permission from Wollman SB, Marx GF: Acute hydration for prevention of hypotension of spinal anesthesia in parturients. Anesthesiology 29:374, 1968.)

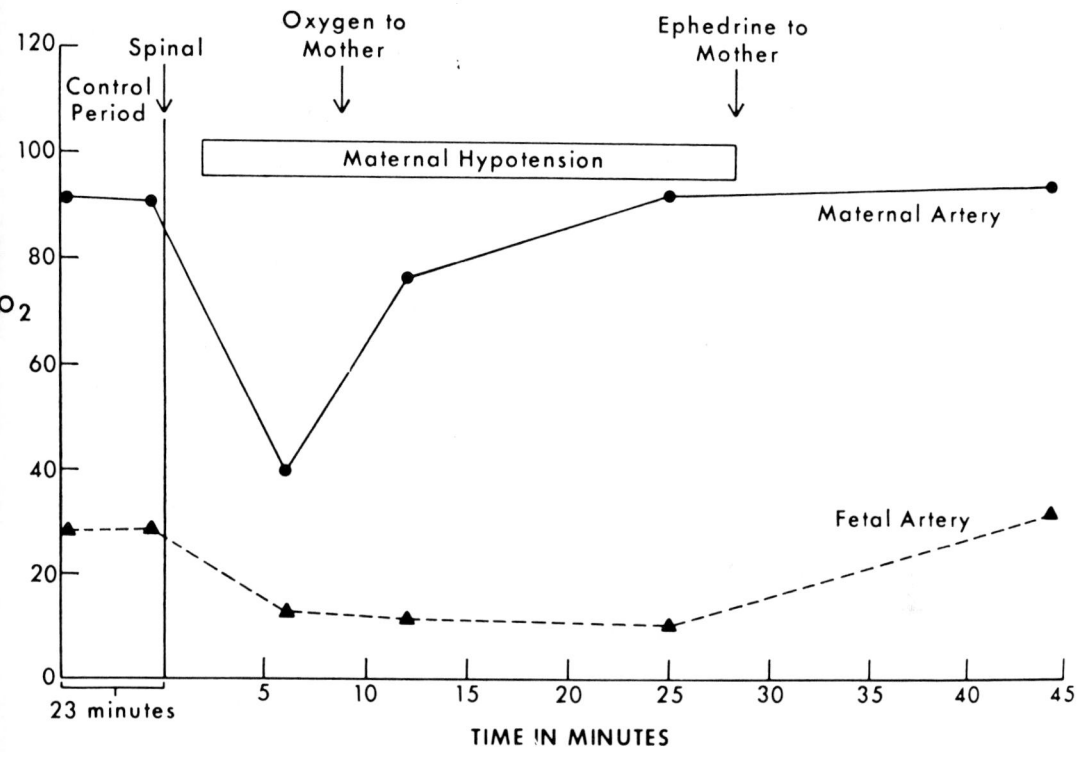

Figure 18.8. Changes in fetal arterial oxygen tension after maternal spinal hypotension, maternal hypoxia, oxygen administration then ephedrine administration to the mother. (Reprinted by permission from Shnider SM, de Lorimier AA, Holl JW, et al.: Vasopressors in obstetrics. I. Correction of fetal acidosis with ephedrine during spinal hypotension. Am J Obstet Gynecol 102:911, 1968.)

ephedrine or mephentermine in doses sufficient to raise the mean arterial blood pressure 40 to 50 per cent above control values had no significant effects on uterine blood flow (Figure 3.8). Although ephedrine may cross the placenta and has been reported to increase fetal heart rate and beat-to-beat variability, no adverse fetal or neonatal effects have been noted.[27]

THERAPY

Therapy for epidural or spinal hypotension includes more left uterine displacement, rapid fluid infusion, Trendelenburg position to increase venous return, intravenous ephedrine and oxygen administration (Table 18.1). Administration of oxygen to the mother may not necessarily raise the fetal PaO_2 until the hypotension is corrected. After spinal hypotension in pregnant ewes, fetal PaO_2 returned to normal only after maternal arterial blood pressure was restored (Figure 18.8).[28]

Vasopressor therapy in obstetrics has been controversial because it may produce uterine vasoconstriction and hypertonus and further deterioration of the fetus.

Table 18.1
Treatment of Hypotension

Increase left uterine displacement
Increase intravenous fluid infusion
Place patient in 10° to 20° Trendelenburg position.
  If no response in 1 minute:
Administer ephedrine 5 to 10 mg I.V.
Administer oxygen by face mask.

However, studies in pregnant sheep made hypotensive with spinal anesthesia show that ephedrine and mephentermine, both primarily centrally acting vasopressors, returned uterine blood flow toward control while restoring maternal arterial blood pressure.[28, 29] Fetal deterioration is, in fact, arrested and often reversed.[28] Vasopressors with primarily peripheral action—such as methoxamine or phenylephrine—may be harmfull to the fetus because they produce further uterine vasoconstriction.[30, 31]

In a prospective study of 60 elective repeat cesarean sections performed under spinal block, Marx and co-workers[32] found better fetal biochemical and neonatal clinical conditions when hypotension was prevented rather than treated. They also found that if hypotension occurred the more rapid the reversal the better the fetal outcome. On the other hand, Ralston and Shnider[33] showed no difference in Apgar scores between neonates of mothers who became hypotensive and those who did not (Table 17.20). In the latter series, maternal blood pressure was monitored at 1-minute intervals, and hypotension was detected early and treated quickly. Thus, with appropriate monitoring and prompt therapy, the deleterious effects of hypotension on the fetus can be prevented.

References

1. Bromage PR: Physiology and pharmacology of epidural analgesia: A review. Anesthesiology 28:592, 1967.
2. Marx GF: Shock in the obstetric patient. Anesthesiology 25:423, 1965.
3. Eckstein KL, Marx GF: Aortocaval compression and uterine displacement. Anesthesiology 40:92, 1974.
4. Goodlin RC: Aortocaval compression during cesarean section: A cause of newborn depression. Obstet Gynecol 37:702, 1971.
5. Holmes F: The supine hypotensive syndrome: Its importance to the anaesthetist. Anaesthesia 15:298, 1960.
6. Bierniarz J, Curuchet E, Crottogini JJ, et al.: Aortocaval compression by the uterus in late human pregnancy: An arteriographic study. Am J Obstet Gynecol 100:203, 1968.
7. Kerr MG, Samuel E: Studies on the inferior vena cava in late pregnancy. Br Med J 1:532, 1964.
8. Greiss FC Jr, Crandell DL: Therapy for hypotension induced by spinal anesthesia during pregnancy. JAMA 191:793, 1965.
9. Greiss FC Jr: Pressure-flow relationship in the gravid uterine vascular bed. Am J Obstet Gynecol 96:41, 1966.
10. Martin CB Jr, Gingerick B: Uteroplacental physiology. J Obstet Gynecol Nurs (Suppl) 5:16, 1976.
11. Adams FH, Assali N, Cushman M, et al.: Interrelationships of maternal and fetal circulations. Pediatrics 27:627, 1961.
12. Adamsons K, Myers RE: Circulation in the intervillous space: Obstetrical considerations in fetal deprivation. In The Placenta, P. Grunewald, ed. University Park Press, Baltimore, 1975, p 158.
13. Lucas WE, Kirschbaum T, Assali NS: Spinal shock and fetal oxygenation. Am J Obstet Gynecol 93:583, 1965.
14. Moya F, Thorndike V: Maternal hypotension and the newborn. In Proceedings of the Third World Congress of Anesthesiology, vol 2. 1964, p 11.
15. Myers RE: Two patterns of perinatal brain damage and their condition of occurrence. Am J Obstet Gynecol 112:246, 1972.
16. Ebner H, Barcohana J, Bartoshok AK: Influence of postspinal hypotension on the fetal electrocardiogram. Am J Obstet Gynecol 80:569, 1960.
17. Hon EH, Reid BL, Hehre FW: The electronic evaluation of the fetal heart rate. II. Changes with maternal hypotension. Am J Obstet Gynecol 79:209, 1960.
18. Bonica JJ, Hon EH: Fetal distress. In Principles and Practice of Obstetric Analgesia and Anesthesia, JJ Bonica, ed. F. A. Davis, Philadelphia, 1964, p 1252.
19. Zilianti SM: Fetal heart rate and pH of fetal capillary blood during epidural analgesia in labor. Obstet Gynecol 36:881, 1970.
20. Moya F, Smith B: Spinal anesthesia for cesarean section: Clinical and biochemical studies of effects on maternal physiology. JAMA 179:609, 1962.
21. Huch A, Huch R: Transcutaneous noninvasive monitoring of pO_2. Hosp Pract 11:43, 1976.
22. Humphrey MD, Chang A, Wood EC, et al.: A decrease in fetal pH during the second stage of labour, when conducted in the dorsal position. J Obstet Gynecol Br Commonw 81:600, 1974.
23. Crawford JS, Burton M, Davies P: Time and lateral tilt at caesarean section. Br J Anaesthesiol 44:477, 1972.
24. Kennedy RL: An instrument to relieve inferior vena cava occlusion. Am J Obstet Gynecol 107:331, 1970.
25. Colon-Morales MA: A self-supporting device for continuous left uterine displacement during cesarean section. Anesth Analg 49:223, 1970. (The device is available from Resuscitation Laboratories, P.O. Box 3051, Bridgeport, CT 06605.)
26. Ralston DH, Shnider SM, deLorimier AA: Effects of equipotent ephedrine, metaraminol, mephentermine, and methoxamine on uterine blood flow in the pregnant ewe. Anesthesiology 40:354, 1974

27. Wright RG, Rolbin SH, Shnider SM, et al.: Maternal administration of ephedrine increases fetal heart rate and variability. In *Abstracts of Scientific Papers*, Annual Meeting, American Society of Anesthesiologists, New Orleans, 1977, p 131.
28. Shnider SM, deLorimier AA, Holl JW, et al.: Vasopressors in obstetrics. I. Correction of fetal acidosis with ephedrine during spinal hypotension. Am J Obstet Gynecol 102:911, 1968.
29. James FM III, Greiss FC Jr, Kemp RA: An evaluation of vasopressor therapy for maternal hypotension during spinal anesthesia. Anesthesiology 33:25, 1970.
30. Shnider SM, deLorimier AA, Asling JH, et al.: Vasopressors in obstetrics. II. Fetal hazards of methoxamine administration during obstetric spinal anesthesia. Am J Obstet Gynecol 106:680, 1970.
31. Greiss FC, Van Wilkes D: Effects of sympathomimetic drugs and angiotensin on the uterine vascular bed. Obstet Gynecol 23:925, 1964.
32. Marx GF, Cosmi RV, Wollman SB: Biochemical status and clinical condition of mother and infant at cesarean section. Anesth Analg (Cleve) 48:986, 1969.
33. Ralston DH, Shnider SM: The fetal and neonatal effects of regional anesthesia in obstetrics. Anesthesiology 48:34, 1978.

CHAPTER 19

Pulmonary Aspiration of Gastric Contents in the Obstetric Patient

Brett B. Gutsche, M.D.

Anesthesia ranks as the fourth leading cause of maternal mortality in the United States and the United Kingdom following hemorrhage, sepsis and toxemia. Pulmonary aspiration of gastric contents is the leading cause of anesthetic maternal mortality; for the most part, it is preventable with proper anesthetic management.[1] Although the exact number of deaths caused by this catastrophe is not available, Mendelson[2] found 66 mothers of 43,000 pregnancies suffered this complication, with 64 showing the symptoms of acid aspiration. Merrill and Hingson[3] estimated there were 100 maternal deaths from pulmonary aspiration yearly, and Phillips et al.[4] proposed that there was one maternal death per year from aspiration in each community of 1 million persons in the United States. Between 1967 and 1969, 50 maternal deaths were reported as the result of anesthesia in England and Wales, 26 of which were secondary to pulmonary aspiration.[5] Crawford,[6] commenting on the above, noted that, while maternal deaths from other causes decreased from the 1964–1966 report, the number of anesthetic deaths remained constant at 50, with nearly 50 per cent being the result of pulmonary aspiration.

The gravid patient during labor and delivery is particularly predisposed to this catastrophe for many reasons. Obviously she frequently goes into labor within a short time of having ingested food. Although many claim pregnancy itself does not delay stomach emptying, Davison and co-workers[7] showed both the half-life of dye instilled into the stomach and gastric emptying time were significantly increased in pregnant women beyond 34 weeks' gestation. Pregnant women with "heartburn" indicative of gastro-esophageal junction dysfunction, very common in late pregnancy, had the longest delay in stomach emptying. In the same study[7] labor clearly retarded stomach emptying, which contradicts the findings of many that labor itself does not affect gastric performance.[8,9] Certainly fear, apprehension and pain can delay gastric emptying. The use of drugs, particularly the narcotics and anticholinergics, may have the same effect. Heavy sedation may obtund protective airway reflexes. Treatment for various conditions of pregnancy may depress upper airway reflexes. Treatment of toxemia resulting in oversedation with anticonvulsants or overdosage with magnesium will increase the risk. Intravenous alcohol, used for the depression of premature labor, not only increases the risk of pulmonary aspiration from central nervous system depression, but it also increases the gastric secretion of acid. The lithotomy position can increase intragastric pressure and make regurgitation more likely, particularly with the application of uterine suprafundal pressure (Figure 19.1). Labor itself is associated with nausea and vomiting. Hypotension, which can be the result of aortocaval compression, sympathetic block from major conduction anesthesia and hemorrhage, may cause nausea and vomiting as well as loss of consciousness that predisposes to pulmonary aspiration. Dehydration and starvation ketosis may retard stomach emptying as well as increase gastric acid secretions.

Increased gastric acid secretion has been demonstrated to occur during pregnancy.[10,11] A possible mechanism is the markedly elevated plasma levels of the hormone gastrin.[12] The major physiologic action of this hormone is the stimulation of acid secretion. The elevated plasma levels of gastrin, together with the very high placental tissue concentration, suggest placental production and/or storage of the hormone.

Roberts and Shirley[13,14] have shown the time from the last ingestion of food or from the onset of labor is of little value in determining the risk of pulmonary aspiration. These same investigators also showed the patient who was fasted before elective cesarean section was still at high risk for this complication (Table 19.1).

Gastric material can reach the lungs following either active vomiting or passive regurgitation. If the protective airway re-

Table 19.1
Percentage of Patients "at Risk" for Aspiration Pneumonitis (Volume of Gastric Aspirate Greater Than 25 ml; pH Less Than 2.5)*

	Cesarean Section		Vaginal Delivery
	Not in Labor	In Labor	
	%	%	%
No antacid (n = 79)	29	18	28
Antacid within 4 hours of delivery (n = 100)	0	3	2.5
Antacid more than 4 hours before delivery (n = 21)		36	10

* Adapted from Roberts RB, Shirley MA: The obstetrician's role in reducing the risk of aspiration pneumonitis with particular reference to the use of oral antacids. Am J Obstet Gynecol 124:611, 1976.

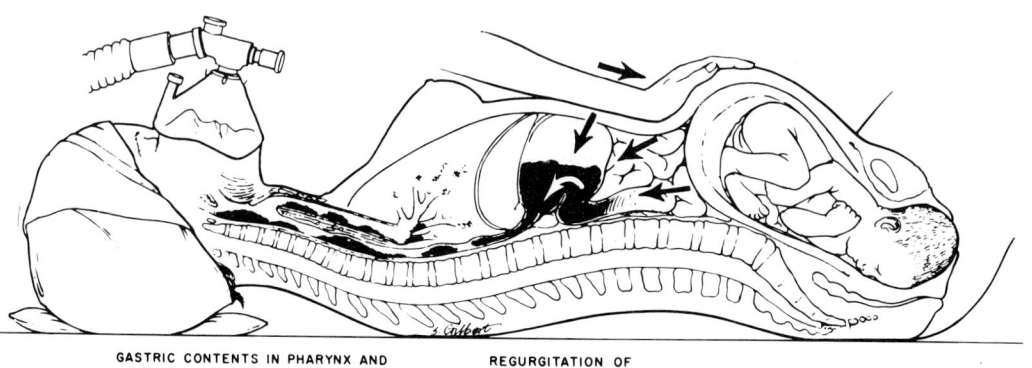

GASTRIC CONTENTS IN PHARYNX AND ASPIRATED INTO TRACHEA AND LUNGS

REGURGITATION OF GASTRIC CONTENTS

Figure 19.1. Regurgitation of gastric contents caused by marked increase in intra-abdominal and intragastric pressure from an attempt to place pressure on the uterus during delivery. (Reprinted by permission from Bonica JJ: *Principles and Practice of Obstetric Analgesia and Anesthesia,* vol 1. F. A. Davis, Philadelphia, 1967, p 676.)

flexes are lost during the process of vomiting or regurgitation due to (1) development of hypotension with cerebral hypoxia, (2) general anesthesia or excessive pre-medication or (3) the onset of muscle paralysis, then aspiration may occur.

PATHOPHYSIOLOGY AND TREATMENT OF PULMONARY ASPIRATION OF GASTRIC CONTENTS

The degree of morbidity and mortality will reflect both the amount of material aspirated as well as the nature of aspirated matter. In general, three types of gastric material can be aspirated, each of which will cause a different clinical picture: (1) fecal or other bacterially contaminated material, usually as a result of intestinal obstruction, perforation or bowel infarct; (2) solid or particulate matter; or (3) material of a pH of less than 2.5, causing a chemical pneumonitis.[2] In the parturient the most common form of pulmonary aspiration is that of acid aspiration; fecal aspiration is rare.

Therapeutic Considerations

Aspiration of gastric material should be suspected if the patient develops, particularly in the presence of central nervous system obtundation, the following signs and symptoms: (1) sudden coughing or laryngospasm; (2) the presence of foreign material in the mouth or posterior pharynx; (3) dyspnea, hyperpnea or apnea; (4) bronchospasm or wheezing; (5) chest retraction or obvious airway obstruction; (6) cyanosis, particularly if not relieved by oxygen; and (7) the development of a pink frothy pulmonary exudate. If aspiration is witnessed or suspected, particularly in an obtunded patient, the patient should be turned on her side and placed head down, the mouth and posterior pharynx should be suctioned and then the trachea should be intubated with a cuffed endotracheal tube. The trachea should be suctioned several times immediately after intubation. Ventilation with 100 per cent oxygen between each suctioning is recommended. Except in the aspiration of particulate matter, tracheal lavage should not be performed, because it will only spread the material and worsen the condition. A specimen of the gastric contents should be obtained and examined for the presence of particulate matter, analyzed for pH and cultured for the presence of bacteria and their antibiotic sensitivities. Arterial blood gas determinations will indicate the need for the increased inspired oxygen concentrations, ventilation and the use of positive end expired pressure (PEEP). Chest x-rays taken as soon as possible after the incident and at regular intervals as the clinical picture indicates will aid in determining the extent and progress of the pathologic process. Continuous central venous pressure (CVP) monitoring and recording of urinary output will aid in fluid management. Any person suspected of aspirating gastric material, particularly if symptoms of aspiration are present, should be placed in an intensive care environment for close monitoring and ventilatory care until resolution of the process. Rapid and early therapy is essential to minimize morbidity and mortality.

Fecal or Bacterial Material

Aspiration of fecal or bacterial contaminated material of any significant amount into the lungs is associated with close to a 100 per cent mortality. A picture of severe generalized pneumonia involving primarily the dependent portion of the lungs develops, along with symptoms of septic or endotoxic shock. Therapy includes massive doses of antibiotics, particularly those effective against gram-negative bacteria. Tracheal cultures for sensitivity may help in choosing appropriate antibiotics. Massive doses of intravenous steroids may be of value. Support of the cardiovascular system with fluids, both colloid and crystalloid, and appropriate inotropic cardiac drugs are indicated. Adequate oxygenation and ventilatory support are required. Fortunately this type of aspiration is rarely seen in the parturient.

Particulate Matter

The clinical picture produced by aspiration of particulate matter depends on the size of the particles and the amount aspirated. Aspiration of large particles or a large amount of particulate material can lead to immediate and complete obstruction of the airway, resulting in suffocation, unless the material can be removed by rapid intubation, suction and possibly bronchoscopy. Instillation of small amounts (3 to 5 ml) of physiologic saline solution before suction may help dislodge particles. Aspiration of a smaller amount of material or material with small particulate size can produce obstruction of bronchi or bronchioles which results in atelectasis of the affected lobe or segment. Clinically this may be accompanied by coughing, tachypnea, cyanosis and tachycardia. Breath sounds may be decreased over the involved areas. Chest x-ray initially shows atelectasis with homogenous densities in affected areas. If involvement is sufficiently great, there will be mediastinal shift. If the condition is untreated, pulmonary abscess may develop. Initial treatment is immediate and repeated tracheobronchial suction, oxygenation, ventilation and tracheal instillation of small amounts of saline to help dislodge material. Encouragement of coughing may help dislodge the material. Except in cases in which only minimal amounts of material are aspirated, bronchoscopy should be performed as soon as possible after the incident to diagnose and remove foreign material. Initially the fiberoptic bronchoscope may be used through the endotracheal tube to diagnose the presence of foreign material and to remove under direct vision small particulate matter. The presence of large particulate matter or the development of atelectasis requires bronchoscopy with a ventilating bronchoscope to remove this material and allow reinflation of the atelectatic area. Tracheal aspirates should be obtained at regular intervals, especially with the development of fever, for gram stain, culture and sensitivity to allow rational antibiotic therapy.

Acid Gastric Secretions

By far the most common form of pulmonary aspiration in the parturient is aspiration of acid gastric contents. The syndrome of acid aspiration was first described by Mendelson[2] in 1946. Teabeaut[15] showed in rabbits that once the pH of the aspirated material fell below 2.5 the typical clinical syndrome developed, whereas a pH above 2.5 produced no more damage than the instillation of water. Both Mendelson[2] and Bosomworth and Hamelberg[16] demonstrated that the pH of the aspirate, not gastric or enteric enzymes, was responsible for the development of the syndrome. Although in Mendelson's original study no patients died, more recent evidence suggests a mortality as high as 70 per cent.[17-21] Obviously the amount and pH of the material aspirated will determine the severity of the lesion. Roberts and Shirley[13,14] have suggested the aspiration of 25 ml (0.4 ml/kg) or more of gastric juice with a pH of 2.5 or less will produce symptoms. Lewis et al.[18] found a 100 per cent mortality in four humans who aspirated gastric contents with a pH of less than 1.75. Aspiration of large volumes of material with a pH greater than 2.5 has also been reported to result in a picture of Mendelson's syndrome.[22]

Symptoms of acid aspiration may have a sudden onset heralded by a sudden bronchospasm or may be delayed for several hours after the insult, particularly if the patient is under the influence of general anesthesia. Coughing may be the only symptom, or this may progress to an asthmatic-like attack with bronchospasm, expiratory wheezing, tachypnea, dyspnea and a decreased pulmonary compliance. Cyanosis frequently develops which may not be relieved by oxygen. There may then be the development of a pink frothy pulmonary exudate or edema with fine rales developing. Despite the clinical picture of pulmonary edema, left heart failure is rarely present, as indicated by a low or normal pulmonary wedge pressure and a decreased plasma volume averaging 500 ml or more accompanied by a hemoconcentration[18,23,24] (Figure 19.2). The CVP may be slightly elevated due to an increased pulmonary vascular resistance.[25]

Blood gases usually show a marked hypoxemia with a PaO_2 of 50 torr or less on room air. With the administration of high inspired oxygen concentrations, a marked alveolar-arterial gradient $P_{(A-a)}O_2$ is found (Figure 19.3). This is thought to represent an impaired diffusion, pulmonary shunting and a pulmonary arteriolar vasoconstriction.[18,24] Initially the $PaCO_2$ may be normal or slightly below normal, but, with the progression of the process, this may become slightly elevated. A metabolic acidosis is often seen as the condition progresses.

The chest x-ray shows soft mottled densities widely distributed over the peripheral areas, but especially pronounced in the dependent lung areas, particularly of the right side. The initial picture resembles that of a "snow storm" over the lung fields (Figure 19.4). There is usually no mediastinal shift. As the process continues an x-ray picture typical of pulmonary edema may develop.

The pathologic picture is best described as that of a severe burn of the lung. Initially there is decreased pulmonary compliance. This is followed by interstitial edema, transudation of a plasma-like substance and disruption of the alveolar-capillary membrane. There is acute bronchitis and bronchiolitis, sloughing of mucosa, intra-alveolar edema and intra-alveolar hemorrhage. Lung weight may be two or three times normal. Initially no signs of infection are present, but with progression there may be an increase in polymorphonuclear leukocytes. When infection becomes pres-

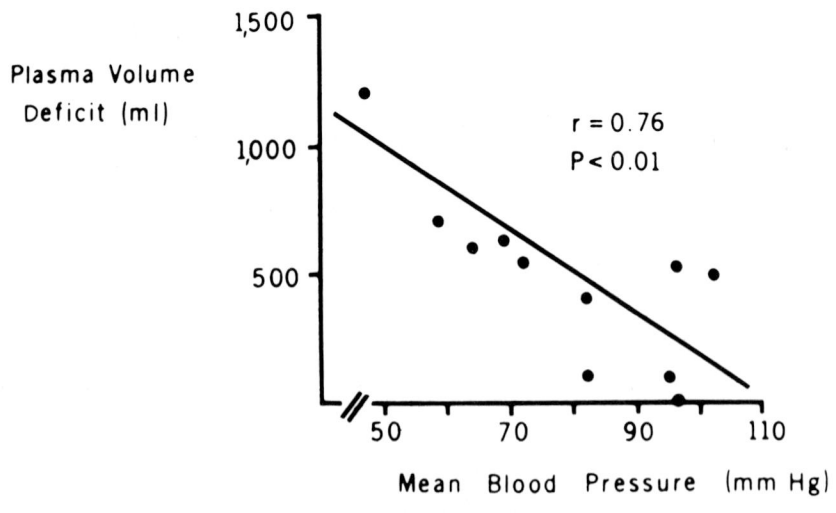

Figure 19.2. Plasma volume deficits 12 to 18 hours after aspiration in 11 patients. There is significant correlation between moderate deficits and mean systemic blood pressure. (Reprinted by permission from Lewis RT, Burgess JH, Hampson LG: Cardiorespiratory studies in critical illness: Changes in aspiration pneumonitis. Arch Surg 103:335, 1971.)

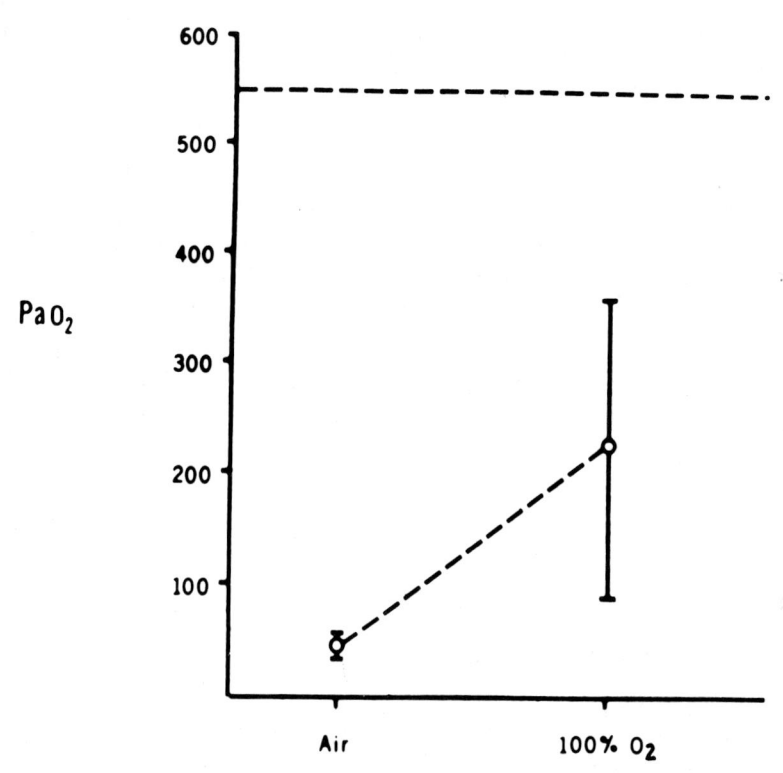

Figure 19.3. Response of mean PaO$_2$ to breathing 100 per cent oxygen for 15 minutes in 12 patients. In all cases the rise fell short of the generally accepted normal value of 500 mm Hg, indicating a right-to-left shunt-like effect. (Reprinted by permission from Lewis RT, Burgess JH, Hampson LG: Cardiorespiratory studies in critical illness: Changes in aspiration pneumonitis. Arch Surg 103:335, 1971.)

ent it may be with either gram-positive or gram-negative bacteria. The pathophysiologic picture of pulmonary acid aspiration has been well reviewed by Morgan[24] and Alexander.[26]

At present therapy is often ineffective at best. Morbidity and mortality are high; however, early initiation of therapy will do much to lessen them. The primary object of therapy is to ensure adequate oxygenation and ventilatory function until the damaged lungs can recover.

In the event that one actually witnesses pulmonary aspiration, as during the induction of anesthesia, the patient should be intubated at once with a cuffed endotracheal tube. This should be followed by immediate tracheal suction. Unless particulate matter is retrieved from the trachea, the instillation of any material into the trachea is not indicated. Hamelberg and Bosomworth[27] observed that 60 ml of material containing methylene blue dye instilled in the trachea of dogs, both *in vivo* and *in vitro*, reached the lung periphery in 12 to 18 seconds. Saline lavage with small quantities of fluid only spread the process and caused further damage. Attempts to dilute or neutralize acid instilled into the lungs of rabbits with saline or sodium bicarbonate solution created more lung damage than the acid instillation alone.[28] Tracheal instillation of steroids in animals subjected to acid aspiration did not de-

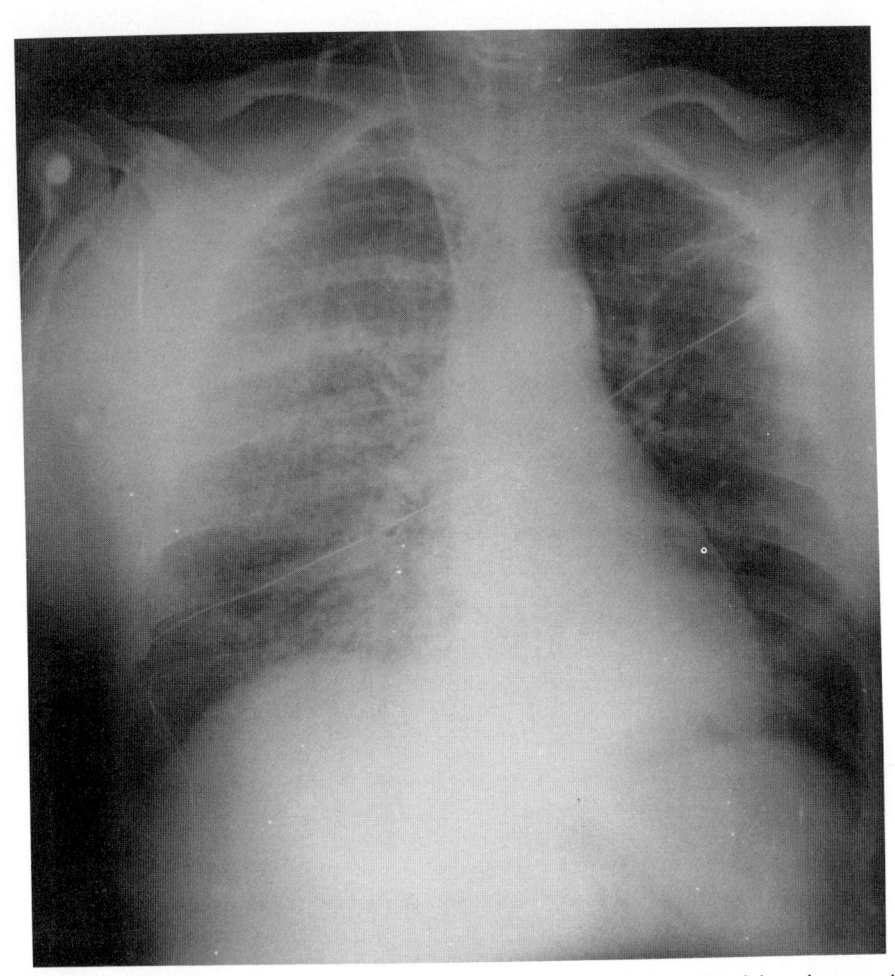

Figure 19.4. Acid aspiration (Mendelson's syndrome) with marked involvement of the right lung. Note the generalized soft, mottled densities and the absence of mediastinal shift.

crease the severity of the lung lesions, and tracheal instillation of steroids alone produced lung lesions.[29]

POSITIVE PRESSURE VENTILATION

Following suction, the patient should be ventilated with high concentrations of oxygen. The questions arise as to (1) who should be ventilated, (2) when it should be started and (3) how long it should be continued. There is abundant evidence from animal studies that positive pressure ventilation markedly decreases mortality from acid aspiration.[16,19,30,31] Cameron and co-workers[32] demonstrated in dogs that the immediate initiation of positive pressure ventilation after an insult of 2 ml/kg of 0.1 N HCl placed in the right main stem bronchus resulted in a 100 per cent survival rate. However, if ventilation was delayed 24 hours, only 40 per cent survived.

From the above data it would appear early ventilation, even perhaps in the absence of severe symptoms, is indicated. If aspiration is suspected, but not witnessed the author believes that ventilation should be begun as soon as any signs or symptoms become apparent, e.g. dyspnea, bronchoconstriction, moist rales or an x-ray which shows a picture of acid aspiration pneumonitis. A PaO_2 less than 50 torr on room air or less than 200 torr with spontaneous respiration and administration of 100 per cent oxygen would be an indication for intubation and ventilatory therapy.[25] One should not wait for the development of pulmonary edema before starting ventilation. Roberts[33] recommends immediate intubation and ventilation with blood gas monitoring of all patients who have aspirated gastric material with a pH of less than 3.0. Ventilation is continued at least 8 hours after the aspiration.

It seems the type of ventilation (i.e. either intermittent mandatory ventilation or PEEP) is not of great importance, provided that adequate oxygenation and carbon dioxide elimination are maintained. The use of PEEP may allow lower inspired oxygen concentrations, decreasing the risk of pulmonary oxygen toxicity, but it increases the chance of pneumothorax and decreases cardiac output, particularly at higher pressures. High humidity of inspired gases and frequent tracheo-bronchial toilet are necessary. Initially control of bronchospasm with bronchodilators such as aminophylline, isoproterenol or terbutaline may be required, remembering that these drugs are associated with uterine relaxation. The time of extubation should be governed by pulmonary function studies, arterial blood gas determinations and the patient's clinical picture. Chapman[25] recommends a 15-minute trial of spontaneous respiration before extubation where (1) a PaO_2 of greater than 60 torr is maintained on 30 per cent inspired oxygen, (2) there is no evidence of a respiratory acidosis, (3) the vital capacity is greater than 15 ml/kg, (4) the inspiratory force is more than 20 cm H_2O and (5) the $P_{(A-a)} O_2$ is less than 300 torr on 100 per cent oxygen.

PULMONARY EDEMA

The development of pulmonary edema is an ominous sign. Therapy includes sedation, tracheal suction, high oxygen administration and positive pressure ventilation with the possible addition of PEEP. Because the plasma volume is low and cardiac failure is rare,[18,19,23,24] rotating tourniquets and diuresis are not usually indicated. By the same token overhydration with crystalloid may add to the fluid outpouring across the damaged alveolar-capillary membrane. In the past recommendations have been made for the use of colloid and/or furosemide.[18,23] Geer and co-workers[34] studied the effect of furosemide and 25 per cent albumin, both alone and in combination, in rabbits subjected to a controlled non-fatal acid aspiration. Lung water, extravascular lung albumin and $P_{(A-a)} O_2$ were significantly decreased (improved) with the combination but were not changed or increased (made worse) with the use of either furosemide or albumin alone. The use of fluids, albumin and diuretics should be monitored with at least a CVP, but a pulmonary artery wedge pressure is more reliable, because the CVP will not be affected by the normally increased pulmonary artery pressure.[25]

STEROID THERAPY

The routine use of steroids has been and is still recommended by many,[15,21,23,27,28,35-37] since the successful use of cortisone was first demonstrated in pulmonary acid aspiration by Hausmann and Lunt in 1955.[38] Dosage recommendations have varied widely. Unfortunately earlier evidence of efficacy was based on uncontrolled clinical studies or on animal studies in which ventilation was combined with steroids.[27,36] Dudley and Marshall[39] showed that very small doses of dexamethasone produced the greatest decrease in lung water in rabbits subjected to standard tracheal instillation of pH 1.5 hydrochloric acid. Larger doses of dexamethasone or methylprednisolone were not effective. Other more recent controlled animal studies, looking at the effect of both ventilation and steroids,[31,40,41] as well as further clinical work[19] have cast great doubt on the effectiveness of steroid therapy. Nevertheless, the author believes that early use of steroids for a short period of time likely causes no harm and recommends the immediate intravenous administration of 200 mg of hydrocortisone at the time of acid aspiration (gastric pH < 3.0) and continuation of 100 mg every 6 to 8 hours by continuous intravenous drip for several days or until there is clinical improvement. Administration would then be rapidly tapered off or even stopped immediately. The equivalent dose of other steroids can be used.

ANTIBIOTIC THERAPY

Immediate treatment with broad spectrum antibiotics following pulmonary acid aspiration has been suggested as prophylaxis against infection, particularly when steroids are used.[27,37] Prophylactic antibiotics were widely used in the past. However, Lewis et al.[18] showed that sputum cultures were negative in 12 of 15 patients at the time of initial aspiration. Despite prophylactic antibiotics, 13 of 15 developed positive cultures with resistant organisms. The majority of opinion today is not to initiate prophylactic antibiotics at the time of acid aspiration.[20,21,24,25] If the material aspirated is grossly contaminated, then initial antibiotics would be indicated. Otherwise, regular cultures should be taken of the tracheal aspirate for gram stain, culture and sensitivity. Appropriate antibiotics can then be rationally started on the basis of this information.

PREVENTION OF PULMONARY ASPIRATION IN THE OBSTETRIC PATIENT

"That which can not be easily treated had better be prevented." These words by the famous British anesthetist, J. Alfred Lee, summarize well the situation in dealing with pulmonary aspiration in the parturient. All parturients must be recognized as having significant amounts of material in the stomach that can be aspirated. Realizing this, the best way to prevent aspiration is to maintain the protective upper airway reflexes during labor and delivery. This would preclude the routine use of general anesthesia in favor of other forms of analgesia. It must be understood that alternative forms of analgesia are also potentially hazardous. Heavy maternal sedation with systemic narcotics, tranquilizers and sedatives may obtund the airway reflexes. Narcotics are associated with nausea and vomiting. Regional anesthesia can lead to (1) local anesthetic toxicity with convulsions, followed by central nervous system depression; (2) hypotension from sympathetic block compounded by aortocaval compression, again causing central nervous system depression; and (3) abdominal and intercostal muscle weakness, depressing the ability of the patient to cough. Inhalation analgesia, although avoiding neonatal depression and maintaining upper airway reflexes, may inadvertently proceed to the stage at which airway obstruction occurs and airway reflexes are obtunded. Furthermore, the anesthetist must be wary that the patient may vomit, and, if the mask is not removed and the mouth suctioned, the vomitus can be inhaled.

Antacid Therapy

Taylor and Pryse-Davies[11] first showed the efficacy of oral magnesium trisilicate BPC* to increase the gastric pH above 2.5.

---

* Many articles from the United Kingdom recommend the use of magnesium trisilicate BPC which is actually 5 gm of magnesium trisilicate, 5 gm of magnesium hydroxide and 5 gm of sodium bicarbonate made to 100 ml with peppermint water. It is not magnesium trisilicate alone, which itself is a poor antacid because of its long latency.

Since then many investigators have recommended the routine administration of various regimens of prophylactic oral antacids every 2 to 4 hours in dosages of 15 to 30 ml given to the parturient throughout labor and delivery. There are much data to prove the efficacy of such prophylaxis. Roberts and Shirley[13] showed that the administration of 15 ml of a suspension of magnesium and aluminum hydroxide (Wingel) every 4 hours maintained a gastric pH above 2.5 in 47 of 48 patients, whereas those not receiving antacids had an incidence of 10 in 43 with a pH of less than 2.5. When the time between subsequent administrations of antacid exceeded 4 hours, four of nine parturients had a gastric pH of less than 2.5, which would indicate a rebound in gastric acid production following use of antacids. The use of antacids was not associated with an increased gastric volume. These investigators also indicated that 30 minutes were required from the time of administration to assure a gastric pH of greater than 2.5. Peskett[42] has also demonstrated the effectiveness of magnesium trisilicate BPC in raising the gastric pH above 2.5 in obstetric patients.

Lahiri and co-workers[43] have suggested the oral use of 15 ml of a 0.3 M solution of sodium citrate when more rapid neutralization of gastric contents is required. A major advantage of this solution is that, unlike most readily available antacids, it is a clear solution free of particulate matter which may cause pulmonary lesions if aspirated.[44,45] Unfortunately, it is not available commercially and must be prepared by the hospital pharmacy. The unpleasant taste of sodium citrate may be masked by mixing it with 20 per cent syrup.[46]

Although helpful, antacid prophylaxis is not a panacea and will not protect all obstetric patients. It will not protect against the aspiration of solid or bacterially contaminated material. It may not effectively neutralize gastric material when large volumes are present.[22] Once begun, unless continued on a regular 3- or 4-hour basis, a rebound in gastric acid production may result.[13] Finally, pulmonary aspiration of suspensions of insoluble antacids, although less dangerous than the aspiration of low pH gastric contents, may be associated with lung damage.[44,45]

Anticholinergic Therapy

It has been suggested that the use of anticholinergics (atropine, scopolamine, glycopyrrolate) protects against acid aspiration by: (1) decreasing the volume of gastric secretions, (2) decreasing the amount of gastric acid secreted and (3) increasing the competence of the gastro-esophageal junction. Human studies have failed to demonstrate effectiveness of anticholinergics in decreasing either the acidity or volume of gastric contents.[13,41,47,48] Whether anticholinergics do improve the effectiveness of the gastro-esophageal junction pinchcock mechanisms as claimed by some requires further elucidation.[49] A possible disadvantage of anticholinergic drugs is that they may decrease gastric motility and hence delay gastric emptying.

Emptying the Stomach

The use of emetics (i.e. apomorphine) or naso-gastric tubes will not guarantee an empty stomach. If the stomach is distended, it may be decompressed by a naso-gastric tube which should be removed before induction. If left in place, it will only serve to make the pinchcock action of the gastro-esophageal junction less competent and will act as a wick.

Routine Endotracheal Intubation

When general anesthesia is required for the obstetric patient, intubation with a cuffed endotracheal tube must be performed. The author strongly disagrees with those who believe general anesthesia in the parturient without intubation may be safer than with intubation, particularly in the hands of an inexperienced or untrained anesthetist. Such inexperienced people have no place giving general anesthesia to any patient, much less to the parturient, who is at high risk for this life-threatening catastrophe. It is rare that general anesthesia is required for vaginal delivery. Even difficult forceps deliveries can usually be accomplished with a pudendal block supplemented by inhalation **analgesia.** If general anesthesia is required, it is in the mother's best interest to delay delivery until a competent anesthetist or anesthesiologist is available, just as this would be insisted on for the surgical patient. General anesthesia for the parturient without intubation, except under the most unusual circumstances, is not acceptable practice in the author's opinion. A rapid intravenous induction of anesthesia with thiopental and succinylcholine followed by immediate intubation of the trachea, as described in chapters 10 and 17, is recommended.

Although awake intubation before the induction of anesthesia may in theory seem ideal, it is impractical in most parturients because it is time consuming and unpleasant to both the mother and anesthetist. On the other hand, the author strongly recommends awake "blind" nasal intubation in any patient in whom a difficult laryngoscopy is anticipated, i.e. morbidly obese, hypoplastic mandible, limited range of neck motion.

POSITION DURING INDUCTION

The author does not recommend the use of any form of a "head-up tilt" as suggested by many,[50-52] because intubation is more difficult and because of concern with the danger of hypotension and almost certain pulmonary aspiration should vomiting occur just before muscle relaxation. The patient is placed supine on the delivery table and the right hip is elevated 10 to 12 cm with folded sheets or the table is tipped 10° to the left to minimize aortocaval compression.

PREVENTION OF FASCICULATIONS

Administration of a depolarizing muscle relaxant such as succinylcholine causes generalized muscle fasciculations and an immediate rise in intragastric pressure.[53,54] Pre-treatment with a small dose of a nondepolarizing muscle relaxant, such as curare 3 mg or pancuronium 0.5 mg, will prevent the fasciculations and associated rise in intragastric pressure, thereby reducing the risk of passive regurgitation.

CRICOID PRESSURE

An assistant pressing the cricoid cartilage against the body of the sixth cervical vertebra will occlude the esophagus and prevent passive regurgitation of stomach contents during intubation[55] (Figure 19.5). Cricoid pressure has been shown to be effective in preventing aspiration with gastric pressures as high as 50 to 94 (mean 74) cm H_2O.[56] Potential hazards of the maneu-

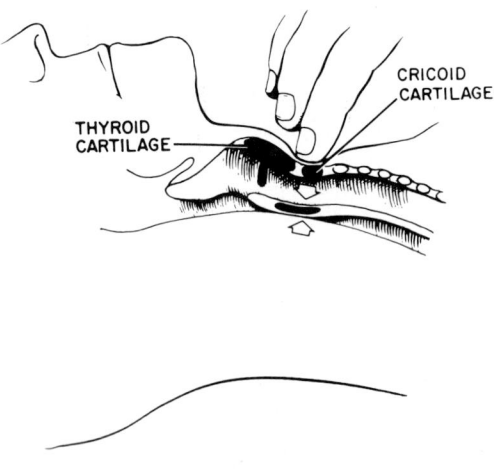

Figure 19.5. The technique of posterior pressure on the cricoid cartilage to occlude the esophagus can be effective in blocking regurgitation but not active vomiting. (Reprinted by permission from Hamelberg W, Bosomworth PB: *Aspiration Pneumonitis.* Charles C Thomas, Springfield, Ill., 1968.)

ver are excessive pressures with possible trauma to the larynx or lateral displacement of the larynx making intubation more difficult. Thus a trained assistant who understands these problems should be used.

AWAKE EXTUBATION

After emergence from anesthesia the endotracheal tube must be left in place until the patient is awake, completely responsive to command and with no signs of muscle weakness. The patient should be placed in the Trendelenburg position with her head to the side. The mouth and posterior pharynx are suctioned. Extubation should take place with the patient breathing 100 percent oxygen. The lungs are inflated, and during inflation the cuff is deflated and the tube immediately removed. Deflation of the cuff and removal of the tube during positive pressure inflation of the lungs will tend to blow material that may have collected above the cuff up and out of the trachea. In the supine position some patients, even when fully reactive, will be unable to protect their airway from vomited or regurgitated gastric contents. Therefore, we recommend placing the patient on her side immediately after extubation.

CONCLUSION

Pulmonary aspiration of stomach contents is a leading cause of maternal morbidity and mortality. Most cases of aspiration in the parturient are avoidable, by careful observation and expert anesthesiologic care during labor and delivery. All parturients must be assumed to have a full stomach. Avoidance of general anesthesia, oversedation and hypotension will do much to eliminate pulmonary aspiration. When general anesthesia is required, a skilled anesthetist and a trained assistant are required. Should pulmonary aspiration occur, prompt and proper therapy are required with continuous monitoring best accomplished in an intensive care situation if high mortality is to be avoided. The parturient requires and deserves the same degree of anesthesiologic competence as the patient undergoing emergency surgery.

References

1. Andrews BF, Apgar V, Chez R, et al.: Reducing the risks of obstetric anesthesia. Patient Care 8: 155, 1974.
2. Mendelson CL: The aspiration of stomach contents into the lungs during obstetric anesthesia. Am J Obstet Gynecol 52:191, 1946.
3. Merrill RB, Hingson RA: Studies of the incidence of maternal mortality from the aspiration of vomitus during anesthesia occurring in major obstetric hospitals in the United States. Anesth Analg 30:121, 1951.
4. Phillips OC, Frazier TM, Davis GH, et al.: The role of anesthesia in obstetric mortality. Anesth Analg 40:557, 1961.
5. Report on Confidential Enquiries into Maternal Deaths in England and Wales, 1967-69. Report of the Health Society Subject No. 1. Stationary Office, London, 1972.
6. Crawford JS: A critical account of the "Confidential Enquiries" report. Proc R Soc Med 67:905, 1974.
7. Davison JS, Davison MC, Hay DM: Gastric emptying time in late pregnancy and labour. J Obstet Gynaecol Br Commonw 77:37, 1970.
8. Hirsheimer A, January DA, Daversa JJ: An x-ray study of gastric function during labor. Am J Obstet Gynecol 36:671, 1938.
9. Crawford JS: Some aspects of obstetric anesthesia. Br J Anaesth 28:201, 1956.
10. Murray FA, Erskine JP, Fielding J: Gastric secretion in pregnancy. J Obstet Gynaecol Br Emp 64: 373, 1957.
11. Taylor G, Pryse-Davies J: The prophylactic use of antacids in the prevention of the acid-pulmonary aspiration syndrome (Mendelson's syndrome). Lancet 1:288, 1966.
12. Attia RR, Eberd AM, Fischer JE: Gastrin: Placental maternal and plasma cord levels, its possible role in maternal residual gastric acidity. In *Abstracts of Scientific Papers*, Annual Meeting, American Society of Anesthesiologists, San Francisco, 1976, p 547.
13. Roberts RB, Shirley MA: Reducing the risk of acid aspiration during cesarean section. Anesth Analg 53:859, 1974.
14. Roberts RB, Shirley MA: The obstetrician's role in reducing the risk of aspiration pneumonitis with particular reference to the use of oral antacids. Am J Obstet Gynecol 124:611, 1976.
15. Teabeaut JR: Aspiration of gastric contents: An experimental study. Am J Pathol 28:51, 1952.
16. Bosomworth PP, Hamelberg W: The etiologic and therapeutic aspects of aspiration pneumonitis: Experimental study. Surg Forum 13:158, 1962.

17. Morton HJV, Wylie WD: Anaesthetic deaths due to regurgitation or vomiting. Anaesthesia 6:190, 1951.
18. Lewis RT, Burgess JH, Hampson LG: Cardiorespiratory studies in critical illness: Changes in aspiration pneumonitis. Arch Surg 103:335, 1971.
19. Awe WC, Fletcher WS, Jacob SW: The pathophysiology of aspiration pneumonitis. Surgery 60:232, 1966.
20. Cameron JL, Mitchell WH, Zuidema GD: Aspiration pneumonitis, clinical outcome following documented aspiration. Arch Surg 106:49, 1973.
21. Bartlett JG, Gorbach SL: The triple threat of aspiration pneumonia. Chest 68:560, 1975.
22. Taylor G: Acid pulmonary aspiration syndrome after antacids: A case report. Br J Anaesth 47:615, 1975.
23. Baggish MS, Hooper S: Aspiration as a cause of maternal death. Obstet Gynecol 43:327, 1974.
24. Morgan JG: Pathophysiology of gastric aspiration. Int Anesthesiol Clin 15:1, 1977.
25. Chapman RL: Treatment of aspiration pneumonitis. Int Anesthesiol Clin 15:85, 1977.
26. Alexander IGS: The ultrastructure of the pulmonary alveolar vessels in Mendelson's (acid pulmonary aspiration) syndrome. Br J Anaesth 40:408, 1968.
27. Hamelberg W, Bosomworth PP: Aspiration pneumonitis: Experimental studies and clinical observations. Anesth Analg 43:669, 1964.
28. Bannister WK, Sattilaro AJ, Otis RD: Therapeutic aspects of aspiration pneumonitis in experimental animals. Anesthesiology 22:440, 1961.
29. Taylor G, Pryse-Davies J: Evaluation of endotracheal steroid therapy in acid pulmonary aspiration syndrome (Mendelson's syndrome). Anesthesiology 29:17, 1968.
30. Booth DJ, Zuidema GD, Cameron JL: Aspiration pneumonia: Pulmonary arteriography after experimental aspiration. J Surg Res 12:48, 1972.
31. Chapman RL, Modell JH, Ruiz BC, et al.: Effects of continuous positive-pressure ventilation and steroids on aspiration of hydrochloric acid (pH 1.8) in dogs. Anesth Analg 53:556, 1974.
32. Cameron JL, Sebor J, Anderson RP, et al.: Aspiration pneumonia. Results of treatment by positive-pressure ventilation in dogs. J Surg Res 8:447, 1968.
33. Roberts RB: Aspiration and its prevention in obstetric patients. Int Anesthesiol Clin 15:49, 1977.
34. Geer RT, Soma LR, Barnes C, et al.: Effects of albumin and/or furosemide therapy on pulmonary edema induced by hydrochloric acid aspiration in rabbits. J Trauma 16:788, 1976.
35. Kennedy RL: General analgesia and anesthesia in obstetrics. Clin Obstet Gynecol 17(2):227, 1974.
36. Lawson DW, DeFalco AJ, Phelps JA, et al.: Corticosteroids as treatment for aspiration of gastric contents: An experimental study. Surgery 59:845, 1966.
37. Ashe JR Jr.: Pulmonary aspiration: A life threatening complication in obstetrics. N C Med J 37:655, 1976.
38. Hausmann W, Lunt RL: The problem of the treatment of peptic aspiration pneumonia following obstetric anaesthesia (Mendelson's syndrome). J Obstet Gynaecol Br Emp 62:509, 1955.
39. Dudley WR, Marshall BE: Steroid treatment for acid-aspiration pneumonitis. Anesthesiology 40:136, 1974.
40. Chapman RL Jr, Downs JB, Modell JH, et al.: The ineffectiveness of steroid therapy in treating aspiration of hydrochloric acid. Arch Surg 108:858, 1974.
41. Downs JB, Chapman RL, Modell JH, et al.: An evaluation of steroid therapy in aspiration pneumonitis. Anesthesiology 40:129, 1974.
42. Peskett WGH: Antacids before obstetric anaesthesia: A clinical evaluation of the effectiveness of mist magnesium trisilicate BPC. Anaesthesia 28:509, 1973.
43. Lahiri SK, Thomas TA, Hodgson RMH: Single-dose antacid therapy for the prevention of Mendelson's syndrome. Br J Anaesth 45:1143, 1973.
44. Kuchling A, Joyce TH III, Cook S: The pulmonary lesion of antacid aspiration. In Abstracts of Scientific Papers, Annual Meeting, American Society of Anesthesiologists, Chicago, 1975, p 281.
45. Gibbs CP, Schwartz DJ, Wynne JW, et al.: Antacid pulmonary aspiration. In Abstracts of Scientific Papers, Annual Meeting, Society for Obstetric Anesthesia and Perinatology, Memphis, 1978, p 26.
46. Abouleish E, Schenle IA: Efficacy of antacid therapy (Correspondence). Br J Anaesth 49:394, 1977.
47. Christensen V, Skovsted P: Effects of general anaesthetics on pH of gastric contents of man during surgery. A survey of halothane, fluroxene and cyclopropane anaesthesia. Acta Anaesth Scand 19:49, 1975.
48. Marks WE Jr, Bullard JR: Effects of glycopyrrolate on gastric volume and pH in patients requiring cesarean section. In Abstracts of Scientific Papers, Annual Meeting, Society of Obstetric Anesthesia and Perinatology, Seattle, 1977, p 14.
49. Abouleish E, Grenvic A: Vomiting, regurgitation and aspiration in obstetrics. Pa Med 77(5):45, 1974.
50. Snow RG, Nunn JF: Induction of anaesthesia in the foot-down position for patients with a full stomach. Br J Anaesth 31:493, 1959.
51. Hodges RJH, Tunstall ME, Bennett JR: Vomiting and the head-up position. Br J Anaesth 32:619, 1960.
52. Stark DCC: Aspiration in the surgical patient. Int Anesthesiol Clin 15:13, 1977.
53. Andersen N: Changes in intragastric pressure following administration of suxamethonium: Preliminary report. Br J Anaesth 34:363, 1962.
54. Miller RD, Way WL: Inhibition of succinylcholine-induced increased intragastric pressure by nondepolarizing muscle relaxants and lidocaine. Anesthesiology 34:185, 1971.
55. Sellick BA: Cricoid pressure to control regurgitation of stomach contents during induction of anaesthesia. Lancet 2:404, 1961.
56. Fanning GL: The efficacy of cricoid pressure in regurgitation of gastric contents. Anesthesiology 32:553, 1970.

CHAPTER 20

Neurologic Complications of Regional Anesthesia for Obstetrics

Philip R. Bromage, M.B., B.S. (Lond) F.F.A.R.C.S., F.R.C.P.(C)

Among the hazards of childbirth lies the remote possibility of neurologic damage from ischemia of spinal nerves, roots or cord due to mechanical or vascular factors associated with the process of labor and delivery. Regional anesthesia also carries certain neurologic risks, some of which are transient and trivial if properly managed, and some of which are grave. This chapter will review the neurologic hazards of regional anesthesia and will stress the importance of distinguishing associated but unrelated complications from those that are causally related to regional anesthetic procedures.

The incidences of natural and iatrogenic complications vary between different series. Precise statistics on the over-all incidence of neurologic complications do not exist, and the reader is cautioned against taking any one statistic as a fixed point of reference, because the ground is constantly changing. For example, until about 15 years ago the incidence of nerve injuries in the absence of regional anesthesia was given as about 1 in 2,100 to 2,600 vaginal deliveries.[1,2] Since then obstetrical practice has become more agressive, and a higher cesarean section rate will probably have saved many cases from foot drop due to compression of the lumbosacral trunk as it crosses the ala of the sacrum. Other complications peculiar to cesarean section will have increased in their place, but these will not be discussed in this chapter.

This review will cover complications due to subarachnoid and epidural blockade (lumbar and caudal approaches), inasmuch as the majority of neurologic sequelae are related to one of these two techniques.

TRANSIENT NEUROLOGIC COMPLICATIONS

Prolonged Neural Blockade

Unduly prolonged blockade lasting 9 to 48 hours may occasionally follow repeated epidural injections of concentrated solutions of very powerful local anesthetic agents. The cause is probably attributable to accumulation of highly lipid-soluble drug in epidural fat near the tip of the epidural catheter, creating a local depot from which local anesthetic is taken up into neighboring neural tissues over a period of many hours. This phenomenon has been reported with 0.5 per cent tetracaine and 0.5 per cent bupivacaine for relief of pain in labor,[3-5] and it is likely to be seen as an occasional complication with concentrated solutions of other highly lipid-soluble agents such as etidocaine. This type of prolonged blockade is reversible, it does not involve any abnormal processes and no lasting untoward effects have been reported. Table 20.1 summarizes nine cases reported from the recent literature. It should be noted that in all the cases in Table 20.1 the epidural solutions used were unnecessarily concentrated for the task of providing pain relief during labor. Pregnant women at term are particularly sensitive to local anesthetic agents, and the author believes that bupivacaine in 0.25 per cent concentration is adequate for relief of pain in childbirth.

Headache

Post-puncture headache is caused by cerebrospinal fluid (CSF) hypotension due to loss of fluid through a patent hole in the dura. Parturient patients are twice as likely to suffer post-puncture headache as normal patients. The incidence of headache is related to the size of the needle hole, being about 70 per cent after puncture with a 16-gauge epidural needle, but only about 2 per cent when a 25-gauge spinal needle is used. Dural puncture holes take 10 to 14 days and sometimes longer to heal. In the meantime headache from loss of CSF can be prostrating and may cause unnecessary prolongation of hospital stay. Treatment is designed to bolster the sagging dural sac, either by pressure from without or by encouraging CSF formation and sealing the dural hole. Epidural saline infusions of 1.5 liters in 24 to 36 hours act as a temporary support for the dura and reduce the incidence of severe headache from 70 per cent to 20 per cent after large-size puncture holes.[6] Alternatively, an epidural blood patch with 10 ml of the patient's own freshly drawn blood affords instantaneous and effective relief.[7,8]

Backache

Backache is not properly a neurologic complication, although it is sometimes considered as one. Backache is a frequent occurrence in an obstetric population, with an incidence of 30 to 40 per cent regardless of whether regional or general anesthesia is used. The cause probably lies in ligamentous strain from lordosis of pregnancy.

Bladder Dysfunction

Lack of bladder sensation during prolonged continuous epidural blockade may cause retention and overstretching of the bladder wall. Long-acting agents are more likely to cause retention than short-acting agents.[9] Strict attention to care of the bladder during labor should avoid this complication.

Shivering

A small proportion of women complain of shivering and shaking after induction of

Table 20.1
Prolonged Blockade after Epidural Analgesia in Labor, followed by Complete Recovery

Author	Drug	No. of Cases	Duration of Residual Analgesia
			hrs
Bromage[3]	Tetracaine 0.5% + epinephrine	3	9–48
	Bupivacaine 0.5% + epinephrine	1	10
Pathy and Rosen[4]	Bupivacaine 0.5% + epinephrine	1	48
Cuerden et al.[5]	Bupivacaine 0.5% + epinephrine	4	23–48

caudal or lumbar epidural blockade; this is seen more frequently after large doses. Shivering usually stops spontaneously in 5 to 15 minutes and is of no serious concern. The causes are speculative and probably due to disturbances of thermal sensory information while the block is becoming established.

Horner's Syndrome

Horner's syndrome has been reported as a relatively frequent complication of caudal and lumbar epidural analgesia in labor, even when sensory blockade has not extended above T7.[10,11] One prospective study at Oxford, England, revealed a 75 per cent incidence of pupillary changes or other manifestations of cervical sympathetic blockade.[12] This benign neurologic oddity is without satisfactory explanation at the present time but is a reminder of the extraordinarily wide analgesic diffusion that characterizes epidural blockade at term.[13]

Overdose

Pregnant women at term require about 30 per cent less subarachnoid and epidural local anesthetic than the normal population. Failure to allow for this reduced requirement will lead to relative overdose and excessively high segmental blockade, with undue vasomotor and muscular paralysis.

Massive Misplaced Injection

The most serious immediate neurologic complication is massive injection of local anesthetic into the wrong place, either subdural, subarachnoid or intravenous.

Massive Subdural Injection

A potential space exists between the dura mater and the pia-arachnoid membranes. Rough handling of the needle or unnecessary rotation of the bevel during induction of epidural blockade are factors that may cause a breach in the dura, with the possibility of injecting solutions or passing a catheter directly into the subdural space. Boys and Norman[14] have documented a case of subdural catheterization where 40 mg of 0.5 per cent bupivacaine led to blockade from C7 to L2.

Massive Subarachnoid Injection

Accidental puncture of the meninges and inadvertent subarachnoid injection of a sizeable epidural dose of local anesthetic are followed by rapid total spinal anesthesia, vascular hypotension, apnea and loss of consciousness. Epidural catheters have been known to puncture the meninges,[15,16] and so a precautionary test dose should always be injected through an epidural catheter before proceeding to large volumes.

Treatment of massive subarachnoid and massive subdural injection is directed towards supporting circulation and respiration until the effects of the block wear off. Endotracheal intubation and ventilation is carried out, and arterial pressure is maintained with fluid administration, left uterine displacement and a suitable vasopressor. Massive subarachnoid blockade is lethal if untreated, but, with prompt and proper management, it is usually no more than a clinical nuisance.

Toxic Intravenous Injection

Accidental intravascular injection is a potential hazard in any form of regional anesthesia. Rapid intravenous injection may result in convulsions and cardiovascular depression. It is standard teaching that needles should be kept moving during infiltration anesthesia to avoid the danger of inadvertent intravenous injection. This precaution is impossible in spinal or epidural analgesia because of the narrowness of the space, and so it is especially important to perform tests to ensure that large bolus doses of local anesthetic are not accidentally injected into the vascular system.

Two sites of accidental intravenous injection are relatively common. First, needles passed into the caudal canal may pierce the cortical layer of a sacral vertebra and enter cancellous bone. Subsequent injections into the marrow cavity enter the circulation as rapidly as by direct intravenous injection, and toxic reactions may result.[17] Second, cannulation of an epidural vein is a relatively common accident in labor, with an incidence of about 0.75 per cent. It is more likely to occur if puncture is made in the lateral part of the space where the veins are more plentiful than in the midline. Due to partial occlusion of the inferior vena cava, pressure and flow in the extradural and azygos system is higher at term than in the normal population. Azygos flow is likely to rise in proportion to the degree of caval obstruction, and this is greatest when the mother is lying on her back. Hence, extradural intravenous injections in the dorsal position travel fast and reach the heart as a bolus, so that quite small quantities of local anesthetic produce disproportionately large effects. Convulsions have arisen from a dose as small as 15 mg of etidocaine, with a toxic equivalence of about 60 mg of lidocaine.[18] Prevention lies in: (1) insertion of the catheter in the midline of the epidural space rather than in the lateral extremities of the space, where epidural veins are most plentiful; (2) careful aspiration through the epidural catheter *before* it is taped in place; (3) use of a test dose through the catheter; and (4) injection of top-up doses in the lateral position, not with the mother lying on her back. Treatment of convulsions from extradural venous injection is along standard lines with: (1) turning of mother into lateral posture; (2) hyperventilation with oxygen; (3) intravenous diazepam; (4) succinylcholine and endotracheal intubation if convulsions do not immediately subside; and (5) vasopressor therapy if arterial hypotension occurs.

CHRONIC NEUROLOGIC COMPLICATIONS

Trauma

Trauma to nerve pathways may occur during labor from causes unrelated to regional anesthesia; these will be reviewed later in the chapter. The incidence of direct neurologic trauma from spinal or epidural needles and catheters is extremely rare. Pressure on the cord or spinal roots by a needle point is accompanied by severe lancinating pain, and this is a signal to withdraw the needle immediately. Trauma to the spinal cord can be avoided by making spinal or epidural puncture below the termination of the conus medullaris. The cord usually ends at the level of the first lumbar intervertebral disc, but occasionally it may extend lower to the level of the disc between the second and third lumbar vertebrae (Figure 20.1). Therefore, selection of the third or fourth interspace is a prudent initial step in performing subarachnoid or epidural puncture.

Epidural catheters have been suspected of causing trauma to spinal roots. However, there have always been alternative and more likely causes in suspected cases, and there is no objective evidence of trauma caused by an epidural catheter. Intrathecal catheters for continuous subarachnoid analgesia are more likely to damage the soft spinal cord. During experiments in dogs where percutaneous intracisternal catheters were passed downwards in the subarachnoid space, it was surprising how easily some catheters could penetrate the cord and travel in it without any appreciable sense of resistance being transmitted to the operator's fingers. There is no indication for using continuous intrathecal analgesia in obstetrics today, and

NEUROLOGIC COMPLICATIONS OF REGIONAL ANESTHESIA

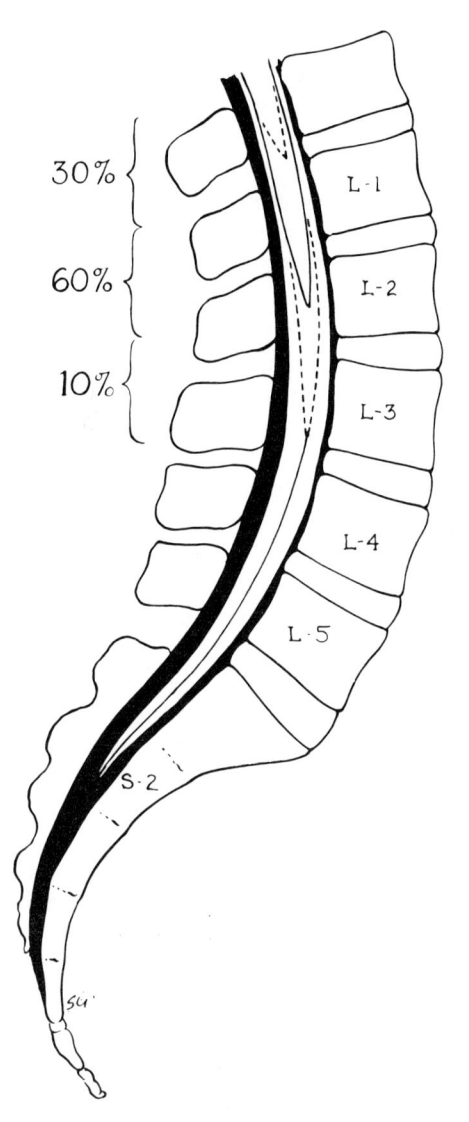

Figure 20.1. Variations of the level of termination of the spinal cord. The figures (*left*) indicate the approximate percentage each level was found among 129 specimens. Extradural space is shown in black and subarachnoid space in white. (Reprinted by permission from Bonica JJ. In: *Principles and Practice of Obstetric Anesthesia*, vol *1*, F. A. Davis, Philadelphia, 1969, p 552 adapted from data by Reimann AE, Anson BJ: Vertebral level of termination of the spinal cord with a report of a case of sacral cord. Anat. Rec. 88:127, 1944.)

the risk of damage from intrathecal catheters should not arise.

Complications of Vascular Origin

EPIDURAL HEMATOMA

Minor degrees of bleeding into the spinal canal are relatively common from injury to the large, thin-walled epidural veins. Under normal circumstances bleeding quickly stops and there are no sequelae. Experience with the epidural blood patch method of treating spinal headaches shows that volumes of 2 to 10 ml of blood in the epidural space do not cause harm. However, abnormalities of the clotting mechanism may permit uncontrolled oozing to continue until a large hematoma has formed, with consequent paralysis from pressure on the spinal cord. Subarachnoid or epidural blockade should be avoided in the presence of clotting abnormalities or a low platelet count, or when anticoagulants are being administered to the mother. Paralysis from epidural hematoma is a dire emergency, and urgent surgical decompression of the cord is indicated. Recovery is likely if this is done within 2 hours, but permanent paralysis will follow if surgery is delayed.[19]

OTHER VASCULAR LESIONS

Other vascular lesions related to regional anesthesia, such as the anterior spinal artery syndrome, are rare possibilities in an elderly population, but they are not likely to be seen in women of childbearing age. Other vascular lesions unrelated to regional anesthesia such as spinal cord angioma will be discussed later in this chapter.

Infection

Infection of the epidural or subarachnoid space is an extremely rare event, but it is devastating when it does occur. Infection in the spinal canal is usually secondary to infection elsewhere in the body, and only very rarely is it introduced from an exogenous source.[20] Nevertheless, there is a temptation to lower aseptic standards in the hurly-burly conditions of a busy delivery suite, and this temptation must be resisted by all concerned. The anesthesiologist and all those in close attendance should wear face masks during performance of subarachnoid or epidural blocks.

Single subarachnoid or epidural injections are extremely unlikely to introduce exogenous infection, but continuous epidural and caudal techniques establish multiple opportunities for contamination. Micropore filters have been recommended as a protection against both particulate and microbial invasion of the epidural space, but the pore size must be 0.22 μm or less to exclude common bacterial contaminants. Some disposable epidural trays include a filter of 1 μm pore size, but false hopes should not be entertained that these large pores will be of any benefit in excluding bacteria, although they will keep out microscopic particles of broken glass that often contaminate solutions from glass ampules.[21,22]

EPIDURAL ABSCESS

Baker and her associates[23] reviewed 39 cases of pyogenic spinal epidural abscess over a period of 27 years at the Massachusetts General Hospital. In 38 of these, abscess was secondary to endogenous infection elsewhere in the body. Only one case was associated with an epidural catheter, and this patient did not suffer any permanent sequelae. Symptoms and signs of acute epidural abscess develop rapidly and inexorably, and anesthesiologists should be familiar with the cardinal signs. Four signs are always present: (1) severe back pain, (2) local overlying tenderness, (3) fever and (4) leukocytosis. Nuchal rigidity is present in 50 per cent of cases. The CSF has markedly elevated protein to over 400 mg/100 ml, and it also shows leukocytosis.

Treatment is by urgent spinal decompression. Paraplegia is almost inevitable unless laminectomy is done at an early stage.

Because there is a risk of metastatic epidural infection from established infectious processes elsewhere in the body, the question arises: Is it safe to induce epidural analgesia in the presence of pre-existing infection and bacteremia? For example, what policy should be adopted in the face of prematurely ruptured membranes and signs of developing amnionitis? Despite the widespread use of epidural and caudal anesthesia in the presence of premature ruptured membranes, no case of chorioamnionitis and associated epidural abscess has been reported. The author believes that epidural analgesia should ***probably*** be avoided, for a bacteremia will be present, and the remote possibility of metastatic epidural infection is heightened, regardless of whether or not an epidural catheter is inserted. This belief is not shared by the editors of this book.

SUBARACHNOID INFECTION

Subarachnoid infection is now an extremely rare complication of regional anesthesia for obstetrics, and the cause may be hard to determine. Cases of chronic adhesive arachnoiditis are probably related to pre-existing chronic infection of the spinal canal[24,25] or to contamination with chemical irritants.

Chemical Contamination of the Subarachnoid and Epidural spaces

The epidural space seems to be remarkably tolerant of some chemical contaminants. For example, epidural injections of 6 per cent aqueous phenol are used by some to relieve terminal cancer pain without any untoward sequelae, and yet the same solution would have disastrous results in the subarachnoid space. Accidental epidural injections of various solutions such as thiopental and 6 per cent potassium chloride have been reported without permanent sequelae. However, other patients have not been so fortunate, and prolonged sequelae have been reported after accidental injection of contaminants such as collodion.[20]

The pia-covered cord and roots in the subarachnoid space are much more vulnerable to the effects of chemical contaminants. A hole in the dura from accidental dural puncture allows epidural solutions to leak into the subarachnoid space, particularly if injection is made rapidly and under pressure. Then contaminants that might have been innocuous when excluded by an intact dura become potentially harmful. Craig and Habib[26] report a case of paraparesis from epidural injection of 1.5 per cent benzyl alcohol under these circumstances:

Accidental dural puncture with a 16-gauge needle occurred during induction of epidural analgesia for pain relief in labor in a 24-year-old primiparous woman. After delivery 40 ml of 0.9 per cent saline were injected into the epidural space as a prophylactic measure against a low CSF pressure headache. Unfortunately the saline contained 1.5 per cent benzyl alcohol as a preservative. Paraparesis of the lower limbs followed. Recovery gradually took place over a period of about 16 months.

In this instance the concentration of benzyl alcohol was not high enough to cause damage in the epidural space, and it must be concluded that the saline and preservative leaked into the subarachnoid space through the large needle hole in the dura.

Traces of detergents used for cleaning reusable spinal needles and syringes have been imputed as a possible cause of myelitis if they are accidentally introduced into the subarachnoid space.[27] This source of contamination may be considered as a possible explanation for six cases of grave neurologic sequelae reported from Porto Alegre in Brazil.[28] Three of the six cases occurred in young women receiving epidural analgesia for childbirth. In all six cases the picture was one of severe adhesive arachnoiditis of a chemical rather than an infective nature, but the cause could not be identified, and detergent contamination is only one of several possibilities.

ASSOCIATED NEUROLOGIC LESIONS UNRELATED TO REGIONAL ANESTHESIA

At the beginning of this chapter it was pointed out that a small number of neurologic accidents may attend the process of childbirth, regardless of whether or not a regional anesthetic is given. Therefore, it is important to have some knowledge of the origin, nature and prevalence of these lesions so that they can be distinguished from accidents that are truly related to the regional anesthetic. Neurologic lesions of obstetric origin can occur at a number of levels. Intracranial lesions do not concern this discussion and we will consider only those of spinal or peripheral origin, at three sites: (1) the cord, (2) spinal roots and (3) plexus trunks and peripheral nerves. The approximate prevalence of these three sites is shown in Table 20.2. Underlying neuropathies from diabetes, porphyria or other causes may increase the incidence of selected populations.

Cord Lesions

Vascular anomalies of the cord are usually associated with a history of some weakness of the legs **before** the onset of labor, but this is not always forthcoming; then diagnosis may be extremely difficult and arrived at by exclusion. Selective arteriography of the cord may be needed to demonstrate a vascular anomaly, but this sophisticated radiologic examination is not likely to be undertaken in the absence of a high index of suspicion.

The Valsalva-like efforts of labor may

Table 20.2
Causes of Postpartum Neural Deficits Unrelated to Regional Anesthesia

Site	Cause	Prevalence (Approximate)
Cord	Hemangioma of spinal cord,	Rare
	Spontaneous epidural hematoma, etc.	1 in 15,000
Roots	Spinal root compression from prolapsed intravertebral disc	1 in 6,000
Peripheral nerves	Compression and injury of peripheral nerves crossing the pelvic brim (e.g. lumbosacral trunk, femoral nerve, lateral femoral cutaneous nerve, etc.)	1 in 4,000 to 1 in 2,100

rupture a small epidural vein, and in patients with clotting deficiencies an epidural hematoma may form, leading to compression of the adjacent cord. Unlike epidural abscess, the process is usually silent and painless, but surgical treatment is just as urgently needed if signs of cord compression arise, and then early laminectomy must be undertaken.

Root Lesions

The muscular efforts of labor may give rise to a prolapsed intervertebral disc, with subsequent root compression. There is usually back pain and numbness of the affected segmental area. The diagnosis is confirmed by myelography.

Trunk and Nerve Lesions

The most common obstetric nerve lesion is caused by compression of the lumbosacral trunk between the descending fetal head and the ala of the sacrum (Figure 20.2). Compression at this site is more likely to occur in platypelloid pelves, where the lumbosacral trunk is relatively unprotected. Kinking and compression of the femoral nerve or the lateral femoral cutaneous nerve can occur at the inguinal ligament from prolonged posture in the lithotomy position. All these peripheral nerve lesions have typical clinical patterns depending on their motor and sensory components. For example, lumbosacral trunk injuries are characterized by foot drop combined with sensory loss over the outer calf and foot, and sometimes over the inner calf (L4) as well. Recovery is to be expected, and restoration of function is usually complete in 12 to 16 weeks.

DIAGNOSIS

Postpartum neurologic deficits inevitably focus suspicion on whatever regional anesthetic may have been used during childbirth. Therefore, the anesthesiologist should have a clear scheme of investigation in his mind so that he can deploy the necessary diagnostic and therapeutic resources. The following questions must be answered:

1. Is the lesion real or imagined?
2. What is the site of the lesion?
3. What is the nature of the lesion?
4. What is the cause?
5. Is there any associated cause, such as diabetes, that requires investigation and treatment?

The following steps are followed in the investigation:

1. History: A careful history is crucial, paying particular attention to the possibility of any antecedent sensory or motor disturbances in the lower limbs.
2. Physical examination: Careful mapping of sensory and motor deficits, with note of any sphincter disturbance, will establish whether the lesion has the characteristics of a segmental or a peripheral injury. Examination of the back will reveal

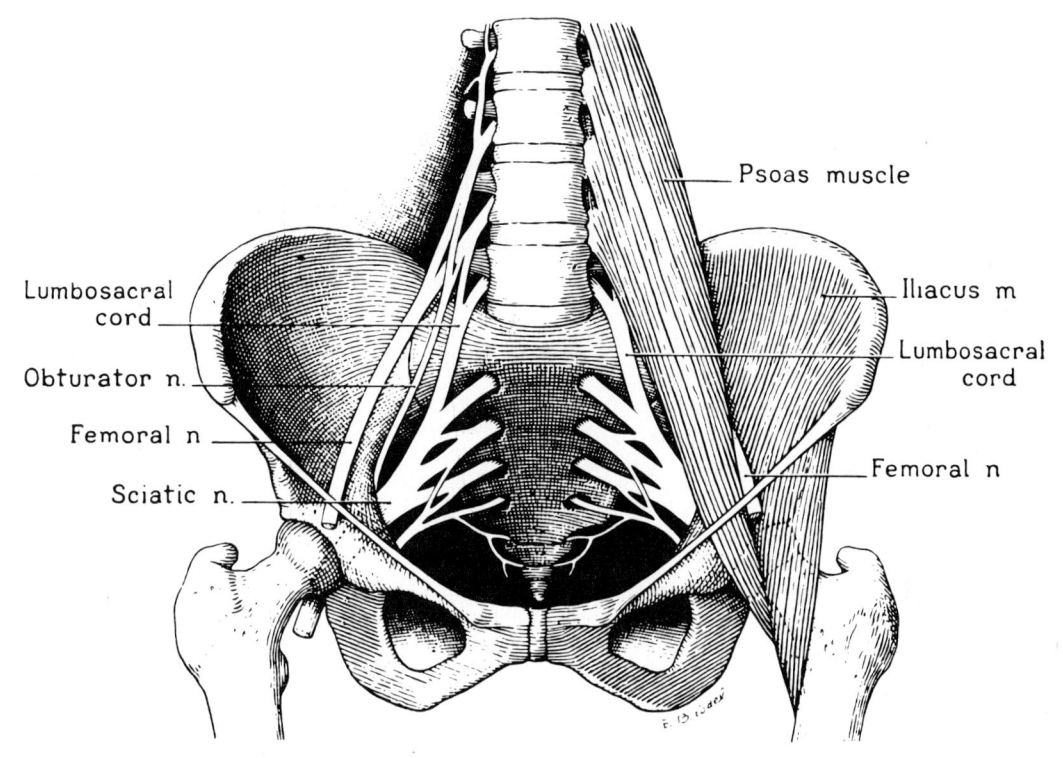

Figure 20.2. The relationship of the lumbosacral cord to the pelvis and the psoas major muscle. (Reprinted by permission from Cole JT: Maternal obstetric paralysis. Am J Obstet Gynecol 52:374, 1946.)

any local tenderness that might raise suspicion of acute spinal infection.

3. Supporting tests: According to the results of the history and physical examination, the following tests should be performed: (1) Spinal x-ray to examine size and shape of lumbar disc spaces. (2) Coagulogram to exclude clotting abnormalities. (3) Lumbar or cisternal puncture for CSF examination if indicated by signs and symptoms of epidural abscess. (4) Myelography if spinal block is suspected. (5) Electromyography of leg and paraspinal muscles in the event of motor loss. Sequential examinations of limb and paraspinal muscles should be carried out to assess the evolution of denervation patterns, and to establish whether the lesion is within the spinal canal and involving both anterior and posterior primary rami or whether it is distal to the intervertebral foramen and involving only the limb muscles supplied by the anterior primary rami.[29-31]

Investigation should also include other systems that may have a casual significance. A glucose tolerance test and an examination of urine or feces should be done to exclude diabetes or porphyria as possible underlying causes of neuropathy.

Statistically, postpartum neurologic lesions are much more likely to arise from obstetric or natural causes than from the results of concomitant regional anesthesia. In a survey of 780,000 epidural blocks for all types of indication, Usubiaga[20] found an incidence of 1 in 11,000 neurologic complications. Other smaller populations at specialist centers have had even lower complication rates. Hellman[32] reported on more than 20,000 cesarean sections and vaginal deliveries under epidural anesthesia without a single major neurologic complication. Between 1956 and 1977 approximately 30,000 deliveries were conducted under epidural blockade at the Royal Victoria Hospital in Montreal. During that time there were several peripheral nerve injuries attributable to obstetric causes, but no permanent neurologic sequelae were caused by the regional anesthesia. The incidence of neurologic complications after well conducted regional anesthesia is extremely low, and well below the naturally occurring incidence of approximately 1 in 3,000 that may be expected in a normal obstetric population.

SUMMARY

The neurologic complications of regional anesthesia for obstetrics may be transient or permanent. The transient complications are relatively common and cover a wide range of possibilities. All are trivial if properly managed, but some are potentially lethal if left untreated. Therefore, it is of paramount importance that all those using regional anesthesia for obstetrics should be prepared to manage the acute complications that may arise. Permanent complications due to regional anesthesia are extremely rare, with an overall incidence of about 1 in 11,000, and an incidence of less than 1 in 20,000 in specialist centers. Neurologic complications due to natural or obstetric causes occur with an incidence of about 1 in 3,000; these are usually trunk or peripheral nerve injuries that tend to recover in 12 to 16 weeks. Therefore, it is very important to be able to distinguish between obstetric and anesthetic causes of neurologic sequelae. The steps to be taken in arriving at this distinction are outlined.

References

1. Tillman AJB: Traumatic neuritis in the puerperium. Am J Obstet Gynecol 29:660, 1935.
2. Hill EC: Maternal obstetric paralysis. Am J Obstet Gynecol 83:1452, 1962.
3. Bromage PR: An evaluation of bupivacaine in epidural analgesia for obstetrics. Can Anaesth Soc J 16:46, 1969.
4. Pathy GV, Rosen M: Prolonged block with recovery after extradural analgesia for labour. Br J Anaesth 47:520, 1975.
5. Cuerden C, Buley R, Downing JW: Delayed recovery after epidural block in labour. A report of four cases. Anaesthesia 32:773, 1977.
6. Moir DD: *Obstetric Anesthesia and Analgesia.* Williams & Wilkins, Baltimore, 1976, p 181.
7. DiGiovanni AJ, Dunbar BS: Epidural injections of autologous blood for postlumbar-puncture headache. Anesth Analg (Cleve) 49:268, 1970.
8. DiGiovanni AJ, Galbert MW, Wahle WM: Epidural injections of autologous blood for postlumbar-puncture headache. II. Additional clinical experience and laboratory investigation. Anesth Analg (Cleve) 51:226, 1972.
9. Bridenbaugh LD: Catheterization after long- and short-acting local anesthetics for continuous caudal block for vaginal delivery. Anesthesiology 46: 357, 1977.
10. Evans JM, Gauci CA, Watkins G: Horner's syndrome as a complication of lumbar extradural block. Anaesthesia 30:774, 1975.
11. Mohan J, Potter JM: Pupillary constriction and ptosis following caudal epidural analgesia. Anaesthesia 30:769, 1975.
12. Carrie LES, Mohan J: Horner's syndrome following obstetric extradural block. Br J Anaesth 48: 611, 1976.
13. Bromage PR: Spread of analgesic solutions in the epidural space and their site of action: A statistical study. Br J Anaesth 24:161, 1962.
14. Boys JE, Norman PF: Accidental subdural analgesia. Br J Anaesth 47:1111, 1975.
15. Gavin R: Continuous epidural analgesia. An unusual cause of dural perforation during catheterization of the epidural space. N Z Med J 64:280, 1965.
16. Moir DD, Hesson WR: Dural puncture by an epidural catheter. Anaesthesia 20:373, 1965.
17. McGowan RG: Accidental marrow sampling during caudal anesthesia. Br J Anaesth 44:613, 1972.
18. Bromage PR, Datta S, Dunford LA: Etidocaine: An evaluation in epidural analgesia for obstetrics. Can Anaesth Soc J 21:535, 1974.
19. Harik SI, Raichle ME, Reis DJ: Spontaneous remitting spinal epidural hematoma in a patient on anticoagulants. N Engl J Med 284:1355, 1971.
20. Usubiaga JE: Neurological complications following epidural analgesia. Int Anesthesiol Clin 13:2, 19, 50, 1975.
21. Ho NFH: Particulate matter in parenteral solutions. I. A review of the literature. Drug Intelligence 1:7, 1967.
22. Somerville TG, Gibson M: Particulate contamination in ampoules: A comparative study. Pharmaceut J August 18, 1973, p 128.
23. Baker AS, Ojemann RG, Swartz MN, et al.: Spinal epidural abscess. N Engl J Med 293:463, 1975.
24. Wadia NH, Datsur DK: Spinal meningitides with

radiculomyelopathy. Part I. Clinical features. J Neurol Sci 8:239, 1969.
25. Alpers BJ, Mancall EJ: *Clinical Neurology.* F. A. Davis, Philadelphia, 1971.
26. Craig DB, Habib GG: Flaccid paraparesis following obstetrical epidural anesthesia: Possible role of benzyl alcohol. Anesth Analg 56:219, 1977.
27. Winkelman NW: Neurologic symptoms following accidental intraspinal detergent injection. Neurology 2:284, 1952.
28. Kliemann FAD: Paraplegia and intracranial hypertension following epidural anesthesia. Report of four cases. Arq Neuro-Psiquiatria 33:217, 1975.
29. Marinacci AA, Courville CB: Electromyogram in evaluation of neurological complications of spinal anesthesia. JAMA 168:1337, 1958.
30. Marinacci AA: Clinical electromyography: A review. Bull Los Angeles Neurol Soc 35:181, 1970.
31. Goodgold J, Eberstein A: *Electrodiagnosis of Neuromuscular Diseases.* Williams & Wilkins, Baltimore, 1972.
32. Hellmann K: Epidural anesthesia in obstetrics: A second look at 26,127 cases. Can Anaesth Soc J 12:398, 1965.

CHAPTER 21

Anesthesia for Operations During Pregnancy

Gershon Levinson, M.D.
Sol M. Shnider, M.D.

The incidence of surgery during pregnancy reportedly ranges from 0.3 to 1.6 per cent.[1-3] Shnider and Webster[1] reported that one in every 116 pregnant women has a major surgical anesthetic. Others have reported that as many as 2 per cent of all operations carried out in women are performed during pregnancy.[3] Based on these reports it has been estimated that each year in the United States up to 50,000 pregnant women may receive an anesthetic for surgery during pregnancy. These women require special attention in their anesthetic management if maternal morbidity and fetal wastage is to be avoided. The basic objectives in the anesthetic management of pregnant women undergoing surgery are: (1) maternal safety; (2) avoidance of teratogenic drugs; (3) avoidance of intrauterine fetal asphyxia; and (4) prevention of premature labor.

MATERNAL SAFETY

The physiologic changes that occur during pregnancy are discussed in chapter 1. Many of these changes are due to hormonal factors as well as to the mechanical effects of the enlarging uterus and occur during the first and second trimesters. The changes of greatest relevance to the anesthesiologist are summarized below.

Alveolar ventilation is increased about 25 per cent by the fourth month of pregnancy and rises progressively to 70 per cent at term (Figure 21.1).[4] End tidal PCO_2 falls to 33 torr by the third month of pregnancy (Figure 21.2).[5] Functional residual capacity is decreased 10 per cent at 6 months and 20 per cent at term (Figure 21.3).[5] Oxygen consumption increases significantly during mid-pregnancy due to the developing placenta, fetus and uterine muscle. Anesthetic requirement for halogenated agents is decreased up to 40 per cent during the second trimester.[6]

Induction of and emergence from anesthesia is more rapid because of the increased ventilation and decreased functional residual capacity. The likelihood of anesthetic overdose is increased. The increased oxygen consumption and decreased functional residual capacity make the pregnant patient more likely to become hypoxic with respiratory obstruction or difficult endotracheal intubation. Even during rapid endotracheal intubation (30 seconds of apnea) arterial PO_2 can fall to 50 to 60 mm Hg in mothers who are not pre-oxygenated.

ANESTHESIA FOR OPERATIONS DURING PREGNANCY

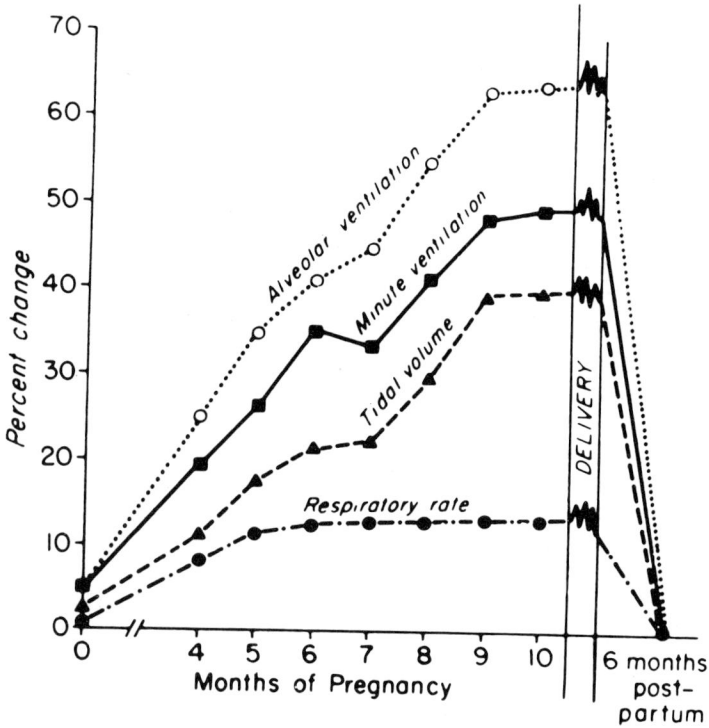

Figure 21.1. Changes in respiratory parameters during pregnancy. (Reprinted by permission from Bonica JJ: *Principles and Practice of Obstetric Analgesia and Anesthesia*, vol 1. F. A. Davis, Philadelphia, 1967.)

Cardiac output and stroke volume are increased 35 to 40 per cent[7-9] (Figure 13.2) and blood volume is increased 20 to 30 per cent by 20 to 24 weeks' gestation.[10,11] Inferior vena caval occlusion, although most pronounced in women near term, is also significant during the second trimester (Figure 21.4) despite the apparently small size of the uterus. Lateral tilt to prevent supine hypotension and uterine hypoperfusion should be used for all surgical procedures if possible.

The increase in femoral venous pressure shown in Figure 21.4 is likely also reflected in the epidural veins and may be relevant in determining the dosage of local anesthetic necessary to achieve a given level of spinal anesthesia. Because of epidural venous engorgement the size of the subarachnoid space is decreased, and the amount of local anesthetic should be reduced by 25 to 30 per cent from mid-pregnancy to term lest an excessively high level of anesthesia occur.

It is unclear precisely at which point in gestation a pregnant woman becomes more susceptible to regurgitation and aspiration under anesthesia. Plasma gastrin levels, believed to be of placental origin, are elevated throughout gestation but are especially high in the second half.[12] During pregnancy the gradually enlarging uterus displaces the stomach, alters the angle of the gastro-esophageal junction and predisposes the patient to passive regurgitation. Symptoms of esophageal reflux (heartburn) are common throughout pregnancy. All patients undergoing anesthesia should be pre-medicated with an oral antacid. The authors believe that any pregnant women

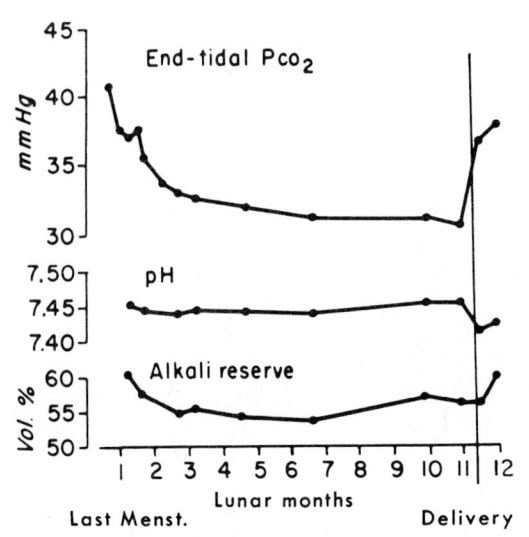

Figure 21.2. Progressive changes of alveolar carbon dioxide tensions, pH and alkali reserve throughout pregnancy. (Reprinted by permission from Bonica JJ: *Principles and Practice of Obstetric Analgesia and Anesthesia,* vol 1. F. A. Davis, Philadelphia, 1967.)

undergoing surgery during the third trimester or **any time during pregnancy if she has symptoms of esophagitis** should be intubated rapidly after induction of general anesthesia.

TERATOGENICITY OF ANESTHETICS

Teratogenicity, either morphologic, biochemical or behavioral, may be induced at any stage of gestation by exogenous agents and detected at birth or later. To produce a defect, a teratogenic drug must be given in an appropriate dosage, during a particular developmental stage of the embryo, in a species or individual with a particular genetic susceptibility (Figure 21.5).

In humans the critical stages of organ development are illustrated in Figure 21.6. Each organ and each system undergoes a critical stage of differentiation during which vulnerability to teratogens is greatest and specific malformations can be produced. For example, the period of sensitivity of the heart is 18 to 40 days and the limbs 24 to 34 days. Variations in genetic susceptibility may make interpretation of teratogenic studies difficult. Drugs may have a marked effect in one species and little teratogenic effect in another. Even in the same species different strains may respond differently. Thalidomide, which produces gross malformations in humans and rabbits, is safe in rats.[13] Of the women who took thalidomide during the susceptible period, over 75 per cent delivered normal babies.[14]

Almost all commonly used anesthetics and pre-medicant drugs are teratogenic in some animal species. However, the applicability of these animal studies to humans has not been determined.

Systemic Medications

ANIMAL STUDIES

Numerous anomalies have been reported after pentobarbital or phenobarbital administration to mice, but not rats or rabbits.[15-17] For example, a single dose of thiamylal caused teratogenic and growth-suppressing defects in the offspring of mice.[16] Chlorpromazine, prochlorperazine, imipramine and amphetamines given to pregnant rats and rabbits have been shown to be teratogenic and produce permanent changes in brain levels of norepinephrine, dopamine, 5-hydroxytryptamine and their metabolites in the offspring.[18-20]

Methadone is teratogenic in mice[21] but not in rats or rabbits.[22] In hamsters the number of abnormal fetuses from females injected with a single dose of diacetylmorphine (heroin), phenazocine, pentazocine, propoxyphene and methadone increased as the maternal dose increased.[23] Morphine and meperidine produced an increase in the number of fetal anomalies only to a certain dose level. With multiple doses of diacetylmorphine and methadone the incidence of anomalies increased further. Curiously, in this study, the narcotic

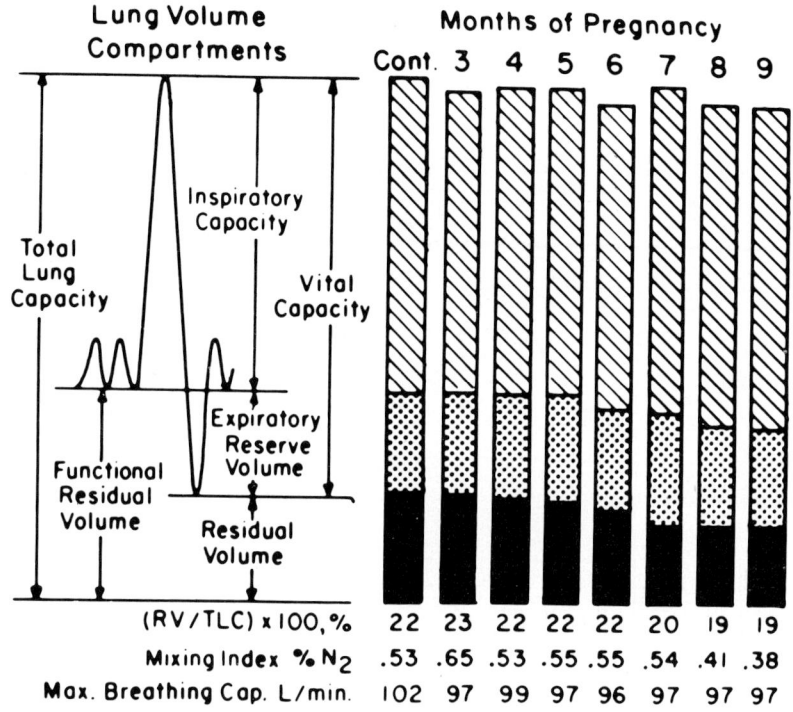

Figure 21.3. Serial measurements of lung compartments, pulmonary mixing index and maximum breathing capacity during normal pregnancy. (Reprinted by permission from Bonica JJ: *Principles and Practice of Obstetric Analgesia and Anesthesia,* vol 1. F. A. Davis, Philadelphia, 1967.)

antagonists nalorphine, naloxone and levallorphan blocked the teratogenic effects. The authors postulate that hypoxia and hypercarbia induced by the unantagonized narcotics may have actually been the teratogens rather than the narcotics per se.

HUMAN STUDIES

Three retrospective studies have suggested an association between ingestion of minor tranquilizers during pregnancy and an increased risk of congenital anomalies.

One study examined the prenatal records of over 19,000 live births to determine the incidence of severe anomalies in children whose mothers had taken either meprobamate (Equanil, Miltown), chlordiazepoxide (Librium), "other drugs" or no drugs.[24] The incidence of anomalies when meprobamate or chlordiazepoxide was prescribed during the first 6 weeks of gestation was significantly higher (12.1 per cent and 11.4 per cent, respectively) than when one of the other drugs (4.6 per cent) or no drug (2.6 per cent) was given. When the tranquilizers were administered later in pregnancy no differences were seen in the incidence of anomalies among the four groups. The study was not controlled for the presence of other risk factors for delivery of a child with congenital anomalies and the findings of chlordiazepoxide were based on only four very different anomalies (duodenal atresia with Meckel's diverticulum, spastic dysplegia with deafness, microcephaly and mental deficiency) and did not reach the 5 per cent level of statistical significance. However, the findings for meprobamate did reach a higher level of significance and, in addition, showed a preponderance of anomalies involving the heart (5 of 8 cases).

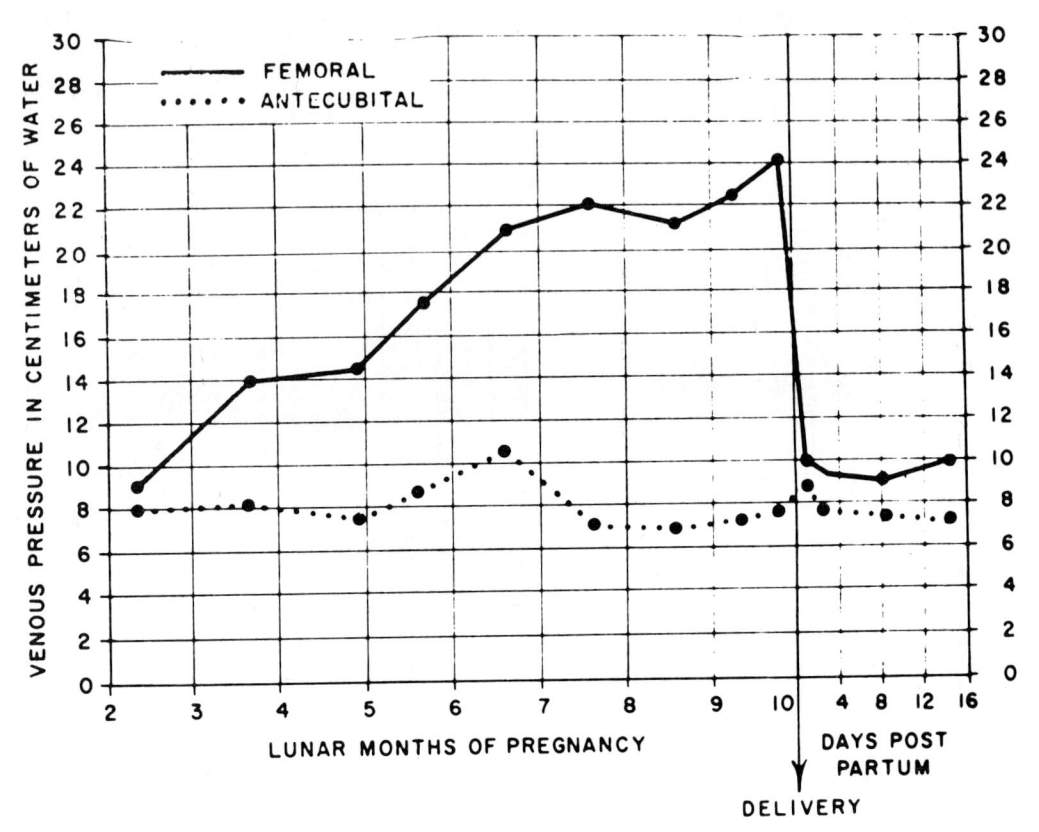

Figure 21.4. Venous pressure during pregnancy in the femoral and antecubital veins. (Reprinted by permission from Bonica JJ: *Principles and Practice of Obstetric Analgesia and Anesthesia,* vol 1. F. A. Davis, Philadelphia, 1967.)

A second study from the Finnish Register of Congenital Malformations (1967 to 1971) reported an association of cleft palate with maternal ingestion of three groups of drugs: tranquilizers (diazepam and meprobamate), salicylates and opiates.[25] The study compared the usage of these drugs during the first trimester in mothers of 590 children with oral clefts and found that intake of these drugs was significantly greater in these mothers than in controls: antianxiety agents—6.2 per cent in study mothers versus 2.9 per cent in control mothers; opiates—6.7 per cent versus 2.2 per cent; and salicylates—14.9 per cent versus 5.6 per cent.

A third study was based on interviews of 278 mothers of children with selected birth defects who had been exposed to a variety of drugs during the first trimester of pregnancy.[26] Mothers of infants with cleft lips with or without cleft palate reported use of diazepam four times more frequently than mothers of infants with other defects.

In contrast to these three studies a fourth investigation failed to find an increased risk of congenital malformation associated with the use of minor tranquilizers during early pregnancy.[27] A total of 50,282 pregnancies were reviewed and the incidence of malformations in 1,870 children exposed in utero to meprobamate or chlordiazepoxide was compared to the incidence in 48,412 unexposed children. No differences in the groups were found.

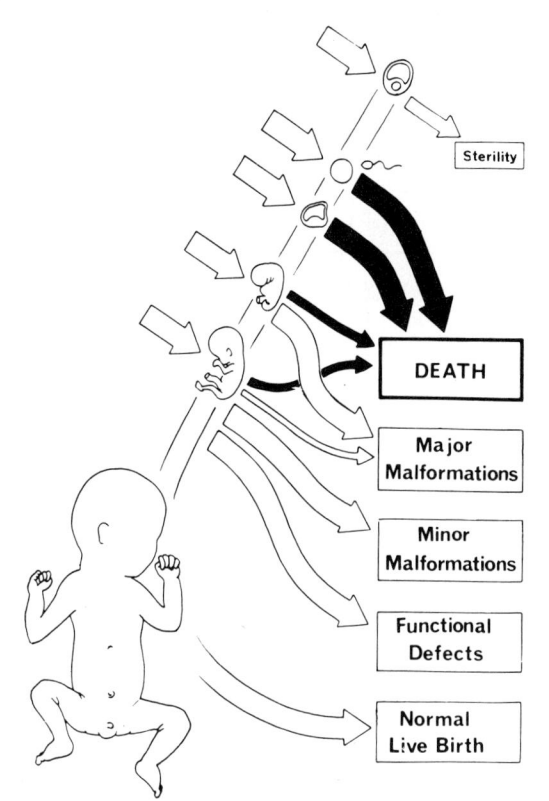

Figure 21.5. Schematic representation of the influence of teratogenic factors on gametogenesis and various stages of embryonic and fetal development. During the preimplantation period strong teratogenic agents kill the embryo. During embryogenesis from day 13 to day 60 teratogenic agents are embryotoxic or produce major congenital malformations. During the following fetal period minor morphologic and functional malformations can be produced. (Reprinted by permission from Tuchmann-Duplessis H: The effects of teratogenic drugs. In *Scientific Foundations of Obstetrics and Gynaecology*, E Phillipp, J Barnes, and M Newton, eds. F. A. Davis, Philadelphia, 1970.)

Nonetheless the Food and Drug Administration (FDA Drug Bulletin September-November 1975) has stated that, "while these data do not provide conclusive evidence that minor tranquilizers cause fetal abnormalities they do suggest an association. Since the use of these drugs during the first trimester of pregnancy is rarely a matter of urgency, benefit-risk considerations are such that their use during this period should almost always be avoided".

Anesthetics

ANIMAL STUDIES

When **nitrous oxide,** 80 per cent, was administered to chicken eggs for the entire course of incubation, only 10 to 20 per cent hatched and these had a high incidence of neurologic defects.[28] The combination of nitrous oxide and mild hypoxia (10 per cent oxygen) for 6 hours produced more anomalies than mild hypoxia alone.[28] When nitrous oxide 50 per cent was administered to pregnant rats for 1 or 2 days a high incidence of intrauterine death and a significant increase in skeletal malformations were found.[29]

Halothane in low concentrations for 12 to 48 hours produced numerous anomalies in rat fetuses.[30] In mice 3 hours of halothane 1.5 per cent markedly increased the incidence of cleft palates and paw defects.[31] In hamsters, 3 hours of halothane 0.6 per cent in mid-gestation increased the number of abortions.[32] Other investigators using rats, rabbits and mice have not shown teratogenic effects of halothane.[33, 34]

Methoxyflurane 0.5 per cent administered for 6 hours to incubating eggs resulted in a high incidence of embryonic deaths and multiple anomalies in the survivors. Methoxyflurane 0.3 per cent given for 3 hours per day for 3 days produced up to a 40 per cent incidence of anomalies.[35]

Diethyl ether, cyclopropane and **fluroxene** have been shown to be teratogenic in chick embryos.[35, 36]

Muscle relaxants do not cross the placenta in significant amounts. **Curare** has been shown to cause musculoskeletal deformities when injected into the incubating chick embryo.[37] Data from other species are not available.

Local anesthetics act by stabilizing cell membranes and conceivably might affect cell mitosis and embryogenesis. These drugs, however, have not been extensively studied. Bupivacaine, etidocaine or prilocaine injected into rats or rabbits have not demonstrated teratogenicity.[38]

HUMAN STUDIES

Large retrospective studies in the United States and Great Britain have suggested that female anesthesiologists and wives of male anesthesiologists have significantly increased rates of spontaneous abortions and their babies are more likely to have congenital defects than the offsprings of non-operating room physicians.[39, 40] In the American study, operating room nurses and nurse anesthetists were also surveyed and also found to have offspring with significantly higher rates of congenital abnormalities.[40] In this study female anesthesiologists working in the operating room had babies with twice the incidence of congenital anomalies as female pediatricians (5.9 versus 3.0 per cent) ($p = 0.07$). Nurse anesthetists working in the operating room had offspring with a higher incidence of anomalies (9.6 per cent) than non-operating room nurses (5.9 per cent) ($p < 0.01$). In addition, there was an increase of 25 per cent in the incidence of anomalies in offspring from wives of male anesthesiologists compared to those of male pediatricians (5.4 versus 4.2 per cent) ($p = 0.04$). Chronic exposure to trace amounts of anesthetic gases or vapors has been suggested as the etiologic factor. Scavenging systems to remove these compounds are currently being introduced into most operating rooms, and future surveys will indicate whether removal of trace con-

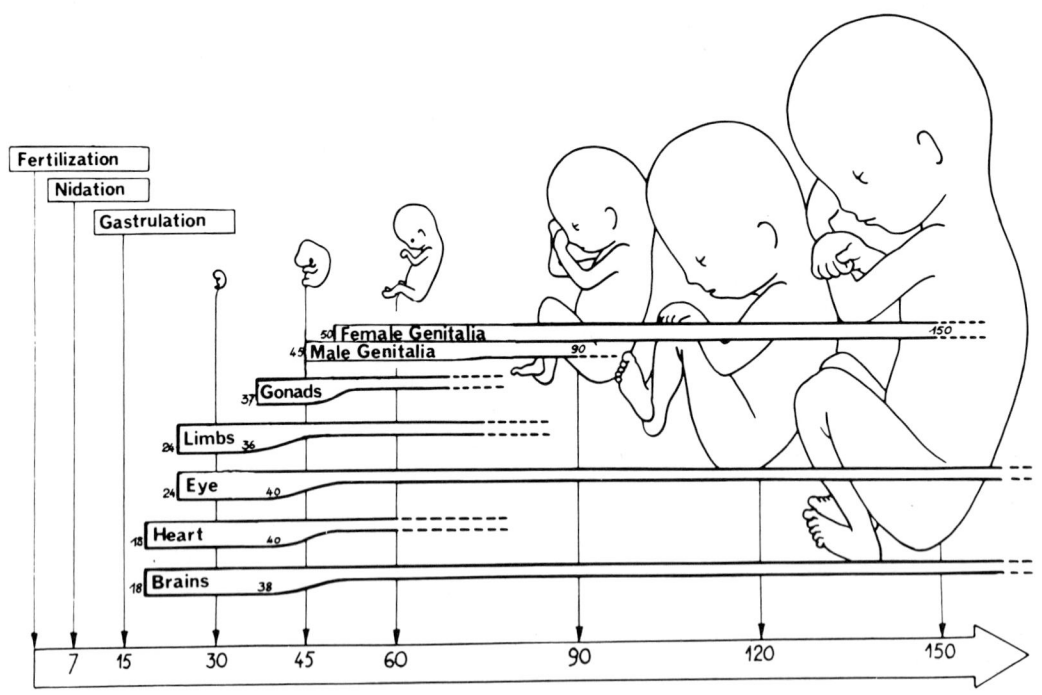

Figure 21.6. Schematic representation of the timing of the morphogenesis of various organs, corresponding to the critical periods of teratogenic susceptibility. (Reprinted by permission from Tuchmann-Duplessis H: The effects of teratogenic drugs. In *Scientific Foundations of Obstetrics and Gynaecology*, E. Philipp, J Barnes, and M. Newton, eds. F. A. Davis, Philadelphia, 1970.)

centrations of drugs has reduced the incidence of abortion and anomalies.

Several surveys of women who had received anesthesia for operations during pregnancy have failed to indict any anesthetic as a teratogen. Smith[2] retrospectively reviewed the neonatal outcomes of 67 women who had undergone surgery during pregnancy. Eleven of these women received an anesthetic during the first trimester. No congenital anomalies were found.

Shnider and Webster[1] reviewed the records of 147 women who received anesthesia for surgery during pregnancy: 47 during the first trimester, 58 during the second and 42 during the third. These women were compared to 8,926 who delivered during this time period. The incidence of congenital anomalies was not significantly different in these groups. These investigators also reviewed the statistics from 61,000 patients who participated in the National Collaborative Study. The incidence of birth defects in women who had not undergone surgery during pregnancy (60,000 women) was 5.02 per cent compared to 6 per cent in the 50 women undergoing appendectomy ($p > 0.05$). In several smaller series the incidence of anomalies with surgery during pregnancy was also not increased.[41-44]

In all studies to date the number of women receiving an anesthetic during their pregnancy is in fact too small to state categorically that anesthetics are not teratogenic. Sullivan[45] has calculated the number of patients that must be exposed to a suspected teratogen in order to prove the drug's teratogenicity. For example, if an anesthetic doubled the incidence of an anomaly such as anencephaly, which has a spontaneous incidence of one per 1,000, then 23,000 women would have to have been exposed to the anesthetic in order to have a statistically significant result.

If, of course, an anesthetic had the teratogenicity of thalidomide, which increases the normal incidence of anomalies by 50,000 to 500,000 times, then a smaller number of anesthetic exposures would demonstrate teratogenicity. Clearly no anesthetic is such a potent teratogen.

Oxygen and Carbon Dioxide

Alterations in arterial blood gases frequently occur under anesthesia. In the experimental animal, hyperoxia, hypoxia and hypercapnia may be teratogenic.

In mice,[46] rabbits,[47] rats[48] and chicks[49] congenital anomalies have been reported after exposure to hypoxia during organogenesis. The possible teratogenicity of hyperoxia is controversial. In hamsters, 100 per cent oxygen at 2 atmospheres pressure for 3 hours, or 3 atmospheres pressure for 2 hours resulted in a significant number of congenital anomalies.[50] These defects included spina bifida, exencephaly and limb defects. Hyperbaric oxygen administered to rabbits during late pregnancy resulted in retrolental fibroplasia, retinal detachment, microphthalmia and stillbirth.[51] Although it is clear from these studies that hyperbaric oxygen is teratogenic, high concentrations of oxygen at normal atmospheric pressure have not been found to be teratogenic in the experimental animal.[52, 53]

Prolonged periods of hypercarbia are associated with congenital anomalies in rats and rabbits. Carbon dioxide 6 per cent and oxygen 20 per cent administered to rats for 24 hours resulted in a high incidence of cardiac anomalies.[54] In rabbits prolonged continuous inhalation of 10 to 13 per cent carbon dioxide resulted in a high incidence of vertebral column malformations.[53]

In humans, brief exposures to hypoxia, hyperoxia, hypercarbia and hypocarbia have not been proven to be teratogenic, although isolated case reports alleging such an association have been published.[55-57] Chronic hypoxemia, as occurs in people living at high altitude, is also not associated with an increased incidence of anomalies.

Maternal Emotional Stress and Trauma

A number of factors that may be encountered in the pregnant patient having surgery have been suggested as being potentially teratogenic. Maternal anxiety and stress,[58-64] maternal immobilization[65] and mechanical trauma—such as falls, blows to the abdomen, automobile accidents and bullet wounds[66-70]—have all been implicated in case reports. The significance of these factors as teratogens is uncertain, as large epidemiologic studies have not been done.

Behavioral Teratology

The term "behavioral teratology" was first used by Werboff and Gottlieb[71] to describe the adverse action of a drug on "the behavior or functional adaptation of the offspring to its environment". Reserpine, chlorpromazine and meprobamate administered to rats produced alterations of behavior in the offspring that persisted during adulthood.[72-75] Other drugs such as bromides,[76] barbiturates[77] and salicylates[78] all impaired maze-learning ability in rat offspring. Recently Smith et al.[79] reported the behavioral effects of halothane in rat offspring. Pregnant female rats were anesthetized with halothane 2.5 per cent for 5 minutes followed by 1.2 per cent for 115 minutes during either the first, second or third trimester. Their offspring were then tested at approximately 75 days post-delivery, which developmentally corresponds to young adulthood in humans. Learning deficits and changes in footshock sensitivity were found in the litters of mothers exposed during the first and second trimesters but not during the third (Figure 21.7).

It seems that in subteratogenic doses some psychoactive compounds produce behavioral deficits while not producing gross morphologic changes. The central nervous system, because of its prolonged period of development—which is not complete at the time of birth—may be susceptible to teratogens over an extended period. It has been alleged that even conventional doses of medications or anesthetics administered during childbirth may produce permanent central nervous system dysfunction in the offspring.[80] These allegations are based on poorly controlled, improperly analyzed studies, but, nevertheless, they are widely quoted. Well designed studies examining the long-range neurobehavioral effects of maternal medication on the offspring are currently under way in several medical centers. At present there is no evidence establishing the validity of the assertion that anesthesia administered to a pregnant woman adversely affects later mental and neurological development of the infant.[81]

Transplacental Carcinogenesis

Concern regarding the potential for anesthetic agents administered to a pregnant woman to induce cancer in her baby is based on a number of observations. Oral administration of large doses of chloroform[82,83] or trichloroethylene[84] produced cancer of the liver or kidney in mice. Halothane has been shown to interfere with the synthesis of DNA[85,86] and may also produce abnormal products of cell division.

Using an in vitro microbial assay system employing two histidine-dependent mutants of **Salmonella typhimurium**,[87] Baden et al.[88,89] showed that fluroxene was mutagenic but that halothane, enflurane, methoxyflurane and isoflurane were not. In the experimental animal more than 30 different chemical compounds have been shown to be capable of inducing cancer in offspring when administered to the mother during gestation.[90] It seems that the fetus is often far more susceptible than the mother to carcinogenic compounds.

In a pilot study, Corbett[91] reported that isoflurane administered to mice during

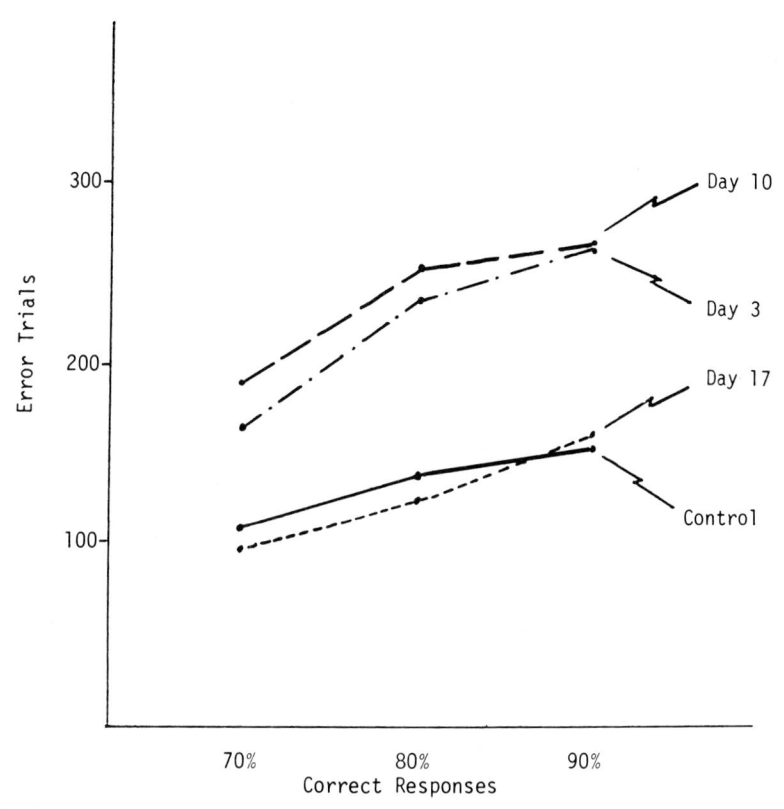

Figure 21.7. Total numbers of error trials on the maze task according to three increasingly difficult criteria. Control animals and animals who had received halothane during the third trimester of gestation behaved similarly. Behavioral abnormalities were seen in animals exposed to halothane during early pregnancy. (Reprinted by permission from Katz J, Smith RF, Bowman RE: Effects of single anesthetic exposure in utero on future nervous system performance. In *Abstracts of Scientific Papers,* Annual Meeting, American Society of Anesthesiologists, San Francisco, 1976, p 148.)

gestation produced hepatic neoplasms in the offspring. Because his studies had methodological flaws (test and control animals were treated differently), the studies were repeated and expanded to include enflurane, halothane, nitrous oxide and methoxyflurane.[92] All treatment and control groups had a similar number of neoplastic lesions. **There was no indication that any anesthetic agent was carcinogenic.**

AVOIDANCE OF INTRAUTERINE FETAL ASPHYXIA

Intrauterine fetal asphyxia is avoided by maintaining normal maternal PaO_2, $PaCO_2$ and uterine blood flow. Fetal oxygenation is directly dependent on maternal arterial oxygen tension, oxygen capacity (hemoglobin content), oxygen affinity and uteroplacental perfusion. Maternal hypoxia will result in fetal hypoxia and, if uncorrected, fetal demise.

Maternal Oxygenation

Common causes of maternal hypoxia during anesthesia for operations during pregnancy as well as during childbirth include laryngospasm, airway obstruction, improperly positioned endotracheal tube, inadequate ventilation and low inspired oxygen in the anesthetic gas mixture.

Common causes of hypoxia during regional anesthesia include severe toxic reactions or excessively high spinal or epidural blocks with maternal hypoventilation. The usual careful anesthetic management should prevent the occurrence or continuation of significant maternal and fetal hypoxia.

Elevated maternal oxygen tensions commonly occur during anesthesia. In studies with isolated preparations of human placental and umbilical vessels, vasoconstriction occurs if high oxygen tensions are administered.[93-95] Therefore, it had been feared that elevated oxygen tensions would decrease utero-placental blood flow and fetal oxygenation. Studies of fetal scalp capillary PO_2, measured by sampling fetal blood[96] or using the transcutaneous oxygen electrode,[97] have shown that increasing maternal PaO_2 will increase fetal PO_2 (Figure 21.8). If the normal placental-fetal circulation has been significantly compromised by conditions such as umbilical cord compression or maternal hypotension, then increasing maternal oxy-

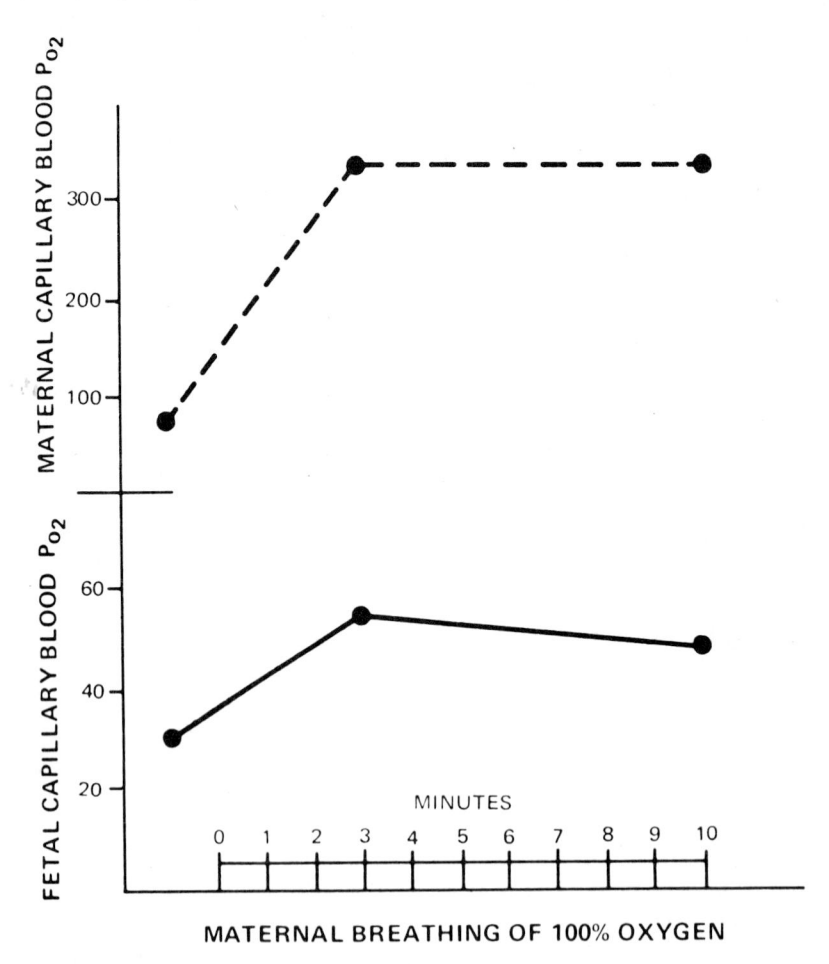

Figure 21.8. Effect of maternal inhalation of 100 per cent oxygen in one case. At 3 and 10 minutes, fetal PO_2 was significantly above the basal level. (Reprinted by permission from Wood C: Use of fetal blood sampling and fetal heart rate monitering, p. 169. In *Diagnosis and Treatment of Fetal Disorders*, K Adamsons, ed. Springer-Verlag, New York, 1968.)

ANESTHESIA FOR OPERATIONS DURING PREGNANCY

genation will not be reflected in the fetus. In no studies has maternal hyperoxia resulted in fetal hypoxia.[96-99]

A rise in maternal PaO₂ even to 600 torr seldom produces a fetal PaO₂ above 45 torr and never above 60 torr. The reasons for this large maternal-fetal oxygen tension gradient are high oxygen consumption of the placenta and uneven distribution of the maternal and fetal blood flow in the placenta. Thus, maternal hyperoxia cannot produce in utero retrolental fibroplasia or premature closure of the ductus arteriosus.

Maternal Carbon Dioxide

Fetal PCO₂ is also directly related to maternal PaCO₂ (Figure 21.9). There is evidence that low maternal PaCO₂ or high maternal pH may be deleterious to the fetus for a number of reasons. Maternal hypocapnea produced by excessive posi-

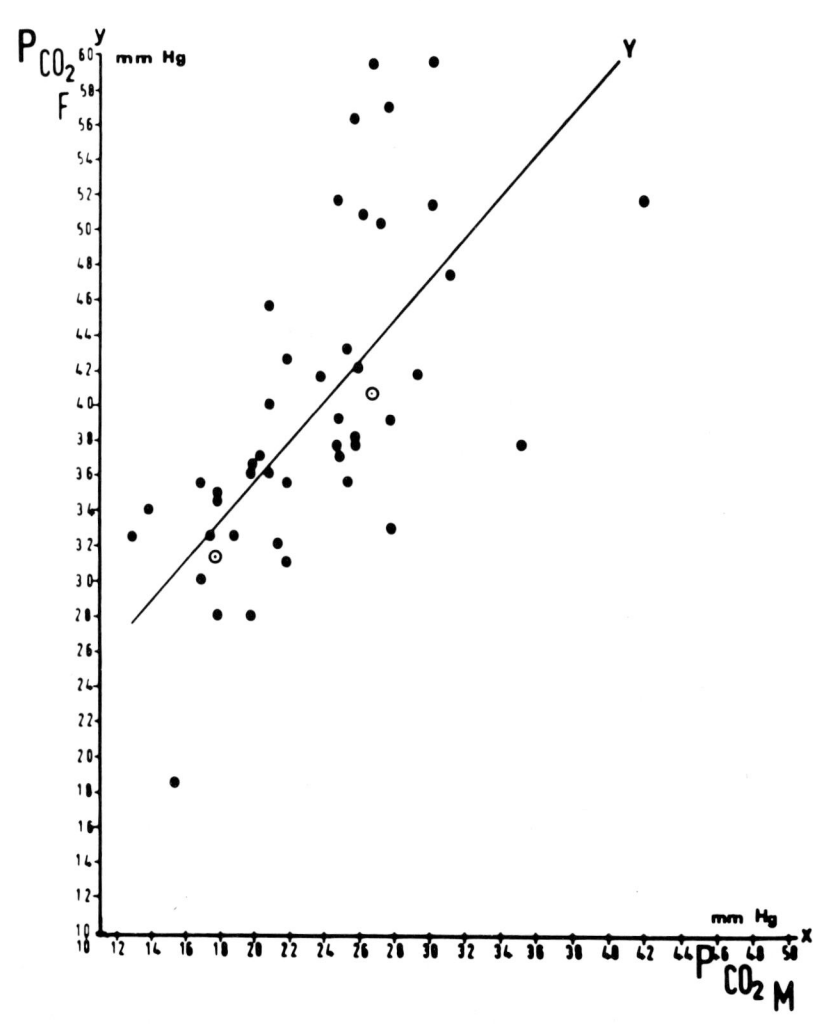

Figure 21.9. Correlation of maternal capillary carbon dioxide tensions with fetal scalp blood carbon dioxide tensions in normal patients. M, maternal; F, fetal. (Reprinted by permission from Lumley J, Wood C: Effect of changes in maternal oxygen and carbon dioxide tensions on the fetus. In *Clinical Anesthesia Parturition and Perinatology,* G Marx, ed, vol 10/2. F. A. Davis, Philadelphia, 1973, p 128.)

tive-pressure ventilation may increase mean intrathoracic pressure, decrease venous return to the heart and lead to a fall in uterine blood flow (Figure 3.12).[100] Maternal respiratory or metabolic alkalosis also decreases umbilical blood flow because of direct vasoconstriction (Figure 21.10).[101] In addition, maternal alkalosis shifts the maternal oxy-hemoglobin dissociation curve to the left, thereby increasing the affinity of maternal hemoglobin for oxygen, resulting in the release of less oxygen to the fetus at the placenta. Thus, fetal hypoxia and metabolic acidosis can occur as a result of maternal hyperventilation during anesthesia.

Maternal hypercapnia, as may occur with spontaneous ventilation and deep levels of anesthesia, will be associated with fetal respiratory acidosis. Moderate elevations of fetal $PaCO_2$ are probably not detrimental, but severe fetal acidosis may produce myocardial depression.

Maternal Hypotension

Maternal hypotension from deep general anesthesia, sympathectomy, hypovolemia or vena caval compression will cause a fall in uterine blood flow and may lead to fetal asphyxia. Hypotension and regional anesthesia have been discussed in chapter 18. With a general anesthetic—for example, halothane—a small fall in blood

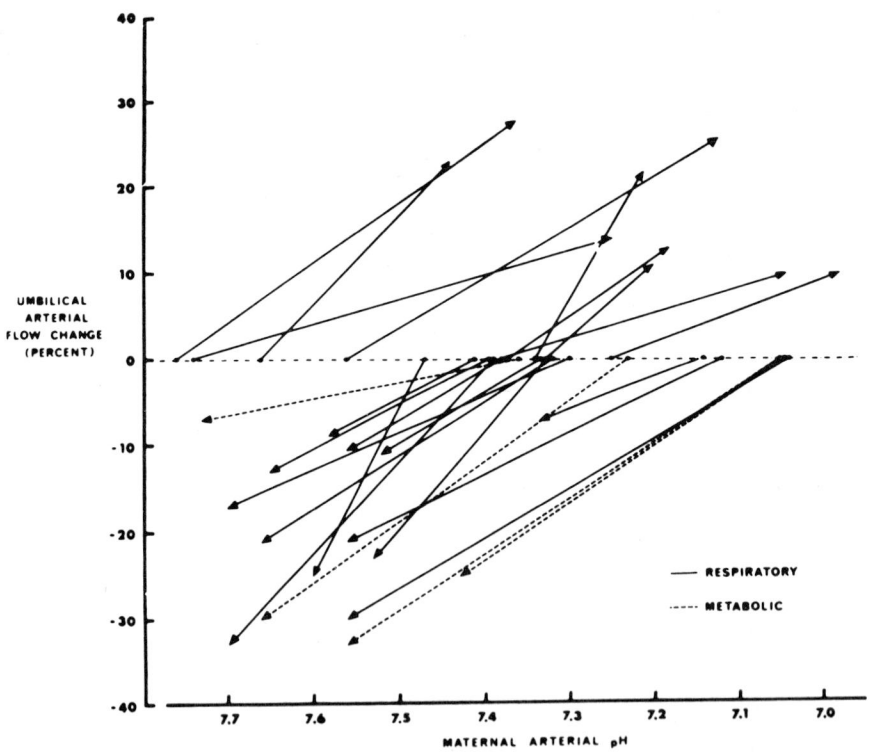

Figure 21.10. Effect of changes in maternal arterial pH on blood flow in one umbilical artery. All changes are expressed as per cent change of initial flow. *Closed circles* and *triangles* represent values before and during changes in maternal pH, respectively. *Solid lines* indicate pH changes produced by respiratory alkalemia and acidemia; *broken lines* indicate pH changes produced by metabolic alkalemia. (Reprinted by permission from Motoyama EK, Rivard G, Acheson F, et al.: The effects of changes in maternal pH and PCO_2 on the PO_2 of fetal lambs. Anesthesiology 28:891, 1967.)

pressure that may occur with light anesthesia is not associated with significant reductions in uterine blood flow because of the concomitant decrease in uterine vascular resistance.[102] Deep levels of halothane anesthesia resulting in significant hypotension (30 to 40 per cent below control) will produce a fall in uterine blood flow and fetal asphyxia. In monkeys, deep halothane anesthesia producing prolonged maternal hypotension to a mean arterial pressure of 40 torr or lower regularly produced fetal asphyxia, brain damage or death.[103] Fetal PaO$_2$ fell from a normal control value of 30 torr to 15 torr, fetal pH fell from 7.30 to 7.10 or lower, fetal bradycardia occurred, and with severe asphyxia (pH 7.0) lasting several hours myocardial failure and fetal death occurred. With less severe asphyxia permanent brain damage occurred with lesions similar to those of human cerebral palsy.

Uterine Vasoconstriction and Hypertonus

Uterine vasoconstriction from endogenous or exogenous sympathomimetics increases uterine vascular resistance and decreases uterine blood flow.[104-106] Sympathetic discharge and adrenal medullary activity may be encountered in the anxious unpre-medicated patient or during light general anesthesia.[107] Vasoactive drugs such as methoxamine, phenylephrine or dopamine will reduce uterine blood flow.[108-111] Systemic absorption of small amounts of epinephrine, as commonly occurs with regional blocks using local anesthetic solutions with epinephrine, may also produce uterine vasoconstriction.[112] Uterine hypertonus is also associated with an increase in uterine vascular resistance and will decrease uterine blood flow. Drugs which increase uterine tone are ketamine in single intravenous doses above 1.1 mg/kg,[113] toxic doses of local anesthetics[114] (Figure 4.4) or α-adrenergic vasopressors.

PREVENTION OF PREMATURE LABOR

Several anecdotal reports have suggested that anesthesia and operations during pregnancy may result in premature labor during the post-operative period.[115-117] In these reports intra-abdominal procedures in which uterine manipulation or retraction was necessary most often resulted in premature labor. Ovarian cystectomy, especially in the first trimester, has a high incidence of abortion. This is not inevitable; in many operations on the ovary, pregnancies have proceeded normally to term. Neurosurgical, orthopaedic, thoracic or plastic surgery procedures were not associated with premature labor. In a review of 147 pregnant patients undergoing surgery, Shnider and Webster[1] reported that 8.8 per cent (13 patients) went into labor shortly after surgery. This incidence was influenced by the number of premature deliveries that occurred after Shirodkar procedures. (A Shirodkar operation is a repair of an incompetent cervix. The primary disease results in premature labor.) In this series 28 per cent of patients undergoing Shirodkar procedures had premature deliveries; in a series reported by Smith[2] 40 per cent of patients had premature labor postoperatively. Therefore, it is apparent that pre-operative pathology plays a prominent role in cases of premature labor.

Whether anesthetics can stimulate or inhibit the onset of premature labor is unknown. There is little information on the effects of anesthesia on oxytocin, prostaglandins, follicular-stimulating hormones, estrogen or progesterone levels in the uterus or blood. Some commonly used anesthetic agents, such as halothane and enflurane, decrease uterine tone and inhibit uterine contractions. On this basis, some have suggested that these agents be used during advanced pregnancy when uterine manipulation is anticipated. However, **in no study has any one anesthetic agent or technique been found to be associated with a higher or lower incidence of premature delivery.**

As previously stated, some anesthetic agents—such as ketamine in doses greater than 1.1 mg/kg—and some vasopressors do increase uterine tone and should probably be avoided when possible. Rapid intravenous injection of anticholinesterase agents, such as neostigmine or edrophonium, may directly stimulate acetylcholine release and theoretically could increase uterine tone and stimulate premature labor. Neostigmine, when used to reverse the effects of muscle relaxants, should be administered slowly and be preceded by adequate doses of atropine.

RECOMMENDATIONS FOR ANESTHETIC MANAGEMENT

1. **Elective surgery** should be deferred until after delivery when the physiologic changes of pregnancy have returned toward normal. Women of childbearing age scheduled for elective surgery should be carefully queried regarding the possibility of pregnancy.

2. **Urgent surgery**—that is, operations that are essential but can be delayed without increasing the risk of permanent disability—should be deferred until the second or third trimester. **At present, no anesthetic drug—pre-medicant, intravenous induction agent, inhalation agent or local anesthetic—has been PROVED to be teratogenic in HUMANS.** However, despite the lack of proof, the authors consider it prudent to minimize or eliminate fetal exposure to drugs during the vulnerable first trimester.

3. **Emergency surgery**—that is, operations that cannot be delayed without increasing maternal morbidity or mortality—may be necessary during the first trimester. They are ideally performed under regional block if the contemplated surgery and maternal condition allow. Teratogenicity of local anesthetics in animals or humans has not been reported.

4. With spinal anesthesia fetal exposure to local anesthetic is much less than with other regional blocks.

5. During the pre-operative visit, great effort should be made to allay maternal anxiety and apprehension. If pharmacologic pre-medication is necessary barbiturates are preferable to minor tranquilizers such as diazepam or meprobamate. Glycopyrrolate, unlike atropine and scopolamine, does not cross the placenta.

6. If general anesthesia is necessary during the first trimester there is no proof that any well conducted technique is superior to any other. The authors believe it is best to choose drugs with a history of safe usage over many years. These include thiopental, succinylcholine, curare, morphine, meperidine, nitrous oxide and halothane. Adequate oxygenation and avoidance of hyperventilation are mandatory.

7. During pregnancy patients may be at increased risk of aspiration, and the usual safeguards to prevent aspiration pneumonitis should be performed.

8. Aortocaval compression during the second and third trimesters should be prevented by avoiding the supine position. Use of the left lateral tilt position should be used whenever possible.

9. Ideally, continuous fetal heart rate monitoring during surgery should be employed after the sixteenth week of gestation. This may provide an indication of abnormalities in maternal ventilation or uterine perfusion (Figure 21.11).

10. Uterine activity should be monitored continuously with an external tocodynamometer during the post-operative period to detect the onset of premature labor.

ANESTHESIA FOR OPERATIONS DURING PREGNANCY

TIME	9:58	10:05	10:32	10:55	13:45
	PRE-INDUCTION	POST-INDUCTION	POST-INCISION	POST-CORRECTION	RECOVERY ROOM
pH			7.25	7.30	7.37
$PaCO_2$ (TORR)			31	28	29
PaO_2 (TORR)			56	382	121
SaO_2			87%	100%	98%
% O_2			50	100	40

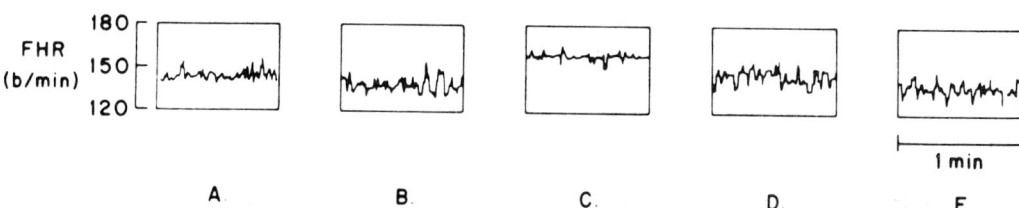

Figure 21.11. Serial samples of fetal heart rate in a patient undergoing eye surgery. *A* and *B*, baseline fetal heart rate at 140 beats per minute with normal beat-to-beat variability. *C*, fetal tachycardia and stabilization of the beat-to-beat interval during inadvertent maternal hypoxemia (maternal PaO_2 = 56 torr). *D*, after correction of maternal ventilation there is a return to baseline fetal heart rate and variability. *E*, normal baseline post-operatively. (Reprinted by permission from Katz JD, Hook R, Barash PG: Fetal heart rate monitoring in pregnant patients undergoing surgery. Am J Obstet Gynecol 125:267, 1976.)

Betamimetic therapy, instituted early, may prevent pre-term delivery.

References

1. Shnider SM, Webster GM: Maternal and fetal hazards of surgery during pregnancy. Am J Obstet Gynecol 92:891, 1965.
2. Smith BE: Fetal prognosis after anesthesia during gestation. Anesth Analg 42:521, 1963.
3. Smith BE: Teratogenic capabilities of surgical anesthesia. Adv Teratol 3:127, 1968.
4. Cugell DW, Frank NR, Gaensler EA, et al.: Pulmonary function in pregnancy. I. Serial observations in normal women. Am Rev Tuberc 67:568, 1953.
5. Prowse CM, Gaensler EA: Respiratory and acid-base changes during pregnancy. Anesthesiology 26:381, 1965.
6. Palahniuk RJ, Shnider SM, Eger El II: Pregnancy decreases the requirement for inhaled anesthetic agents. Anesthesiology 41:82, 1974.
7. Lees MM, Taylor SH, Scott DB et al.: A study of cardiac output at rest throughout pregnancy. J Obstet Gynaecol Br Commonw 74:319, 1967.
8. Lees MM, Scott DB, Kerr MG, et al.: The circulatory effects of recumbent postural changes in late pregnancy. Clin Sci 32:453, 1967.
9. Ueland K, Novy MJ, Peterson EN, et al.: Maternal cardiovascular dynamics. IV. The influence of gestational age on the maternal cardiovascular response to posture and exercise. Am J Obstet Gynecol 104:856, 1969.
10. Pritchard JA: Changes in blood volume during pregnancy and delivery. Anesthesiology 26:393, 1965.
11. Ueland K: Maternal cardiovascular dynamics. VII. Intrapartum blood volume changes. Am J Obstet Gynecol 126:671, 1976.
12. Attia RR, Eberd AM, Fischer JE: Gastrin: Placental, maternal and plasma cord levels, its possible role in maternal residual gastric acidity. In *Abstracts of Scientific Papers*, Annual Meeting, American Society of Anesthesiologists, San Francisco, 1976, p 547.
13. Tuchmann-Duplessis H: Influence of certain drugs on the prenatal development. Int J Gynaecol Obstet 8:777, 1970.
14. Eriksson M, Catz CS, Yaffe SJ: Drugs and pregnancy. Clin Obstet Gynecol 16:199, 1973.
15. Setala K, Nyyssonen O: Hypnotic sodium pentobarbital as a teratogen for mice. Naturwissenschaften 51:413, 1964.
16. Tanimura T: The effect of thiamylal sodium administration to pregnant mice upon the de-

velopment of their offspring. Acta Anat Nippon 40:323, 1965.
17. Goldman AS, Yakovac WC: Prevention of salicylate teratogenicity in immobilized rats by certain central nervous system depressants. Proc Soc Exp Biol Med 115:693, 1964.
18. Roux C: Action tératogène de la prochlorpérazine. Arch Franc Pédiatr 16:968, 1959.
19. Robson JM, Sullivan FM: The production of foetal abnormalities in rabbits by imipramine. Lancet 1:638, 1963.
20. Tonge SR: Permanent alterations in catecholamine concentration in discrete areas of brain in the offspring of rats treated with methylamphetamine and chlorpromazine. Br J Pharmacol 47:425, 1974.
21. Jurand A: Teratogenic activity of methadone hydrochloride in mouse and chick embryos. J Embryol Exp Morphol 30:449, 1973.
22. Markham JK, Emmerson JL, Owen NV: Teratogenicity studies of methadone HCl in rats and rabbits. Nature 233:342, 1971.
23. Geber WF, Schramm LC: Congenital malformations of the central nervous system produced by narcotic analgesics in the hamster. Am J Obstet Gynecol 123:705, 1975.
24. Milkovich L, van den Berg BJ: Effects of prenatal meprobamate and chlordiazepoxide hydrochloride on human embryonic and fetal development. N Engl J Med 291:1268, 1974.
25. Saxén I, Saxén L: Association between maternal intake of diazepam and oral clefts. Lancet 2:498, 1975.
26. Safra MJ, Oakley GP: Association between cleft lip with or without cleft palate and prenatal exposure to diazepam. Lancet 2:478, 1975.
27. Hartz SC, Heinomen OP, Shapiro S, et al.: Antenatal exposure to meprobamate and chlordiazepoxide in relation to malformations, mental development, and childhood mortality. N Engl J Med 292:726, 1975.
28. Smith BE, Gaub MI, Moya F: Teratogenic effects of anesthetic agents: Nitrous oxide. Anaesth Analg 44:726, 1965.
29. Fink BR, Shepard TH, Blandau RJ: Teratogenic activity of nitrous oxide. Nature 214:146, 1967.
30. Basford AB, Fink BR: The teratogenicity of halothane in the rat. Anesthesiology 29:1167, 1968.
31. Smith BE, Usubiaga LE: Lehrer SB: Cleft palate induced by halothane anesthesia in C-57 black mice. Teratology 4:242, 1971.
32. Bussard DA, Stoelting RK, Peterson C, et al.: Fetal changes in hamsters anesthetized with nitrous oxide and halothane. Anesthesiology 41:275, 1974.
33. Kennedy GL, Smith SH, Keplinger ML, et al.: Reproductive and teratologic studies with halothane. Toxicol Appl Pharmacol 35:467, 1976.
34. Warton RS, Mazze RI, Baden JM, et al.: Fertility, reproduction and postnatal survival in mice chronically exposed to halothane. Anesthesiology 48:167, 1978.
35. Smith BE, Gaub MI, Moya F: Investigations into the teratogenic effects of anesthetic agents: The fluorinated agents. Anesthesiology 26:260, 1965.
36. Anderson NB: The teratogenicity of cyclopropane in the chicken. Anesthesiology 29:113, 1968.
37. Drachman DB, Coulombre AJ: Experimental clubfoot and arthrogryposis multiplex congenita. Lancet 2:523, 1962.
38. *Physicians Desk Reference*, ed 32. Medical Economics, Oradell, N J, 1978, pp 581 and 1791.
39. Spence AA, Cohen EN, Brown BW Jr, et al.: Occupational hazards for operating room-based physicians: Analyses of data from the United States and the United Kingdom. JAMA 238:955, 1977.
40. Cohen EN, Brown BW, Bruse DL, et al.: Occupational disease among operating room personnel: A national study. Anesthesiology 41:321, 1974.
41. Lloyd TS: The safety of surgical operations during pregnancy. South Med J 58:179, 1965.
42. Braunwald NS: Personal communication. Cited in Ueland K: Cardiac surgery in pregnancy. Am J Obstet Gynecol 92:148, 1965.
43. Jacobs WM, Cooley D, Goen GP: Cardiac surgery with extracorporeal circulation during pregnancy: Report of 3 cases. Obstet Gynecol 24:167, 1965.
44. Meffert WG, Stansel HC Jr: Open heart surgery during pregnancy. Am J Obstet Gynecol 102:1116, 1968.
45. Sullivan FM: General discussion. Pediatrics 53:798, 1974.
46. Ingalls TH, Curley FJ, Prindle RA: Anoxia as a cause of fetal death and congenital defect in the mouse. Am J Dis Child 80:34, 1960.
47. Degenhardt KH: Durch O_2-Mangel induzierte fehlbildungen der axialgradienten bei kaninchen. Z Naturforsch 9:530, 1954.
48. Haring OM: The effects of prenatal hypoxia on the cardiovascular system in the rat. Arch Pathol 80:351, 1965.
49. Grabowski CT: Teratogenic significance of ionic and fluid imbalance. Science 142:1064, 1963.
50. Ferm BH: Teratogenic effects of hyperbaric oxygen. Proc Soc Exp Biol Med 116:975, 1964.
51. Fujikura T: Retrolental fibroplasia and prematurity in newborn rabbits induced by maternal hyperoxia. Am J Obstet Gynecol 90:854, 1964.
52. Smith BE: Personal communication.
53. Grote W: Storung der Embryonalentwicklung bei erhohtem CO_2-und O_2-Partialdruck und bei Unterdruck. Z Morphol Anthropol 56:165, 1965.
54. Haring OM: Cardiac malformations in rats induced by exposure of the mother to carbon dioxide during pregnancy. Circ Res 8:1218, 1960.
55. Ballabriga A, Samso Dies J, Bado JV: Estudios electro-encefalogradicos sobre la anoxia fetal y neonatal en los animales de experimentacion. Med Clin 3:164, 1957.
56. Pitt DB: A study of congenital malformations. Part II. Aust N Z J Obstet Gynaecol 2:82, 1962.
57. Warkany J, Kalter H: Congenital malformations. N Engl J Med 265:1046, 1961.
58. Abramson JH, Ansuyah RS, Mbambo V: Antenatal stress and the baby's development. Arch Dis Child 36:42, 1961.
59. Davis A, DeVault S, Talmadge M: Anxiety, preg-

nancy and childbirth abnormalities. J Consult Psychol 25:74, 1961.
60. Davids A, DeVault S: Maternal anxiety during pregnancy and childbirth abnormalities. Psychosom Med 24:464, 1962.
61. Crist T, Hulka JF: Influence of maternal epinephrine on behaviour of offspring. Am J Obstet Gynecol 106:687, 1970.
62. Ferreira AJ: Emotional factors in prenatal environment. J Nerv Ment Dis 141:108, 1965.
63. Geber WF: Developmental effects of chronic maternal audiovisual stress on the rat fetus. J Embryol Exp Morphol 16:1, 1966.
64. Geber WF, Anderson TA: Abnormal fetal growth in the albino rat and rabbit induced by maternal stress. Biol Neonate 11:209, 1967.
65. Goldman AS, Yakovac WC: The enhancement of salicylate teratogenicity by maternal immobilization in the rat. J Pharmacol Exp Ther 142:351, 1963.
66. Hinden E: External injury causing foetal deformity. Arch Dis Child 40:80, 1965.
67. Ozan HA, Gonzalez AA: Post-traumatic fetal epilepsy. Neurology 13:541, 1963.
68. Torpin R, Miller GT, Culpepper BW: Amniogenic fetal digital amputations associated with clubfoot. Obstet Gynecol 24:379, 1964.
69. Turner EK: Teratogenic effects of the human foetus through maternal emotional stress: Report of a case. Med J Aust 2:502, 1960.
70. Wiedemann HR: Schadigungen der frucht in der schwangerschaft. Med Monatsschr 9:141, 1955.
71. Werboff J, Gottlieb JS: Drugs in pregnancy: Behavioral teratology. Obstet Gynecol Surv 18:420, 1963.
72. Werboff J: Effects of prenatal administration of tranquilizers on maze learning ability. Am Psychol 17:397, 1962.
73. Hoffield DR, McNew J, Webster RL: Effect of tranquillizing drugs during pregnancy on activity of offspring. Nature 218:357, 1968.
74. Clarke CVH, Gorman D, Vernadakis A: Effects of prenatal administration of psychotropic drugs on behavior of developing rats. Dev Psychobiol 3:225, 1970.
75. Young RD: Effects of differential early experiences and neonatal tranquillisation on later behavior. Psychol Rep 17:675, 1965.
76. Harned BK, Hamilton HC, Cole BB: The effect of administration of sodium bromide to pregnant rats on the learning ability of the offspring. II Maze test. J Pharmacol Exp Ther 82:215, 1974.
77. Armitage SG: The effects of barbiturate on the behavior of rat offspring as measured on learning and reasoning situations. J Comp Physiol Psychol 45:146, 1952.
78. Butcher RE, Voorhees CV, Kimmel CA: Learning impairment from maternal salycylate treatment in rats. Nature New Biol 236:211, 1972.
79. Smith RF, Bowman RE, Katz J: Behavioral effects of exposure to halothane during early development in the rat: Sensitive period during pregnancy. Anesthesiology 49:319, 1978.
80. Kolata GB: Behavioral teratology: Birth defects of the mind. Science 202:732, 1978.
81. Committee on Drugs of the American Academy of Pediatrics and the Committee on Obstetrics: Maternal anf Fetal Medicine of the American College of Obstetricians and Gynecologists: Effect of medication during labor and delivery on infant outcome. Pediatrics 62:402, 1978.
82. Eschenbrenner AB, Miller E: Induction of hepatomas in mice by repeated oral administration of chloroform with observations on sex differences. J Natl Cancer Inst 5:251, 1945.
83. Report of Carcinogenesis Bioassay of Chloroform. Carcinogenesis Program, Division of Cancer Cause and Prevention. National Cancer Institute, Bethesda, 1976.
84. Carcinogenesis: Bioassay of trichloroethylene CAS No. 90-01-6, NCI-CG-TR-Z, National Cancer Institute, Bethesda, February, 1976.
85. Jackson SH: The metabolic effect of halothane on mammalian hepatoma cells in vitro. II. Inhibition of DNA synthesis. Anesthesiology 39:405, 1973.
86. Sturrock J, Nunn JF: Effects of halothane on DNA synthesis and the presynthetic phase (G1) in dividing fibroblasts. Anesthesiology 45:413, 1976.
87. Ames BN: The detection of chemical mutagens with enteric bacteria. In *Chemical Mutagens: Principles and Methods for Their Detection*, A Hollaender, ed. Plenum Publishing Corp., New York, 1971, p 267.
88. Baden JM, Brinkenhoff BS, Wharton RS, et al.: Mutagenicity of volatile anesthetics: Halothane. Anesthesiology 45:311, 1976.
89. Baden JM, Kelley M, Wharton RS, et al.: Mutagenicity of halogenated ether anesthetics. Anesthesiology 46:346, 1977.
90. Tomatis L: Transplacental carcinogenesis. In *Modern Trends in Oncology*. RW Raven, ed. Butterworths, London, 1973, p 99.
91. Corbett TH: Cancer and congenital anomalies associated with anesthetics. Ann NY Acad Sci 271:58, 1976.
92. Eger EI II, White AE, Brown CL: A test of carcinogenicity of enflurane, isoflurane, halothane, methoxyflurane, and nitrous oxide in mice. Anesth Analg 57:678, 1978.
93. Nyberg R, Westin B: The influence of oxygen tension and some drugs on human placental vessels. Acta Physiol Scand 39:216, 1957.
94. Panigel M: Placental perfusion experiments. Am J Obstet Gynecol 84:1664, 1962.
95. Tominaga T, Page EW: Accommodation of the human placenta to hypoxia. Am J Obstet Gynecol 94:687, 1966.
96. Khazin AF, Hon EH, Hehre FW: Effects of maternal hyperoxia on the fetus. I. Oxygen tension. Am J Obstet Gynecol 109:628, 1971.
97. Walker A, Madderin L, Day E, et al.: Fetal scalp tissue oxygen measurements in relation to maternal dermal oxygen tension and fetal heart rate. J Obstet Gynaecol Br Commonw 78:1, 1971.
98. Neuman W, McKinnon L, Phillips L, et al.: Oxygen transfer from mother to fetus during labor. Am J Obstet Gynecol 99:61, 1967.
99. Gare DJ, Shime J, Paul WM, et al.: Oxygen

administration during labor. Am J Obstet Gynecol 105:954, 1969.
100. Levinson G, Shnider SM, de Lorimier AA, et al.: Effects of maternal hyperventilation on uterine blood flow and fetal oxygenation and acid-base status. Anesthesiology 40:340, 1974.
101. Motoyama EK, Rivard G, Acheson F, et al.: The effect of changes in maternal pH and PCO_2 on the PO_2 of fetal lambs. Anesthesiology 28:891, 1967.
102. Palahniuk RJ, Shnider SM: Maternal and fetal cardiovascular and acid-base changes during halothane and isoflurane anesthesia in the pregnant ewe. Anesthesiology 41:462, 1974.
103. Brann AW, Myers RE: Central nervous system finding in the newborn monkey following severe *in utero* partial asphyxia. Neurology 25:327, 1975.
104. Adamsons K, Mueller-Heubach E, Myers RE: Production of fetal asphyxia in the rhesus monkey by administration of catecholamines to the mother. Am J Obstet Gynecol 109:148, 1971.
105. Rosenfeld CR, Baron MD, Meschia G: Effects of epinephrine on distribution of blood flow in the pregnant ewe. Am J Obstet Gynecol 124:156, 1976.
106. Shnider SM, Wright RG, Levinson G, et al.: Uterine blood flow and plasma norepinephrine changes during maternal stress in the pregnant ewe. Anesthesiology 50:30, 1979.
107. Shnider SM, Wright RG, Levinson G, et al.: Plasma norepinephrine and uterine blood flow changes during endotracheal intubation and general anesthesia in the pregnant ewe. In *Abstracts of Scientific Papers,* Annual Meeting, American Society of Anesthesiologists, Chicago, 1978, p 115.
108. James FM III, Greiss FC Jr, Kemp RA: An evaluation of vasopressor therapy for maternal hypotension during spinal anesthesia. Anesthesiology 33:25, 1970.
109. Shnider SM, de Lorimier AA, Asling JH, et al.: Vasopressors in obstetrics. II. Fetal hazards of methoxamine administration during obstetric spinal anesthesia. Am J Obstet Gynecol 106:680, 1970.
110. Ralston DH, Shnider SM, de Lorimier AA: Effects of equipotent ephedrine, metaraminol, mephentermine and methoxamine on uterine blood flow in the pregnant ewe. Anesthesiology 40:354, 1974.
111. Callender K, Levinson G, Shnider SM, et al.: Dopamine administration in the normotensive pregnant ewe. Obstet Gynecol 51:586, 1978.
112. Wallis KL, Shnider SM, Hicks JS, et al.: Epidural anesthesia in the normotensive pregnant ewe: Effects on uterine blood flow and fetal acid-base status. Anesthesiology 44:481, 1976.
113. Galloon S: Ketamine for obstetric delivery. Anesthesiology 44:522, 1976.
114. Greiss FC Jr, Still J, Anderson SG: Effects of local anesthetics on the uterine vasculatures and myometrium. Am J Obstet Gynecol 124:895, 1976.
115. Levine W, Diamond B: Surgical procedures during pregnancy. Am J Obstet Gynecol 81:1046, 1961.
116. Bronstein ES, Friedman M: Acute appendicitis in pregnancy. Am J Obstet Gynecol 86:514, 1963.
117. Bassett JW: Appendicitis in pregnancy. Am J Obstet Gynecol 82:828, 1961.
118. Katz JD, Hook R, Barash PG: Fetal heart rate monitoring in pregnant patients undergoing surgery. Am J Obstet Gynecol 125:267, 1976.

CHAPTER 22

Obstetric Anesthesia and Lawsuits

David Karp, M.A.
Marrs Craddick, LL.B., J.D.

With some exceptions, malpractice law suits against anesthesiologists usually involve catastrophic injuries, including cardiac arrest and death, brain damage, paralysis and infection. Anesthesiology is clearly one of the highest risk specialties for liability insurance, and understandably so. No other specialty in medicine asks the physician to render a patient unconscious and insensate, in a physical state still barely understood by medical science, to keep the patient suspended and stable while the surgeon or obstetrician performs his operation, and then to return the patient to consciousness without ill effect. There is an ever-present risk of injury to patients undergoing anesthesia because of the unknown and infinitely variable responses of each patient's body. In obstetric anesthesia, there is an added risk of injury to the fetus or newborn which the anesthesiologist must anticipate and avoid. Actual injury to a patient caused by the mismanagement of anesthesia is infrequent when measured against the total number of local and general anesthetics given each year in this country. However, because of the severity of the injuries associated with anesthesia, it is not surprising that many of the highest malpractice verdicts involve anesthetic complications.

PHYSICIAN-PATIENT RELATIONSHIP

Due to the nature of his specialty, there are two considerable disadvantages with which the anesthesiologist is burdened, when compared to a surgeon or obstetrician, which increase his chances of being sued. First, the anesthesiologist generally has only a short-term and superficial personal contact with the patient. Aside from brief periods during the pre-anesthesia interview, in the operating or delivery room or later on in the recovery room, the anesthesiologist's relationship with his patient ordinarily is a silent one. Second, the anesthesiologist seldom has an opportunity to personally correct a problem which may have resulted from anesthesia. If surgery is unsuccessful, the surgeon may be able to redo the operation and maintain rapport with the patient. The anesthesiologist, on the other hand, seldom has the opportunity himself to treat his patient for injuries related to anesthesia, but must rely on others to do so. As a consequence, his patient may be inclined to regard a complication from anesthesia with an attitude more critical than might have been the case had she known her doctor better.

The obstetric anesthesiologist frequently has the opportunity to broaden his communication with his patient during labor while administering epidural or caudal anesthesia. The anesthesiologist is more than a consultant to the surgeon, more than an assistant at delivery or during an operation, and his contacts with the patient can be improved if he makes a greater effort to establish an independent relationship. Many anesthesiologists now consider it a part of their treatment to make at least one post-operative visit to the patient's room to learn if there are any problems which might have resulted from anesthesia, such as damage to teeth secondary to intubation, sore throat, back pain or other complaints. In this brief visit, the anesthesiologist can reassure the patient and, when applicable, decide whether specific treatment for a complaint is necessary. The visit should be documented in the chart, and recommendations for treatment should be coordinated with the obstetrician. When problems do exist, a second visit, demonstrating the anesthesiologist's concern, may help to strengthen his rapport with the patient even more.

CAPTAIN OF THE SHIP DOCTRINE INAPPLICABLE

The captain of the ship doctrine, under which surgeons or obstetricians could be considered liable for the conduct of all members of the surgical or obstetric team, including the physician-anesthesiologist, does not apply in situations when injury occurs solely as a consequence of the anesthesiologist's professional negligence. The anesthesiologist's independent expertise in his field makes him a co-equal member of the obstetric team, and the obstetrician is ordinarily responsible only for his own decisions. It is anticipated that the obstetrician will consult with the anesthesiologist on matters outside the obstetrician's scope of expertise, and the law takes cognizance of the fact that an obstetrician has to rely on the anesthesiologist to make major decisions concerning choice of anesthetic agent, monitoring vital signs during surgery and delivery and administering peri-anesthetic drugs. Therefore, because the obstetrician is entitled to rely on the judgment of the anesthesiologist in matters relating to anesthesia, he is not liable if it is the judgment of the anesthesiologist which is defective; only the anesthesiologist would be liable in such a case. Nevertheless, some plaintiffs' attorneys believe they are protecting their clients' interests by suing all persons present during a surgery even though it is apparent that some may not be liable. For this reason, an obstetrician may sometimes be sued as a defendant in a law suit in which an anesthesiologist, a co-defendant, is the actual target, and vice versa.

In cases in which the actual cause of injury to the patient is not easily identifiable, such as post-operative infections, adverse reaction to a drug or anesthetic agent, perinatal injuries of the newborn or idiopathic complications, the anesthesiologist is likely to be included in the law suit along with the obstetrician and virtually all members of the operating or delivery team. It is often only through the discovery process in litigation that the actual cause of injury can be determined and the person responsible identified.

RESOLUTION OF THE LITIGATION

It is a mistake to assume, as many doctors do, that judges and juries are unfavorably disposed toward physicians in malpractice actions. Although everyone has heard or read about large verdicts rendered in malpractice cases, the overwhelming majority of actions tried in court against doctors and other health care providers end with vindication of the defendant. Defense verdicts, however, are not newsworthy, and are rarely publicized. On the other hand, awards of large sums of money to the plantiff have news value and are publicized, thus, perhaps, creating an erroneous impression in the public mind that physicians are losing more often in court than actually is the case. Past experience has been that doctors win against their patients in a very large majority of the law suits. An over-all analysis of suits closed between 1960 and 1973 by the American Mutual Insurance Company in northern California indicated that 42 per cent of the law suits against its insureds were dismissed, 34.1 per cent were settled, 20.4 per cent were tried in court and resulted in defense verdicts, and 3.5 per cent resulted in a plaintiff's verdict.[1]

A more recent study, published by the National Association of Insurance Commissioners (N.A.I.C.) in May, 1977, summarized claims experience nationwide. The N.A.I.C. Closed Claim Study examined 24,158 claims and found that the plaintiff won only 20 per cent of the trials, whereas defendant-doctors won 80 per cent. It is interesting to note that only about 10 per cent of all the claims reported in the N.A.I.C. study were disposed of by trial, binding arbitration or a review panel. Almost 22,000 cases were disposed of in some other manner, with favorable results for the plaintiff in 36 per cent of these cases and favorable results for the doctor-defendant in 64 per cent of the cases.[2]

The California Board of Medical Quality Assurance reported that in 1977 the number of malpractice awards against physicians declined by 10 per cent, but that the amount of awards (on the average) increased 30 per cent over the previous year.[3]

Some of the reasons for the success of the defendant-doctors, which is expected to continue in the future, are that it is recognized in the law applicable to physicians that medicine is not an exact science and that human judgment, which is fallible and also variable, is involved to such an extent that it is difficult to establish clearly in some cases that the judgment exercised by an individual physician was wrong. A trial juror usually is a person who has in his past experience always been satisfied with and grateful for services rendered to himself and to his family by a member or members of the medical profession. In addition, the legal representation of members of the medical profession involved with malpractice litigation usually is conducted by experienced trial attorneys who are themselves specialists in litigation of this type and who thoroughly familiarize themselves with medical issues in individual cases and know the applicable law. Moreover, when a jury does impose liability on a member of the medical profession, it is not usually because the jury was confused or because they acted on whim. With rare exceptions, there has been testimony by members of the medical profession given at the trial which has supported the finding of the jury which has voted to impose liability on a physician or physicians.

Whatever the reason for which a doctor has been sued, the final determination of his culpability or lack of it will depend on a determination being made, usually by a jury, whether he followed or failed to follow the **standards of care** for his specialty. Many factors which can affect this determination—e.g. the credibility of witnesses, the weight of evidence, the demeanor of the defendant and the issue of proximate cause (the relationship between the treatment rendered or omitted and the injury)—are considered by the jury, or in arbitration cases by the arbitrator, in reaching a verdict, but it is this determination, i.e. whether the defendant adhered to applicable standards of care, which is the crux of the case.

The main controversy between the opposing parties in a law suit which involves allegations of medical malpractice usually arises from their conflicting efforts to identify and to specify standards (i.e. requirements) of practice which were applicable to the defendant-physician during the period of time that he provided professional services to the patient who subsequently brought the law suit against him. Once the jury has determined what standard applied, which is often very difficult for them to do, it is usually a relatively easier task for them to decide whether the conduct of the defendant conformed to the standard. The rules of law which define the duties of the jurors and the methods they must follow in their efforts to determine the standard which applied have crucial importance and should be fully understood by every member of the medical profession, although experience suggests that this is hardly the case.

DEFINING STANDARDS OF PRACTICE

The law itself is sympathetic to physicians; this circumstance has given rise to constant criticism from members of the Bar who represent patients who desire to sue their doctors. **The law recognizes that physicians must make judgments and that all human judgment is fallible.** Therefore, liability is not imposed for mere error in judgment, but rather only for conduct constituting a **departure from standard practice** which results in injury to a patient. The law defers to physicians themselves to identify and to define the standards of their profession. The law does not prescribe, much less dictate, to members of the medical profession how injuries and illnesses of patients are to be treated. The *only* evidence that may be taken in court regarding the existence of a standard of practice in the community applicable to a given set of circumstances involving a physician-patient relationship is the opinion of a knowledgeable physician who gives testimony in court relevant to the subject. The function of the jury is restricted and they are not permitted to set up an arbitrary standard of their own to be applied to the conduct of physicians. Their function is limited to weighing and considering the testimony given by members of the medical profession in their effort to determine what was or was not required of the defendant-physician by applicable standards of practice in the medical community.

It is recognized that medicine is not an exact science and that physicians and surgeons can and do differ with each other regarding treatment for particular problems. There is no limit set in the law regarding the number of different approaches to treatment of any given problem which would be acceptable. The only requirement is that any given approach to treatment, to be acceptable, must be supported by physicians in good standing in the community. Neither does the law prescribe the number of physicians who must support a given approach in order to qualify that particular approach as one of the methods accepted in the community.

The inquiry of a jury in a malpractice case, therefore, is required to be directed toward a determination of whether the method or approach selected by the individual defendant-physician under the circumstances of the case presented was one accepted at least by some, even if not by all, physicians in good standing in the community. If it was, then it is there that the inquiry ends and the physician has a complete defense to a charge that he departed from standard practice. It is not relevant to continue the inquiry to see what type of result was obtained from treatment selected by the defendant. It may well be that, viewed in the light of later events, a different method of treatment should have been chosen or that a method other than the one selected by the defendants would have been better suited to bring about the result desired from treatment. Hindsight, however, is not the test, and the judgment of the defendant-physician is to be evaluated on the basis of what was presented to him at the time it was made and not on the basis of how things turned out subsequently.

EFFECT OF COMPARATIVE NEGLIGENCE DOCTRINE

Some states have adopted the concept of comparative negligence in adjudicating personal injury law suits. This doctrine permits a jury to apportion damages based on the degree of negligence, if any, among all parties (including the plaintiff), which contributed to the injury. Thus, although there is still a risk that the anesthesiologist may be included in a law suit based on an injury which is clearly not related to his administration of anesthesia, hopefully, through the concepts of comparative negligence and equitable apportionment of damages, his minimal responsibility for causation of negligent injury will be reflected in an assessment of damages which is minimal, if any.

In some states, the concept of joint and several liability applied in malpractice cases can lead to a judgment against both the obstetrician and the anesthesiologist for which each is equally liable even though the fault of one or the other may be minimal.

PREVENTING THE LAWSUIT

Adhere to Standards of Care

From the cases in which issues involving the practice of anesthesia have been judicially decided, some basic guidelines have emerged. Some of these minimum practice requirements are:

1. Conduct a pre-anesthetic interview and examination of the patient. How extensive an interview and examination depends on how much information the patient needs in order to give her informed consent (see below) and how much the doctor needs to know in order to be prepared to handle problems which might reasonably be expected to occur in view of the history and findings.

2. Review the medical chart for the current surgery and, when available and relevant, the charts for prior surgeries.

3. Record the review of history, findings and proposed anesthetic management in the patient's chart. Charting such data is imperative, because studies show many patients cannot recall pre-operative discussions with the anesthesiologist.

4. Consult, as appropriate, with the surgeon and, as needed, with other specialists.

5. Discuss the risks and hazards of anesthesia with the patient so that she can freely give her consent to be anesthetized.

The required minimums itemized above seem from the authors' standpoint to be nearly universal in the practice of anesthesia. When it comes to evaluating the effort of a physician to fulfill these and other requirements of anesthetic practice, the law is flexible and indulgent. In general, the level of proficiency required of the anesthesiologist is that of other anesthesiologists in the community, or a similar community, who have **average** training and skill. The proficiency of the exceptional or gifted anesthesiologist is not used as a guideline in determining the standard of performance required by law. Although the anesthesiologist himself may not be satisfied to aspire only to practice average medicine, the law requires no more; if the anesthesiologist demonstrates proficiency at the level which is average for the community, he has a defense to a charge of negligence. It must be kept in mind, however, that standards of competence change, and, through educational seminars, continuing education programs and medical literature, the anesthesiologist should keep abreast of what is being done by his colleagues.

Monitor the Patient

The types of malpractice suits which have more than any other, called attention to the anesthesiologist are cardiac arrest cases and cases in which the patient has suffered brain injury secondary to hypoxia or anoxia. It is commonly accepted among anesthesiologists that such complications can occur in the hands of the most proficient and attentive anesthesiologist and that medical science has not yet perfected methods by which the physician can anticipate or even identify all of the reasons why a patient might arrest or become hypoxic under the administration of a "routine" anesthetic. Therefore, the emphasis among anesthesiologists has been to develop methods for detecting these problems so that they can be reversed before injury to the patient occurs.

Monitoring the patient during anesthesia has in the past been a controversial subject. The number and types of monitors acceptable to anesthesiologists as a group have been the subject of considerable debate, especially in states where many large awards in malpractice cases have been rendered against anesthesiologists for failure to monitor or for inadequate monitoring, rather than for acts which might be described as negligent. The standards for monitoring during anesthesia vary throughout the country, and it is still possible to find reputable anesthesiologists who would attempt to defend digital pulse monitoring and the lack of continuous and electronic pulse monitoring as accepted in the community as standard practice. There are indications, however, that juries, exercising common sense rather than technical knowledge, are less willing to accept what some physicians say is the standard in this regard. Because most anesthesiologists agree that hypoxia or anoxia can exist for up to 4 minutes in most cases without injury to the patient and that continuous monitoring increases the anesthesiologist's chances of detecting a problem before injury occurs during this 4-minute period, it is apparent why a jury might conclude that, if continuous monitoring is not standard, it should be. Obviously if it can be argued that continuous monitoring provides greater protection for the patient, anesthesiologists will be hard pressed to defend decisions not to monitor, except perhaps in emergencies.

Obtain an Informed Consent

Few issues in the realm of malpractice litigation have angered and confused physicians as has the "doctrine of informed consent." The product of a series of appellate court decisions, the doctrine of informed consent deals with the questions of how much information a patient needs to receive in order to be sufficiently informed before consenting to proposed surgery or treatment and how much information can be given to the patient without frightening her and making her a greater anesthetic risk. At present, the law in several states generally provides that, as an integral part of the physician's over-all obligation to the patient, there is a duty of reasonable disclosure of the available options with respect to proposed therapy or surgery and of the dangers inherently and potentially involved in each.

The purpose of the law can be simply stated. A physician who recommends a particular course of therapy for his patient always has in mind the benefits which he hopes will be achieved. In seeking the patient's consent for the treatment, fairness demands that the patient be informed of both the contemplated benefits and potential risks so that she can make a knowledgeable decision as to whether for her the benefits outweigh the risks. All information which might reasonably affect her decision should be provided to the patient. The requirement of disclosure has been judicially qualified, however, by acknowledgment that the patient's interest in information does not extend to a lengthy polysyllabic discourse of all possible complications and by recognition that in electing a procedure the patient is most concerned with the risk of death or serious bodily injury.

When required to adjudicate a claim by a patient that she did not give an informed consent, the jury ordinarily is instructed by the judge that a physician must advise his patient of the potential of death or serious harm, if it exists, explain in lay terms the complications which might possibly occur and provide any additional information which would be provided by reputable physicians in the community under similar circumstances. The jury is further instructed that the plaintiff must then prove that, had she been so advised, a reasonable person in the patient's position would have refused the proposed surgery or treatment. In cases in which the sole issue involves informed consent and the evidence indicates that the medical treatment administered to the patient was appropriate, experience has shown that juries generally conclude that a reasonable person, who was adequately informed, would have consented to the proposed procedure.

In anesthesiology, the physician's duty to disclose risks to the patient does not extend to reviewing the choices for anesthetic agents, because the patient is not expected to understand the pharmacologic variations of anesthetic agents. But a disclosure of the relevant types of anesthesia and the known general risks, including death, paralysis, infection and idiopathic encephalopathy, cannot be withheld from the patient, except when the patient is in no condition to withstand or understand such disclosure, when she requests that she not be so advised or when there is no opportunity for the physician to make the disclosure, such as in emergencies.

The prudent anesthesiologist can probably discharge his professional obligations to the patient and comply with the requirements of the law by:

1. Discussing his choice of anesthetic agent and techniques with the patient and his general reasons for the selection.

2. Advising the patient that the administration of any anesthesia involves some risks.

3. Inquiring whether the patient wishes to know the risks of the anesthesia planned. If the patient states she wishes to know the risks, the anesthesiologist should tell the patient the most common complications—such as sore throat, transient backache, hypotension, headache when applicable—as well as rare complications—including death, paralysis, infection and any other apparent problems which a particular patient may be at risk for—bearing in mind that the purpose is to adequately inform the patient and not to frighten her. At the end of the discussion questions should be elicited and answered and the fact and nature of the conversation should be charted with an entry which indicates "Major and minor risks discussed; questions answered; patient consents." Some patients prefer not to know the risks of anesthesia; if the patient declines the discussion, the chart should be noted: "Patient declines discussion of risks." Discussions of risks for incompetent patients should be held with a spouse or next of kin, who will probably be the person who authorizes the surgery or treatment. In those cases in which no next of kin or responsible party is available and

the physician believes the patient is not in suitable condition to discuss the risks, the physician may elect to forego such discussion but should list his reasons for doing so in the patient's chart. Used *judiciously and fairly,* this approach has been held acceptable by the courts.

Although the patient should be afforded the opportunity to make an informed decision, she should not be permitted to dictate medical decisions to the physicians or to force the physician to render or fail to render treatment he deems is advisable based on his professional judgment. If the patient's dictates are contrary to good medical practice, the physician would be well advised to encourage the patient to find another doctor. It is doubtful that the anesthesiologist who agrees to administer a local anesthetic for a procedure for which a general anesthetic would clearly provide better protection against injury to the patient will be able later to fashion a successful defense that the type of anesthetic, although contrary to his best medical judgment, was the choice of the patient. Where either method is considered reasonable and acceptable, however, the anesthesiologist should impart to the patient the reasons for his recommendation and document the reasons if his first choice is not accepted by the patient.

Maintain Equipment and Medical Records

The anesthesiologist has the responsibility for determining that all equipment related to the administration of anesthesia is in proper working order prior to and during the surgery. Equipment, whether owned by the hospital or the physician, should be regularly serviced and a service record maintained. The selection of equipment is left to the anesthesiologist, and the law does not require that a hospital (or private contractor-physician) select one piece of machinery over another. However, some older equipment may be less helpful to the doctor in detecting anesthetic problems and may impose a greater burden for attentiveness on the doctor. The task of testing all parts of the equipment should not be delegated to a nonphysician, because calibrations for warning devices and gas flow indicators should be attuned to the needs of each particular case in accordance with the physician's judgment.

The medical record has been and always will be one of the firmest foundations on which the defense of a malpractice case is based. In addition to the notes the anesthesiologist makes of his pre- and postoperative visits and examinations, the anesthesia record for the labor, delivery or surgery is an essential part of the medical record. Notations of monitored signs, the instillation of drugs and significant patient response during anesthesia become a permanent record which will help to identify the actions of the anesthesiologist if a law suit occurs many months or years after memories have faded. In order to prevent subsequent misinterpretation or misunderstanding, the anesthesiologist should not try to chart an inordinate amount of information in abbreviated form in the anesthesia record. Entries should be legible, concise and properly timed. As an example, in cardiac arrest cases, the careless or inaccurate charting of the time and nature of resuscitative treatment or medications can mean the difference between a defensible and an indefensible case.

Under no circumstances should the anesthesia record (or any other part of the medical chart, for that matter) be altered after an entry has been made. If there is a need for a correction or amendment, the original, incorrect entry should not be obliterated but simply crossed out with a single line so that the original entry can be read. All changes, additions or amendments should be initialed, timed and dated, so that no one can draw the inference the chart was altered for self-serving purposes. Moreover, the anesthesiologist should never pre-chart the anesthetic record for his own convenience. Although he is confident he will be administering specific medications and/or changing the flows of anesthetic agent and oxygen, no entries should be made in the chart until these acts are accomplished.

CONCLUSION

It would be understandable if anesthesiologists, and indeed other medical specialists, were disheartened by the liability risks they face each time a patient is anesthetized or treated. The malpractice crisis which swept the United States in the spring of 1975 highlighted the complexity of the professional liability problem. The publicity generated at the time, however, did not accurately reflect the true state of affairs, and it is anticipated that in the future, as in the past, physicians will prevail in the vast majority of law suits brought by patients.

It should also be kept in mind that the occurrence of an injury associated with anesthesia or other medical treatment does not in itself establish negligence and, as a consequence, liability. The plaintiff must still prove that the defendant-physician failed to follow standard practice in treating the patient and that this failure caused the injury of which she complains. The anesthesiologist who understands his relationship to the patient and to other physicians involved in the treatment and who remains vigilant to the standards he and his colleagues have acknowledged to be operative in their medical community significantly reduces his exposure to malpractice liability.

References

1. American Mutual Insurance Company: *Analysis of Suits Closed since November 1, 1960 to November 1, 1973, American Mutual Insurance Company Physicians Only*. American Mutual Insurance Company, San Francisco, 1974.
2. National Association of Insurance Commissioners: *NAIC Malpractice Claims,* vol 1, no 4. May 1977.
3. American Medical Association: *American Medical News*. American Medical Association, Chicago, February 20, 1978.

SECTION FIVE

FETUS AND NEW-BORN

CHAPTER 23

Evaluation of the Fetus

Russell K. Laros, Jr., M.D.

A number of laboratory studies and tests are currently available which can be used to aid the clinician in assessing fetal well-being, function and maturity. The obstetric anesthesiologist should be aware of the fetal status before undertaking care of the mother. Problems such as intrauterine growth retardation, prematurity and fetal asphyxia will influence his choice of anesthesia. Fetuses at risk can now be identified with much greater precision than in the past. All available tests will not be reviewed in this chapter; rather, discussion will be limited to several techniques which have found the widest clinical acceptance. In each instance the physiologic basis for the particular study will be briefly reviewed, and the author will indicate those clinical situations where it is of greatest value.

URINARY AND PLASMA ESTROGENS

During the first few weeks of pregnancy the corpus luteum produces most of the circulating estrogens. With regression of the corpus luteum maternal estrogens do not decrease, but rather there is a sharp rise in maternal plasma estrone (E_1) and estradiol (E_2). This rise is due to increased placental production of E_1 and E_2 utilizing estrogen precursors. Approximately half of the maternal E_1 and E_2 arise from conversion of maternal dehydroisoandrosterone sulfate (DS) and half from fetal DS. Estriol (E_3), in contrast, is synthesized largely through placental conversion of 16-OH-dehydroisoandrosterone sulfate (16-OH-DS). In the latter half of pregnancy approximately 90 per cent of maternal E_3 arises from conversion of the fetal precursor 16-OH-DS by the placenta. The 16-OH-DS in turn comes from conversion of DS produced by the fetal adrenal and the fetal liver.[1]

Thus, in summary: (1) the placenta is the site of production of the majority of estrogens during all but the early weeks of human pregnancy; (2) placental production consists largely of bioconversion of externally supplied precursors; (3) the high levels of E_3 in pregnancy are largely a result of placental bioconversion of fetal 16-OH-DS; (4) circulating estrogens in the maternal plasma are dependent on the rate of production, conjugation, metabolism and excretion.

There are both practical and theoretical considerations for choosing either plasma or 24-hour urinary E_3 as a measure of fetal well-being. The disadvantages and advantages of each method of collection are detailed in Table 23.1. At present the major disadvantages of using plasma E_3 are the question of diurnal variation and the lack of a large body of clinical data substantiating the equivalence of plasma and urinary values. However, studies suggest that diurnal variations of plasma conjugated or

Table 23.1
Advantages and Disadvantages of Estriol Methods

	Advantages	Disadvantages
24-Hour urine	Large amount of clinical data No diurnal variation Widely available E_3 to creatinine ratio monitors improper collection	24 hr collection: inconvenient, errors in collection Delay in obtaining results Acute changes masked Falsely low levels with renal disease
Plasma	Ease of obtaining sample Rapid results	Diurnal variation False elevation with renal disease Less clinical data

unconjugated E_3 do not exceed 30 per cent and, thus, are no greater than the diurnal variations found with urinary E_3.[2] Renal disease also has an effect on both methods of collection. In severe renal disease only simultaneous plasma and urinary E_3 values overcome the falsely abnormal values shown when either method is used alone.[3]

Serial E_3 determinations (either urinary or plasma) are valuable in assessing fetal well-being in three disorders. These are diabetes mellitus; hypertension and pre-eclampsia-eclampsia; and placental insufficiency states, including intrauterine growth retardation (IUGR) and postmaturity. A significant fall in E_3 is that change which exceeds day-to-day variation. In a series of some 1,300 daily 24-hour urinary E_3 values determined in 60 hospitalized pregnant diabetics, Goebelsmann et al.[4] found this critical change to be a drop of greater than 35 per cent. Similarly, in a series of 58 complicated pregnancies, Mathur and associates[5] found that a fall of 50 per cent or more in plasma E_3 was critical. Either a downward trend or a precipitous fall in E_3 may be a sign of fetal deterioration (Figure 23.1). Prompt delivery should be considered in the context of the total clinical picture; that is, fetal maturity, cervical ripeness and the underlying disease must be considered before reaching a decision for delivery or continuation of the pregnancy.

Other conditions besides fetal distress causing low E_3 values are summarized in Table 23.2. E_3 levels are decreased in the presence of fetal anencephaly because of the marked hypoplasia of the fetal adrenal which leads to subnormal production of E_3 precursors. The adrenal hypoplasia is secondary to reduced or absent ACTH production by the abnormal central nervous system. Fetal adrenal disorders leading directly to low levels of E_3 precursors include primary congenital adrenal hypoplasia and adrenal hypoplasia secondary to maternal corticosteroid administration.

Fetal liver cirrhosis is a rare cause of low E_3 production. Likewise, placental sulfatase deficiency is an uncommon disorder inherited as a rare sex-linked recessive trait. E_3 levels are exceedingly low in this entity in the face of apparent normal fetal growth and activity. Frequently these pregnancies will go post-term.[7]

Finally, the administration of antibiotics which decrease or eliminate normal intestinal flora can result in low E_3 values. The altered bacterial flora decreases the rate of

Table 23.2
Causes of Low E_3 Other Than Placental Dysfunction

Fetal CNS abnormalities
Fetal adrenal disorders
Fetal liver dysfunction
Placental abnormalities
Maternal renal disease
Hepatointestinal circulation interruption

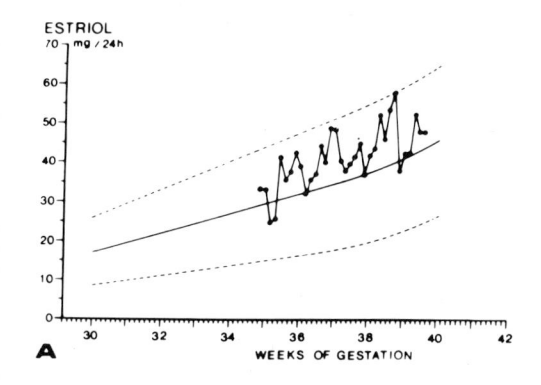

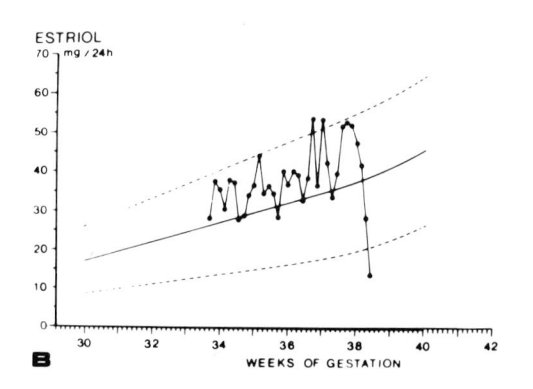

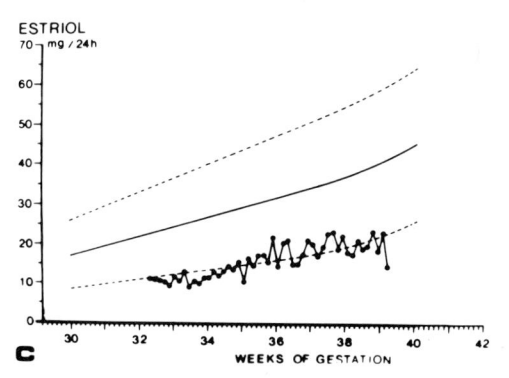

Figure 23.1. Maternal urinary estriol excretion during the last trimester of pregnancy (mean ± 2 S.D.). Examples of serial measurements in three patients. *A*, normal estriol pattern. *B*, falling estriol pattern. Sudden changes such as this are most often seen in diabetes. *C*, chronically low estriol pattern. (Reprinted by permission from Freeman RK, Kreitzer MS: Current concepts in antepartum and intrapartum fetal evaluation. Curr Probl Pediatr 2(9):1, 1972.)

hydrolysis of E_3 conjugates, leading to an increased loss of E_3 in the stool rather than normal reabsorption into the maternal circulation.[8]

HUMAN PLACENTAL LACTOGEN

Human placental lactogen (HPL) is a protein hormone (molecular weight 21,600 daltons) produced by the placental syncytiotrophoblast in large amounts. The hormone has a half-life of less than 30 minutes and, thus, theoretically should accurately reflect acute changes in placental function. There is no diurnal variation in HPL production and the levels appear not to be affected by maternal activity, the presence of fetal congenital anomalies, fetal sex, maternal smoking habits or the maternal administration of corticosteroids. There is a strong positive correlation of HPL levels with both placental and fetal weight and a negative correlation with maternal plasma glucose concentration.[9] There is a gradual rise in maternal HPL levels throughout the first half of gestation. During the second half, values either continue a gradual rise to term or a rise to 36 weeks' gestational age, then remain stable or decrease slightly to term.[10]

Elevated levels of HPL have been documented in association with multiple gestations, diabetes mellitus, Rh sensitization, maternal liver disease and maternal hemoglobinopathy. However, in none of these conditions is the elevated HPL value of specific diagnostic value, nor does it aid in the management of the pregnancy. The elevation is merely the reflection of an increased placental mass. The mechanism of the elevated HPL associated with maternal liver disease is not clear.

Low HPL levels have been documented in association with hypertensive disorders of pregnancy, intrauterine growth retardation and post-maturity. Spellacy[9] reviewed 21 studies describing the HPL patterns in pregnancies complicated by either acute or chronic hypertension. These data suggest that HPL levels correlate with placental function and, by extension, are a predictor of fetal risk. In a similar review of nine studies, most authors found low HPL values in association with IUGR. An exception was those instances where IUGR was secondary to fetal abnormalities such as infection or genetic defects. In these situations, placental growth was frequently normal and HPL levels were normal despite abnormal growth of the fetus. In seven studies correlating HPL values with post-maturity, most authors found low levels of HPL in association with post-maturity.[9] Berkowitz and Hobbins,[11] however, do not believe that HPL levels are useful in following post-term pregnancies. Spellacy and associates have reported two studies which indicate that the measurement of HPL is of value in screening for fetuses at increased risk for intrauterine asphyxia either prior to or during labor. In a retrospective study[12] of 506 pregnant women, they were able to define a "fetal danger zone" where the incidences of intrauterine fetal death were significantly increased (Figure 23.2). They defined the fetal danger zone as a serum HPL level of less than 4 μg/ml in pregnancies of 30 or more weeks' gestational age. In a subsequent study[13] of 2,733 pregnancies, they confirmed the validity of the fetal danger zone and showed that the use of HPL measurements coupled with appropriate obstetric intervention significantly lowered the fetal death rate.

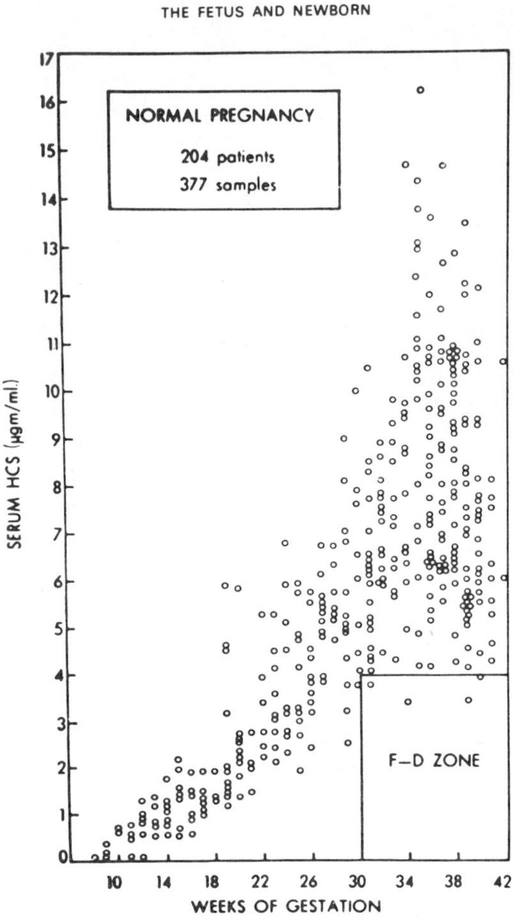

ULTRASONOGRAPHY

In the last 10 years diagnostic ultrasound has rapidly established its place in clinical obstetrics. The apparatus consists of a piezoelectric crystal transducer which comes in direct contact with the maternal abdomen. When the crystal is excited by a pulsating electric current, it produces ultrasonic waves. As the sound waves pass through interfaces of different densities, echoes return to the crystal, where they are detected and translated into new electrical signals.

Four types of ultrasound are now in clinical use. In the amplitude mode (A-mode) the presence and character of interface is studied. A second method is the

Figure 23.2. Serum human placental lactogen (frequently referred to as human chorionic somatomammotropin (HCS)) values in women during normal pregnancy. The F-D zone indicates fetal danger. (Reprinted by permission from Spellacy WN, Teoh ES, Buhi WC, et al.: Value of human chorionic somatomammotropin in managing high-risk pregnancies. Am J Obstet Gynecol 109: 588, 1971.)

brightness mode (B-mode), where the strength of the echoes determine the brightness of dots on an oscilloscope screen. The gray scale is simply an extension of the B-mode which allows more gradation of lightness or darkness. The motion mode (M-mode) is used to measure position and time for objects in motion. When an object's position changes in relation to the transducer, the position of the displayed echo will change correspondingly. Finally, a continuous beam or real-time device is now available which produces a continuous moving image of the objects under the transducer.

Although there are many uses for ultrasound during early pregnancy, this discussion shall only consider applications in the second and third trimesters, namely assessment of fetal age, fetal growth, fetal weight, the presence of anomalies and definition of placental location.

Fetal Age

The fetal biparietal diameter (BPD) can be measured with great accuracy using either A-mode or B-mode scanning and relates fairly precisely to fetal age (Figure 23.3). Campbell[14] obtained sonar BPD's between 20 and 28 weeks' gestation and showed that 84 per cent of gravidas with uncertain dates delivered within ± 9 days of the due date predicted by sonar. Sabbagha and associates[15] found that fetal dating using the BPD measurement was most accurate between 20 and 28 weeks of gestation. During this interval, fetal age as determined by BPD measurements varied by ± 11 days for 95 per cent of the population studied.

Fetal Weight

There are now a number of reports presenting nomograms which allow estimation of fetal weight. The nomograms use BPD alone or in conjunction with other fetal measurements. Unfortunately, to date all methods have large standard errors at either extreme of weight and are only precise over the middle weight range.

Fetal Growth

Sonography is frequently used to evaluate a fetus suspected of having IUGR. As a first step, sonographic measurement of the BPD can confirm or assign a fetal age. Then serial sonography can be used to establish a BPD growth pattern. Other sonographic measurements of the fetus which alone or in combination may be useful in detecting IUGR are the abdominal circumference at the level of the umbilical vein and the intrauterine volume. Campbell and Wilkin,[16] using a second-degree polynomial regression formula, were able to identify infants weighing less than 5 per cent below their expected weight for gestational age with a 95 per cent confidence at 32 weeks' gestation; this accuracy decreased to 63 per cent at 38 weeks. Their false positivity rate was just over 1 per cent at all gestational ages.

Placental Localization

Ultrasound can be used very effectively to locate the placenta. Such localization can be accomplished with 95 per cent accuracy during the latter part of gestation and thus is very useful in the management of patients with antepartum hemorrhage. Additionally, placental localization is useful in managing patients with abnormal fetal lies and prior to amniocentesis.[17]

Congenital Anomalies

Ultrasound can also be used to evaluate a fetus suspected of having a congenital anomaly. It is most useful in detecting hydramnios, fetal ascites, anencephaly, hydrocephaly and anomalies of the fetal spine. Unfortunately, a negative finding does not definitively rule out these abnormalities.

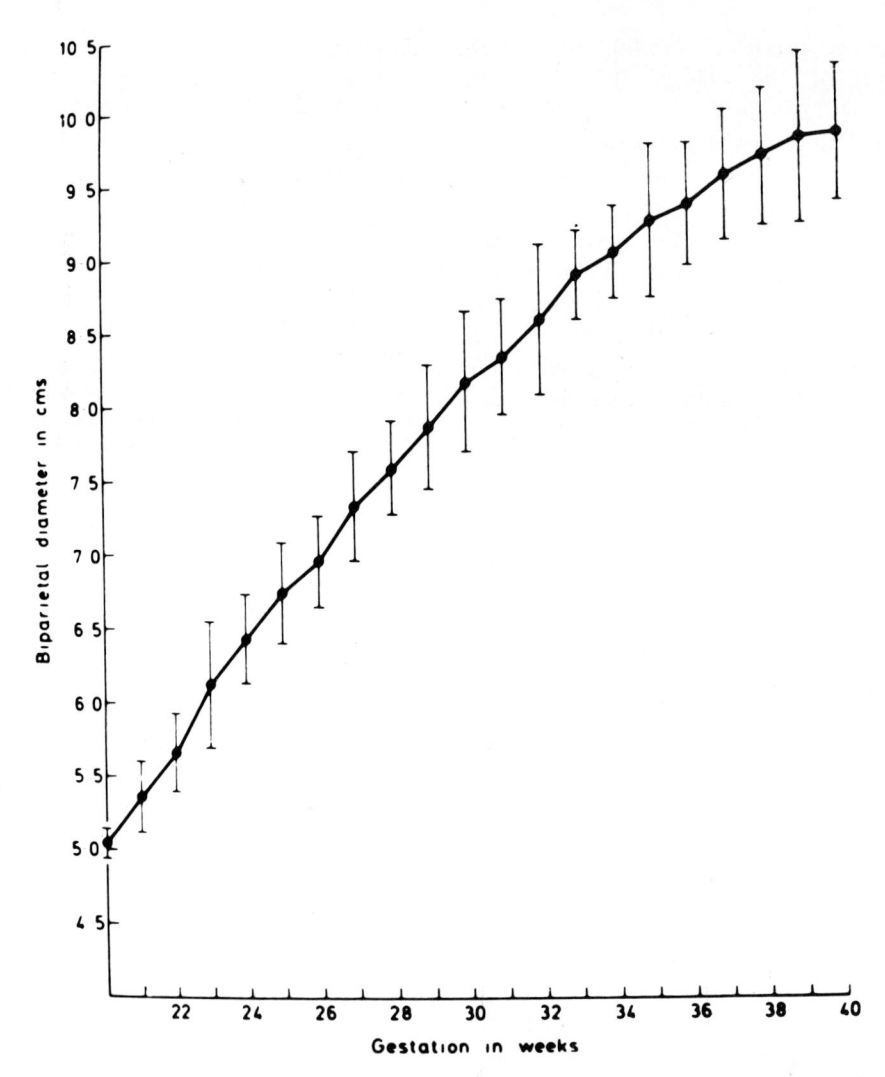

Figure 23.3. Fetal biparietal measurements for each week's gestation from 20 to 40 weeks (mean ± 2 S.D.). Measurements made using A-mode and B-mode ultrasonic techniques. (Reprinted by permission from Campbell S: The prediction of fetal maturity by ultrasonic measurement of the biparietal diameter. J Obstet Gynaecol Br Commonw 76:603, 1969.)

Fetal Breathing

Finally, evaluation of fetal breathing using either real-time imaging or a special A-mode scanning device promises to be a sensitive indicator of intrauterine fetal hypoxia. In 1971 Boddy and Robinson described recording fetal chest wall movements in both lambs and in human fetuses.[18] These observations have been extended, and it is now recognized that there are distinct patterns of fetal breathing. These include times of low breathing activity (midnight, 8 a.m. and 4 p.m., with less than 10 per cent of the fetuses breathing) and peaks of breathing rate (4 a.m., noon and 8 p.m., with greater than 80 per cent breathing).[19] Using A-scan technology, Boddy and Dawes[20] have noted patterns of prolonged apnea or gasping and apnea prior to fetal death. In contrast, the observation of normal fetal breathing patterns was a reassuring sign and correlated with normal fetal outcome.

AMNIOTIC FLUID ANALYSIS

Amniotic fluid can be obtained by transabdominal amniocentesis. It is most commonly used to assess fetal lung maturity. The hazards of delivering an immature infant are multiple and include difficulties in nutrition, problems in biochemical homeostasis, vulnerability of the immature fetal brain and the development of idiopathic respiratory distress syndrome (IRDS) or hyaline membrane disease. Because IRDS leads to so much morbidity and mortality, its avoidance whenever possible is most desirable.

Amniotic Fluid Surfactant Determination

Gluck[21] has recently reviewed the pathophysiology of IRDS and the measurement of amniotic fluid surfactant activity in detail. In this discussion only several facets of clinical relevance will be reviewed. The surfactant complex is made up primarily of phospholipids, the most abundant of which is lecithin. Lecithin is secreted by type II alveolar cells and is excreted into the fetal trachea and thence into the amniotic fluid. During early gestation only a small amount of surfactant activity is present; however, with maturation of the appropriate enzyme system between 34 and 36 weeks of gestation, there is an abrupt rise in amniotic fluid surfactant activity (Figure 23.4). This rise in activity above a critical level is accompanied by a virtual absence of IRDS in the neonate.

Surfactant activity can be measured directly using the amniotic fluid **foam test** or shake test described by Clements and associates[22] or by measuring the ratio of the major phospholipids, **lecithin and sphingomyelin (L/S ratio)** as described by Gluck[21] and others. The L/S ratio is measured using thin-layer chromatography; a positive ratio is generally considered to be one greater than 2.0 to 3.5 and assures a very low risk that the fetus will develop IRDS. Additional information can be added by measuring the minor **phospholipids phosphatidylinositol (PI)** and **phosphatidylglycerol (PG)**.[23] The relative percentage of phospholipid represented by PI and PG at varying gestational ages is depicted in Figure 23.5. When the L/S ratio is less than one, the PG and PI are vitually absent. PG, the unique phospholipid of lung surfactant, first appears when the L/S ratio exceeds two and indicates secretion of mature lung surfactant. Analysis of PG in amniotic fluid serves as an additional index of lung maturity and is especially useful when the specimen is contaminated by blood.

The foam test is based on the ability of lecithin to stabilize foam produced by mechanical agitation of a solution of amniotic fluid and alcohol. In order to perform the test, amniotic fluid in three dilutions with saline is mixed with 95 per cent ethanol as indicated in Table 23.3. The test solution, having 47.5 per cent volume fraction of ethanol, excludes interfering substances (protein, bile salts, fatty acids) from the surface of the amniotic fluid but permits double-chain phospholipids, such as lecithin, to compete for the surface film. When the solution is shaken with air, stable bubbles form if a sufficient number of double-chain phospholipids are present. The tubes are capped and shaken vigorously and then placed in a rack, undisturbed for 15 minutes. The air-liquid interface of each tube is then examined for the presence of stable bubbles. A tube is recorded as positive (+) when there are enough bubbles present to form a complete ring around the air-liquid interface. A tube is recorded as intermediate (±) when small bubbles are present but not in sufficient numbers to

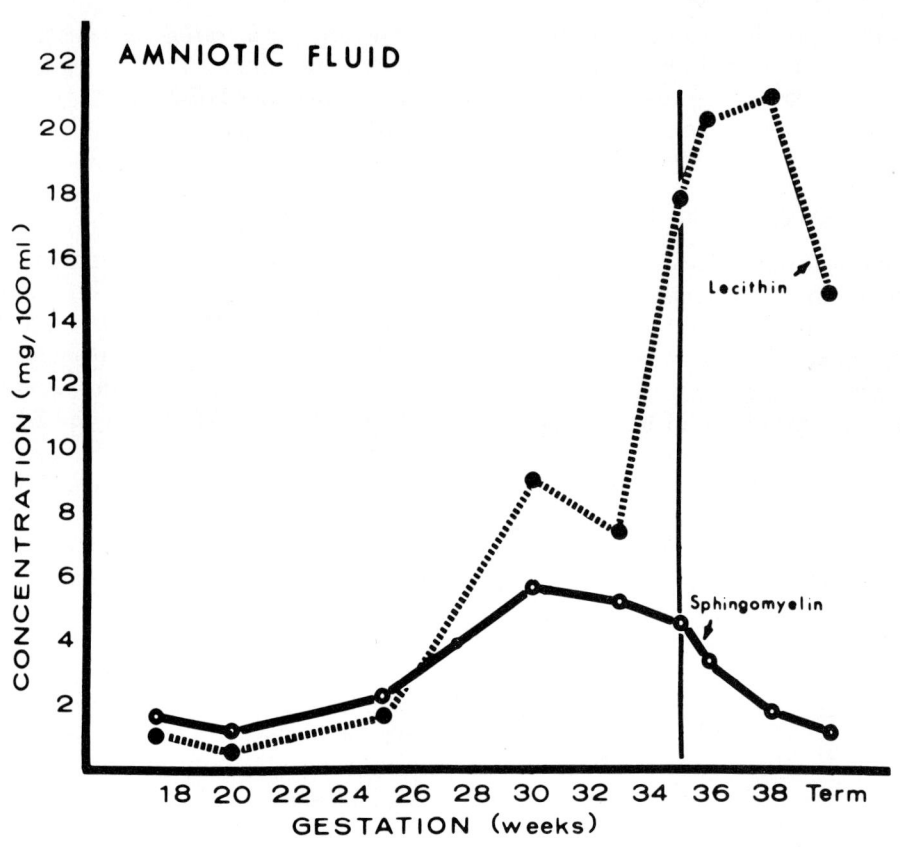

Figure 23.4. Levels of lecithin and sphingomyelin in amniotic fluid at increasing gestational ages. An acute rise in lecithin at 35 weeks marks pulmonary maturity. (Reprinted by permission from Gluck L, Kulovich MV, Borer RC, et al.: The diagnosis of the respiratory distress syndrome (RDS) by amniocentesis. Am J Obstet Gynecol 109:440, 1971.)

Table 23.3
Preparation of Tube Dilutions for a Rapid Test of Amniotic Fluid Surfactant

	Tube Dilutions		
	1/1	1/1.3	1/2
		ml	
Amniotic fluid	1.0	0.75	0.50
NaCl	0.0	0.25	0.50
95% ethanol	1.0	1.0	1.0

form a complete ring and negative when no bubbles are present. There is a progressive increase in incidence of hyaline membrane disease with decreasing reaction. Schlueter and associates[24] have defined five risk groups based on the degree of foam stability as outlined in Table 23.4. Infants at low risk (groups I and II) were heavier and more mature than those at high risk (groups III, IV and V). However, among infants of equivalent gestational age or birth weight, the incidence of IRDS still correlated significantly with the foam test results (Figure 23.6).

The advantage of the foam test is its rapidity and simplicity; the disadvantage is a high level of false negatives and the fact that it cannot be performed on specimens contaminated by meconium or blood. The author has used the foam test as the first method of laboratory assessment of lung maturity. If the amniotic fluid

EVALUATION OF THE FETUS

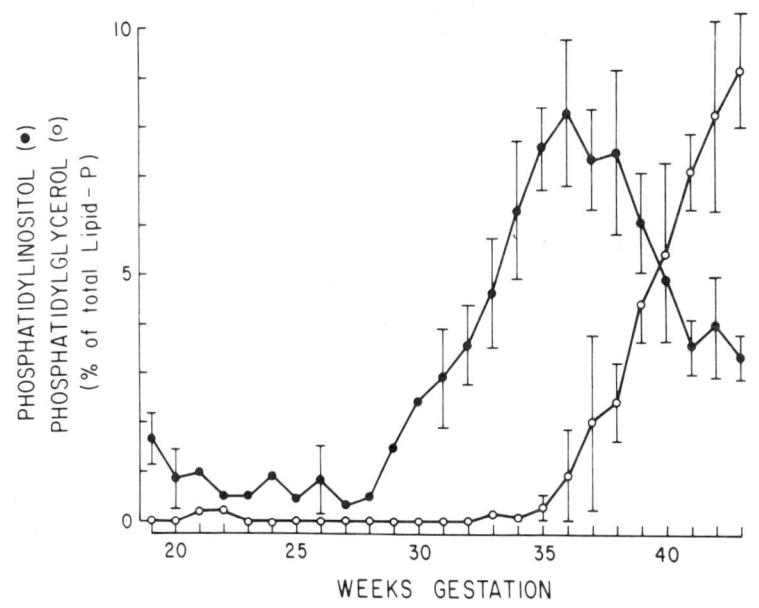

Figure 23.5. The content of PI(●) and PG(○) in amniotic fluid during normal gestation. The phospholipids were quantified by measuring the phosphorus (P) content and expressed as percentages of total lipid phosphorus. Means ± standard deviations of three to five samples are shown for each *point*. (Reprinted by permission from Hallman M, Kulovich M, Kirkpatrick E, et al.: Phosphatidylinositol and phosphatidylglycerol in amniotic fluid: Indices of lung maturity. Am J Obstet Gynecol 125:613, 1976.)

Table 23.4
Risk of Developing Hyaline Membrane Disease (HMD) if Delivered within 24 Hours of Shake Test

Risk Group	Amniotic Fluid Dilution			Incidence of HMD
	1/1	1/1.3	1/2	%
I	+	+	+	<1
II	+ +	+ ±	± ±	10
III	+ ±	± ±	— ±	25
IV	±	±	—	41
V	± —	— —	— —	79

is found to indicate risk group I, no further study is necessary. However, if the risk group is II or higher, an L/S ratio and PG level are performed on the fluid.

Measuring surfactant activity will aid the clinician in timing deliveries in a variety of situations. Hack and associates[25] found that 12 per cent of all infants admitted to their intensive care nursery with IRDS were the products of elective interventions (cesarean sections or inductions). These findings suggest that some study of lung maturity should be used before elective repeat cesarean section or induction of labor in almost every case. This is especially true when there is the slightest doubt as to the actual fetal age.

Amniotic fluid analysis is also valuable in the early diagnosis of hereditary disorders and congenital anomalies and in managing fetuses with hemolytic disease.

Amniotic Cell Culture

Chromosomal abnormalities such as Down's syndrome or trisomy-21 can be diagnosed from fetal cells obtained from the amniotic fluid and grown in culture.[26,27]

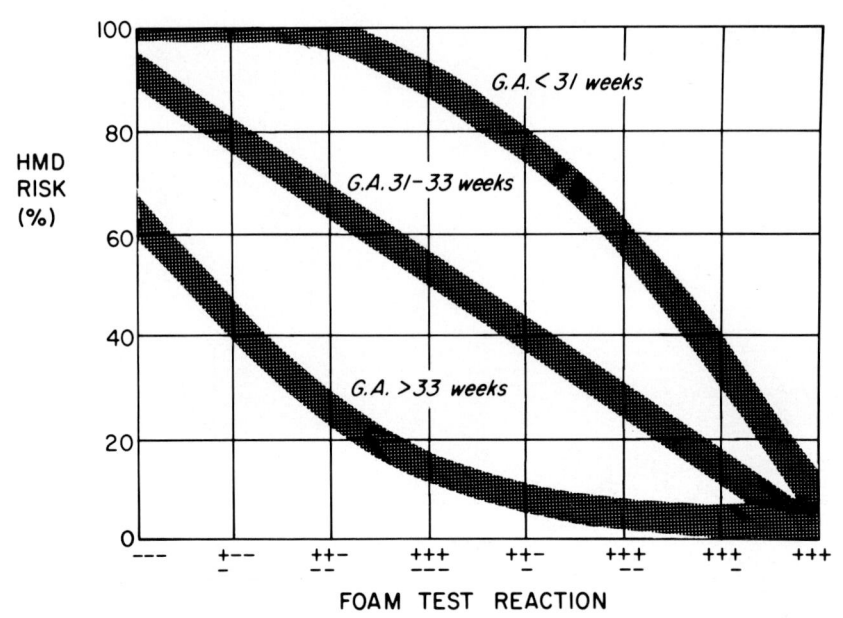

Figure 23.6. Scheme for antenatal prediction of hyaline membrane disease (*HMD*) from amniotic fluid foam test reaction plus gestational age. Foam test reaction is on the *longitudinal axis* and risk of HMD on the *vertical axis*. The risk is predicted from the *shaded band* appropriate for the gestational age. The width of each band approximates the error of the estimate. For example with a foam test reaction of ± ± ± the risk of HMD is approximately 15% if gestational age is > 33 weeks, 65% if the gestational age is 31 to 33 weeks and approximately 90% if it is < 31 weeks. (Reprinted by permission from Schleuter M, Phibbs RH, Creasy RK, et al.: Antenatal prediction of graduated risk of hyaline membrane disease by amniotic fluid foam test for surfactant. Am J Obstet Gynecol. In press, 1979.)

These cells may also be used to determine the enzyme deficiencies present in Tay-Sachs disease or galactosemia.

α-Fetoprotein

α-Fetoprotein is synthesized primarily in the fetal liver and is present in both maternal plasma and amniotic fluid.[28] In early gestation elevated amniotic fluid levels suggest central nervous system anomalies such as spina bifida, anencephaly or hydrocephaly.[29,30] During late pregnancy high levels suggest congenital nephrosis,[31] esophageal atresia or fetal death.[32]

Fetal Hemolytic Anemia

Bilirubin is found in the amniotic fluid of normal pregnancies between the twelfth and thirty-sixth week of gestation. The analysis for bilirubin is done spectrophotometrically by scanning the absorbance of amniotic fluid at wave lengths between 300 and 600 mµ.[33] The presence of bilirubin is indicated by increased optical density between 375 and 525 mµ with a peak at 450 mµ. The height of this peak is expressed as the ΔO.D. at 450 mµ (Figure 23.7). A ΔO.D. of less than 0.01 indicates fetal maturity.

The concentration of bilirubin in the amniotic fluid also accurately reflects the increased hemoglobin degradation found in erythroblastosis fetalis and, thus, serves as an index of the severity of the disease.[35-37] The bilirubin level provides the indication for intrauterine fetal transfusion, early delivery or no therapeutic intervention.[33,38-40] (Figure 23.8).

EVALUATION OF THE FETUS

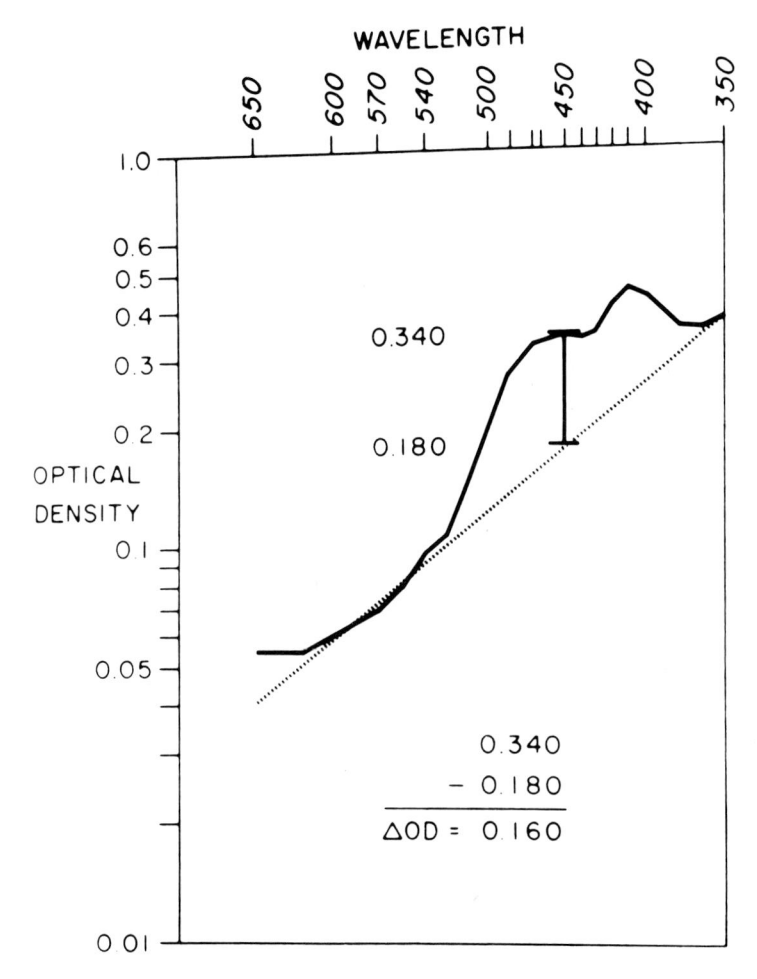

Figure 23.7. Determination of ΔO.D. 450 in amniotic fluid. An arbitrary *broken line* has been drawn connecting the spectrophotometric readings obtained at 375 and 600 mμ. The *straight line* represents the ΔO.D. at 450 mμ. (Reprinted by permission from Merkatz IR, Aladjem S, Little B: The value of biochemical estimations on amniotic fluid in management of the high-risk pregnancy. Clin Perinatol 1:301, 1974.)

STRESS AND NON-STRESS MONITORING

During a uterine contraction there is a significant fall in utero-placental blood flow and, thus, a decrease in the amount of oxygen delivered to the fetus. The normal feto-placental unit has sufficient respiratory reserve to withstand uterine contractions without production of transient episodes of fetal asphyxia. However, in situations of placental insufficiency, the added stress of contractions may cause transient asphyxia which is reflected by changes in the fetal heart rate pattern (chapter 24).

The **oxytocin challenge test** (OCT) is performed during the last trimester of pregnancy by stimulating uterine contractions with an intravenous infusion of dilute oxytocin solution. The uterine contractions and fetal heart rate are monitored with an external recording device. The methodology of performing an oxytocin challenge test has been detailed elsewhere.[41] A positive OCT requires consistent and persistent hypoxic-type fetal heart rate patterns (late decelerations) occurring repeatedly with most uterine contractions.[42-44]

The author wishes to emphasize the importance of obtaining adequate uterine activity, that is, at least three contractions of moderate intensity as determined by palpation in a 10-minute interval.

Indications for use of the oxytocin challenge test include hypertensive-renal disease, chronic hypertension, diabetes mellitus, cyanotic heart disease, hemoglobinopathy, hyperthyroidism, collagen disease, prolonged gestation (greater than 42 weeks), suspected intrauterine growth retardation, history of previous stillbirth, low E_3 excretion, meconium-stained amniotic fluid and Rh sensitization. Relative contraindications include previous classical cesarean section, placenta previa and patients believed to be at risk for premature labor, that is those with premature ruptured membranes, multiple pregnancies or an incompetent cervix.

There now seems ample experience with the oxytocin challenge test to confirm that it does, in fact, allow rapid evaluation

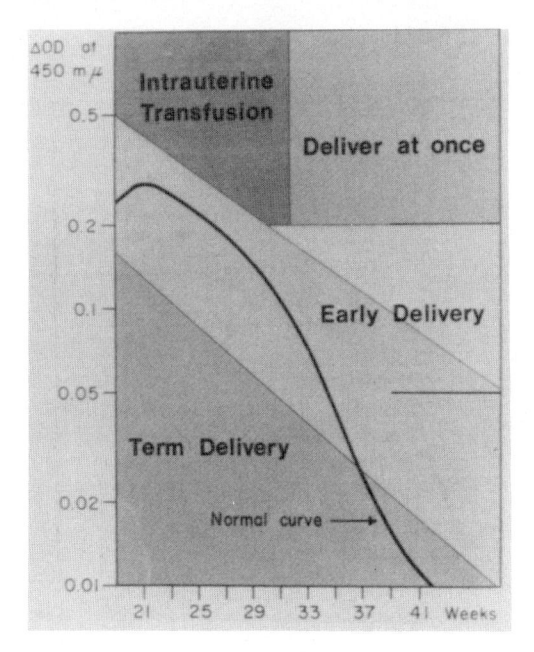

Figure 23.8. Suggested management of Rh-sensitized pregnancies based on level of ΔO.D. 450 and gestational age. (Reprinted by permission from Merkatz IR, Aladjem S, Little B: The value of biochemical estimations on amniotic fluid in management of the high-risk pregnancy. Clin Perinatol 1:301, 1974.)

Table 23.5
Scoring System for Evaluating the Non-stress Test*

Fetal Heart Rate Observation	Score 0	Score 1	Score 2
Baseline rate (beats per min)	< 100 or > 180	100–119 or 161–180	120–160
Fetal activity (movements per 30 min)	0	1–4	≥ 5
Accelerations (per 30 min)	0	Periodic or 1–4 sporadic	≥ 5 sporadic
Baseline Variability			
Oscillatory amplitude (beats per min)	< 5	5–9 or > 25	10–25
Oscillatory frequency (per min)	< 3	3–6	> 6
Decelerations	Severe variable or repetitive late	Mild variable or non-repetitive late	None or early

* Reprinted by permission from Krebs HB, Petres RB: Clinical application of a scoring system for evaluation of antepartum fetal heart rate monitoring. Am J Obstet Gynecol 130:765, 1978.

of placental respiratory function.[43] A positive oxytocin challenge test may signify fetal compromise; however, there is an incidence of false positives of approximately 25 per cent. Therefore, the finding of a positive OCT dictates repetition of the study or the collection of other studies which allow evaluation of placental function, such as E_3, HPL and analysis of the amniotic fluid for presence of meconium. In contrast, a negative OCT is excellent evidence of continued fetal well-being for at least 7 days. The oxytocin challenge test is particularly useful in cases in which the level of E_3 is chronically low. The combination of a positive OCT and abnormally low estriols (chronically low or falling) is an ominous sign and suggests that prompt delivery may be appropriate.

Finally, the use of the **non-stress test** must be considered. In reviewing a large number of OCT's, Trierweiler and associates[45] concluded that variability of the fetal heart rate appeared to be characteristic of fetal well-being. Additionally, they supported the observation that a reactive fetus was characterized by acceleration of the fetal heart rate in response to external stimuli or during fetal movement.[46] The ability to derive equal information from observation of the fetal heart rate without the necessity of stimulating uterine contractions with oxytocin is obvious. Many authors have now confirmed the value of the non-stress test in high-risk patients.[47-50] They were able to demonstrate a close correlation between non-stress patterns and neonatal outcome. Those fetuses with a reactive pattern (baseline variability greater than six beats per minute and accelerations of at least 15 beats per minute with fetal movement) had good outcomes. Krebs and Petres[50] have developed a scoring system for evaluation of the non-stress test which is summarized in Table 23.5. In their experience, a score of 9 to 12 was a reliable sign of fetal well-being and an OCT did not provide additional information. However, if the score was less than 9, an OCT should be performed.

CONCLUSIONS

There are now available a number of studies which aid the clinician in management of both normal and abnormal pregnancies. Thoughtful use of these studies does improve perinatal outcome. As new studies are developed and those presently available (fetal breathing and non-stress monitoring) become better defined, even more accurate fetal surveillance and lower fetal morbidity and mortality rates can be anticipated.

References

1. Siiteri PK, MacDonald DC: Placental estrogen biosynthesis during human pregnancy. J Clin Endocrinol Metab 26:751, 1966.
2. Klopper A, Wilson G, Masson G: The variability of plasma hormone levels in late pregnancy. In Hormonal Investigations in Human Pregnancy, R Scholler, ed. Editions Sept, Paris, 1974, p 77.
3. Carrington ER, Oesterling MJ, Adams FM: Renal clearance of estriol in complicated pregnancies. Am J Obstet Gynecol 106:1131, 1970.
4. Goebelsmann V, Freeman RK, Mestman JH, et al.: Estriol in pregnancy. Am J Obstet Gynecol 115:795, 1973.
5. Mathur RS, Chestnut SK, Leaming AB, et al.: Application of plasma estriol estimations in the management of high risk pregnancies. Am J Obstet Gynecol 117:210, 1973.
6. Freeman RK, Kreitzer MS: Current concepts in antepartum and intrapartum fetal evaluation. Curr Probl Pediatr 2(9):1, 1972.
7. Oakey RE, Marion L, MacDonald RR: Biochemical and clinical observations in a pregnancy with placental sulfatase and other enzyme deficiencies. Clin Endocrinol 3:131, 1974.
8. Boehm FM, DiPietro DL, Goss DA: The effect of ampicillin administration on urinary estriol and serum estradiol in the normal pregnant patient. Am J Obstet Gynecol 119:98, 1974.
9. Spellacy WN: Monitoring of high-risk pregnancies with human placental lactogen. In Management of the High-risk Pregnancy, WN Spellacy, ed. University Park Press, Baltimore, 1976, p 107.
10. Spellacy WN, Buhi WC, Berk SA, et al: Distribution of human placental lactogen in the last half of normal and complicated pregnancies. Am J Obstet Gynecol 120:214, 1974.
11. Berkowitz RK, Hobbins JC: A reevaluation of the value of hCS determination in the management of prolonged pregnancy. Obstet Gynecol 49:156, 1977.

12. Spellacy WN, Teoh ES, Buhi WC, et al.: Value of human chorionic somatomammotropin in managing high-risk pregnancies. Am J Obstet Gynecol 109:588, 1971.
13. Spellacy WN, Buhi WC, Birk SA: The effectiveness of human placental lactogen measurements as an adjunct in decreasing perinatal deaths. Am J Obstet Gynecol 121:835, 1975.
14. Campbell S: The prediction of fetal maturity by ultrasonic measurement of the biparietal diameter. J Obstet Gynaecol Br Commonw 76:603, 1969.
15. Sabbagha RE, Turner HJ, Chez RA: Sonar BPD and fetal age—definition of the relationship. Obstet Gynecol 121:371, 1975.
16. Campbell S, Wilkin D: Ultrasonic measurement of fetal abdominal circumference in the estimation of fetal weight. Br J Obstet Gynaecol 82:689, 1975.
17. Kabayashi M, Hillman LM, Fillisti L: Placental localization. Am J Obstet Gynecol 106:279, 1970.
18. Boddy K, Robinson JS: External methods for detection of fetal breathing *in utero.* Lancet 2:1231, 1971.
19. Fox HE, Hohler CW: Fetal evaluation by real-time imaging. Clin Obstet Gynecol 20:339, 1977.
20. Boddy K, Dawes GS: Fetal breathing. Br Med Bull 31:3, 1975.
21. Gluck L: Fetal maturity and amniotic fluid surfactant determinations. In *Management of the High-risk Pregnancy.* WN Spellacy, ed. University Park Press, Baltimore, 1976, p 189.
22. Clements JA, Platzker ACG, Tierney DF, et al.: Assessment of the risk of the respiratory distress syndrome by a rapid test for surfactant in amniotic fluid. N Engl J Med 286:1077, 1972.
23. Hallman M, Kulovich M, Kirkpatrick E, et al.: Phosphatidylinositol and phosphatidylglycerol in amniotic fluid: Indices of lung maturity. Am J Obstet Gynecol 125:613, 1976.
24. Schlueter M, Phibbs RH, Creasy RK, et al.: Antenatal prediction of graduated risk of hyaline membrane disease by amniotic fluid foam test for surfactant. Am J Obstet Gynecol. In press, 1979.
25. Hack M, Fanaroff AA, Klaus M, et al.: Neonatal respiratory distress following elective delivery: A preventable disease? Am J Obstet Gynecol 126:43, 1976.
26. Milunsky A: *The Prenatal Diagnosis of Hereditary Disorders.* Charles C Thomas, Springfield, Ill., 1973, pp 1–135.
27. Golbus MS, Conte FA, Schneider EL, et al.: Intrauterine diagnosis of genetic defects, results, problems, and follow-up of 100 cases in a prenatal genetic detection center. Am J Obstet Gynecol 118:897, 1974.
28. Bergstrand CG, Czar B: Demonstration of a new protein fraction in serum from the human fetus. Scand J Clin Lab Invest 8:174, 1956.
29. Brock DJH, Sutcliffe RG: Alpha fetoprotein in the antenatal diagnosis of anencephaly and spina bifida. Lancet 2:197, 1972.
30. Harris R, Jennison RF, Barson AJ, et al.: A comparison of amniotic fluid and maternal serum alpha fetoprotein levels, the early antenatal diagnosis of spina bifida and anencephaly. Lancet 1:429, 1974.
31. Seppala M, Tallberg P, Ehnholm C: Studies on embryo-specific protein. Physiological characteristics of embryo-specific alpha globulin. Ann Med Exp Biol Fenn 45:16, 1967.
32. Seppala M, Ruoslahti E: Alpha fetoprotein in antenatal diagnosis. Lancet 1:155, 1973.
33. Queenan JT: Amniotic fluid analysis. Clin Obstet Gynecol 14:505, 1971.
34. Merkatz IR, Aladjem S, Little B: The value of biochemical estimations on amniotic fluid in management of the high-risk pregnancy. Clin Perinatol 1:301, 1974.
35. Bevis DCA: Blood pigment in haemolytic disease of the newborn. J Obstet Gynaecol Br Commonw 63:68, 1956.
36. Liley AW: Liquor amnii analysis in management of pregnancy complicated by Rhesus sensitization. Am J Obstet Gynecol 82:1359, 1961.
37. Queenan JT: Amniotic fluid analysis. Clin Obstet Gynecol 14:505, 1971.
38. Freda VJ: The Rh problem in obstetrics and a new concept of its management using amniocentesis and spectrophotometric scanning of amniotic fluid. Am J Obstet Gynecol 92:341, 1965.
39. Queenan JT, Goetschel E: Amniotic fluid analysis for erythroblastosis fetalis. Obstet Gynecol 32:120, 1968.
40. Whitfield CR: A three year assessment of an action line method of timing intervention in rhesus isoimmunization. Am J Obstet Gynecol 108:1239, 1970.
41. Ray M, Freeman R, Pine S, et al.: Clinical experience with the oxytocin challenge test. Am J Obstet Gynecol 114:1, 1972.
42. Ewling D, Farina J, Otterson W: Clinical application of the oxytocin test. Obstet Gynecol 43:563, 1974.
43. Farahani G, Vasudeva K, Petrie RH, et al.: Oxytocin challenge test in high risk pregnancy. Obstet Gynecol 47:159, 1976.
44. Freeman RK: The use of the oxytocin challenge test for antepartum clinical evaluation of respiratory function. Am J Obstet Gynecol 121:481, 1975.
45. Trierweiler MW, Freeman RK, James J: Baseline fetal heart rate characteristics as an indicator of fetal status during the antepartum period. Am J Obstet Gynecol 125:618, 1976.
46. Lee CY, DiLoreto FC, O'Lane JM: A study of fetal heart rate acceleration patterns. Obstet Gynecol 45:142, 1975.
47. Rochard F, Schifrin BS, Goupil F, et al.: Non-stressed fetal heart rate monitoring in the antepartum period. Am J Obstet Gynecol 126:699, 1976.
48. Fox HE, Steinbrecher M, Ripton B: Antepartum fetal heart rate and uterine activity studies. Am J Obstet Gynecol 126:61, 1976.
49. Nichimson DJ, Turbeville JS, Perry JE, et al.: The non-stress test. Obstet Gynecol 51:419, 1978.
50. Krebs HB, Petres RB: Clinical application of a scoring system for evaluation of antepartum fetal heart rate monitoring. Am J Obstet Gynecol 130:765, 1978.

CHAPTER 24

Diagnosis and Management of Fetal Asphyxia

Julian T. Parer, M.D., Ph.D.*

Intrauterine asphyxia is probably the most common cause of stillbirths and newborn depression. Asphyxia is most likely to occur in the intrapartum period when transient decreases in uterine blood flow occur with each uterine contraction. A placenta with borderline function before the onset of contractions will be unable to provide adequate gas exchange during labor because uterine blood flow is an important determinant of placental function. Fetal asphyxia during pregnancy and labor can most effectively be predicted and, therefore, avoided by fetal monitoring. After approximately 15 years of clinical use, it seems that electronic fetal heart rate monitoring is the most accurate technique currently available.

There is little physiologic information available on the etiology of the various fetal heart rate patterns and variability, and this has significantly retarded a rational approach to heart rate pattern interpretation. Initially, the interpretation was purely empirical, with a pattern being described as abnormal when a depressed fetus resulted. Transient decelerations of fetal heart rate were noted in some cases with depressed fetuses,[1,2] whereas others noted that variability of fetal heart rate seemed to be a positive sign of fetal health.[3] A major source of confusion in interpretation has been the fact that the so-called ominous patterns are actually associated with healthy fetuses in a significant number of cases.[4,5] This difficulty has been at least partially solved by the combination of electronic heart rate monitoring and fetal blood sampling during the intrapartum period. Scalp sampling is used to detect the false abnormal pattern.[6-8] It is not possible to use this technique in **antepartum** fetal evaluation when approximately one in four oxytocin challenge tests (see chapter 23) which are "positive," a so-called ominous finding, are in fact falsely positive.[9]

Despite these drawbacks, fetal heart rate monitoring is a valuable aid in diagnosing fetal asphyxia. The following approach to the interpretation of fetal heart rate pattern has been found valuable and is becoming widely accepted.[10] It is admittedly still empirical, and its prime aims are: (1) to recognize the fetus which is becoming asphyxiated and (2) to minimize unnecessary obstetric interference for "fetal distress" except when it is in fact needed.

THE FETAL HEART RATE MONITOR

The fetal heart rate monitor is an instrument with two input components, one to

---
* Supported by Grant HD 09980 from the National Institutes of Health, United States Public Health Service.

recognize and process heart rate and the other to recognize uterine contractions.

Fetal heart rate (FHR) is determined from the R wave of the fetal electrocardiogram complex, a signal generated by the movement of a cardiovascular structure (using ultrasound and the Doppler principle) or cardiac sounds picked up by a microphone. Uterine contractions are detected either by an open-ended catheter inserted transcervically into the amniotic cavity and attached to a strain gauge transducer or an external device called a tokodynamometer placed on the maternal abdomen which recognizes the tightening of the maternal abdomen during a contraction.

Devices which are attached directly to the fetus or placed within the uterine cavity are termed direct, internal or invasive. These devices are the fetal electrode (generally a stainless steel spiral) and the intraamniotic catheter. Devices which do not require direct connection with the fetus are called non-invasive or external. These consist of the Doppler ultrasound device, phonocardiogram, or external abdominal ECG for detecting heart rate, and the tokodynamometer for uterine contractions. The most accurate device for detecting heart rate is that which gives the most discrete signal and has the least external interference. The R wave of the fetal ECG complex detected by a fetal spiral electrode is generally the most accurate for the intrapartum period.

An understanding of the mode of action of the cardiotachometer is essential for appreciating FHR variability. The cardiotachometer consists of three components, one for recognizing the cardiac event, another which measures the time interval between the events and another which rapidly divides the time interval in seconds into 60 to give a rate for each interval between beats. These individual rates are then traced on a strip chart recorder moving at a specific speed. An example of several heart beats and the resulting recording is shown in Figure 24.1. When the paper moves slowly, instead of a plateau-like pattern, it appears as a jittery line, and

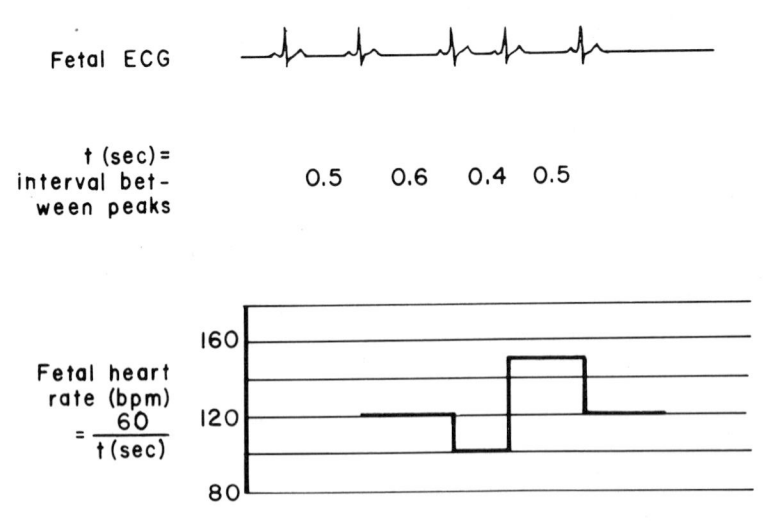

Figure 24.1. The operation of the cardiotachometer. The peaks of the R waves are detected and the time interval between them is measured. This is electronically divided into 60, and the resulting rate is traced on a strip chart recorder. This example shows the normal situation, where there are slight differences in the intervals between adjacent heart beats, giving rise to heart rate "variability."

this is described as variability. If each interval between heart beats were identical then the line would be flat. This is termed absent variability, or a flat or silent baseline.

The ability of the cardiotachometer to depict variability accurately is dependent on the discreteness of the signal which is portraying heart events. The peak of the R wave is discrete and occupies a short distance. However, the Doppler signal is broad and slurred and the machine is not always able to select accurately and consistently a point on this slurred curve representing the exact time of a cardiac event. Hence, an artificial variability tends to be portrayed by this device.

Variability is described as short-term, representing the beat-to-beat differences in heart rate or at most differences between several adjacent beats, and long-term, representing crude fluctuations which occur generally three to six times per minute.[11]

Variability of the fetal heart rate is thought to denote the physiologic integrity of the pathway from the fetal cerebral cortex through the cardiac integratory center in the medulla oblongata, the vagus nerve and the cardiac conduction system.[12] Any factor which alters the integrity of this pathway will cause a decrease in variability. Cerebral or cardiac asphyxia will affect the pathway and, hence, is associated with the decrease in variability.

In experimental animals the initial response to acute hypoxia is not a decrease in variability. This may be because of the compensating mechanism operating during fetal hypoxia, i.e. redistribution of blood flow to vital organs (e.g. heart, brain and placenta), decreased total oxygen consumption, and dependence of some vascular beds on anaerobic metabolism.[13] Prolonged hypoxia will result, however, in breakdown of these compensations with cerebral and myocardial hypoxia and decreased heart rate variability.

In addition to asphyxic causes of decreased variability there are a number of non-asphyxic causes. These are listed in Table 24.1.

FETAL SCALP SAMPLING

Fetal scalp sampling was introduced initially as an independent means of fetal surveillance during labor.[14] However, most authorities now agree that a combination of heart rate monitoring and fetal scalp sampling is the preferred method of fetal evaluation during labor.[6-8] Fetal scalp sampling is used when abnormal heart rate patterns occur (see below), which cannot readily be abolished.

Scalp sampling is carried out by placing an endoscope against the fetal presenting part and puncturing the fetal skin using a small blade device, until a droplet of blood wells up. This is collected anaerobically and analyzed for pH and PCO_2 (and other factors if necessary). The bicarbonate or base excess can be calculated by means of the Henderson-Hasselbalch equation. It has been noted that at pH's above 7.20 to 7.25 the fetus is generally vigorous at birth, whereas at pH's below 7.20 the fetus is usually depressed.[6,15,16] However, there is a considerable overlap in the groups, and a single figure such as 7.20 cannot be relied on entirely. Numerous other factors must be taken into account, such as the maternal acid-base status, the relationship of the

Table 24.1
Non-asphyxic Causes of Decreased Variability

Drugs
   Central depressants, e.g. narcotics, tranquilizers
   Parasympatholytics, e.g. atropine, scopolamine
Tachycardia
Prematurity
"Sleep"
Bradyarrhythmias
Some anencephalics

sampling to uterine contractions, the permanence of the placental insult, the influence of in utero treatment, the type of acidosis (i.e. respiratory versus metabolic), the stage of labor and the various other clinical aspects of the particular case.

TREATMENT OF THE FETUS IN UTERO

It is only since the advent of heart rate monitoring and fetal scalp sampling that it has been possible to treat the fetus in utero effectively. Previously, treatment could not be used because there was no way of knowing whether fetal condition improved.

Placental respiratory function is determined by adequacy of blood flow on each side of the placenta and adequate delivery of oxygen to and removal of carbon dioxide from the fetal circulation. Maneuvers used to treat the fetus in utero are directed toward correcting deficiencies in these functions. These treatments are listed in Table 24.2 together with the supposed insult and the expected mechanism of correction of the defect.

FETAL HEART RATE PATTERNS

The characteristics of the fetal heart rate pattern are divided into baseline and periodic features. The baseline features, heart rate and variability, are those which are recorded between uterine contractions. Periodic changes occur in association with uterine contractions.[1]

The baseline rate is described as normal if it is within the range of 120 to 160 beats per minute. Values above 160 are defined as tachycardia and those below 120 as bradycardia. Both tachycardia and bradycardia have been associated with fetal asphyxia.[7]

The baseline variability is described as normal if it has an amplitude range greater than 5 beats per minute.[17] Baseline variability is described as absent if there is no fluctuation in either beat-to-beat variability or long-term variability and is described as decreased if it is persistently below 5 beats per minute in amplitude. The significance of baseline variability has been discussed above.

There are four periodic changes occurring in association with uterine contractions:

Table 24.2
Treatment of the Fetus in Utero

Events Inciting Abnormal Patterns	Corrective Maneuver	Mechanism
Hypotension, e.g. supine hypotension, conduction anesthesia	Intravenous fluids; position change; ephedrine	Restores uterine blood flow toward normal
Excessive uterine activity	Decrease oxytocin; lateral position	Restores uterine blood flow toward normal
Transient umbilical cord compression (variable decelerations)	Change maternal position e.g. left lateral, right lateral, Trendelenburg	Restores umbilical blood flow
Decreased uterine blood flow associated with uterine contractions (late decelerations)	Change position to lateral and Trendelenburg	Restores uterine blood flow
Prolonged asphyxia (decreasing variability)	Position change; maternal hyperoxia	Restores uterine or umbilical blood flow; increases maternal-fetal O_2 gradient

1. **Early decelerations** occur concomitantly with the uterine contraction. They are smooth and mirror images of the contraction. Their onset is with the onset of the contraction. They are persistent from contraction to contraction, and they are mild in nature, never being more than about 20 beats per minute below the baseline. They are thought to be caused by vagal reflex and are not associated with compromised fetuses. They can be reproduced by compressing the fetal head.

2. **Late decelerations** have their onset delayed after the onset of the contraction, generally 10 to 30 seconds (Figure 24.2). They are also mirror images of the uterine contractions, smooth in configuration, and persistent from contraction to contraction. The degree of deceleration is related to the intensity of the contraction. They are partially vagal in origin, probably being caused by baro- and chemoreceptor influence. They may also have a non-vagal component of myocardial hypoxia which cannot be abolished by atropine. They are associated with fetal compromise, particularly when associated with lack of variability and when they are profound. They have been classified by Kubli et al.[18] as mild, moderate or severe depending on the amplitude of drop in FHR from the baseline rate: *mild*, less than 15 beats per minute; *moderate*, 15 to 45 beats per minute; *severe*, more than 45 beats per minute fall from baseline (Table 24.3). The duration of the deceleration is not a consideration in this classification.

3. **Variable decelerations** are variable in duration, profundity and appearance from contraction to contraction (Figure 24.3). They are most commonly abrupt in onset and cessation, reflecting a reflex, presumably vagal, origin. They are also classified as mild, moderate or severe, not depending on the amplitude of drop from baseline but rather on absolute rate at the nadir of the deceleration and the duration of the drop in FHR[18] (Table 24.3). For instance, a severe variable deceleration is one which has a heart rate of below 70 beats per minute for longer than 60 seconds. Another classification of variable deceleration has been suggested by Goodlin.[19] He considers a variable deceleration to be se-

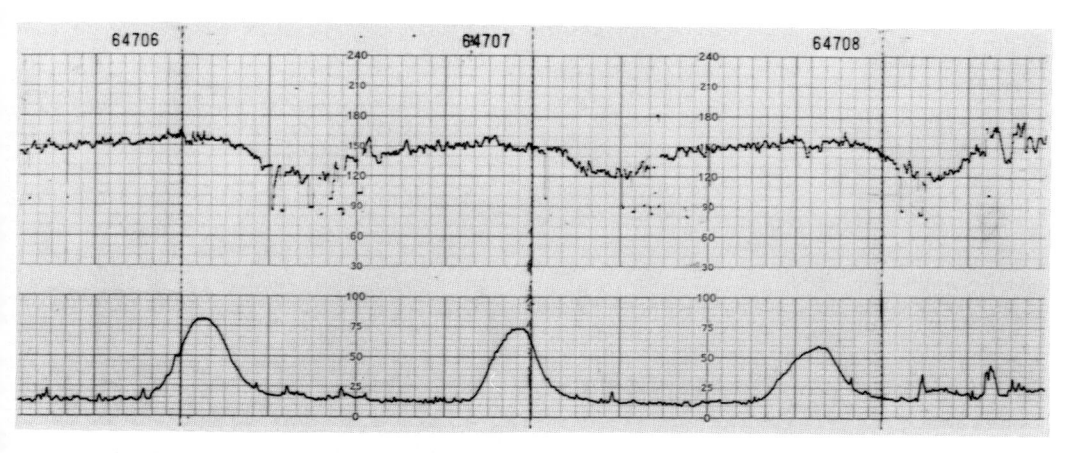

Figure 24.2. Late decelerations. This is an antepartum recording with ultrasound device for heart rate detection and tokodynamometer for uterine activity. The mother was hypertensive, and the infant was severely growth-retarded, being 1700 gm at 38 weeks' gestation. Paper speed = 3 cm per minute.

Table 24.3
Grading of Late and Variable Decelerations[18]

Deceleration	Mild	Moderate	Severe
Late	Drop in FHR of less than 15 beats per min.	Drop in FHR of 15 to 45 beats per min.	Drop in FHR of more than 45 beats per min.
Variable	Duration shorter than 30 seconds regardless of heart rate *or* Heart rate greater than 80 beats per min regardless of duration *or* Heart rate greater than 70 beats per min with duration shorter than 60 seconds	Heart rate less than 70 beats per min with a duration of 30 to 60 seconds *or* Heart rate greater than 70 beats per min with a duration of longer than 60 seconds.	Heart rate less than 70 beats per min with a duration longer than 60 seconds

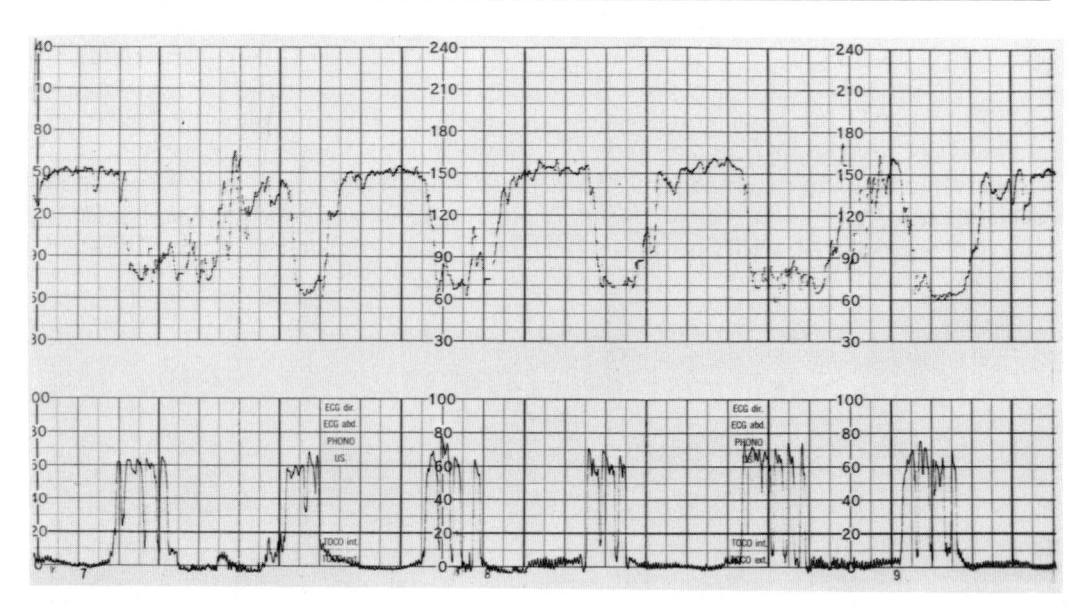

Figure 24.3. Variable decelerations. Intrapartum recording using fetal scalp electrode and tokodynamometer. The spikes on the uterine activity channel represent maternal pushing efforts in the second stage of labor. Note normal baseline variability between contractions. Paper speed = 3 cm per minute.

vere if it is greater than 60 seconds in duration or below 60 beats per minute or 60 beats per minute below the baseline. Variable decelerations are associated with fetal compromise when they are severe but generally only when they have been occurring for prolonged periods, that is 15 to 30 minutes.

4. **Accelerations** with contractions are sometimes seen (Figure 24.4). These have not been associated with fetal compromise, but some believe that they are pre-

DIAGNOSIS AND MANAGEMENT OF FETAL ASPHYXIA

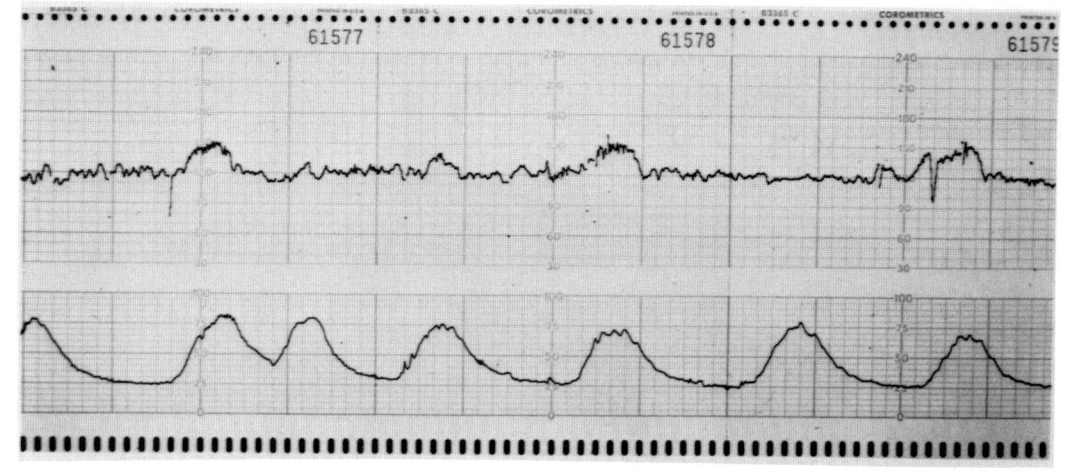

Figure 24.4. Accelerations with contractions.

cursors of variable decelerations. Their significance is not the same as that of accelerations with fetal movement in the antepartum period. The latter is a definite positive sign of a healthy fetus.

Uterine Activity

Uterine activity as determined by the intrauterine catheter is described by frequency and intensity. Adequate uterine activity is described as that which achieves acceptable cervical dilation per unit time, generally regarded as at least 1 cm per hour dilation in the active phase.[20] When cervical dilation is less than this, uterine activity measurements can be used to determine whether such activity is adequate; if not, oxytocin augmentation may be used. Adequate uterine activity is generally described as approximately 250 to 300 Montevideo units, or contractions occurring every 2 or 3 minutes of 50 to 70 mm Hg intensity (chapter 4).

Pattern Interpretation

NORMAL HEART RATE PATTERN

Table 24.4 contains the baseline and periodic pattern characteristics of the normal fetal heart rate pattern. A typical pattern is illustrated in Figure 24.5. A fetus born

Table 24.4
Characteristics of Normal Fetal Heart Rate Patterns

Baseline rate	120 to 160 beats per min
Baseline variability (amplitude range)	> 5 beats per min
Periodic pattern	Absent or early decelerations or accelerations
Fetal outcome	Vigorous; Apgar score > 7
Scalp sampling	Not useful
Treatment of fetus	Not necessary

demonstrating this pattern will be vigorous, with greater than 99 per cent reliability.[4,5] Scalp sampling is not useful with this pattern and need not be carried out. No treatment of the fetus is necessary. The woman may labor in any position she chooses provided the fetus remains well oxygenated as illustrated by the normal heart rate pattern.

There are, however, three provisos that this pattern will predict a normal fetus. First, delivery must be accomplished within a few minutes of the pattern recording. In theory the fetal storage to utilization ratio of oxygen is about 2 minutes, although as noted above, various physiologic compensations will usually enable

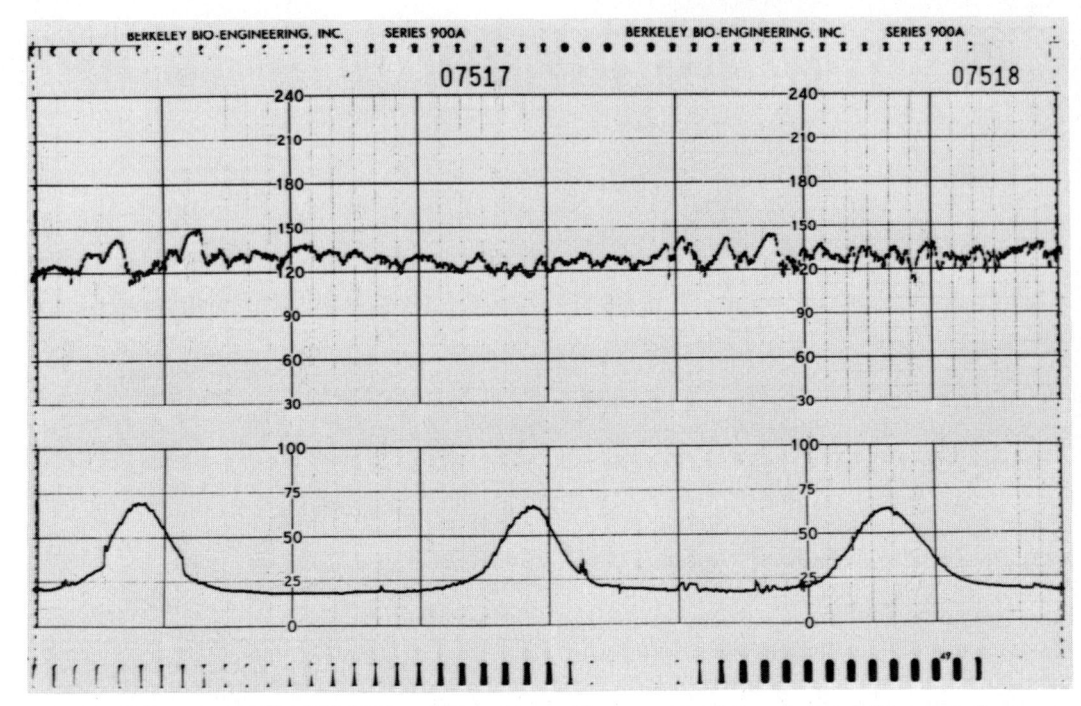

Figure 24.5. Normal fetal heart rate pattern with normal rate and variability and absence of periodic changes. This pattern illustrates a normally oxygenated fetus. Paper speed = 3 cm per minute.

the fetus to survive without brain damage for possibly up to 10 minutes in the event of total cessation of oxygen supply, such as with a total prolapse of the cord or a complete abruptio placentae. Hence, the guarantee for fetal vigor only lasts a few minutes after the end of the recording. The second proviso is that the fetus not be subjected to a traumatic delivery, for example cervical spine fracture during a difficult midforceps delivery or breech extraction. The third proviso for vigor at birth is that the fetus have no serious congenital anomalies inconsistent with extrauterine life.

Although one can be confident that a fetus with normal fetal heart rate patterns will be born vigorous and with a good Apgar score, the converse does not hold true for the fetus with an abnormal or so-called ominous heart rate pattern.

ABNORMAL FETAL HEART RATE PATTERNS

It has been noticed by various authorities that despite the fact that certain FHR patterns were described as ominous, a number of babies born with such patterns are actually vigorous at birth.[4-8] This was believed to be an error in the diagnosis of fetal distress using this tool. Furthermore, it was believed that the range of fetal vigor and acidosis seen with the various abnormal patterns represented a normal distribution within the group of infants demonstrating the pattern.[18] With further empirical experience, however, it has become obvious that this is not so, but that the "abnormal" group can be dichotomized.[17] Some changes in heart rate occur before the fetus is severely asphyxiated and before the loss of fetal vigor. It is now ob-

DIAGNOSIS AND MANAGEMENT OF FETAL ASPHYXIA

vious that the ***presence of heart rate variability*** is a valuable feature in enabling us to determine which of those infants with "abnormal" heart rate patterns are not yet seriously asphyxiated (Figure 24.6).

The term "ominous" was previously used to include all of the abnormal patterns and, because of this, has lost a great deal of its usefulness. Accordingly, the author proposes characterizing the previously considered ominous patterns into (1) the "stress" pattern and (2) the "sinister" pattern. There is an intermediate group within the stress pattern, indicating an evolution between the two. The characteristics of each of these patterns are shown in Table 24.5.

The fetus with the "acute stress" pattern may have a baseline rate outside the normal range, that is, tachycardia or bradycardia may be present. The variability, however, is still within normal limits. There may be late or variable decelerations. Wide clinical experience has shown that the fetal outcome with such patterns is almost invariably a vigorous fetus at

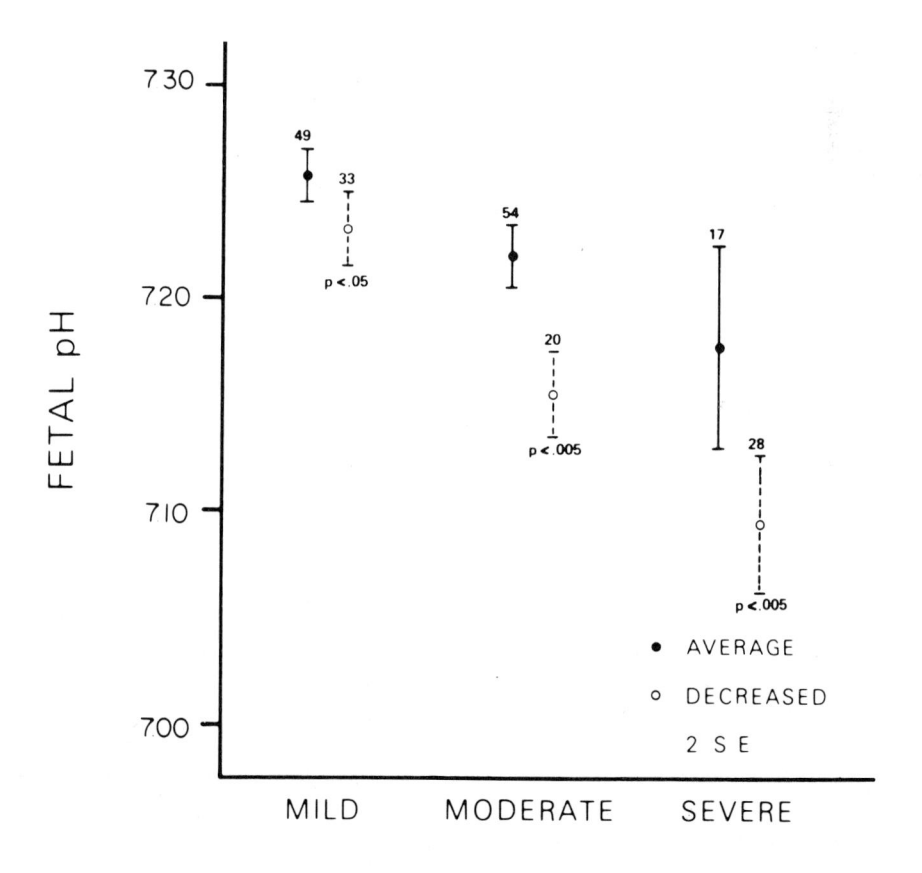

Figure 24.6. As late deceleration patterns become more marked, the mean pH value falls. However, when FHR variability is present in association with late deceleration patterns, the mean pH is consistently higher than when it is absent. (Reprinted by permission from Paul RH, Suidan AK, Yeh SY, et al.: Clinical fetal monitoring. VII. The evaluation and significance of intrapartum baseline FHR variability. Am J Obstet Gynecol 123:206, 1975.)

least at 5 minutes of age (Figures 24.3, 24.7, 24.8). The 1-minute Apgar score may be depressed, possibly due to CO_2 narcosis, but prolonged or extensive metabolic acidosis is rarely present. If the abnormal periodic heart rate pattern is abolished, scalp sampling is not useful in this pattern. In fact, acidosis may persist in such fetuses some time after the abolition of the insult and the stress pattern, but it is progressively resolved. Vigorous treatment by the maneuvers outlined in Table 24.2 is necessary with this sort of pattern. It usually follows an acute problem such as hypotension or excessive oxytocin-induced uterine activity superimposed on a previously normally oxygenated fetus and normally functioning placenta. Hence, it is usually readily abolished.

If it is not abolished and the patterns are severe, that is, the bradycardia is profound and prolonged or the late or variable decelerations are severe, then it may evolve into a stress pattern termed the "chronic stress" pattern. The prime characteristic of this is that variability decreases below 5 beats per minute and may even become absent (Figure 24.9). Furthermore, the pe-

Table 24.5
Characteristics of Abnormal Fetal Heart Rate Patterns

	Stress Pattern		Sinister Pattern
	Acute	Chronic	
Baseline rate	Normal or abnormal	Normal or abnormal	Normal or abnormal
Baseline variability	> 5 beats per min	< 5 beats per min	Absent
Periodic pattern	Late or variable decelerations	Late or variable decelerations or absent	Severe late or variable decelerations
Fetal outcome	Apgar score > 7 at 5 min	Possibly depressed	Usually depressed
Scalp sampling	Not necessary if abnormality is abolished	Mandatory for management	Rapid delivery preferred
Treatment of fetus	Vigorous treatment necessary	Vigorous treatment necessary while evaluating fetus	Rapid delivery preferred

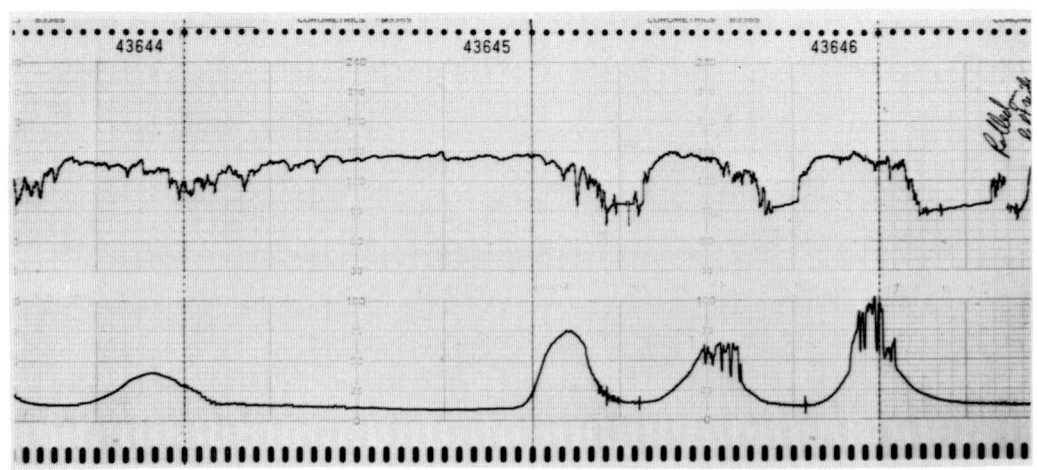

Figure 24.7. This pattern was previously normal, but late decelerations occur coincident with hypotension following a caudal anesthetic. Note maintenance of normal variability. This stressed fetus was delivered vaginally, shortly after this tracing, with Apgar scores of 2 (1 minute) and 7 (5 minutes). Paper speed = 3 cm per minute.

DIAGNOSIS AND MANAGEMENT OF FETAL ASPHYXIA

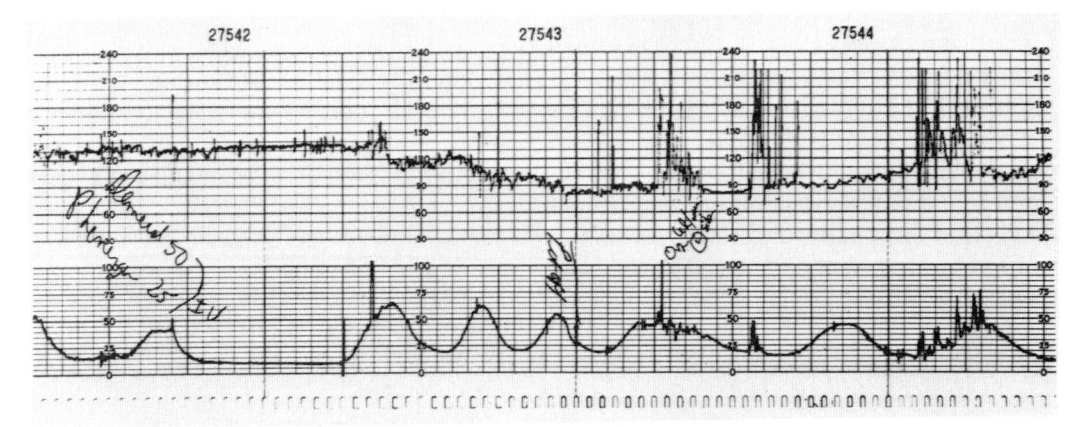

Figure 24.8. Prolonged fetal bradycardia probably caused by excessive oxytocin-induced hyperstimulation of the uterus following intravenous IV Demerol and Phenergan. The hyperstimulation and heart rate are returning to normal at the end of the tracing. Note that variability was maintained throughout this stress.

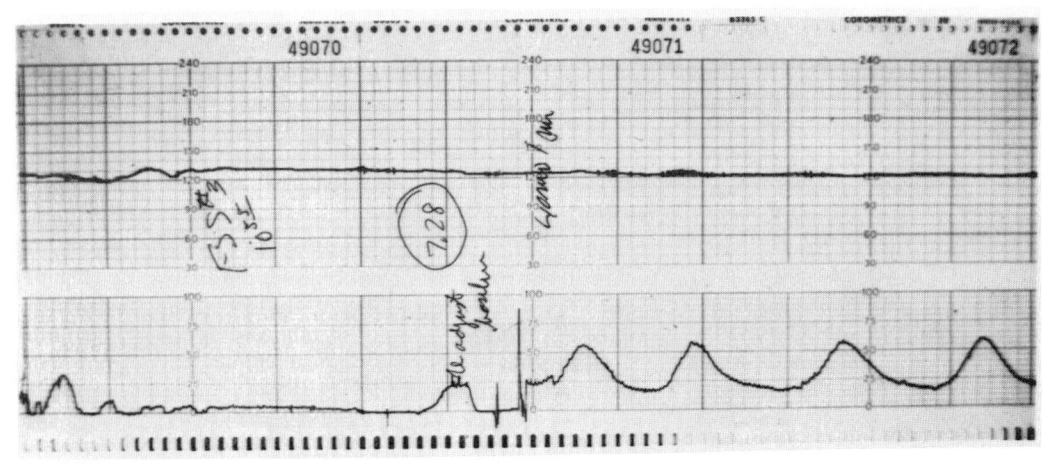

Figure 24.9. Absent variability of fetal heart rate. The patient was a severe preeclamptic on magnesium sulfate and narcotics. Only the normal scalp pH (7.28) assures one that the absent variability is non-asphyxic in origin and, therefore, not a chronically stressed, decompensating fetus.

riodic changes may be absent. It has been noted in a number of fetuses which have died in utero while being monitored that death can occur without periodic changes.[21] It is thought that the fetus has gone through a stage of periodic changes and the heart has lost its ability to respond to the transient hypoxia with contractions. The author believes that fetuses exhibiting the chronic stress pattern are impossible to manage during labor unless scalp sampling is available or unless one can be sure that the cause of the decreased variability is non-asphyxic, e.g. due to a recent large dose of narcotic or parasympatholytic drug.

The "sinister pattern" has absent heart rate variability, the rate may be within or outside the normal range, and the periodic changes, either late or variable decelerations, are severe in nature (that is, the dip is approaching 60 beats per minute below the baseline or persists for 60 seconds). There is a smooth, rather than abrupt, decrease in heart rate and recovery. Such a heart rate pattern almost invariably results in a depressed fetus (Figures 24.10, 24.11). It is generally the result of persistent insults in a previously borderline oxygenated fetus with borderline placental function. It is extremely unlikely that such a pattern can be reversed, and, because such fetuses are either already severely acidotic or soon to become so, fetal scalp sampling is generally of little use in managing this pattern. Expeditious delivery is indicated. Various fetal treatment maneuvers may be used while the patient is being readied for rapid delivery.

In summary, electronic fetal heart rate monitoring has emerged as an effective technique for detecting the fetus which is

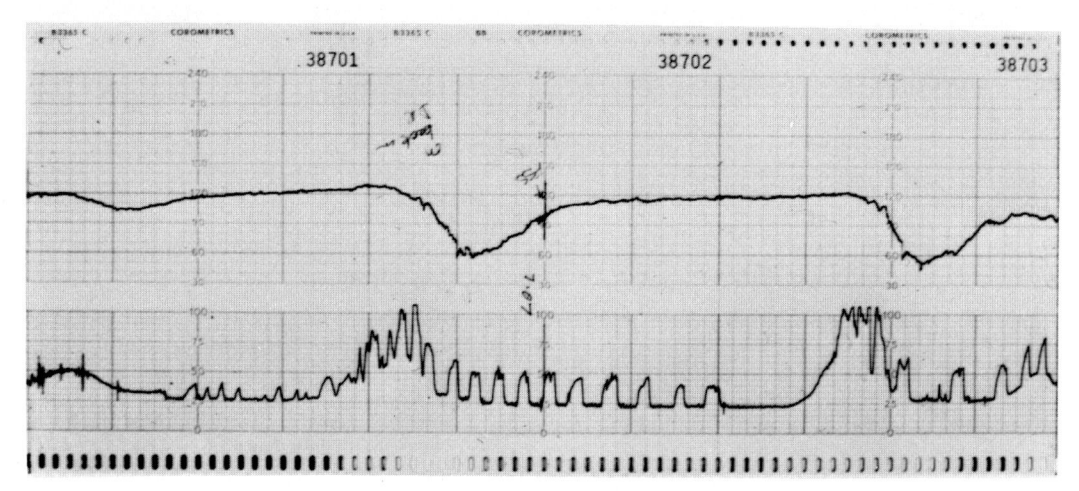

Figure 24.10. A sinister heart rate pattern with absent variability and severe late decelerations. Same patient as Figure 24.9, 11 hours later; 3340-gm female with Apgar scores of 3 (1 minute) and 4 (5 minutes). Cesarean section was considered contraindicated due to a severe maternal coagulopathy.

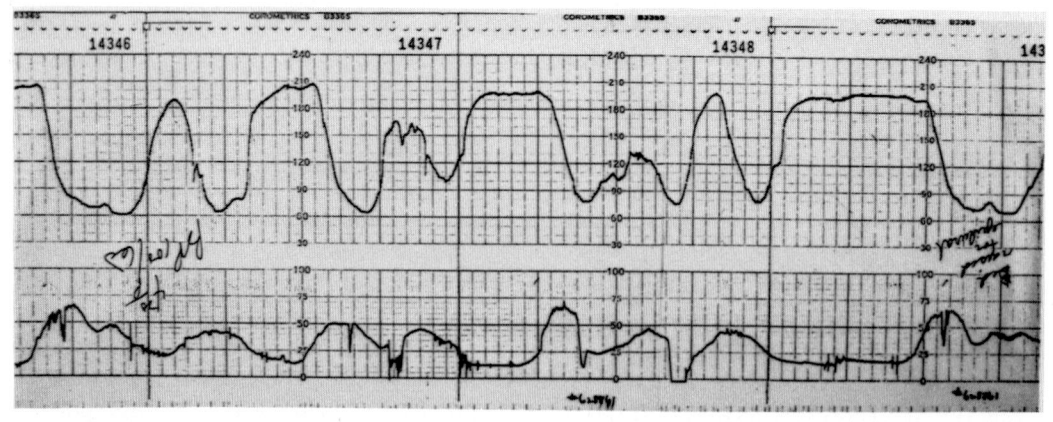

Figure 24.11. A sinister heart rate pattern in 28-week gestation fetus (determined after delivery) with baseline tachycardia, absent heart rate variability, and severe periodic changes. The scalp pH was 7.0, and the fetus died in utero shortly after this tracing. Cesarean section was not done because it was believed that the fetus was previable, although, in fact, it was 1100 gm.

either already asphyxiated or soon likely to become so. Heart rate pattern interpretation can be divided into "normal" and "abnormal" patterns. The strength of the normal pattern is that it invariably signifies a well oxygenated fetus. The abnormal patterns are not so readily interpreted, because in a number of cases the fetus with "abnormal" patterns is, in fact, born in a vigorous state. Certain patterns signify a stress to the fetus and, if the stress is acute and fetal heart rate variability remains, such fetuses are also born vigorous. In the face of a stress pattern with decreasing variability the fetus decompensates, and management of this pattern can only be accomplished with fetal scalp sampling or delivery. A third abnormal pattern with absent heart rate variability and profound decelerations is termed a sinister pattern; because such fetuses are generally depressed at birth, immediate delivery is indicated with little additional information being gained by scalp sampling.

By following the above approach to interpretation, it is seen that only one small group, the chronic stress pattern with decompensation, requires fetal scalp sampling for ideal management. This group usually includes such a small number of fetuses that if scalp sampling cannot be carried out or is not available, it is believed that immediate delivery is indicated.

References

1. Hon EH: *An Atlas of Fetal Heart Rate Patterns.* Harty Press, New Haven, Conn., 1968.
2. Caldeyro-Barcia R, Mendez-Bauer C, Poseiro JJ, et al.: Control of human fetal heart rate during labor. In *The Heart and Circulation in the Newborn and Infant,* DE Cassels, ed. Grune & Stratton, New York, 1966, p 7.
3. Hammacher K, Huter KA, Bokelmann J, et al: Foetal heart frequency and perinatal condition of the foetus and newborn. Gynaecologia 166:349, 1968.
4. Hon EH: Detection of fetal distress. In *Fifth World Congress of Gynecology and Obstetrics,* C Wood, ed. Butterworth, London, 1967, p 58.
5. Shifrin BS, Dame L: Fetal heart rate patterns: Prediction of Apgar score. JAMA 219:1322, 1972.
6. Wood C, Newman W, Lumley L, et al.: Classification of fetal heart rate in relation to fetal scalp blood measurements and Apgar score. Am J Obstet Gynecol 105:942, 1969.
7. Beard RW, Filshie GM, Knight CA, et al.: The significance of the changes in the continuous fetal heart rate in the first stage of labour. J Obstet Gynaecol Br Commonw 78:865, 1971.
8. Tejani N, Mann LI, Bhakthavathsalan A, et al.: Correlation of fetal heart rate-uterine contraction patterns with fetal scalp blood pH. Obstet Gynecol 46:392, 1975.
9. Freeman RK, Goebelsman U, Nochimson D, et al.: An evaluation of the significance of a positive oxytocin challenge test. Obstet Gynecol 47:8, 1976.
10. Boehm FR: FHR variability: Key to fetal well-being. Contemp OB/GYN 9:57, 1977.
11. Laros RK, Wong WS, Heilbron DC, et al.: A comparison of methods for quantitating fetal heart rate variability. Am J Obstet Gynecol 128:381, 1977.
12. Parer JT: Physiological regulation of fetal heart rate. J. O. G. N. Nursing 5:26s, 1976.
13. Fetal oxygen uptake and umbilical circulation during maternal hypoxemia in chronically catheterized sheep. In: Fetal and Newborn Cardiovascular Physiology, Vol. 2. *Fetal and Newborn Circulation,* LD Longo and DD Reneau, eds. Garland Press, New York, 1978, p. 231.
14. Saling E, Schneider D: Biochemical supervision of the foetus during labour. J Obstet Gynaecol Br Commonw 74:799, 1967.
15. Beard RW, Morris ED, Clayton SG: pH of foetal capillary blood as an indicator of the condition of the foetus. J Obstet Gynaecol Br Commonw 74:812, 1967.
16. Mendez-Bauer C, Arnt IC, Gulin L, et al.: Relationship between blood pH and heart rate in the human fetus during labor. Am J Obstet Gynecol 97:530, 1967.
17. Paul RH, Suidan AK, Yeh SY, et al.: Clinical fetal monitoring. VII. The evaluation and significance of intrapartum baseline FHR variability. Am J Obstet Gynecol 123:206, 1975.
18. Kubli FW, Hon EH, Khazin AF, et al.: Observations on heart rate and pH in the human fetus during labor. Am J Obstet Gynecol 104:1190, 1969.
19. Goodlin RC: Inappropriate fetal bradycardia. Obstet Gynecol 48:117, 1976.
20. Laros RK Jr, Margules M: Patterns of uterine activity and cervical dilatation in normal and abnormal labour. J. O. G. N. Nursing 5:61s, 1976.
21. Cetrulo C, Schifrin BS: Fetal heart rate patterns preceding death *in utero.* Obstet Gynecol 48:521, 1976.

CHAPTER 25

Evaluation of the Neonate

Sheila E. Cohen, M.B., Ch.B., F.F.A.R.C.S.

Evaluation of the fetus and neonate is of vital importance in order to prevent and treat problems which result in increased perinatal morbidity and mortality. Factors which may modify infant outcome and survival include complications occurring during pregnancy or labor, perinatal asphyxia, anesthetic medications and the presence of congenital abnormalities. Evaluation prior to delivery is primarily aimed at determining optimal obstetric management, whereas the importance of assessment immediately after birth lies in promptly identifying severely depressed infants who require active resuscitation. In the first hours of life it is imperative that infants who need special observation and therapy are identified and placed in intensive care nurseries. Such management has considerably reduced neonatal mortality, particularly with regard to premature infants. Further evaluation over the early days and months of life enables a prognosis to be formulated as to the long-term physical, neurologic and psychologic well-being of the infant. In addition, most of these methods of evaluation are widely utilized to assess outcome in obstetric and anesthetic research.

EVALUATION OF THE NEONATE IN THE DELIVERY ROOM

Breathing Time, Crying Time and Time to Sustained Respiration

After delivery, the infant's condition must be rapidly assessed to determine the need for immediate resuscitation. Before the introduction of the Apgar score, the time interval between delivery and the "first gasp" (breathing time) or "first cry" (crying time) was used to identify asphyxiated infants. The underlying hypothesis was that infants who breathed very shortly after birth, i.e. in the first 60 to 90 seconds, were healthy and did not require resuscitation, whereas infants in whom respiration was delayed were asphyxiated. It was demonstrated subsequently by James et al.[1] that the mere onset of respiration did not bear a constant relationship to oxygenation. In a group of 63 newborns with varying degrees of asphyxia, 26 had extremely low oxygen saturations or even a total absence of oxygen. In spite of this, 14 of these infants spontaneously initiated respiration or made respiratory efforts. Although most infants who initiate respiration are healthy and will make satisfactory progress without resuscitation, some severely hypoxic infants who are moderately depressed will make initial respiratory efforts but will deteriorate in the absence of supplemental oxygen. Thus, as an index designed to discriminate which infants require resuscitation, the time of the first gasp or first cry is not wholly satisfactory. As most severely depressed infants fail to breathe, it will usually identify this group as needing resuscitation. However, because of the expectant nature of the measurements, delay in intervention may occur. On the other hand, the time interval between delivery and the estab-

EVALUATION OF THE NEONATE

lishment of **sustained** respiration is widely used to identify the vigorous or depressed neonate. A time to sustained respiration greater than 90 seconds invariably indicates a depressed or asphyxiated neonate and correlates well with a baby with an Apgar score of 6 or less.

Apgar Score

It was not until 1953 when Dr. Virginia Apgar developed her now universally accepted scoring system[2] that evaluation of the newborn immediately after birth was standardized into a simple, reproducible form which all personnel could easily be trained to perform. To ensure objectivity, it was intended that the score be performed by a pediatrician or some other individual not directly involved in care of the patient. The score was designed to clearly identify depressed infants requiring resuscitation and thereafter to follow their progress over the first minutes of life. The score directs the attendant's attention to five vital signs: heart rate, respiratory effort, muscle tone, reflex irritability and color. Each sign is given a numerical value as shown in Figure 25.1.

HEART RATE

Heart rate is determined by auscultation of the chest or less commonly by observation of the epigastrium or precordium for visible heart beat or palpation of the cord at the umbilicus. As with the fetus, the neonate at birth usually has a heart rate of over 100 beats per minute. A heart rate less than 100 usually signifies asphyxia. Another very common cause in an otherwise healthy baby is reflex bradycardia from enthusiastic efforts to aspirate the pharynx or empty the stomach. Rarely bradycardia is due to congenital heart block or propranolol therapy to the mother.[3]

RESPIRATORY EFFORT

An infant who is breathing and crying lustily receives a 2 rating, whereas an apneic infant receives a score of 0. All other types of respiratory effort—such as irregular, shallow ventilation or weak cry—are scored 1. The respiratory rate, per se, is

	A Appearance	P Pulse	G Grimace	A Activity	R Respiration
Score	Color	Heart Rate	Reflex Irritability	Muscle Tone	Respiratory Effort
0	Blue, pale	Absent	No response	Limp	Absent
1	Body pink, Extremities blue	Below 100	Grimace	Some flexion of extremities	Slow, irregular
2	Completely pink	Over 100	Cough, sneeze, or cry	Active motion	Good, crying

Figure 25.1. Apgar score is based on five signs, each scored 0, 1 or 2.

not considered, *only the quality of the respiratory efforts.*

MUSCLE TONE

A baby with active movement or spontaneously flexed arms and legs which resist extension is rated 2, whereas a completely flaccid infant receives a 0 score. Anything in between receives a value of 1. Some maternally administered drugs such as diazepam may selectively depress muscle tone without affecting circulation or respiration,[4] whereas others, such as ketamine in large doses (> 2 mg/kg), may increase tone while depressing respiration.[5]

REFLEX IRRITABILITY

This is tested by either inserting a nasal catheter, flicking the soles of the feet or drying the baby vigorously. A sneeze or lusty cry is scored 2, a grimace or weak cry 1 and no response 0.

COLOR

All infants are cyanotic at birth because of their high hemoglobin concentrations and low PaO_2. The disappearance of cyanosis is usually rapid when ventilation and circulation are normal. Many healthy, vigorous infants still have generalized or acrocyanosis at 1 minute due in part to peripheral vasoconstriction in response to the cold delivery room. A completely pink baby receives a score of 2, a pale or blue baby a score of 0 and a neonate with acrocyanosis a score of 1. If an infant seems to be breathing well and does not become pink despite administration of 100 per cent oxygen, the most common cause is acidosis and pulmonary vasoconstriction. Other causes include cyanotic congenital heart disease, methemoglobinemia, polycythemia or pulmonary disease such as hypoplastic lungs. The very pale infant may be hypovolemic and hypotensive. Some maternally administered drugs such as alcohol or magnesium may cause peripheral vasodilation and a pink color in a hypotonic lethargic baby.

Of the five criteria in the Apgar score, heart rate and respiratory effort are most important in identifying a distressed newborn, and color is of least value. Modifications of this scoring system with relative weight values for each sign or elimination of the color evaluation have been suggested.[6] However, the Apgar score as originally described has achieved its universal acceptance and popularity due in large part to its simplicity and reproducibility. The Apgar score has prognostic significance in regard to development of respiratory distress syndrome,[7] neurologic abnormalities[8] and indeed death.[9] Thus, it quickly identifies those infants requiring active resuscitation, which, by its early initiation, will reduce neonatal morbidity and mortality.

The Apgar score is usually measured at 1 and 5 minutes after birth. If the infant's condition continues to change in response to resuscitative efforts, the score should be repeated at 10 and 20 minutes of life. In addition to its simplicity, this measure has the effect of forcing the birth attendants to focus attention on the neonate at a time when care of the mother may also be demanding their attention. Although it has been used for over 25 years as an evaluative and prognostic tool, it is useful to review its value and limitations in light of knowledge acquired since its inception.

Apgar Score and Resuscitation

On the basis of 1-minute scores, neonates may be divided into three groups which relate to the degree of depression and, thus, to the need for active resuscitation. The Apgar score has been shown to correlate well with acid-base measurements performed immediately after birth[1]. Infants with scores greater than 7 have either normal values or, more commonly, a mild respiratory acidosis; infants with scores of 4 to 6 are moderately depressed and have a respiratory acidosis with some slight depression of buffer base; those with low scores (0 to 3) usually have a combined metabolic and respiratory acidosis. This last group has usually experienced a period of prolonged or severe asphyxia.

The degree of intervention required during resuscitation relates to the extent to which the score is lowered. For example, essentially healthy neonates scoring 8 to 10 need no respiratory assistance, mild to moderately depressed infants (scores 3 to 7) frequently improve rapidly in response to oxygen administered by mask (with positive pressure when necessary), whereas those who are severely depressed (scores 0 to 2) merit immediate active intervention, including endotracheal intubation and, perhaps, cardiac massage. A detailed description of resuscitation of the newborn based on the Apgar score is described in chapter 26. A second evaluation of the score at 5 minutes forces the resuscitation team to assess their progress, and better enables them to decide whether to continue their attempts. As a guide to identifying and treating the depressed neonate, the Apgar score has not yet been surpassed by any other index.

Prognostic Value of the Apgar Score

Apgar and James[10] and the Collaborative Study of Cerebral Palsy[11] investigated the correlation between neonatal mortality and Apgar score. The distribution of 1- and 5-minute scores for the first 17,221 infants in the collaborative study is shown in Table 25.1. There was a strong positive correlation between Apgar scores and birth weight.

In Apgar's study the mortality in the first 28 days of life, in both full-term and premature infants, was inversely related to the score at 1 minute. In very low birth weight infants, mortality tended to be high at all scores, although, as in all birth weight groups considered, there was a significant difference in survival in infants whose scores were poor (0 to 3), fair (4 to 6) or good (7 to 10).[10] In an attempt to establish a more accurate predictive index, the Collaborative Study evaluated scores at both 1 and 5 minutes. They confirmed Apgar's results for 1-minute scores, finding mortality in the first 27 days to be 23 per cent for infants having scores of 0 or 1, decreasing to 0.1 per cent for infants with 1-minute scores of 10. The 27-day mortality of infants with 5-minute scores of 0 or 1 was 49 per cent; it decreased with increasing scores. The Collaborative Study also demonstrated that Apgar scores more accurately predicted mortality during the first 2 days of life, rather than the period from 2 to 27 days, and that the 5-minute score was more useful in this respect (Figure 25.2). In spite of a smaller incidence of low scores at 5 minutes, such scores were much more likely to be associated with increased mortality. When birth weight was considered in conjunction with Apgar score, the highest mortality occurred in infants with both low birth weight and low Apgar scores. There was also a trend to increased mortality in infants weighing over 4,000 gm, perhaps because these infants were the offspring of diabetic mothers or because they had sustained birth trauma during a difficult delivery.

Table 25.1
Percentage Distribution of 1- and 5-minute Apgar Scores*

Apgar Score	0–3	4–6	7–10
	%	%	%
1 Minute	6.4	14.5	78.9
5 Minutes	1.8	3.5	94.8

* Data from Drage JS, Kennedy C, Schwarz BK: The Apgar score as an index of neonatal mortality. A report from the Collaborative Study of Cerebral Palsy. Obstet Gynecol 24: 222, 1964.

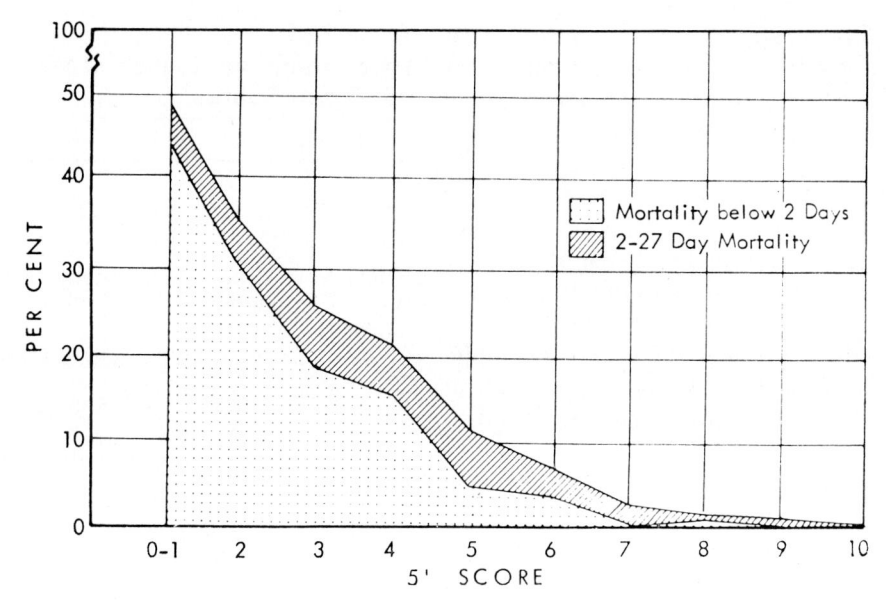

Figure 25.2. Percentage of neonatal mortality within each 5-minute score. (Reprinted by permission from Drage JS, Berendes H: Apgar scores and outcome of the newborn. Pediatr Clin North Am 13:635, 1966.)

Thus, the Apgar score is useful as a general prognostic tool in predicting short-term mortality in groups of infants, particularly those of low birth weight. It has little value, however, when attempting to predict the likelihood of survival in any individual case.

The Collaborative Study further investigated the value of this score as a predictor of neonatal morbidity.[8] Neurologic examinations were performed at 1 year of age and were related to 1- and 5-minute Apgar scores and to birth weight. Of the 14,115 infants examined, 1.9 per cent were discovered to have definite neurologic abnormalities. When considered in conjunction with Apgar scores at 1 minute, an incidence of 3.6 per cent of neurologically abnormal infants was found in the group who had scores of 0 to 3, whereas the incidence was only 1.6 per cent in infants who had scored 7 to 10. When grouped according to 5-minute score, the disparity was even greater; the incidence of abnormal infants in the "low score" group was four times as high as in the "high score" group. Again, birth weight was an extremely significant factor, with a more than 6-fold increase in neurologic abnormalities in infants weighing 1,001 to 2,000 gm at birth compared with those weighing over 2,500 gm (Figures 25.3 and 25.4). As Scanlon has emphasized, however, the pessimism which has been associated with low scoring infants as a result of these data is ill deserved.[12] The vast majority of full-term infants, even in the poorest scoring group, were neurologically normal, i.e. 96.4 per cent had no neurologic deficit. Therefore, the predictive accuracy of the Apgar score alone in this respect is low, and other factors such as low birth weight and prematurity must be taken into account.

Limitations of the Apgar Score

Several problems become apparent when the Apgar score is critically examined as an evaluative index. The intended objectivity of the score may be threatened

EVALUATION OF THE NEONATE

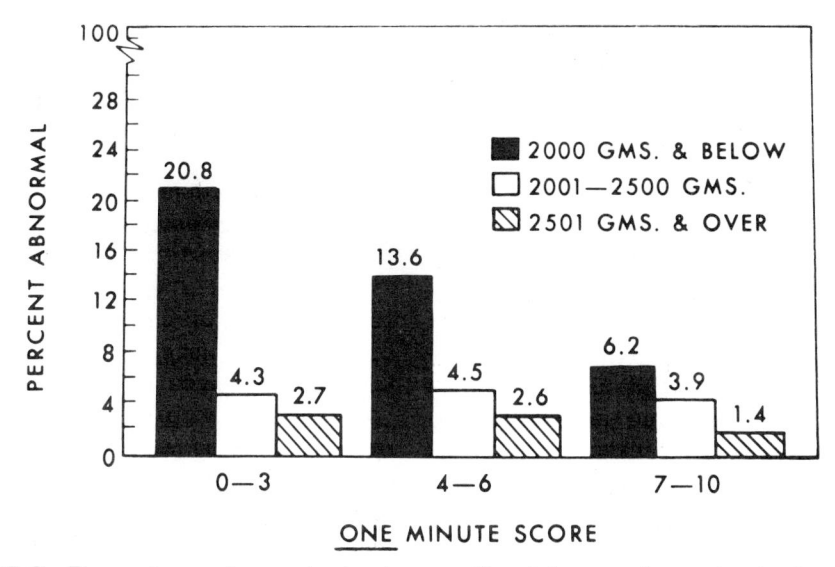

Figure 25.3. Percentage of neurologic abnormality at 1 year of age, by 1-minute Apgar score and birth weight groups. (Modified from Drage JS, Kennedy C, Berendes H, et al.: The Apgar score as an index of infant morbidity. Dev Med Child Neurol 8:141, 1966.)

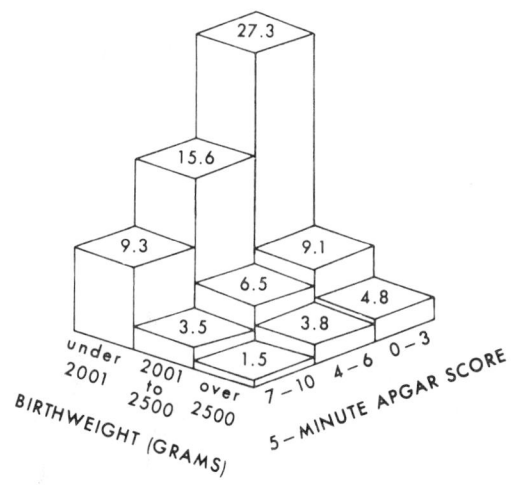

Figure 25.4. Percentage of neurologic abnormality at 1 year of age, by 5-minute Apgar score and birth weight groups. (Modified from Drage JS, Kennedy C, Berendes H, et al.: The Apgar score as an index of infant morbidity. Dev Med Child Neurol 8: 141, 1966.)

by lack of personnel available to measure it who are not involved with care of the patient. However, this criticism of subjectivity can be leveled equally justifiably at most other indices used to assess neonatal condition. Perhaps a more important limitation is the relative crudeness of the measurement, which looks only at the vital functions necessary to sustain life and continues observation for only a very brief period. Many serious neonatal problems do not present until after the infant has left the delivery room, and Apgar herself commented that the score "is no substitute for a careful physical examination and careful observation over the first few hours of life." As the infant has to be considerably affected to significantly lower the score, subtle effects of perinatal asphyxia or maternal medication may be missed entirely. Newer and more sophisticated techniques of examining the neurologic and behavioral aspects of the newborn have repeatedly demonstrated profound and sometimes prolonged depression in infants who have perfectly normal Apgar scores. Thus, studies using this index as an outcome measure which have judged drug regimens as "safe" must be reinterpreted in the light of more recent data.

LATER EVALUATION OF THE NEONATE

General Examination of the Newborn

As soon as the infant's condition has stabilized after delivery, a careful and thorough examination must be performed to look for abnormalities which may require special management. Developmental anomalies of the nervous system, such as spina bifida or myelomeningocele, are usually obvious, but congenital cardiac disease may be asymptomatic at this stage. An infant who remains cyanosed or whose lungs are difficult to inflate should immediately arouse suspicion of a diagnosis of diaphragmatic hernia, whereas the presence of bubbling secretions would suggest tracheo-esophageal fistula. If either of the latter conditions is suspected, further diagnostic measures must be undertaken immediately. Examination of the mouth may reveal cleft lip or palate, a large tongue as in cretinism or micrognathia as in the Pierre-Robin syndrome. It is especially important to recognize these abnormalities, as dangerous respiratory obstruction may develop, particularly during feeding.

Continued Observation of the Neonate

In most centers, for the first few hours of life the infant is intensively observed in a special nursery. During the first 24 hours the infant undergoes massive physiologic adjustments from intrauterine to extrauterine life. Desmond and associates[13] observed a number of physical signs during the first 10 hours of life in essentially healthy neonates (Figure 25.5). A period of great activity is seen immediately after birth, which subsides after the first 30 minutes, giving way to sleep for subsequent hours. The infant then once more becomes active and aroused and may pass meconium and cry. Respiratory difficulties such as grunting or intercostal retraction, signifying the presence of respiratory distress syndrome, may not become obvious until this time. Central nervous system damage may manifest itself by irritability, "jitteriness" or seizures; in such cases, a full neurologic examination is indicated.

The biochemical status of the infant is also changing during this period. In normal infants the respiratory acidosis which is usually present at birth is rapidly corrected during the first hours of life, and by 24 hours blood gases are similar to those found in utero.[14] In sick neonates, serial evaluation of acid-base status using an umbilical arterial catheter may reveal abnormalities which point to the need for oxygen or bicarbonate therapy or ventilatory support. Asphyxiated infants or those severely depressed by anesthetic medication frequently demonstrate a prolonged respiratory acidosis in addition to a metabolic acidosis. The metabolic derangements in these and in premature infants resolve much more slowly than in healthy infants.

Assessment of Weight and Gestational Age

Morbidity and mortality are high in low birth weight infants. It is important to recognize that this group comprises two distinct subgroups: (1) infants who are small because they have been born prematurely and (2) infants who are of lower birth weight than would be expected from knowledge of their gestational age. Intrauterine growth standards have been constructed which permit classification of an infant as small, appropriate or large for gestational age (Figure 25.6).[15] Deviation from normal growth occurs in a variety of pathologic conditions. Intrauterine growth retardation may occur in conjunction with chronic maternal hypertension, toxemia or placental insufficiency and, occasionally, in severe malnutrition. The distinction between premature but appropriate for gestational age infants and full-term infants of similar weight who are small for gestational age is important, because different

EVALUATION OF THE NEONATE

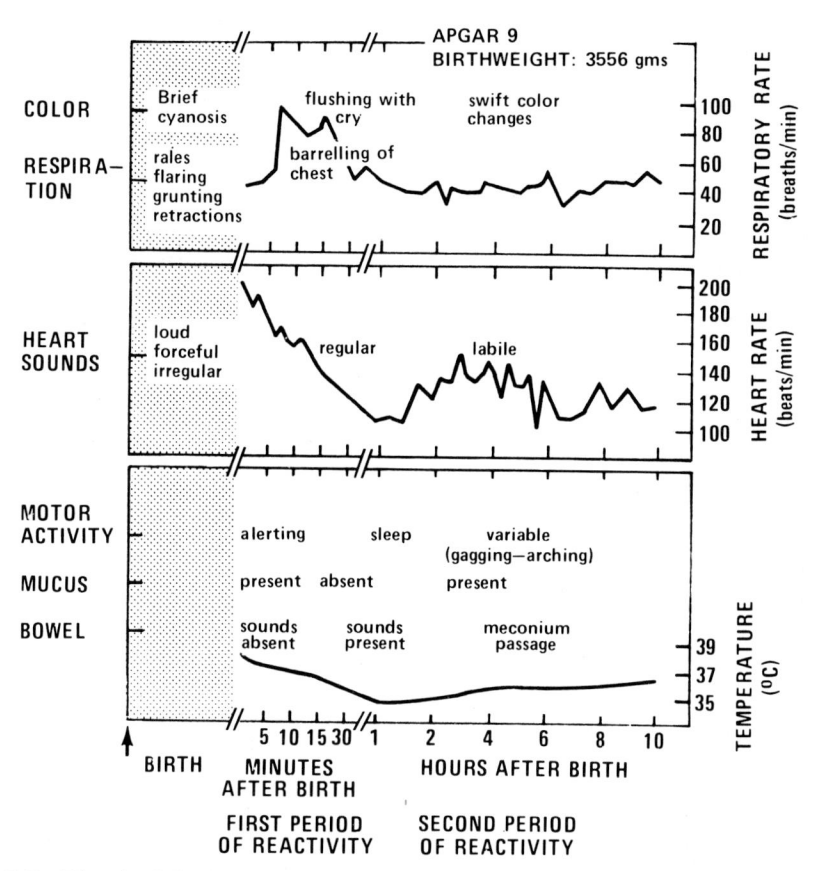

Figure 25.5. Physical findings noted during the first 10 hours of life in a high Apgar score infant delivered under spinal anesthesia without prior pre-medication. (Modified by permission from Desmond MM, Rudolph AJ, Phitaksphraiwan P: The transitional care nursery. Pediatr Clin North Am 13:651, 1966.)

problems may be anticipated in each group. Premature infants are susceptible to respiratory distress, jaundice, hypothermia, intracranial hemorrhage and retrolental fibroplasia. Small for gestational age infants are more likely to suffer from hypoglycemia and infection, as well as requiring a greater caloric intake which is associated with a higher oxygen consumption.[16] Congenital and chromosomal abnormalities occur more frequently in small for gestational age infants.

The prognosis of small for gestational age infants is generally poorer than premature appropriate for gestational age infants of the same weight, as judged by the results of developmental testing. It can be postulated that the nutritional deficiency or chronic hypoxia which results in low birth weight is also responsible for poor neurologic development. Both morbidity and mortality in the newborn are related to gestational age, following a similar pattern to the relationship with birth weight, i.e. rates are highest in infants of lowest birth weight and earliest gestational age and diminish as normal values are approached. Morbidity and mortality are also increased when excessive birth weight or post-maturity is present; large birth weight is often associated with maternal diabetes or difficult deliveries, and in post-maturity

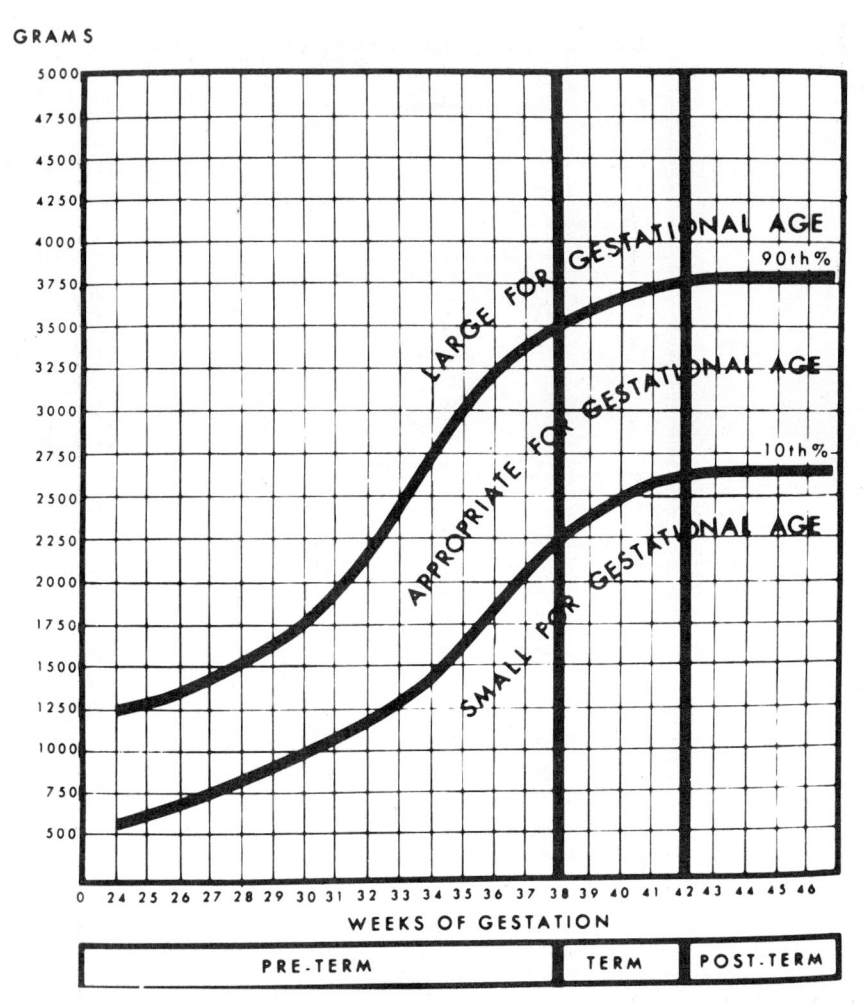

Figure 25.6. University of Colorado Medical Center classification of newborns by birth weight and gestational age. (Reprinted by permission from Lubchenco LO: Assessment of weight and gestational age. In *Neonatology,* GB Avery, ed. J. B. Lippincott, Philadelphia, 1975, p 127.)

the fetus tends to have outgrown its placental supply. Consideration of gestational age with respect to birth weight is, of course, only possible if the former can be accurately determined. Although the date of the last menstrual period provides valuable information, bleeding early in pregnancy frequently cannot be distinguished from a normal period and, thus, the date of conception is unknown. Several schemes have been developed for assessing gestational age, which relate development to either the appearance of certain neurologic signs or to external characteristics in the newborn. Although either of these parameters give a fair estimate of gestational age, the best approximation is provided by the Dubowitz score,[17] which utilizes both sets of criteria. As modified by Ballard (Figure 25.7), a graded score is awarded for the presence of six neurologic signs which predominantly reflect muscle tone and which are related to maturation of the nervous system. The signs selected

EVALUATION OF THE NEONATE

Neuromuscular Maturity

	0	1	2	3	4	5
Posture						
Square Window (wrist)	90°	60°	45°	30°	0°	
Arm Recoil	180°		100°–180°	90°–100°	<90°	
Popliteal Angle	180°	160°	130°	110°	90°	<90°
Scarf Sign						
Heel to Ear						

Physical Maturity

	0	1	2	3	4	5
Skin	gelatinous red, transparent	smooth pink, visible veins	superficial peeling, &/or rash few veins	cracking pale area rare veins	parchment deep cracking no vessels	leathery cracked wrinkled
Lanugo	none	abundant	thinning	bald areas	mostly bald	
Plantar Creases	no crease	faint red marks	anterior transverse crease only	creases ant. 2/3	creases cover entire sole	
Breast	barely percept.	flat areola no bud	stippled areola 1–2mm bud	raised areola 3–4mm bud	full areola 5–10mm bud	
Ear	pinna flat, stays folded	sl. curved pinna; soft c̄ slow recoil	well-curv. pinna; soft but ready recoil	formed & firm c̄ instant recoil	thick cartilage ear stiff	
Genitals ♂	scrotum empty no rugae		testes descending, few rugae	testes down good rugae	testes pendulous deep rugae	
Genitals ♀	prominent clitoris & labia minora		majora & minora equally prominent	majora large minora small	clitoris & minora completely covered	

Adapted from: Devel. Med. Child. Neurol. 8:507–511, 1966
Arch. Dis. Child. 43:89–93, 1968
J. Ped. 77:1, 1970
By: J. Ballard, M.D. August, 1971
Revised: February, 1972

Apgars ___ 1 min ___ 5 min
Age at Exam ___ hrs
Race ___ Sex ___
B.D. ___
LMP ___
EDC ___
Gest. age by Dates ___ wks
Gest. age by Exam ___ wks
B.W. ___ gm. ___ %ile
Length ___ cm. ___ %ile
Head Circum. ___ cm. ___ %ile
Clin. Dist. None ___ Mild ___
Mod. ___ Severe ___

MATURITY RATING

Score	Wks.
5	26
10	28
15	30
20	32
25	34
30	36
35	38
40	40
45	42
50	44

Figure 25.7. Assessment of gestational age. (Reprinted by permission from Sweet AY: Classification of the low-birth-weight infant. In *Care of the High Risk Neonate,* MH Klaus and AA Fanaroff, eds. W. B. Saunders, Philadelphia, 1973, p 47.)

are those least affected by the state of arousal of the infant or the presence of neurologic abnormality. Both of these factors had affected previous assessments based on neurologic criteria. Seven external characteristics (including skin texture, color and opacity, nipple formation, ear form, etc.) are similarly considered, and a composite score is obtained. Dubowitz found that the total score could be reliably reproduced by different observers, could be performed at any time during the first 5 days of life and was able to accurately assess gestational age to within 1 week.

Neurobehavioral Testing

The inability of the Apgar score to detect subtle or delayed effects of perinatal events led pediatricians, psychologists and, more recently, anesthesiologists to seek more sensitive methods of evaluating the neonate. Although traditional neurologic examination is undoubtedly of diagnostic value in infants with frank neurologic problems, it is of limited value for recognizing the sequelae of lesser perinatal insults and for predicting their influence on future development. For a complete description of the neurologic examination of the neonate and the abnormalities associated with neurologic disorders, the reader is referred to Volpe's review of the subject.[18]

Dissatisfaction with existing techniques has caused attention to be directed toward other aspects of newborn behavior. As far back as 1957, Graham and co-workers[19] correlated decreased performance in a series of neonatal behavior tests with the severity of perinatal hypoxia. Infants with a history of hypoxia could clearly be distinguished from a control group of "normal" infants. Drugs administered to the mother may also result in subtle and prolonged effects on the newborn, in spite of normal Apgar scores at birth. Kron et al.[20] demonstrated that a single injection of 200 mg of secobarbital given to the mother immediately before delivery was associated with poorer sucking responses in the infant for as long as 4 days after birth. Brazelton[21] similarly found a lag of 2 days in the establishment of breast feeding and 1 day in weight gain in babies of mothers who were heavily medicated in labor, as compared with those who were not. Visual attentiveness of the newborn was also depressed for as long as 4 days after the administration of narcotics or barbiturates to the mother within 1½ hours of delivery.[22]

Various neurobehavioral tests have been developed which have modified and extended the classical newborn neurologic examination. For many years the infant had been regarded as functioning only reflexly at a spinal or brain stem level. When subjected to closer scrutiny it was appreciated that the newborn is capable of quite organized behavior in the first days of life.

Brazelton's realization that maternal medication exaggerated and prolonged the period of relative disorganization which occurs for some period following "normal" delivery led him to develop a more exact way of quantitating the psychophysiologic adaptive changes occurring during the first week after birth. The Brazelton Neonatal Behavioral Assessment Scale[23] has formed the basis of many other such scales and examines various aspects of newborn behavior which are thought to involve the CNS at a cortical level. Such functions include the newborn's ability to alter its state of arousal, suppress meaningless or intrusive stimuli and respond appropriately to a spectrum of external events in its environment. Central nervous system integrity is also evidenced by the newborn's motor behavior, both in initiating complex motor acts and in reflex motor responses. In the normal infant, smooth arcs of limb movements are present, whereas jerky hypertonic activity signifies imbalance between flexor and extensor muscle groups and reflects a poorly organized CNS. The Brazelton assessment is a comprehensive evaluation of newborn behavior, but it is time consuming and must be performed by a trained observer.

Neonatal behavioral tests have proved sensitive in demonstrating depression of the neonate after perinatal asphyxia, illness, maternal medication and a variety of other influences. Repeated assessments are most valuable, because they allow recovery from such effects to be monitored and permit formulation of a long-term prognosis. The Brazelton scale proved superior to routine neurologic examinations in predicting which infants would be neurologically abnormal at 7 years of age.[24] Although both tests succeeded in identifying most of the infants who were ultimately considered to be impaired, the neurologic examination had a higher "false

EVALUATION OF THE NEONATE

alarm" rate and mislabeled more normal children than the Behavioral Assessment.

The obstetric anesthesiologist is, of course, most interested in the effects on the neonate of maternally administered drugs. Conway and Brackbill[25] claimed that both maternal analgesia and anesthesia could affect newborn behavior for as long as 4 weeks after birth, although it was difficult in their study to separate the effects of individual drugs, dosages and anesthetic techniques. Behavioral effects have been correlated with electroencephalographic records of newborns and have confirmed that heavy maternal medication may cause transient CNS depression until the third day of life.[26]

With the intention of studying primarily the effects on the neonate of maternal medication and anesthetic techniques, Scanlon and associates[27] devised a neurobehavioral test, the Early Neonatal Neurobehavioral Scale (ENNS), based on the Prechtl and Beintema Neurological Examination and the Brazelton Behavioral Scale (Figure 25.8). This examination has proved to be relatively simple and rapid to perform, with a high degree of reproducibility between observers. It was initially designed to assess infants during the first 8 to 12 hours of life, this period of time corresponding with the half-life of local anesthetics used for epidural anesthesia. The test must be conducted when the in-

```
Name _____ Unit Number _____
Time _____ Blood Gases Po₂ _____ Pco₂ _____ pH _____
Anesthetic Level _____ Type _____ Body Temp _____
Apgar      HR ___ Resp Eff ___ Tone ___ Irrit ___ Color ___ Total ___
           NEURO EXAM:
STATE _____  1. Response to pinprick   0  1  2  3
                 Habituation no. _____
       _____  2. Resistance against passive motion
                 A. Pull to sitting      0  1  2  3
                 B. Arm recoil           0  1  2  3
                 C. Truncal tone         0  1  2  3
                 D. General body tone    0  1  2  3
       _____  3. Rooting                0  1  2  3
       _____  4. Sucking                0  1  2  3
       _____  5. Moro response          0  1  2  3
                 Threshold (# of attempts)
                 Extinguishment
       _____  6. Habituation to light in eyes        No. _____
       _____  7. Response to sound      0  1  2  3
                 Habituation no. _____
       _____  8. Placing                0  1  2  3
              9. Alertness               0  1  2  3
             10. General assessment      A  B  N  S†
                    (circle)
                 Reasons
                 State _____
                 Lability of state _____
COMMENTS:
```

Figure 25.8. Protocol for Early Neonatal Neurobehavioral Scale (ENNS) or Scanlon Score. *A,* abnormal; *B,* borderline; *N,* normal; *S,* superior. (Reprinted by permission from Scanlon JW, Brown WU, Weiss JB, et al.: Neurobehavioral responses of newborn infants after maternal epidural anesthesia. Anesthesiology 40:121, 1974.)

fant is awake but resting quietly in a room without other distracting influences. The observer assesses the infant's state of wakefulness on several occasions, reflex responses (rooting, sucking, Moro's maneuver), muscle tone and power and responses to light, pinprick and sound. Decrement behavior or "habituation" after repetition of these stimuli is also recorded. The ability of the infant to decrease and eventually abolish its response to stimuli which are meaningless to it seems to represent the earliest example of processing of information by the cerebral cortex, memory and perhaps even learning. This property, commonly referred to as habituation, seems to be particularly sensitive to the effects of anesthetic drugs. Even small amounts of maternal systemic medication such as meperidine 50 mg, have been shown to depress such "higher" CNS functions, as reflected by a slower rate of habituation to a redundant sound stimulus. This parameter and responsiveness to external stimuli were found by Brackbill et al.[28] to be the most sensitive elements of a variety of evaluative tests.

An increasing mass of information is accumulating relating newborn behavior to the effects of anesthesia. Scanlon et al.[27] have demonstrated that infants of mothers who received epidural anesthesia with either lidocaine or mepivacaine had significantly lower scores than "non-epidural" infants on tests of muscle strength and tone but behaved normally with respect to habituation to repetitive stimuli. They concluded that these infants were "floppy but alert," and that higher CNS functions had not been depressed by the medication. These effects were present only in the first 8 hours of life, which corresponds with the period during which significant concentrations of local anesthetics were found in the newborn circulation; lidocaine was detected in the neonatal blood stream for 8 hours and mepivacaine for as long as 24 hours after birth.[29]

Epidural anesthesia using bupivacaine has been shown by the same authors to be free from the motor depression seen with lidocaine and mepivacaine.[30] Such babies were indistinguishable from controls (Table 5.3). Bupivacaine is present only in very small amounts in the newborn circulation after epidural anesthesia and disappears much more rapidly from the fetal circulation than the other agents. The mechanism by which local anesthetics exert their effects in the newborn is unknown, although an effect on the neuromuscular junction has been postulated.

The effects of general anesthesia for elective cesarean section in normal pregnancies have also been studied. Infants whose mothers had undergone general rather than spinal anesthesia exhibited global depression of neurobehavioral performance, in spite of there being no difference in Apgar scores between the groups.[31] Palahniuk et al.[32] compared three anesthetic techniques for cesarean section: (1) methoxyflurane with high inspired oxygen, (2) nitrous oxide with low inspired oxygen and (3) lumbar epidural anesthesia. Although all infants appeared clinically normal, those in the nitrous oxide group were less alert and had lower scores on neurobehavioral testing (ENNS) than the other groups for a period of 24 hours. A different study compared the results of the ENNS in infants whose mothers had received ketamine-nitrous oxide or thiopental-nitrous oxide general anesthesia or chloroprocaine epidural anesthesia for vaginal delivery.[33] Epidural anesthesia was associated with the greatest percentage of high scores on the first and second days of life. The infants performed least well after thiopental, with ketamine producing an intermediate effect. In general, maternal administration of central nervous system depressants seems to cause a transient depression of newborn behavior, which is probably related to the presence of drugs in the neonatal circulation.

It is appropriate at this juncture to question the significance, as regards well-being and future development, of abnormalities revealed by neurobehavioral testing. Tronick et al.[34] studied the effects of different analgesic regimens for labor on the behavior of normal neonates, attempting to control for other stress factors. Techniques included maternal local and regional anesthesia, and in some cases additional light systemic medication was administered. Only minimal effects were found in all groups. These proved to be transient, and all effects progressively improved over the first 10 days of life. These data do not negate the findings by other authors of more profound depression following heavier medication. In other series infants may have been included who had suffered depression from other stresses.

There is no evidence as yet of prolonged adverse effects being associated with neurobehavioral depression caused by maternal medication. However, the interaction between the newborn and its mother, "maternal-infant bonding,"[35] and the environment in general is thought by many to be vital for the establishment of healthy behavior patterns. Inconsolability or excessive sleepiness may induce negative feelings in the mother toward her child, so that early bonding is impaired. On a more tangible level, it is easy to see that successful establishment of breast feeding may be threatened by undue drowsiness in the infant. It is perhaps of greater prognostic significance when neurobehavioral depression occurs which cannot be attributed to medication and which, therefore, might be the result of perinatal asphyxia or brain damage. If the results of such assessments are to be used to predict further development, the history must be made known to the person interpreting the test.

Neurobehavioral assessment techniques have so far been used predominantly in the research area and are still probably too cumbersome to be applied routinely as a clinical diagnostic tool. Like most of the other evaluative indices, they can be criticized as being subjective and are regarded with scepticism by many as being less meaningful than "hard" scientific data. At the present time, neurobehavioral testing is only one method of evaluating the newborn and must not be used in isolation. It must take its place along with the history, Apgar score, neurologic and biochemical investigations in the continuum of evaluation procedures in the newborn. Until further knowledge is gained of long-term effects of drug administration on the newborn, it is perhaps prudent to choose anesthetic or analgesic techniques which have the least observable effects, especially if their analgesic efficacy is indistinguishable from drugs with a more profound effect. With continuing efforts being directed toward assessing the effects of iatrogenic influences, not restricted to anesthesia, on the newborn, it is hoped that an improvement in perinatal care will result.

References

1. James LS, Weisbrot IM, Prince CE, et al.: The acid-base status of human infants in relation to birth asphyxia and the onset of respiration. J Pediatr 52:379, 1958.
2. Apgar V: A proposal for a new method of evaluation of the newborn infant. Anesth Analg 32:260, 1953.
3. Gladstone GR, Hordof A, Gersony WM: Propranolol administration during pregnancy: Effects on the fetus. J Pediatr 86:962, 1975.
4. Flowers CE, Rudolph AJ, Desmond MM: Diazepam (Valium) as an adjunct in obstetric analgesia. Obstet Gynecol 34:68, 1969.
5. Chang T, Chucot L: Study of ketamine as an obstetric anesthetic agent. Am J Obstet Gynecol 113:247, 1972.
6. Crawford JS: Anesthesia for caesarean section: Proposal for evaluation with analysis of a method. Br J Anaesth 34:179, 1962.
7. Rudolph AJ, Desmond MM, Pineda RG: Clinical diagnosis of respiratory difficulty in the newborn. Pediatr Clin North Am 13:669, 1966.
8. Drage JS, Kennedy C, Berendes H, et al.: The Apgar score as an index of infant morbidity. Dev Med Child Neurol 8:141, 1966.

9. Drage JS, Berendes H: Apgar scores and outcome of the newborn. Pediatr Clin North Am 13:635, 1966.
10. Apgar V, James LS: Further observations on the newborn scoring system. Am J Dis Child 104:419, 1962.
11. Drage JS, Kennedy C, Schwarz BK: The Apgar score as an index of neonatal mortality. A report from the Collaborative Study of Cerebral Palsy. Obstet Gynecol 24:222, 1964.
12. Scanlon JW: How is the baby? The Apgar score revisited. Clin Pediatr 12:61, 1973.
13. Desmond MM, Rudolph AJ, Phitaksphraiwan P: The transitional care nursery. Pediatr Clin North Am 13:651, 1966.
14. Weisbrot IM, James LS, Prince CE, et al.: Acid-base homeostasis of the newborn infant during the first 24 hours of life. J Pediatr 52:395, 1958.
15. Lubchenco LO: Assessment of weight and gestational age. In Neonatology, GB Avery, ed. J. B. Lippincott, Philadelphia, 1975, p 127.
16. Brazelton TB, Parker WB, Zuckerman B: Importance of behavioral assessment of the neonate. Curr Probl Pediatr 7(2):34, 1976.
17. Dubowitz LM, Dubowitz V, Goldberg C: Clinical assessment of gestational age in the newborn infant. J Pediatr 77:1, 1970.
18. Volpe JJ: Neurological disorders. In Neonatology, GB Avery, ed. J. B. Lippincott, Philadelphia, 1975, p 729.
19. Graham FK, Pennoyer MM, Caldwell BM, et al.: Relationship between clinical status and behavior test performance in a newborn group with histories suggesting anoxia. J Pediatr 50:177, 1957.
20. Kron RE, Stein M, Goddard KE: Newborn sucking behavior affected by obstetric sedation. Pediatrics 37:1012, 1966.
21. Brazelton TB: Psychophysiologic reactions in the neonate. II. Effect of maternal medication on the neonate and his behavior. J Pediatr 58:513, 1961.
22. Stechler G: Newborn attention as affected by medication during labor. Science 144:315, 1964.
23. Brazelton TB: Neonatal Behavioral Assessment Scale. J. B. Lippincott, Philadelphia, 1973.
24. Brazelton TB, Parker WB, Zuckerman B: Importance of behavioral assessment of the neonate. Curr Probl Pediatr 7(2):71, 1976.
25. Conway E, Brackbill Y: II. Delivery medication and infant outcome: An empirical study. Monogr Soc Res Child Dev 35:24, 1970.
26. Borgstedt AD, Rosen MG: Medication during labor correlated with behavior and EEG of the newborn. Am J Dis Child 115:21, 1968.
27. Scanlon JW, Brown WU, Weiss JB, et al.: Neurobehavioral responses of newborn infants after maternal epidural anesthesia. Anesthesiology 40:121, 1974.
28. Brackbill Y, Kane J, Manniello RL, et al.: Obstetric meperidine usage and assessment of neonatal status. Anesthesiology 40:116, 1974.
29. Brown WU, Bell GC, Lurie AO, et al.: Newborn blood levels of lidocaine and mepivacaine in the first postnatal day following maternal epidural anesthesia. Anesthesiology 42:698, 1975.
30. Scanlon JW, Ostheimer GW, Lurie AO, et al.: Neurobehavioral responses and drug concentrations in newborns after maternal epidural anesthesia with bupivacaine. Anesthesiology 45:400, 1976.
31. Scanlon JW, Shea E, Alper MH: Neurobehavioral responses of newborn infants following general or spinal anesthesia for cesarean section. In Abstracts of Scientific Papers, Annual Meeting, American Society of Anesthesiologists, Chicago, 1975, p 91.
32. Palahniuk RJ, Scatliff J, Biehl D, et al.: Evaluation of methoxyflurane, nitrous oxide, and lumbar epidural anesthesia for elective cesarean section. In Abstracts of Scientific Papers, Annual Meeting, American Society of Anesthesiologists, San Francisco, 1976, p 249.
33. Hodgkinson R, Marx GF, Kim SS, et al.: Neonatal neurobehavioral tests following vaginal delivery under ketamine, thiopental and extradural anesthesia. Anesth Analg 56:548, 1977.
34. Tronick E, Wise S, Als H, et al.: Regional obstetric anesthesia with lidocaine for vaginal delivery. Acta Obstet Gynecol Scand (Suppl 34)53:3, 1974.
35. Klaus MH, Kennell JH: Maternal-Infant Bonding. C. V. Mosby, St. Louis, 1976.

CHAPTER 26

Resuscitation of the Newborn

Gershon Levinson, M.D.
Sol M. Shnider, M.D.

Immediately after delivery, as the fetus becomes a neonate, major changes in the pulmonary and circulatory systems must occur. The lungs must now assume the role of the placenta in the exchange of oxygen and carbon dioxide. This requires pulmonary expansion, aeration and perfusion. In the vast majority of instances these changes occur spontaneously. Some infants, however, require resuscitation to make the transition from dependent fetal to independent neonatal existence. This chapter will discuss the normal changes at birth, pathophysiology of asphyxia and recommended techniques for resuscitation of the newborn.

CHANGES AT BIRTH

In utero, blood is oxygenated in the placenta and returns to the fetal heart via the umbilical vein, hepatic veins, the ductus venosus and the inferior vena cava[1,2] (Figure 5.9). At the junction of the inferior vena cava and right atrium the caval blood divides into two streams. Approximately 40 per cent enters the right heart where it mixes with venous blood returning via the superior vena cava from the upper part of the body. This blood is ejected by the right ventricle into the pulmonary arteries. However, because the pulmonary vascular resistance is so high, only 5 to 10 per cent actually perfuses the fetal lungs, the remainder being shunted across the ductus arteriosus into the thoracic aorta. About 60 per cent of the well oxygenated blood returning via the inferior vena cava is deflected by the crista dividens through the foramen ovale into the left atrium. Although this blood undergoes admixture with the small amount of venous blood returning from the lungs, it is relatively well oxygenated and provides the heart and brain with somewhat better oxygenation than the lower half of the body.

With clamping of the cord and vasoconstriction of the umbilical vessels at birth, systemic vascular resistance increases markedly, left atrial pressure rises and flow through the foramen ovale ceases; the lungs expand, pulmonary vascular resistance falls and 90 to 100 per cent of the right ventricular output now perfuses the lungs.[3,4]

As arterial oxygen and pH rise, the pulmonary vessels dilate, pulmonary vascular resistance falls further, pulmonary blood pressure falls below systemic and right-to-left shunting of blood through the ductus arteriosus ceases. In the normal newborn the rise in arterial oxygen to above 60 torr will cause vasoconstriction of the ductus arteriosus and aid in functional closure.[5,6]

ASPHYXIA

If immediately after birth adequate ventilation is not established then the ensuing hypoxemia and respiratory and metabolic acidosis will prevent establishment of a normal adult circulation. Pulmonary vascular resistance will remain high and pulmonary blood flow low, and the ductus arteriosus and foramen ovale will remain widely patent with a large right-to-left shunt through both. With progressive hypoxemia and acidosis, myocardial failure and brain damage will occur.

In the extreme case when no pulmonary ventilation occurs in a newborn mammal, by 5 minutes the PaO₂ will fall to under 2 torr, the PaCO₂ will rise to 100 torr and the pH will fall to 7.0 or less units (Figure 26.1).[1] Heart rate and blood pressure will fall and, after a period of gasping, apnea will occur. In the monkey, by 7 minutes there will be irreversible brain damage. After the cessation of gasping, nothing will reinitiate breathing other than artificial ventilation.

ESTABLISHMENT OF VENTILATION

In utero, the fetal lung is filled with an ultra-filtrate of plasma, approximately 30 ml per kg of body weight.[7,8] This fluid produced in the lungs must be removed during and immediately after birth. During a vaginal delivery the thorax of the fetus is squeezed while passing through the birth canal. This helps push out approximately two-thirds of the fluid from the lung, and the remainder is removed after birth by capillaries and lymphatics.[9] Infants delivered by cesarean section do not benefit from the vaginal squeeze, which may account for their increased difficulty in establishing normal ventilation.[10]

Normal infants make their first respiratory movements within seconds of delivery of the thorax. This is due in part to the elastic recoil of the chest wall following expulsion. During the first breath a negative pressure of 60 to 100 cm of water is generated and up to 80 ml of air inspired[11] (Figure 26.2). The breath is generally held for about 2 seconds and then partly ex-

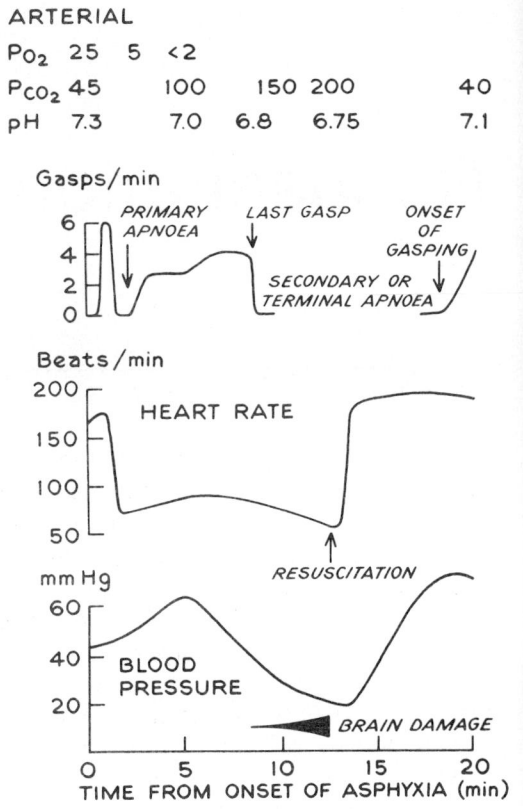

Figure 26.1. Schematic diagram of changes in Rhesus monkeys during asphyxia and resuscitation by positive pressure ventilation. Brain damage was assessed by histologic examination some weeks or months later. (Reprinted by permission from Dawes GS: *Foetal and Neonatal Physiology.* Year Book Medical Publishers, Chicago, 1968, pp 91–105.)

haled. Approximately 75 per cent of the first breath is retained in the lung as part of the developing functional residual capacity. The next few breaths are similar to the first, with lesser amounts of air retained each time. Once ventilation is established the normal mature infant has a tidal volume of 10 to 30 ml, a vital capacity of over 100 ml, a breathing frequency of 30 to 60 times per minute, a minute ventilation of over 500 ml and a lung compliance of 5 ml per centimeter of water.[11]

RESUSCITATION OF THE NEWBORN

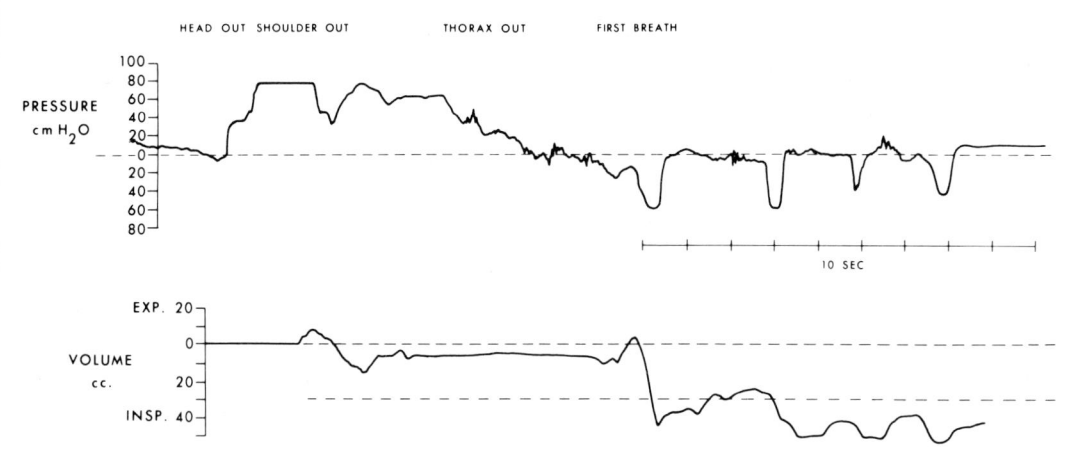

Figure 26.2. Intrathoracic pressures during and immediately after delivery. (Reprinted by permission from Karlberg P: The adaptive changes in the immediate postnatal period, with particular reference to respiration. J Pediatr 56:585, 1960.)

By 90 seconds after delivery most infants have begun rhythmic respirations. Initiation of breathing depends on the condition of the respiratory center, including peripheral chemoreceptors responsive to low pH and low PO_2.

CAUSES OF NEONATAL DEPRESSION

A number of factors may depress the respiratory center of the neonate, including drugs administered to the mother—such as anesthetics, narcotics, barbiturates and magnesium—severe intrauterine fetal hypoxia and acidosis, high or low environmental temperature or central nervous system trauma associated with the birth process.

In addition, there are various situations in which serious neonatal morbidity may occur. Identifying these high-risk fetuses prior to birth allows the anesthesiologist, obstetrician and neonatologist to prepare for immediate resuscitation of the newborn. Some of the factors which should alert the anesthesiologist that the fetus is at high risk are listed in Table 26.1.

The mechanism for the adverse effect on the neonate is obvious in conditions like preeclampsia and anemia which are associated with decreased utero-placental blood flow or oxygenation. In conditions such as diabetes mellitus, neonatal morbidity and mortality are very high but the precise etiology is not known. Nevertheless, in all these conditions aggressive management of the newborn is indicated.

UMBILICAL CORD BLOOD SAMPLING

At delivery the acid-base status and oxygenation of the fetus may be easily ascertained by sampling from a doubly clamped segment of umbilical cord. Babies who have demonstrated fetal distress in utero or who are clinically depressed at 1 minute of age should be studied. Blood is drawn separately with heparinized syringes from both an umbilical artery and the umbilical vein. It should be recalled that the umbilical vein blood is the best oxygenated blood. The normal blood gas values are shown in Table 26.2. If both umbilical venous and umbilical artery blood show low PO_2 and high PCO_2 then utero-placental insufficiency was present. If umbilical artery blood shows signs of asphyxia but umbilical venous blood is relatively nor-

Table 26.1
Factors Which May Help to Identify High-risk Fetuses

Maternal conditions
    Toxemia of pregnancy
    Hypertension
    Diabetes mellitus
    Elderly (> 35 years) or young (< 15 years) primigravida
    Chronic renal disease
    Maternal malnutrition or severe obesity
    Sickle cell disease
    Anemia (< 9 gm hemoglobin)
    Rh or ABO incompatibility
    Heart disease
    Pulmonary disease
    Third trimester bleeding
    Drug or ethanol abuse
    Maternal infection
    Uterine or pelvic anatomic abnormalities
    Prolonged rupture of membranes
    Previous fetal or neonatal deaths

Fetal conditions
    Premature delivery
    Post-maturity (43 weeks)
    Intrauterine growth retardation
    Multiple births
    Polyhydramnios
    Meconium-stained amniotic fluid

Labor and delivery conditions
    Breech or other abnormal presentations
    Forceps delivery (other than low elective)
    Cesarean section
    Prolapsed umbilical cord
    Nuchal cord
    Prolonged general anesthesia
    Excessive sedation or analgesia
    Anesthetic complications (such as hypotension or hypoxia)
    Prolonged or precipitous labor
    Uterine hypertonus (spontaneous or oxytocin-induced)
    Abnormal heart rate or rhythm

mal, that is, a wide venous-arterial difference exists, then umbilical cord compression has likely occurred during delivery. With partial compression of the umbilical cord, the transit time of fetal blood through the placenta is increased, thus allowing more time for equilibration with the maternal blood. The umbilical venous blood becomes well oxygenated, but, because of the obstruction of blood flow from the placenta to the fetus, an inadequate amount of oxygen is delivered to the fetal tissues and the umbilical arterial blood will demonstrate a low PO_2 and pH. A depressed neonate with normal umbilical venous oxygen and acid-base values may, in fact, be asphyxiated. It is obvious, therefore, that both the umbilical vein and artery blood should be analyzed for correct diagnosis of etiology and significance of depression. If umbilical cord blood gases are normal but the neonate is depressed at birth, common causes include drug depression or acute birth trauma.

IMMEDIATE CARE OF THE NEWBORN

Equipment for Resuscitation

Each delivery room should contain the basic equipment for resuscitating the depressed newborn (Table 26.3, part A). This includes infant laryngoscope, supply of batteries and bulbs, endotracheal tubes, infant airways and suction bulbs and catheters. In addition, each room should have a mobile or portable (delivery room to

Table 26.2
Normal Values of Blood Gas and Acid-Base Variables in Human Maternal and Fetal Blood Sampled at the Time of Delivery

	PO_2	O_2 Saturation	PCO_2	pH	Base Excess
	mm Hg	%	mm Hg	units	mEq/L
Maternal artery	100	98	30	7.40	−4
Fetal scalp capillary	25	55	45	7.28	−6
Umbilical vein*	30	65	40	7.32	−5
Umbilical artery*	15	20	50	7.24	−7

* Blood from a segment of umbilical cord.

Table 26.3
Equipment for Neonatal Resuscitation

A. For each delivery room
    Radiantly heated, mobile resuscitation crib
    Suction devices: sterile bulb suction *or* DeLee suction trap and vacuum suction with sterile catheters
    Stethoscope
    Oxygen source
    Positive pressure device such as Ayres T piece or infant self-inflating bag
    Infant face masks
    Infant oropharyngeal airways
    Laryngoscope with Miller number 0 and number 1 blades
    Sterile endotracheal tubes sizes 2.0, 2.5, 3 and 3.5 mm (8, 10, 12 and 14 French) with stylets
    Plastic 10-ml syringes with sizes 8 and 5 French sterile feeding tube for gastric suction
    Infrasonde or Doppler device for neonatal blood pressure
    Sterile umbilical vessel catheterization tray including 3.5 and 5 French umbilical vessel catheters, cord tie and small iris scissors
    Drug tray including neonatal naloxone, epinephrine 1/10,000, sodium bicarbonate, 10% glucose solution, calcium chloride

B. For special neonatal treatment room: all of the above **plus**
    Source of oxygen *and* air with oxygen-air blender
    Heated nebulizer
    Anaeroid manometer for observing airway pressures during controlled ventilation
    Oxygen analyzer
    Pressure transducers and monitor for intra-arterial and venous pressures
    ECG and heart rate monitor
    Blood gas and pH electrodes and machine
    Drug tray including cardiac emergency drugs: epinephrine 1/10,000, sodium bicarbonate, isoproterenol, dopamine, Priscoline, atropine, furosemide, low-salt albumin or plasmanate
    Thoracocentesis tray including size 10 to 16 French red rubber catheters for treatment of pneumothorax

nursery) resuscitation crib. This apparatus should provide a simple but sufficiently large non-slippery surface on which to place the baby with easy access to oxygen and suction, and it should be adaptable to various modes of resuscitation, including simultaneous positive pressure ventilation and placement of umbilical vessel catheters for acid-base control and blood sampling. A source of radiant heat should be mounted above each resuscitation unit. The energy output should be servo-controlled by a sensor taped to the infant's abdomen.

In addition, a special neonatal treatment room located immediately adjacent to the delivery room is desirable for intensive care of the immature or severely asphyxiated newborn in need of prolonged resuscitation. More sophisticated ventilatory and monitoring equipment and a variety of cardiac emergency drugs should be immediately available (Table 26.3, part B).

Establishment of an Airway

As the infant's head is delivered, the mouth and nose are gently suctioned to remove the lung fluid as well as amniotic fluid, blood, mucous and meconium that might be in the pharynx (Figure 26.3). Babies born through meconium require more extensive airway management as will be described subsequently. The infant is placed in the head-down position to allow gravity drainage of this fluid. Suctioning of the pharynx and nose should be brief and gentle, because prolonged or too vig-

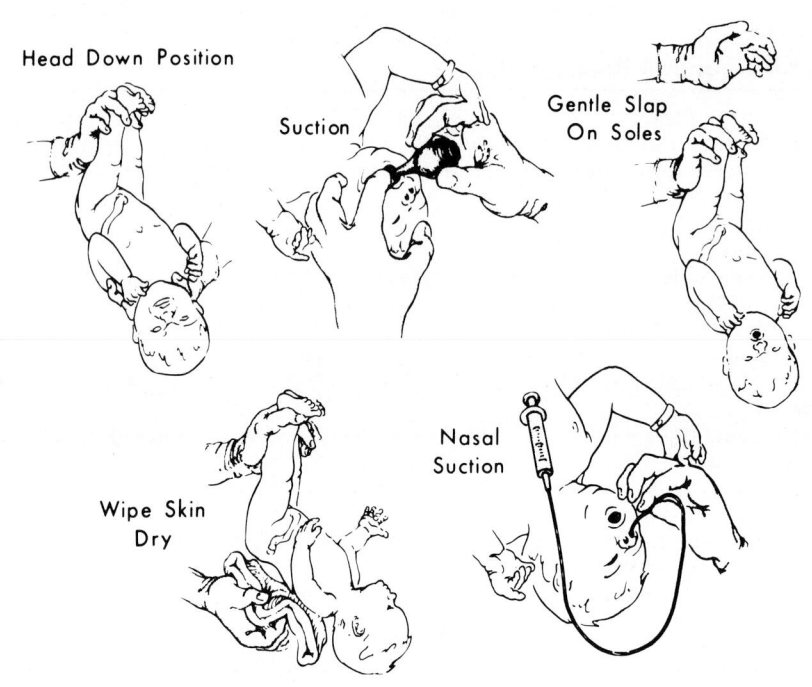

Figure 26.3. Establishment of patency of upper airway by gravity drainage, suctioning and stimulation to cry by rubbing the infant with a towel. (Reprinted by permission from Gregory GA: Cardiopulmonary resuscitation of the newborn. In *The Anesthesiologist, Mother and Newborn,* SM Shnider and F Moya, eds. Williams & Wilkins, Baltimore 1974, p 20.)

orous suctioning may produce breath holding, laryngospasm or profound bradycardia and other arrhythmias. In addition to removing debris from the airway with nasal suctioning, anatomic abnormalities such as choanal atresia may be noted. Babies are obligatory nasal breathers and will develop severe hypoxia if unable to breathe through their nose.

Routine Tracheal Suctioning for Meconium

Meconium aspiration pneumonitis is the leading respiratory cause of death in the full-term newborn. Treatment of meconium aspiration should begin in the delivery room. With suctioning of the airways there is a significant reduction in morbidity and mortality rates[12, 13] (Figure 26.4).

If thick (pea soup) particulate meconium in the amniotic fluid is present, the infant's mouth and nose should be suctioned, preferably with a DeLee trap, as the baby's head is delivered and prior to delivery of the thorax. Immediate endotracheal intubation should then be performed after delivery. The endotracheal tube is used as a suction catheter. The resuscitator, wearing a face mask, should apply mouth-to-tube suction and withdraw the tube. This technique will remove particulate material which is impossible to dislodge with smaller suction catheters. If meconium is aspirated from below the vocal cords, the endotracheal tube is reinserted and the airway is suctioned until no meconium is retrieved; then the lungs are gently re-expanded.

Ideally this is all done before the infant takes his first spontaneous breath. The neonate, vigorous at birth despite the presence of thick meconium, should also be

RESUSCITATION OF THE NEWBORN

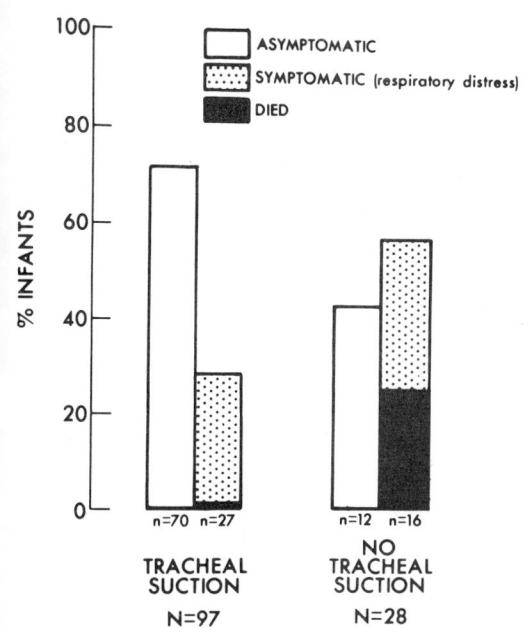

Figure 26.4. Comparison of percentage of incidence of respiratory distress and percentage of mortality in 97 infants who received tracheal suction in the delivery room and 28 infants who did not (numbers of infants below columns); note that one infant died in the tracheal suction group and seven died in the no tracheal suction group. (Reprinted by permission from Ting P, Brady JP: Tracheal suction in meconium aspiration. Am J Obstet Gynecol 122:767, 1975.)

intubated and suctioned. Further therapy for meconium aspiration consists of chest physiotherapy, ultrasonic mist, steroids and antibiotics.

Infants with thick meconium have a high incidence of pneumothorax and pneumomediastinum.[12,14] A chest x-ray should be obtained routinely during the first hour of life. Should the infant's condition suddenly deteriorate, tension pneumothorax should be considered. Management of this condition will be described subsequently.

Tactile Stimulation of the Baby

Many babies must be stimulated at birth to arouse them sufficiently to breathe effectively. This may be accomplished by drying the baby's skin with a warm towel. This maneuver not only stimulates respiration but also reduces heat loss from the infant due to evaporation. Gently flicking the soles of the feet may also produce a cry and rhythmical respiration. Vigorous slapping of the feet, buttocks or costovertebral angles may cause ecchymoses and kidney and adrenal damage.

Maintenance of Body Temperature

Immediately after birth particular attention must be given to the prevention of heat loss by the infant. The naked, wet baby delivered into a room at 25°C will rapidly lose heat by conduction, convection, evaporation and radiation. Catecholamine-mediated, non-shivering thermogenesis by metabolism of brown fat is the principal mechanism utilized by the neonate in his usually futile attempt to maintain normal body temperature.[15-17] This leads to a dramatic increase in oxygen consumption[18] (Figure 26.5). If the neonate's temperature falls, his pulmonary vessels constrict, there is an increased right-to-left shunt and hypoxemia, metabolic acidosis, tachypnea and grunting occur.

Heat conservation techniques must be used. In addition to drying the skin, the baby should be placed under a radiant heater, preferably one servo-controlled by a sensor placed on the baby's skin.

Clinical Assessment of the Neonate

The most widely used method for evaluating the condition of the infant in the delivery room is a score devised by Virginia Apgar in 1953.[19, 20] It is fully described in chapter 25. This easily performed assessment is usually made 1 and 5 minutes after birth. There are five signs: heart rate, respiratory effort, muscle tone, response to stimulation and skin color. A score of 0,

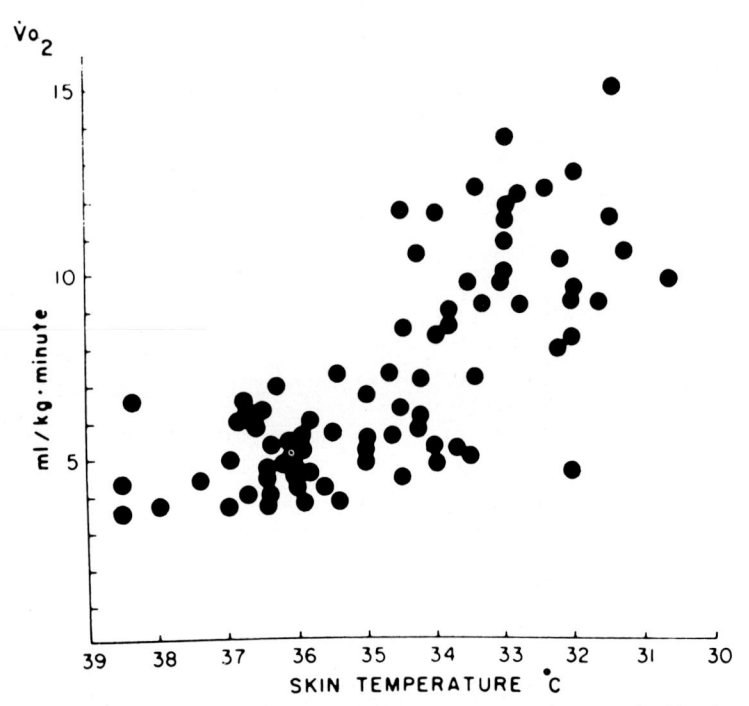

Figure 26.5. The relationship between oxygen consumption and skin temperature of newborn infants under a variety of thermal environmental conditions. (Reprinted by permission from Adamsons K Jr, Gandy GM, James LS: The influence of thermal factors upon oxygen consumption of the newborn infant. J Pediatr 66:495, 1965.)

1 or 2 is assigned according to the presence or absence of each of the signs.

A popular scheme of resuscitation of the newborn based on the 1-minute Apgar score will be described. However, when an infant is known to be severely asphyxiated or depressed, active resuscitation should always be started without waiting for 1 minute to elapse.

VIGOROUS NEONATES (APGAR SCORE 8 to 10)

The vast majority of newborns fall into this category. They require only the usual upper airway suctioning, drying of the skin and a warm ambient environment. Occasionally a baby vigorous at 1 minute of age will deteriorate shortly thereafter. Possible causes are drug depression becoming apparent after stimulation of the baby ceases, persistent naso-pharyngeal suctioning resulting in reflex bradycardia and laryngospasm, hypoxia due to spontaneous pneumothorax, regurgitation and aspiration of gastric contents or congenital anomalies such as a diaphragmatic hernia, which makes adaptation to extrauterine life difficult. A brief physical examination for obvious congenital anomalies should be performed on every newborn. Ideally this includes a measurement of blood pressure by doppler-shift sphygmomanometer or similar external device. Normal systolic pressure in a full-term baby is 65 to 75 mm Hg.[21] A pressure below 50 mm Hg is considered hypotensive.

Routinely at approximately 5 minutes of age a naso-gastric tube is passed and the stomach is aspirated. This procedure will prevent aspiration of gastric contents in the immediate neonatal period and help in the diagnosis of choanal atresia, esophageal atresia and small bowel obstruction. A soft plastic catheter (8 French) is passed into the stomach. Its position **must** be confirmed by injecting 2 to 3 ml of air while auscultating or palpating the left upper abdominal quadrant. It is possible to aspirate a small amount of fluid from an esophageal pouch of an atretic esophagus and fail to diagnose the anomaly. The volume of gastric contents should be measured. The average amount is 4 to 8 ml, but larger quantities are frequently found after cesarean sections. If 25 to 50 ml of fluid are present, a small bowel obstruction should be suspected; amounts greater than 50 ml indicate the need for immediate x-ray examination of the abdomen.[22]

MILDLY DEPRESSED NEONATES (APGAR SCORE 5 to 7)

These infants are minimally depressed either from a brief episode of birth asphyxia or slight drug depression. They usually respond to a combination of tactile stimulation and oxygen-enriched air to breathe. After they become vigorous they are managed as described above. If the baby does not rapidly improve with oxygen blown over the face, then oxygen should be administered by positive pressure (Figure 26.6).

MODERATELY DEPRESSED NEONATES (APGAR SCORE 3 to 4)

These babies are usually more hypoxic and acidotic or have received a larger amount of depressing drugs than the babies who score 5 to 7. They require oxygen by positive pressure ventilation. This can usually be accomplished with a face mask and rebreathing bag, providing the upper airway is clear and an adequate mask fit can be obtained. The infant's head should be in a neutral position, and care must be taken not to occlude the trachea with the fingers supporting the mandible. A small oral airway may be helpful in preventing upper airway obstruction by the tongue. Pressures of 25 to 30 cm H_2O administered for 1 to 2 seconds are usually necessary. Higher pressures may rupture the lungs. Once the lungs have been inflated, pressures of 10 to 15 cm H_2O are usually sufficient to deliver an adequate volume. As with the adult, positive pressure ventilation via a face mask may result in gaseous distension of the stomach, occular damage due to pressure applied to the eyes or abrasions to the face. Gastric distension can be prevented by maintaining an open airway, placement of a naso-gastric tube with the upper end open to the atmosphere or by gentle manual pressure in the left

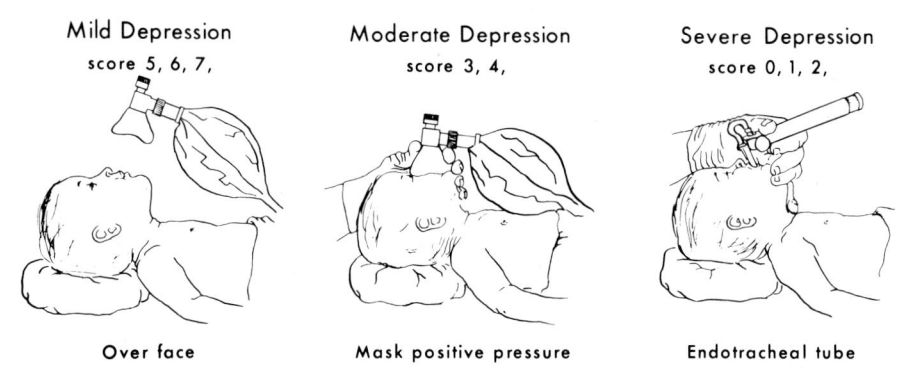

Figure 26.6. A plan for oxygen delivery during resuscitation of the newborn. (Reprinted by permission from Shnider SM, ed: *Obstetrical Anesthesia: Current Concepts and Practice.* Williams & Wilkins, 1970.)

upper quadrant during controlled ventilation. In addition to correcting hypoxia, positive pressure ventilation may stimulate sensitive stretch receptors in the pulmonary tree and initiate a gasp.[23]

If there is no immediate improvement in the clinical condition of the neonate, then positive pressure with the face mask is likely ineffective and prompt endotracheal intubation for ventilation is indicated.

SEVERELY DEPRESSED NEONATES (APGAR SCORE 0 to 2)

These infants are usually severely hypoxic, acidotic and apneic. They require immediate ventilation with oxygen via an endotracheal tube. The infant's head should be placed in the neutral "sniffing position" rather than hyperextended. The larynx of the neonate is more anterior than in the adult and at the level of the second cervical vertebra rather than the sixth. Thus a small straight blade, such as a Miller 0 to 1, provides the best visualization of the larynx. As the laryngoscope is introduced into the right-hand corner of the mouth, the tongue is moved toward the left and the epiglottis is located (Figure 26.7). Gentle pressure over the hyoid bone with the little finger of the hand holding the laryngoscope will move the larynx posteriorly to help expose the epiglottis. The tip of the laryngoscope blade may either be placed in the vallecula or posterior to the epiglottis, and with gentle upward pressure the cords are visualized. If unable to visualize the larynx or insert the endotracheal tube after 30 seconds of trying, the neonate should be ventilated with a bag and mask before a subsequent attempt.

The sterile endotracheal tube should be of such a size that with positive pressure ventilation there is a small air leak. Too large a tube may cause subglottic stenosis, and too small a tube will not permit adequate ventilation and may become plugged easily. Depending on the size of the neonate, a size 2.0 to 3.5 mm (8 to 14 French) is chosen. The tube should be inserted about 2 cm past the cords, and ventilation with 100 per cent oxygen should be begun. Although a pressure of 25 to 30 cm H_2O is usually sufficient to ventilate most asphyxiated infants, those with low compliance, as is found in erythroblastosis or pulmonary hypoplasia, may require higher pressures.

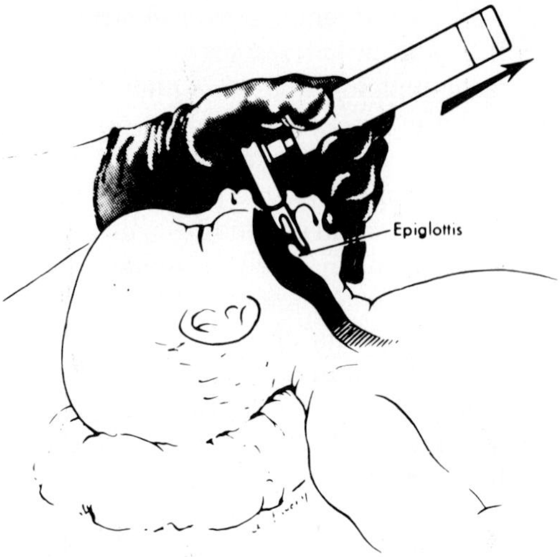

Figure 26.7. Technique for laryngoscopy. Left hand holds the laryngoscope and steadies the head and the little finger depresses the hyoid bone to help bring the larynx into view. (Reprinted by permission from Gregory GA: Resuscitation of the newborn. Anesthesiology 43:225, 1975.)

The correct placement of the endotracheal tube, and the adequacy of ventilation must be immediately ascertained (Figure 26.8). This is done by observation and auscultation of the chest. Both sides of the chest should seem to expand equally, breath sounds auscultated in the mid-axillary line should be equal bilaterally and louder over the chest than the stomach, and the heart rate, color and body tone should improve. Inadvertent esophageal or endobronchial intubations may occur and must be immediately recognized. Esophageal ventilation will also produce chest

RESUSCITATION OF THE NEWBORN

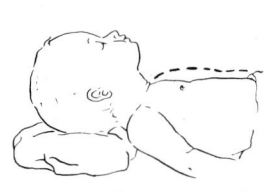

See chest expand

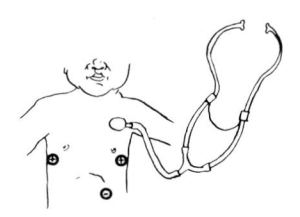

Hear bilateral breath sounds

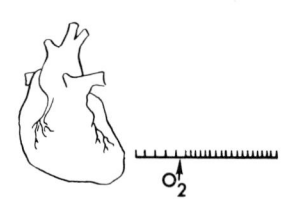

Hear pulse rate increase

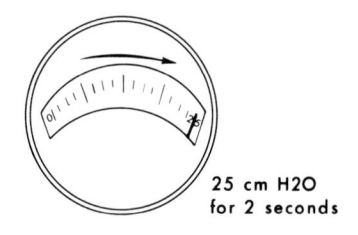

Avoid excessive pressures
25 cm H2O for 2 seconds

Figure 26.8. Means of determining adequacy of ventilation clinically. (Reprinted by permission from Shnider SM, ed: *Obstetrical Anesthesia: Current Concepts and Practice.* Williams & Wilkins, Baltimore, 1970.)

movement and sounds. The sounds, however, will be louder over the abdomen than the chest, and no chest movement will occur at the apices. Clinically the infant will continue to deteriorate. An endobronchial intubation may be recognized by asymmetric movement of the chest and absent or decreased breath sounds over the unventilated lung. It is noteworthy that auscultation for breath sounds even by the experienced resuscitator may be misleading, because sound is well transmitted in these small infants. Thus relying on this sign alone for diagnosis of correct placement of the endotracheal tube is dangerous.

If despite adequate ventilation with 100 per cent oxygen the infant fails to improve and has an Apgar score of 2 or less at 2 minutes or 5 or less at 5 minutes then umbilical artery catheterization is indicated. This will allow measurement of oxygenation, acid-base status and systemic blood pressure and will permit administration of fluids, blood or appropriate drugs.

Umbilical Vessel Catheterization

Using sterile technique a 3.5 or 5 French catheter is inserted into the umbilical artery at the stump of the umbilical cord.[24] The catheter is advanced 2 cm beyond the point at which blood can first be aspirated. This should place the tip of the catheter just above the bifurcation of the aorta and below the celiac, renal and mesenteric arteries. The location of the catheter tip is important because improper placement may be associated with thrombosis or embolism in these major aortic tributaries. Immediately after catheterization blood is sampled for PO_2, PCO_2 and pH, and blood pressure is measured with an appropriate strain gauge.

The umbilical vein is larger and easier to cannulate than the artery. However, using this vessel will not permit assessment of oxygenation or systemic blood pressure. In addition, administration of drugs or hypertonic solutions through this catheter may be hazardous. The catheter can become wedged in a venous radicle of the liver or enter the portal vein. The wedged catheter tip may cause hepatic injury or portal vein thrombosis.[25] Consequently, before injecting a drug through the umbilical vein, the catheter tip must be advanced through the ductus venosus into the inferior vena cava near the right atrium. The precise location of the catheter should be checked by x-ray. It is possible, however, to determine whether the catheter tip has bypassed the liver and is above the diaphragm by noting that the venous pressure decreases with each spontaneous inspiration.[24]

Correction of Acidosis

Severe acidosis, that is a pH less than 7.05 or a base deficit of 15 mEq/L or more, must be promptly corrected by alkali administration to assure normal pulmonary perfusion and oxygenation.[3] If the base excess is known then the dose of sodium bicarbonate needed can be calculated by the formula:

$$\text{mEq of NaHCO}_3 = 0.3 \times \text{weight (kg)} \times \text{base excess in mEq/liter}$$

A 1 molar solution is administered at a rate of 1 mEq/kg per minute or slower. If blood gas analysis is not readily available and the neonate is severely depressed with an Apgar score of 5 or less at 5 minutes despite endotracheal oxygenation, then a dose of bicarbonate of 2 to 3 mEq/kg may be given at the rate described above.

Recent investigations have suggested that there is an association between intracranial hemorrhage and sodium bicarbonate administration.[26] Because intracranial hemorrhage is a common finding in very small, premature infants, particularly those with asphyxia, it is not clear whether the high incidence of intracranial hemorrhage reported following **rapid** bicarbonate administration was due to an acute increase in osmolarity, a rise in arterial PCO_2 or the asphyxia for which the bicarbonate was given. Others have reported that if bicarbonate administration is slow and ventilation is controlled, a rapid improvement in neonatal oxygenation can be expected to occur with no neonatal complications.[27]

Until more information is available, sodium bicarbonate should not be infused unless metabolic acidosis or neonatal depression is severe and then only if the bicarbonate is slowly administered and ventilation is controlled.

Moderate or mild metabolic and respiratory acidosis—that is, a pH between 7.05 and 7.30 and a base deficit of 5 to 15 mEq/L—will usually be corrected spontaneously or by assisted ventilation and volume expansion if indicated.

Treatment of Shock

The most common cause of shock in the newly born infant is hypovolemia. It frequently follows severe intrapartum asphyxia during which a greater than normal portion of fetal blood is shunted to the placenta and remains there following cord clamping and delivery.[28] Hypovolemia is also commonly associated with umbilical cord compression in vertex and especially breech vaginal deliveries. Aside from the consequences of asphyxia, acute compression of the umbilical cord during delivery may result in trapping of fetal blood in the placenta due to occlusion of the compliant umbilical vein when there is flow through the more rigid and muscular umbilical arteries. Ruptured placental or umbilical vessels, although occurring far less frequently than intrapartum asphyxia and cord compression, may result in severe hypovolemic shock.

Hypovolemia should be suspected if the neonate is pale, has poor capillary refill, tachycardia and tachypnea. Precise diagnosis and treatment require constant monitoring of arterial and central venous pressures, and heart rate and repeated measurements of PaO_2, $PaCO_2$, pH and hematocrit. Normal aortic blood pressure measured with the umbilical artery catheter varies with birth weight.[21] Figure 26.9 shows the normal mean arterial blood pressure for each birth weight and the 95 per cent confidence limits of this relationship. Newborns with blood pressures below the lower confidence line are hypotensive and most likely hypovolemic. Intrathoracic venous pressures measured with the umbilical venous catheter are normally 5 to 12 cm H_2O when measured at end-expiration.[24] If pressure is less than 5 cm H_2O then hypovolemia is likely.

Hypovolemic shock requires immediate therapy. Because whole blood is not always immediately available, an infusion of isotonic saline 5 to 10 ml/kg body weight over a 2- to 3-minute period should be given and the response evaluated to determine whether the dose should be repeated immediately. Then salt-poor albumin 1 gm/kg body weight should be administered over a 2- to 5-minute period. An equivalent amount of plasmanate (5 to 10 ml/kg body weight) may be substituted for the isotonic saline and albumin. Repeated infusions of fluid or whole blood should be given as needed to establish and maintain adequate intravascular pressure.

Frequently a hypovolemic asphyxiated neonate will have a relatively normal arterial blood pressure and hematocrit due to intense peripheral vasoconstriction. When the acidosis is corrected with bicarbonate and hyperventilation the blood vessels dilate and hypotension occurs, unmasking the presence of hypovolemia (Figure 26.10). Alternately, when severe hy-

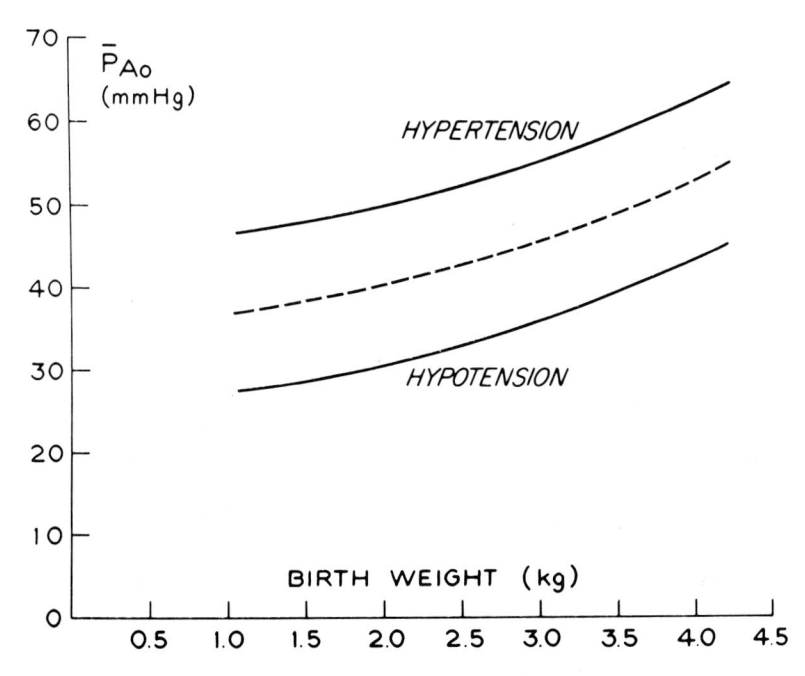

Figure 26.9. Mean aortic blood pressure obtained from an umbilical artery catheter. The *dashed line* is the average blood pressure at each birth weight, and the *solid lines* represent the 95 per cent confidence limits. (Reprinted by permission from Kitterman JA, Phibbs RH, Tooley WH: Aortic blood pressure in normal newborn infants during the first 12 hours of life. Pediatrics 44:959, 1969.)

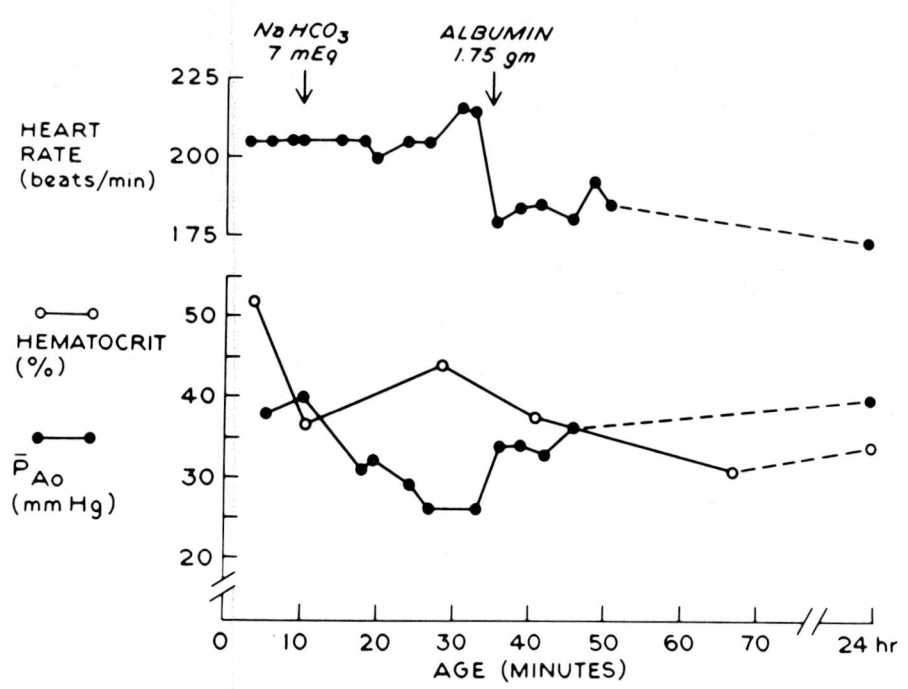

Figure 26.10. Heart rate, hematocrit and mean aortic pressure in a 1370-gm, 30-weeks' gestation infant with asphyxia at birth and respiratory distress. At 12 minutes of age severe metabolic acidosis was treated with NaHCO$_3$. Hypovolemia then became apparent by the progressive fall in blood pressure. Albumin administration restored blood pressure and alleviated tachycardia. (Reprinted by permission from Phibbs RH: What is the evidence that blood pressure monitoring is useful? In *Problems of Neonatal Intensive Care Units. Report of 59th Ross Conference on Pediatric Research*, JF Lucey, ed. Ross Laboratories, Columbus, 1969, p 81.)

povolemia is corrected a marked metabolic acidemia may reappear after systemic circulatory status and peripheral perfusion improves.

Treatment of Hypoglycemia

Infants with intrauterine growth retardation (post-mature), or with diabetic mothers, or born following severe intrapartum asphyxia may be hypoglycemic (less than 30 mg/100 ml in full-sized infant and less than 20 mg/100 ml in low birth weight infant). Hypoglycemia results in reduced cardiac output, hypotension, and, when severe, tremors, convulsions and apnea. It should be treated with 5 to 10 ml/kg body weight of 10 per cent dextrose administered slowly.

Treatment of Cardiac Arrest

If after 15 to 30 seconds of positive pressure ventilation the heart beat is absent or barely detectable with a rate less than 100 beats per minute, closed-chest cardiac massage should be started (Table 26.4). Both thumbs are placed on the sternum at the junction of the lower and middle thirds, and the back is supported with the fingers[29] (Figure 26.11). The sternum should be compressed to a point about two-thirds the distance from the sternum to the vertebral column at a rate of 80 to 100 per minute. The chest compression should be coordinated with ventilation at a rate of five compressions to one breath. An adequate cardiac output with massage can be ascertained by an improvement in

RESUSCITATION OF THE NEWBORN

Table 26.4
Cardiac Arrest

Ventilate with oxygen
Confirm diagnosis
Closed-chest cardiac massage
  Mid-sternum
  80 to 100 compressions per minute
  Five compressions to one breath
Place ECG leads
Immediate umbilical artery catheterization
  Sodium bicarbonate: 5 mEq/kg
  Dextrose 10%: 5 to 10 ml/kg
  Epinephrine: 0.1 to 0.3 ml of 1/10,000 dilution
  Repeat bicarbonate: 5 mEq/kg
  Calcium chloride: 10 to 20 mg
  Dopamine: 5 μg/kg/min
If ECG shows activity but less than 80 beats per minute
  Atropine 0.03 mg/kg
  Isoproterenol 16 μg/ml, I.V. drip

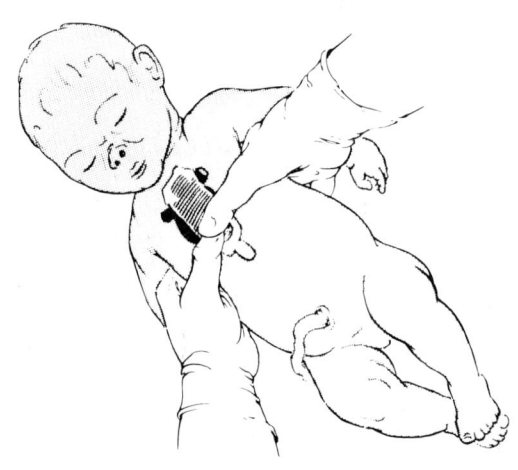

Figure 26.11. Closed-chest cardiac massage in the newborn. Location of the thumbs for sternal compression in the infant. For simplification ventilation of the infant is not shown. (Reprinted by permission from Gregory GA: Cardiopulmonary resuscitation of the newborn. In *The Anesthesiologist, Mother and Newborn*, SM Shnider and F Moya, eds. Williams & Wilkins, Baltimore, 1974, p 207.)

the neonate's color, constriction of the pupils and palpable arterial pulses. Umbilical vessels should be catheterized immediately, and an electrocardiogram should be obtained to monitor heart rate and rhythm. Sodium bicarbonate (5 mEq/kg) and 10 per cent dextrose (5 ml/kg) are administered. If there is no spontaneous rhythm, epinephrine (0.1 to 0.3 ml of a 1/10,000 solution) should be injected into the umbilical artery or vein. Epinephrine should be preceded by the sodium bicarbonate, because it is ineffective in an acidic medium. Calcium chloride (10 to 20 mg/kg administered over a 3- to 5-minute period) may improve myocardial contractility and output. If the heart rate remains below 100 beats per minute atropine (0.03 mg/kg) or an infusion of isoproterenol (16 μg/ml) should be administered until heart rate increases and cardiac output improves. The high concentration of isoproterenol is necessary to prevent fluid overload. If blood volume is adequate an infusion of dopamine, starting with 5 μg/kg/min, may be infused to increase cardiac output. Cardiotonic drugs used during resuscitation, their indications, doses, expected responses and complications are listed in Table 26.5.

SPECIAL PROBLEMS IN RESUSCITATION

Narcotic Depression

When narcotics are administered for pain relief during labor and delivery the infant may be born mildly to moderately depressed. As with the adult the usual sign of narcotic depression in a neonate is hypoventilation and poor response to stimuli. If respiratory depression is thought to be due to narcotic overdose, these infants should be oxygenated and then treated with a narcotic antagonist. Naloxone 0.01 mg/kg is the antagonist of choice. Because normal circulation is usually present in these infants the drug may be given intramuscularly. If the mother is a narcotic addict the use of naloxone is contraindicated in the neonate because acute withdrawal symptoms may be precipitated.

Table 26.5
Cardiac Drugs Used during Resuscitation

Drug	Indication	Dose*	Route	Response	Complication
Atropine	Bradycardia	0.03 mg/kg	I.V.†	Increased heart rate	Marked tachycardia, diminished cardiac output
Calcium gluconate	Low cardiac output	100 mg/kg over 5-10 minutes (ECG monitoring)	I.V.	Improved cardiac output	Bradycardia, dysrhythmias
Epinephrine	"Flat line" ECG	0.1 ml/kg of a 1/10,000 solution	I.V.	"Flat line" ECG converted to some rhythmic response	Hypertension, ventricular fibrillation
Isoproterenol	Bradycardia, hypotension, low cardiac output	4 mg/250 ml of 5% dextrose in water until heart rate increases	I.V.	Increased heart rate, improved cardiac output	Dysrhythmias, low cardiac output if heart rate more than 180-200/min
Dopamine‡	Low cardiac output	5 µg/kg/min, increased to 50 µg/kg/min as necessary	I.V.	Improved cardiac output, slightly increased heart rate	Dysrhythmias

* In general, doses given are starting doses and may have to be increased. Most drugs tend to be more effective when pH > 7.15.
† Intravascular — ideally umbilical artery, if necessary, umbilical vein.
‡ Useful only when blood volume is adequate.

Magnesium Intoxication

Babies born to parturients treated with large doses of magnesium for toxemia of pregnancy may display signs of hypermagnesemia. These infants are peripherally vasodilated, pink, hypotensive and hypotonic. Calcium chloride is an effective antidote.

Local Anesthetic Toxicity

Fetal intoxication with local anesthetics may occasionally occur inadvertently during the maternal administration of caudal or paracervical blocks.[30,31] The infants are severely depressed with bradycardia, hypotension, apnea, hypotonia and convulsions. Careful examination of the baby's head often discloses the needle puncture site. In addition to the usual resuscitation of a severely depressed neonate these babies should be detoxified by gastric lavage with isotonic saline and exchange transfusion.

Pneumothorax

Pneumothorax in the delivery room may occur spontaneously, often associated with meconium aspiration (in which ball-valve air-trapping occurs) or with other diseases associated with poor lung compliance (such as diaphragmatic hernia and pulmonary hypoplasia). When it occurs in a normal lung it is usually caused by excessive airway pressures administered in the resuscitation of a depressed newborn. Tension pneumothorax, in which high intrapleural pressure prevents venous return to the heart, is catastrophic and life-threatening. When the diagnosis is suspected a 22-gauge needle connected to a three-way stopcock and syringe is inserted in the second intercostal space in the midclavicular line. If air is aspirated then the needle should be replaced by an adequately sized catheter (10 to 16 French) and connected to underwater seal and continuous suction.

CONCLUSION

Rapid, organized and skillful resuscitation of the depressed newborn is mandatory. The obstetrician, anesthesiologist and neonatologist must work as a team in evaluating the newborn, establishing a patent airway, providing adequate ventilation and restoring normal blood volume, cardiac output and acid-base status.

References

1. Dawes GS: *Foetal and Neonatal Physiology.* Year Book Medical Publishers, Chicago, 1968, pp 91–105.
2. Rudolph AM, Heymann MA: Fetal and neonatal circulation and respiration. Annu Rev Physiol 36:187, 1974.
3. Rudolph AM, Yuen S: Response of the pulmonary vasculature to hypoxia and H$^+$ ion concentration changes. J Clin Invest 45:399, 1966.
4. Cassen S, Dawes GS, Mott JC, et al.: The vascular resistance of the foetal and newly ventilated lung of the lamb. J Physiol 171:61, 1964.
5. Assali NS, Morris JA, Smith EW, et al.: Studies on ductus arteriosus circulation. Circ Res 13:478, 1963.
6. Boreus LO, Malmfors T, McMurphy DM, et al.: Demonstration of adrenergic receptor function and innervation in the ductus arteriosus of the human fetus. Acta Physiol Scand 77:316, 1969.
7. Adams FH, Moss AJ, Fagan L: The tracheal fluid of the foetal lamb. Biol Neonate 5:151, 1963.
8. Ross BB: Comparison of foetal pulmonary fluid with foetal plasma and amniotic fluid. Nature 199:1100, 1963.
9. Karlberg P: The adaptive changes in the immediate postnatal period, with particular reference to respiration. J Pediatr 56:585, 1960.
10. Usher RH, Allen AC, McLean FH: Risk of respiratory distress syndrome related to gestational age, role of delivery and maternal diabetes. Am J Obstet Gynecol 111:826, 1971.
11. Karlberg P: The first breaths of life. In *Modern Perinatal Medicine,* L Gluck, ed. Year Book Medical Publishers, Chicago, 1974, pp 391–408.
12. Gregory GA, Gooding C, Phibbs RH, et al.: Meconium aspiration in infants: A prospective study. J Pediatr 85:848, 1974.
13. Ting P, Brady JP: Tracheal suction in meconium aspiration. Am J Obstet Gynecol 122:767, 1975.
14. Steele RW, Metz JR, Bass JW, et al.: Pneumothorax and pneumomediastinum in the newborn. Radiology 98:629, 1971.
15. Aherne W, Hull D: The site of heat production in the newborn infant. Proc R Soc Med 57:1172, 1964.
16. Karlberg P, Moore RE, Oliver TK: The thermogenic response of the newborn infant to noradrenaline. Acta Paediatr Scand 51:284, 1962.
17. Dawkins MJR, Scopes JW: Non-shivering thermogenesis and brown adipose tissue in the human newborn infant. Nature 206:201, 1965.
18. Adamsons K Jr, Gandy GM, James LS: The influence of thermal factors upon oxygen consumption of the newborn infant. J Pediatr 66:495, 1965.
19. Apgar V: A proposal for a new method of evaluation of the newborn infant. Curr Res Anesth 32:260, 1953.
20. Apgar V, James LS: Further observations on the newborn scoring system. Am J Dis Child 104:419, 1962.
21. Kitterman JA, Phibbs RH, Tooley WH: Aortic blood pressure in normal newborn infants during the first 12 hours of life. Pediatrics 44:959, 1969.
22. Moya F, Apgar V, James LS, et al.: Hydramnios and congenital anomalies. JAMA 173:1552, 1960.
23. Cross K, Klaus M, Tooley WH, et al.: The response of the newborn baby to inflation of the lungs. J Physiol 151:551, 1960.
24. Kitterman JA, Phibbs RH, Tooley WH: Catheterization of umbilical vessels in newborn infants. Pediatr Clin North Am 17:895, 1970.
25. Erkan V, Blankenship W, Stahlman MT: The complications of chronic umbilical vessel catheterization. Pediatr Res 2:317, 1968.
26. Simmons MA, Adcock EW, Bard H: Hypernatremia and intracranial hemorrhage in neonates. N Engl J Med 291:6, 1974.
27. Tooley WH: Alkali therapy in the asphyxiated newborn infant. In: *Obstetrical Anesthesia,* SM Shnider, ed. Williams & Wilkins, Baltimore, 1970, p 230.
28. Ballard R, Kitterman JR, Phibbs RH, et al.: Observations on hypovolemia in the newborn. Clin Res 20:278, 1972.
29. Gregory GA: Cardiopulmonary resuscitation of the newborn. In *The Anesthesiologist, Mother and Newborn,* SM Shnider and F Moya, eds. Williams & Wilkins, Baltimore, 1974, p 20.
30. Finster M, Poppers PJ, Sinclair JC, et al.: Accidental intoxication of the fetus with local anesthetic drug during caudal anesthesia. Am J Obstet Gynecol 92:922, 1965.
31. Dodson WE, Hillman RE, Hillman LS: Brain tissue levels in a fatal case of neonatal mepivacaine poisoning. J Pediatr 86:624, 1975.

CHAPTER 27

Unusual Causes of Neonatal Respiratory Failure in the Delivery Room

George A. Gregory, M.D.

In the previous chapter, Levinson and Shnider have outlined the usual causes of neonatal respiratory failure in the delivery room. However, other less common conditions may also be encountered. In this chapter these anatomic and physiologic causes of respiratory failure in the delivery room will be described (Table 27.1).

CONGENITAL DEFECTS OF THE RESPIRATORY SYSTEM

Embryology of the Upper Airway

At approximately 9 weeks' gestation, the respiratory diverticulum arises as a medium ventral diverticulum of the foregut. Shortly thereafter, the foregut caudal to the respiratory diverticulum lengthens and a median groove bounded by ridges develops. With growth, the groove deepens and the caudal portions fuse to form the esophagus. Fusion of the ridges extends cranially, dividing the respiratory primordium from the foregut until only the laryngeal aditus is left immediately behind the hypopharyngeal eminence (Figure 27.1). Incomplete fusion of the ridges leads to abnormal openings in the larynx, trachea and esophagus (e.g. laryngeal cleft and tracheo-esophageal fistula), which become sites for post-natal aspiration.

Choanal Stenosis and Atresia

Choanal atresia and stenosis occur approximately once in every 8,000 live births when the bucco-nasal membrane fails to regress as it should. In these cases anomalies of the pharynx and palate are also frequent. Forty per cent of the choanal lesions are unilateral; 13 per cent of affected infants die of respiratory failure.[1]

RECOGNITION IN THE DELIVERY ROOM

Bilateral choanal atresia is easily recognized in the delivery room.[2] Affected infants make breathing efforts but have absent breath sounds and become cyanotic if they breathe with their mouths closed. In fact, the author has found that most normal infants will continue to make respiratory motions and will develop cyanosis and asphyxia if their nose is obstructed. If neonates with choanal atresia breathe through their mouths, breath sounds are normal and the cyanosis disappears. When the mouth is opened, air entry is normal. Infants with partial choanal obstruction have labored breathing, including retractions and discoordinate movements of the chest and abdomen. Inspiratory stridor is present if the extrathoracic trachea collapses during inspiration.

Table 27.1
Unusual Causes of Neonatal Respiratory Failure in the Delivery Room

Congenital defects of respiratory system
  Nose: choanal stenosis and atresia
  Upper airway: Pierre Robin syndrome
  Larynx:
    Webs
    Fusions
    Atresia
    Vocal cord paralysis
    Subglottic stenosis
  Trachea:
    Tracheal agenesis
    Tracheal rings
      Cartilage
      Vascular
    Hemangiomas
    Webs
    Tracheo-esophageal fistula
    Tumors
  Bronchi: congenital bronchial stenosis
Aspiration syndrome
  Meconium aspiration
  Blood aspiration
Diaphragmatic hernia

Nasal obstruction should be suspected in any infant who has good respiratory efforts but in whom air entry is poor or absent. Diagnosis can be made by failing to pass a soft rubber or plastic catheter (8 or 5 French) through each nostril into the posterior pharynx. To rule out choanal obstruction, this maneuver should be done in **every** infant as part of the routine delivery room management of the newborn. Otherwise a unilateral choanal obstruction may go undetected until the infant contracts a respiratory tract infection or lies on the unoccluded nostril, producing total airway obstruction and possibly death. If the catheter passes easily, choanal atresia is ruled out. If it does not, an oral airway should be inserted, a small amount of contrast media should be instilled into the nostril and an x-ray should be obtained. Prior to obtaining x-rays a few drops of ⅛ per cent Neosynephrine should be instilled into both nostrils to rule out edema of the nasal mucosa as the cause of obstruction. The nose should also be examined with an otoscope.

TREATMENT

The initial treatment of choanal atresia or stenosis is to establish an airway.[2] An oral airway or a cut-off rubber nipple can be inserted into the mouth and taped in place. If these procedures fail to maintain an airway, an orotracheal tube should be inserted and left in place until the diagnosis is made and the lesion has been surgically corrected. Even though surgical correction is done in the neonatal period and hypoxia and bradycardia are prevented, the incidence of brain damage is high, probably because of congenital factors. Therefore, the extent of central nervous system damage should be defined as quickly as possible so that care can be withdrawn if profound damage is present.

OTHER CAUSES OF CHOANAL ATRESIA

Functional choanal atresia is more common than congenital anatomic obstruction. Blood, meconium or mucus often obstruct the nose, but gentle nasal suctioning will remove the offending material. Maternally administered drugs such as veratrum alkaloids, reserpine and narcotics (especially heroin) often cause congestion of the nasal mucosa and obstruction. This congestion can be treated with ⅛ per cent Neosynephrine nose drops or by bypassing the nose with an oral airway. Either or both may be required for several days.

Anomalies of the Upper Airway

Anomalies of the upper airway can be divided into those caused by aplasia or hypoplasia of the airway or supporting structures; those related to dysplasia or anomalies of the airway; and those related to extramural lesions compressing the airway. Inspiratory stridor occurs when extrathoracic airways are obstructed (Figures 27.2 and 27.3), and expiratory wheezing occurs when small airways are obstructed. Stridor during both inspiration and expiration is usually caused by problems in the trachea or main stem bronchi.

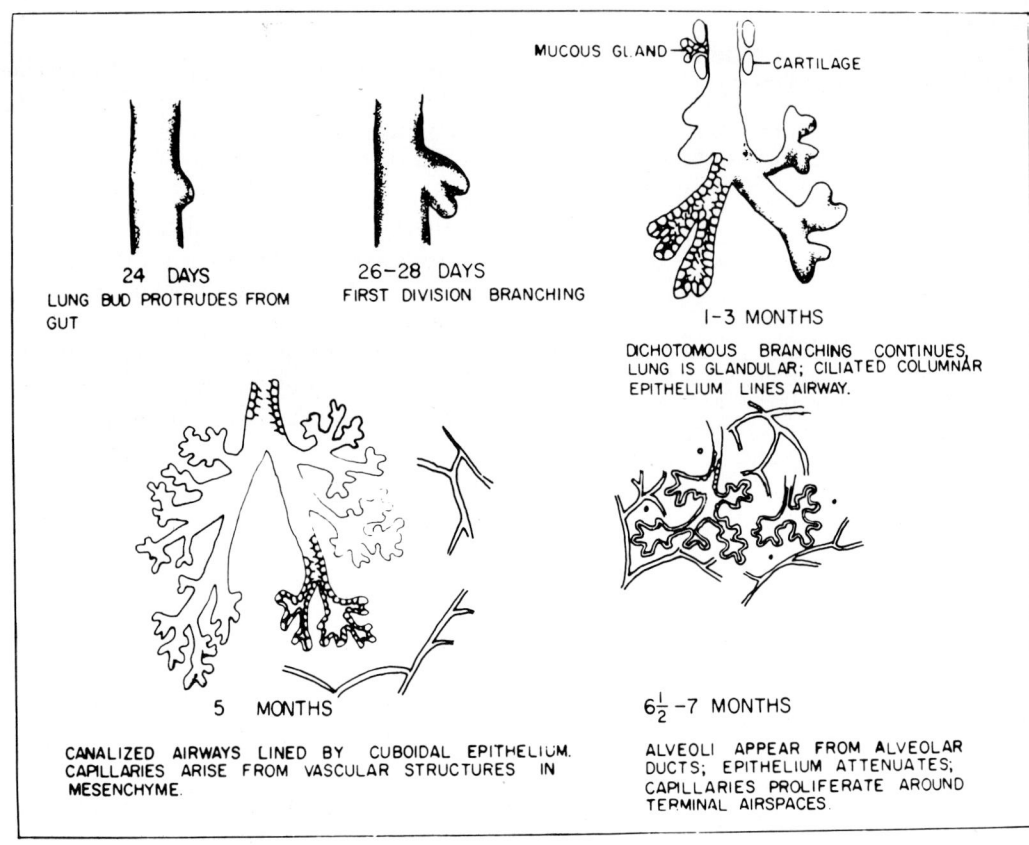

Figure 27.1. Diagrammatic representation of the stages of lung development. (Reprinted by permission from Avery ME, Fletcher BD: *The Lung and Its Disorders in the Newborn Infant,* ed 3. W. B. Saunders, Philadelphia, 1974, p 6.)

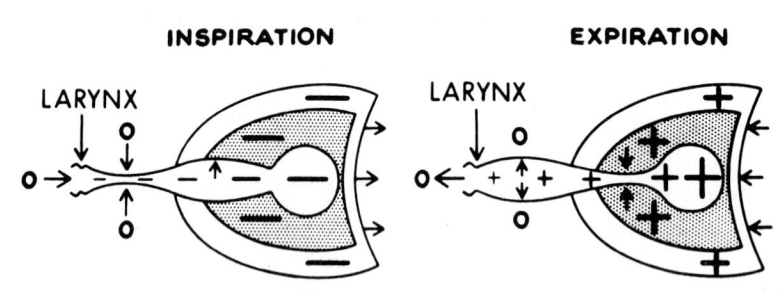

Figure 27.2. The effects of inspiratory and expiratory pressures on the intra- and extrathoracic airways of infants. The pressures along the airway are indicated by plus (+) and minus (−) signs and the magnitude of the pressure by the size of the plus or minus sign. 0 indicates atmospheric pressure. During inspiration there is a gradual change from atmospheric to subatmospheric pressures in the alveoli. The extrathoracic trachea tends to collapse, because the pressure within the trachea is less than that of the surrounding tissues. The intrathoracic airways tend to dilate. During expiration the opposite occurs. The pressure around the intrathoracic airways is greater than that within. The intrathoracic airways tend to collapse. The pressure within the extrathoracic trachea is enlarged. (Reprinted by permission from Rudolph AM: *Pediatrics*, ed 16. Appleton-Century-Crofts, New York, 1977, p 1547.)

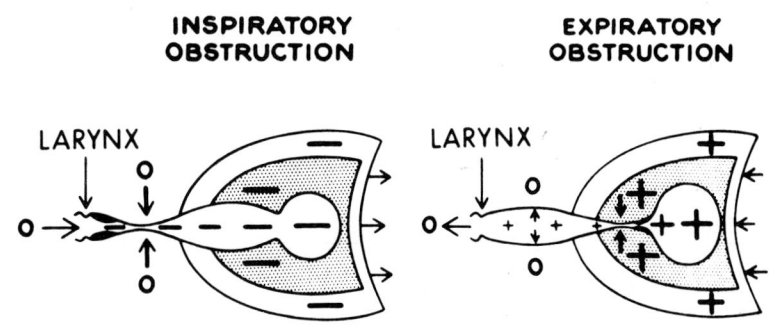

Figure 27.3. The effect of airway obstruction on thoracic and airway pressures. Extrathoracic airway obstruction decreases the pressure within the trachea, which exaggerates the normal tendency for extrathoracic airways to collapse on inspiration. With obstruction of the small airways, the transbronchial pressure gradient is large. During expiration the extrathoracic airways expand, and the normal tendency for intrathoracic airways to collapse is exaggerated. (Reprinted by permission from Rudolph AM: *Pediatrics*, ed 16. Appleton-Century-Crofts, New York, 1977, p 1547.)

PIERRE ROBIN SYNDROME

Pierre Robin syndrome occurs once in 2,000 live births and is associated with glossoptosis and micrognathia in all patients and cleft palate in 57 per cent of patients. Respiratory insufficiency occurs when the tongue is sucked against the posterior pharyngeal wall by intrapharyngeal negative pressures (up to 60 torr) during swallowing and breathing efforts.[3,4] Hypoxia is common, which may be why brain damage occurs with high frequency.

Diagnosis. The diagnosis of Pierre Robin syndrome is made by the characteristic physical findings and upper airway obstruction.

Treatment. Treatment in the delivery room includes establishing an airway by whatever means necessary. An oral airway can usually be inserted acutely, or the tongue can be grasped with a clamp and pulled anteriorly, although the latter maneuver often fails to relieve the obstruction. If the obstruction still persists, a small endotracheal tube can be inserted through the nose into the posterior pharynx to relieve the tremendous negative intraoral pressures. If necessary, an orotracheal tube can usually be inserted, although often with great difficulty. Placing the infant in the prone position helps displace the tongue away from the posterior pharyngeal wall. The infant should **not** be paralyzed when trying to establish an airway because paralysis may make ventilation impossible.

Laryngeal Anomalies

Laryngeal anomalies include webs, fusions, atresia and vocal cord paralysis. Stridor is the hallmark of these lesions and is present at birth. The associated respiratory distress may be severe. Hypoxemia, cyanosis and carbon dioxide retention are frequent; if unrelieved, brain damage may occur. Inspiration and expiration may be prolonged, and breathing may be labored; these signs and symptoms should arouse suspicion of airway obstruction at the vocal cord level. Insertion of an endotracheal tube beyond the vocal cords alleviates these symptoms. Laryngeal webs are often associated with congenital heart disease and other anomalies.[5]

Subglottic Stenosis

The trachea of a normal newborn is 5 to 7 mm in diameter. Stridor usually occurs when the diameter is reduced to less than 4 mm.[6] Congenital subglottic stenosis or edema may produce severe airway obstruction and respiratory failure in the delivery room. Inspiratory stridor, retractions, decreased air entry and, occasionally, apnea are common. Insertion of a *small* (2.5-mm) endotracheal tube beyond the obstruction alleviates the symptoms. Care must be taken to ensure the presence of a small leak between tube and trachea when a positive pressure of 10 cm H_2O is generated. Otherwise the problem may become worse. It may be necessary, and beneficial, to ventilate the infants with racemic epinephrine (Vaponefrin), 2.25 per cent diluted one to five with saline, for 15 minutes if edema is the cause of the obstruction; this will be of no benefit if stenosis is the cause.

Tracheal Agenesis Syndromes

Complete tracheal agenesis is a rare condition at birth. It is incompatible with survival.

Congenital Tracheal Rings

Complete tracheal rings or the "napkin ring" trachea are uncommon but may cause severe respiratory distress when present. The symptoms are similar to subglottic stenosis. Incomplete tracheal rings may also cause upper airway obstruction when the trachea collapses during inspiration (extrathoracic lesion) or exhalation (intrathoracic lesion) (Figure 27.3).[7]

Subglottic Tracheal Hemangiomas and Webs

Hemangiomas in the subglottic area are uncommon but may be disastrous when present. They may be diffuse or localized, and inspiratory stridor and retractions are usual. These lesions often obstruct the trachea. Insertion of an endotracheal tube may tear the hemangiomas and cause pulmonary hemorrhage. If pulmonary hemorrhage occurs, infants should be mechanically ventilated with 100 per cent oxygen and 5 to 10 cm H_2O positive end expiratory pressure should be maintained to tamponade the bleeding. The infant should be paralyzed with muscle relaxants and mechanically ventilated to reduce oxygen consumption and venous return to the heart. An umbilical arterial catheter should be inserted to measure arterial blood pressure and to administer blood and fluids. One milligram of vitamin K and frozen plasma should be given as soon as possible, because these infants often have bleeding disorders as well.

Esophageal Atresia and Tracheo-esophageal Fistula

During the third week of embryonic life the esophagus separates from the ventral trachea. Failure to do so causes esophageal atresia (Figure 27.4). Eighty-five per cent of those without a distal fistula have polyhydramnios. Therefore, tracheo-esophageal fistula should always be suspected when there is polyhydramnios. Because they are often premature (35 per cent), these infants may also develop hyaline membrane disease.

The diagnosis of esophageal atresia usually can be made when a catheter is inserted into the esophagus and cannot be advanced into the stomach. Copious amounts of oropharyngeal secretions are usually found. A roentgenogram of the neck and chest with the catheter in place will confirm the diagnosis. Intermittent or low suction should be applied continuously to the catheter to remove the secretions and to reduce the likelihood of aspiration and pneumonia.

Extramural Lesions of the Trachea

TUMORS

Congenital tumors of the chest include teratomas, hemangiomas and those of neurogenic origin. These lesions are rare but when present may compress the airway and cause respiratory distress. Gas trapping distal to the obstruction may further compromise ventilation.

VASCULAR RINGS

Vascular rings arise from anomalies of the aorta and the major arteries of the thorax. If they compress the trachea, both inspiratory and expiratory obstruction may occur. It may be difficult to insert an endotracheal tube beyond the obstruction.

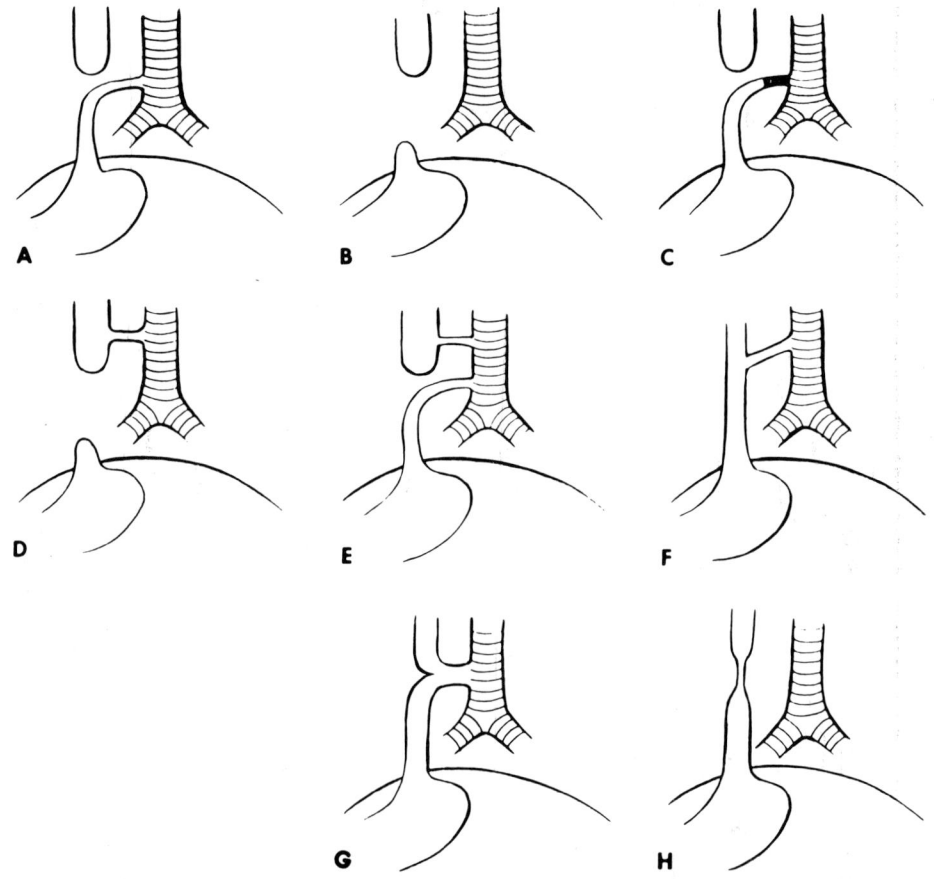

Figure 27.4. Types of tracheo-esophageal fistulas. The type labeled A is overwhelmingly the most common, accounting for over 85 per cent of esophageal malformations. B is next most common, and can be distinguished from A by the absence of air in the intestinal tract on roentgenogram. All of the other types have been noted sporadically. (Reprinted by permission from Avery ME, Fletcher BD: *The Lung and Its Disorders in the Newborn Infant*, ed 3. W. B. Saunders, Philadelphia, 1974, p 134.)

Congenital Bronchial Stenosis

Congenital stenosis of the major bronchi are unusual but cause severe respiratory distress. Gas usually enters the chest easily but has difficulty exiting from the lung. Lobar emphysema and hyperinflation of the lung result. A clue to the diagnosis of bronchial stenosis is that the child breathes normally for the first few breaths and then develops respiratory distress.

Aspiration Syndromes

MECONIUM ASPIRATION

Infants who aspirate blood, mucus, secretions, meconium or cells in utero often have airway obstruction and severe asphyxia immediately after birth. The best studied example is the meconium aspiration syndrome.

Meconium is the breakdown product of swallowed amniotic fluid and gastrointestinal cells and secretions. It seldom occurs prior to 34 weeks' gestation, but infants older than this often respond to stress (hypoxia) with increased gut motility, relaxation of the sphincters and defecation.[8, 9] The gasping associated with asphyxia causes the infant to inhale as much as 60 ml of amniotic fluid (and debris) into the lung where it is situated in the trachea, mouth and main stem bronchi.[10] If birth is delayed, the meconium will be broken down and excreted from the lung in the 50 to 150 ml of lung fluid produced each day. However, if birth is less than 24 hours after the aspiration occurred, the meconium will still be present in the major airways and will progressively move into the lung periphery with the onset of breathing. Obstruction of small airways causes mismatching of ventilation and perfusion. Ventilation becomes rapid (100 to 150 breaths per minute) and shallow, and lung compliance decreases to a level similar to that seen in infants who have hyaline membrane disease (0.8 ml/cm H_2O).[11]

The respiratory failure seen in infants who aspirate meconium can be prevented in more than 99 per cent of cases by removing the meconium from the lung at birth. To do so, the procedure outlined in Table 27.2 is followed. **Immediately** after birth a 12 French (3.0-mm) endotracheal tube is inserted, and suction is applied by the physician's mouth. (A paper face mask prevents inhalation of the aspirate by the physician). Any meconium present in the tube is immediately blown out of the tube, and the infant's trachea is immediately reintubated and the procedure repeated. If no meconium is recovered, the trachea is not reintubated. The infant is then allowed to breathe or is ventilated with oxygen. Excessive airway pressures must be avoided, because pulmonary gas leaks are frequent after meconium aspiration.[12] The air leaks are not related to the suctioning procedure, because they occur at any time during the first 3 days of life. If this suctioning procedure is followed scrupulously, the mortality from meconium aspiration is 0.06 per 1,000 live births (un-

Table 27.2
Treatment of Meconium Aspiration

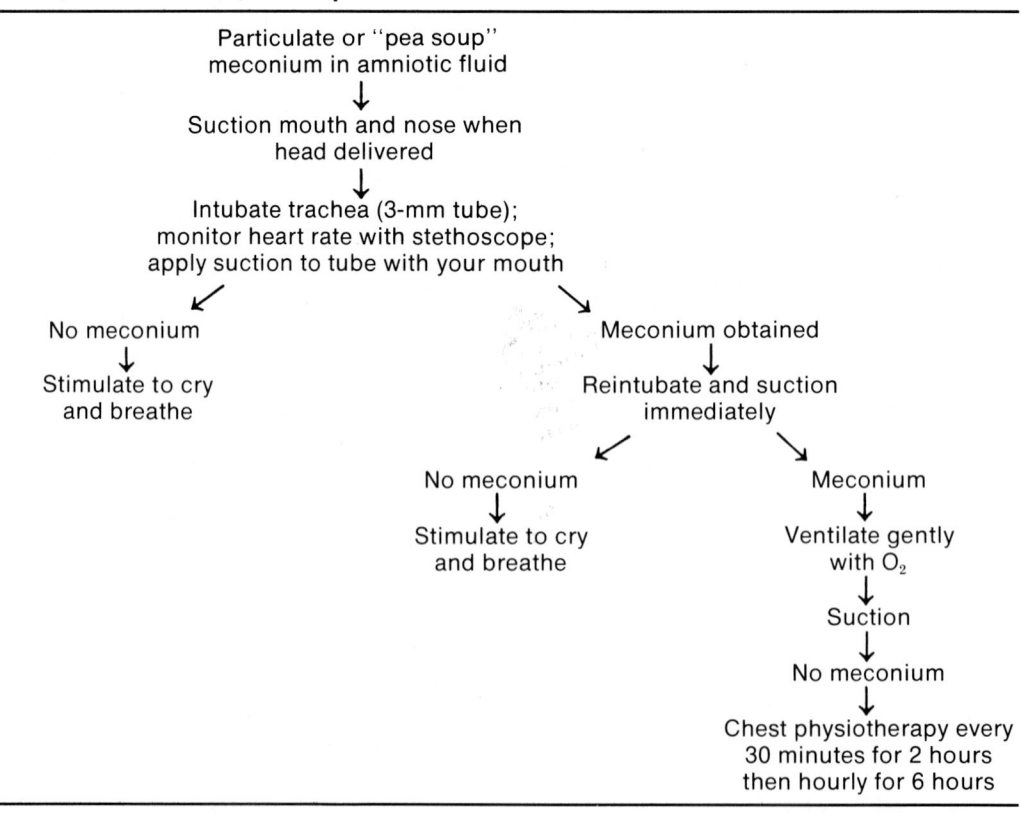

```
           Particulate or "pea soup"
           meconium in amniotic fluid
                     ↓
           Suction mouth and nose when
                 head delivered
                     ↓
           Intubate trachea (3-mm tube);
         monitor heart rate with stethoscope;
         apply suction to tube with your mouth
              ↙                    ↘
       No meconium              Meconium obtained
            ↓                         ↓
       Stimulate to cry         Reintubate and suction
       and breathe                   immediately
                              ↙                   ↘
                        No meconium            Meconium
                             ↓                    ↓
                      Stimulate to cry       Ventilate gently
                      and breathe              with O₂
                                                ↓
                                              Suction
                                                ↓
                                           No meconium
                                                ↓
                                     Chest physiotherapy every
                                     30 minutes for 2 hours
                                     then hourly for 6 hours
```

published data), whereas it is 2.2 per 1,000 live births when no suctioning is applied. In addition, infants rarely require assisted ventilation if tracheal suctioning is done.

If the airway is not suctioned and the meconium is allowed to obstruct the airway, the infant develops cyanosis, retractions, tachypnea and often grunting respiration. The PaO_2 falls below 50 torr with the infant breathing room air, and the $PaCO_2$ decreases to less than 30 torr. A rise in $PaCO_2$ above normal is an indication of impending severe respiratory failure. Hypoxia should be treated with an increased environmental oxygen. If, despite increasing the environmental oxygen to 80 per cent, PaO_2 remains less than 50 torr, an endotracheal tube should be inserted and 3 to 5 cm H_2O continuous positive airway pressure applied. If PaO_2 is still less than 50 torr, mechanical ventilation should be instituted and 3 to 5 cm H_2O positive end expiratory pressure maintained. Fifty per cent of ventilated infants develop a pneumothorax. All infants with meconium aspiration should be well hydrated and receive chest physiotherapy every 30 minutes for the first 2 hours and hourly thereafter for the next 6 hours.

Many infants who have aspirated meconium have pulmonary hypertension and right-to-left shunting of blood through the foramen ovale and ductus arteriosus. If severe, the treatment is mechanical ventilation, pulmonary vasodilation with tolazoline (Priscoline) and fluid replacement.[13]

OTHER ASPIRATION SYNDROMES

The net result of aspirating blood or debris is similar to that of meconium as-

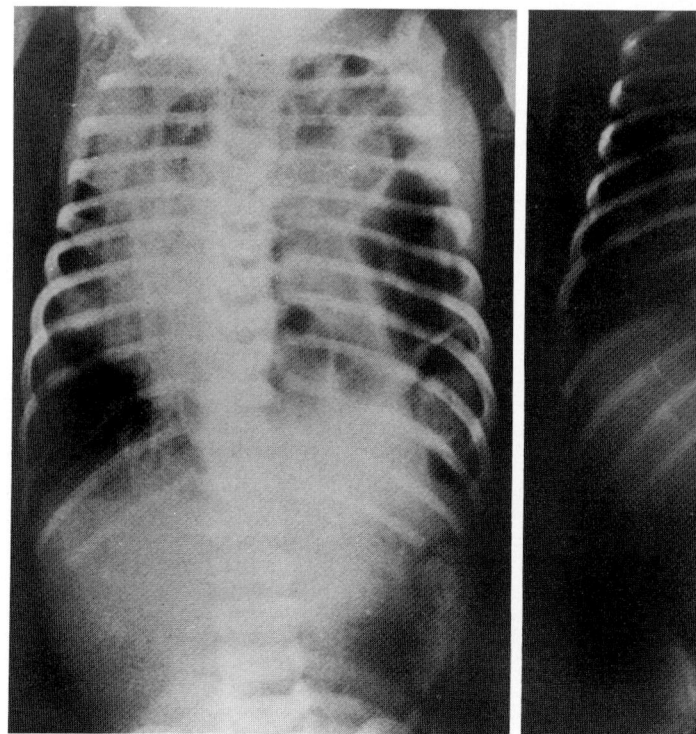

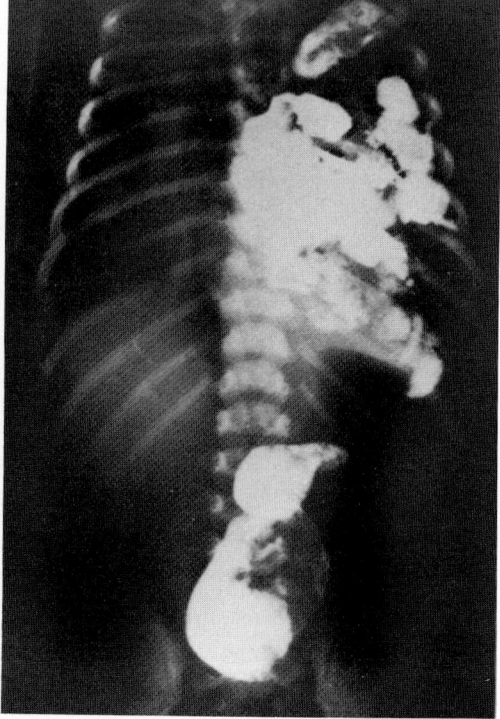

Figure 27.5. Films of the chest and abdomen of a 2-week-old infant with herniation of the bowel into the left hemithorax. Roentgenogram on *left* indicates the cyst-like radiolucencies in the chest and the lack of abdominal bowel pattern. In the roentgenogram on the *right*, the same infant is seen after a gastrointestinal series. (Reprinted by permission from Avery ME, Fletcher BD: *The Lung and Its Disorders in the Newborn Infant*, ed 3. W. B. Saunders, Philadelphia, 1974, p 166.)

piration. Therefore, the treatment is similar, i.e. suctioning of the airway at birth and chest physiotherapy afterwards.

Diaphragmatic Hernia

At about 12 weeks' gestation the diaphragm is normally complete. Failure of all parts to grow together normally allows gut to enter the chest when it returns to the abnormal cavity from the umbilical cord. deLorimier and associates[14] showed that the ipsilateral lung stops growing at whatever gestational age the gut enters the chest and that the contralateral lung is somewhat hypoplastic.

At birth these infants usually have severe respiratory failure. On physical examination they are cyanotic, retract, have grunting respiration and usually have a scaphoid abdomen. Breath sounds may or may not be reduced on the affected side, because they may be transmitted from one side to the other.

The diagnosis is usually made by physical examination and chest roentgenogram (bowel is seen in the left chest) (Figure 27.5). A large difference in PO_2 is often found between temporal or right radial artery and the umbilical artery blood due to right-to-left shunting at the ductus arteriosus. The difference in PaO_2 may be as great as 200 torr.

Treatment includes endotracheal intubation, ventilation with 100 per cent oxygen, insertion of an umbilical or radial artery catheter, correction of blood volume to normal if necessary and correction of the acid-base status. The $PaCO_2$ may be greater than 100 torr due to a large wasted ventilation. Five to 10 times normal ventilation may be required to maintain the $PaCO_2$ in a normal range. Care should be taken **not** to try to expand the small lung on the affected side or a pneumothorax will occur, often on the non-affected, gas-exchanging side. Rapid rate ventilation (80 to 100 breaths per minute) with peak proximal airway pressures of less than 25 cm H_2O are usually adequate. The infant should be transferred to the operating room as soon as its condition is stable.

References

1. Fearon B, Dickson J: Bilateral choanal atresia in the newborn: Plan of action. Laryngoscope 78:1487, 1968.
2. Erickson DJ, Lodge JL, Tomsovic EJ: Medical management of bilateral choanal atresia. Pediatrics 63:561, 1963.
3. Fletcher MM, Blum SL, Blanchard CL: Pierre Robin syndrome: Pathophysiology of obstructive episodes. Laryngoscope 79:547, 1969.
4. Gershanik JJ, Nervez C: Nasoesophageal intubation in the Pierre Robin syndrome. Clin Pediatr 15:173, 1976.
5. Shearer WT, Biller HF, Ogura JH, et al.: Congenital laryngeal web and intraventricular septal defect. Am J Dis Child 123:605, 1972.
6. Hollinger PH, Johnston KC, Zoss AR: Tracheal and bronchial obstruction due to congenital cardiovascular anomalies. Ann Otol 57:808, 1948.
7. Landing BH, Wells TR: Tracheobronchial anomalies in children. In *Perspectives in Pediatric Pathology*, Vol 1. HS Rosenberg and RB Bolande, eds. Year Book Medical Publishers, Chicago, 1973, p 1.
8. Sell EJ, Harris TR: Association of premature rupture of membranes with idiopathic respiratory distress syndrome. Obstet Gynecol 49:167, 1977.
9. Mansfield PB, Graham CB, Beckwith JB, et al.: Pneumopericardium and pneumomediastinum in infants and children. J Pediatr Surg 8:691, 1973.
10. Boddy K, Dawes GS: Fetal breathing. Br Med Bull 31:3, 1975.
11. Rudolph AM: *Pediatrics*, ed 16. Appleton-Century-Crofts, New York, 1977.
12. Gregory GA, Gooding GA, Phibbs RH, et al.: Meconium aspiration in infants: A prospective study. J Pediatr 85:848, 1974.
13. Levin D, Kitterman JA, Gregory GA, et al.: Persistent pulmonary hypertension in the newborn. J Pediatr 89:626, 1976.
14. deLorimier AA, Tierney DF, Parker HR: Hypoplastic lungs in fetal lambs with surgically produced congenital diaphragmatic hernia. Surgery 62:12, 1967.

CHAPTER 28

Retrolental Fibroplasia: Anesthetic Implications

Roderic H. Phibbs, M.D.

Retrolental fibroplasia (RLF) is a destructive vascular proliferation that occurs in the eyes of some prematurely born infants who receive oxygen therapy within the first months after birth.[1] It has long been a major concern of pediatricians who have cared for prematures and has recently emerged as a problem for anesthesiologists as well.

Methods for intensive care of the newborn have improved remarkably during the past decade. The survival rate among very premature infants, who are at greatest risk for developing RLF, has risen. Increasingly often, anesthesiologists are called on to administer oxygen to these infants under two circumstances. First, vigorous, complex and prolonged resuscitation at birth is a major component of the successful care of these newborns (see chapter 26), and the anesthesiologist is often the member of the resuscitation team who delivers oxygen and assisted ventilation during these first hours. Secondly, many of these infants now undergo surgery for such procedures as a patent ductus arteriosus, insertion of cerebrospinal fluid shunts or intra-atrial catheters for parenteral alimentation or laparotomy for bowel obstruction and perforation. They may require inhalation anesthesia, often with increased concentrations of oxygen, because of pulmonary disease. Oxygen administration during resuscitation, surgery or in the post-anesthetic recovery period can be lifesaving and prevent brain damage. However, if not carefully controlled, it can produce severe eye damage, even total blindness.[2]

The pathogenesis of RLF relates to the fact that the retinal vasculature is incompletely developed in the prematurely born infant; it grows from the optic disc peripherally and does not reach the more peripheral region of the retina until nearly the end of gestation. The pathology of RLF occurs at or near the leading edge of this growing vascular bed, usually on the temporal side of the retina. Hyperoxia of the blood in the arterioles causes prolonged vasoconstriction so that normal peripheral growth stops. Arteriovenous shunts then develop at the outer limit of the vasculature and, just proximal to this, most of the capillary network disappears. Still later, new abnormal vascular tufts form by budding from the region where the capillaries had disappeared; these may grow up off the retina and penetrate the vitreous humor.[3] This sequence is called the vascular phase of RLF and may or may not arrest and revert.

Some cases of RLF progress to the cicatricial phase, in which scar tissue forms where the vascular lesions had been. If the scar is small, it deforms the retina to a variable degree as it contracts, usually pulling it temporally. If the scar is large and extends into the vitreum, however, it detaches the retina as it contracts; the degree of visual loss depends on the extent of the lesion. The mildest cases have virtually no functional handicap, whereas the most severe cases can be totally blinded.

Animal studies have shown that the initiating process, retinal vasoconstriction, is dependent on hyperoxia of the arterial blood. Inspired oxygen is important only to the extent that it raises PaO_2 to a dangerous level. Extensive clinical studies also have clearly demonstrated that oxygen therapy is the cause of RLF.[1] Most of the cases have occurred when the ambient oxygen exceeded 40 per cent, usually for several days and often for weeks; however, any increase in inspired oxygen carries some risk of RLF for the premature.

The risk of RLF is related directly to the degree of prematurity. Most cases occur in infants who weigh 1500 gm or less at birth, but any prematurely born infant is at increased risk.[1] These early clinical studies were done 20 years ago when it was impossible to measure PaO_2 systemically in premature infants. Therefore, there could be no definition of a safe upper limit or a minimal period of elevation of PaO_2 necessary to produce RLF, nor could they explain the very puzzling group of infants who were very premature but yet survived prolonged exposure to high concentrations of oxygen without any eye damage. Two possible explanations are (1) that there was extreme variation in susceptibility so that some were unharmed by a level of PaO_2 that blinded others of equivalent maturity and (2) that these infants were unharmed because they had lung disease severe enough so that PaO_2 remained at a safe level despite the high ambient oxygen.

Following these studies oxygen use was curtailed and in the ensuing years there were almost no new cases of RLF; however, neonatal mortality in the first hours of life increased dramatically.[1] By the 1960's, when regular measurement of PaO_2 in sick newborns became possible, the association between hyperoxia and RLF seemed so clear that no one was willing to repeat the clinical trials and intentionally produce hyperoxia in order to define safe limits of PaO_2. Instead, pediatricians assumed they could use increased inspired oxygen safely, guided by measurements of PaO_2, and accepted the guideline of giving no more oxygen than needed to raise the PaO_2 to the normal range of 50 to 90 torr.[4] Nonetheless, new cases of RLF began to appear.[5]

Documented episodes of hyperoxia occurred because pulmonary perfusion and effective ventilation change so rapidly in some sick infants that it is impossible to keep PaO_2 within the presumed safe range, and some hyperoxic infants developed RLF later. Through the accumulation of these isolated experiences with documented hyperoxia, some idea of the quantitative relationship between PaO_2 and RLF has emerged. As might be expected from the older clinical studies, most cases still occur in the most premature infants.[6,7] As suspected, there is extreme variability in sensitivity—some infants tolerate a hyperoxic exposure 10 times as long as that which blinds other infants of equivalent birth weight and maturity.[6,8] This suggests that other factors influence the risk of RLF, but there is no information to suggest what these factors might be.[9,10]

The danger level appears to be a PaO_2 greater than 100 torr; in the most susceptible infants, serious injury can be done by a cumulative exposure of 1 to 2 hours. The current recommendation of the American Academy of Pediatrics stipulates that "when giving supplemental oxygen the arterial oxygen tension should be maintained at a level not higher than 80 to 90 torr. Usually, infants who require oxygen therapy do not need an arterial PO_2 higher than 50 torr, and do well with an arterial PO_2 between 50 and 70 torr."[4]

There are six practical guidelines for the anesthetist who gives oxygen and assisted ventilation to a prematurely born infant:

1. Infants at risk. Although most cases of RLF occur in very premature infants, any infant born before 36 weeks' gestation or weighing less than 2500 gm is at increased risk for RLF.[4] Prematurely born infants remain at risk until their retinal vasculature completes its growth, which probably occurs at 36 to 40 weeks. For example, an infant who comes to surgery at 6 weeks of age, but was born at a gestational (post-conception) age of 26 weeks, has only reached 32 weeks and is still at risk for RLF.

2. When and where to measure PaO_2. Oxygen therapy must be guided by measurements of PaO_2. The clinician cannot rely on skin color, because infants with poor peripheral perfusion may have cyanosis despite a PaO_2 of 200 torr or more. To detect hyperoxia reliably, blood must be sampled directly from an artery, not from "arterialized" capillary blood drawn from a skin puncture in an area previously warmed to produce vasodilation. The latter method does not permit frequent enough sampling to follow the rapid changes in PaO_2 in an infant whose pulmonary status is unstable, and it is invalid if there is poor skin blood flow or when PaO_2 exceeds 90 to 100 torr even though skin perfusion is good.

PaO_2 is most often and easily measured in the newborn by sampling through a catheter passed into the descending aorta via the umbilical artery. Under certain conditions, PaO_2 measured in this manner will be lower than that of blood going to the eyes. In many sick newborn infants, the ductus arteriosus remains patent for hours to weeks after birth. If pulmonary artery pressure exceeds aortic pressure, venous blood will flow from the pulmonary artery through the ductus into the descending aorta (Figure 28.1). This can occur with severe pulmonary hypertension or systemic hypotension, or a combi-

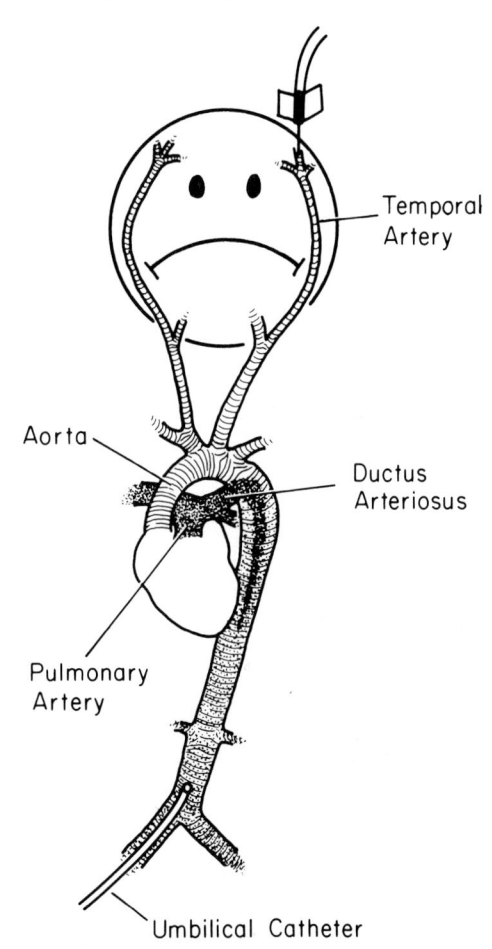

Figure 28.1. Right-to-left shunt of blood through a patent ductus arteriosus causes a lower PaO_2 in the descending aorta, where the sampling catheter is located, than in the ascending aorta which supplies the retinal arteries. The mixed venous blood is indicated by the *dark stippling*. This condition can be detected by simultaneously sampling blood from the needle inserted into a temporal artery, as shown, and from the umbilical artery catheter with its tip in the descending aorta and comparing the PaO_2's of the two samples.

nation of the two. Severe pulmonary hypertension can occur in a variety of conditions which are usually found in more mature infants who are at a lower risk for RLF. Hypoplastic lungs with diaphragmatic hernia is the condition most likely to confront an anesthesiologist. In less mature infants with respiratory distress, such a shunt is usually small or absent unless there is systemic hypotension. Thus, if the PaO_2 in the descending aorta is kept below 80 torr in infants with respiratory distress who weigh less than 1500 gm, PaO_2 in the ascending aorta will rarely exceed 100 torr so long as the infant is normotensive.[11] In such infants, this means that systemic pressure must be monitored closely because hypotension is a common complication of their disease. The presence of this kind of shunting can be detected clinically by simultaneously sampling blood from above and below the ductus arteriosus (Figure 28.1). Good sites for sampling preductal blood include the right radial or either temporal artery. The left radial artery is not good because the left subclavian artery often originates very near the level of the ductus. Unless one is confident that there is little or no chance of a shunt, based on the clinical condition of an infant, a set of paired samples should be taken for comparison.

It would seem that the sampling problem could be avoided by advancing the umbilical artery catheter up the aorta until the tip is above the ductus, but this is generally impractical. A catheter advanced in this manner usually passes through the ductus into the pulmonary artery, so that samplings from it would provide misleading information. Occasionally, the advanced catheter will go into the arch of the aorta, but it may then enter the left carotid artery and obstruct blood flow to the brain. To minimize thrombotic complications, the tip of the umbilical artery catheter should be kept below the origin of the inferior mesenteric artery.

3. Changing PaO_2. The cardiopulmonary status of sick newborn infants is so labile that PaO_2 often changes rapidly, requiring frequent measurements and rapid adjustment of inspired oxygen or ventilator settings. Major changes are particularly likely after the institution of assisted ventilation, change in ventilatory pressure or rates, or after any other therapy which is likely to alter pulmonary ventilation or perfusion. Following such changes, PaO_2 must be remeasured frequently—as a general rule, every 10 to 20 minutes during resuscitation and about 10 minutes after each change in therapy.

During resuscitation of the asphyxiated newborn, PaO_2 rises rapidly, but this does not occur at a predictable time after the onset of assisted ventilation with high oxygen concentrations. Figure 28.2 shows time of PaO_2 rise in a group of asphyxiated premature infants, all of whom had been ventilated continuously with high concentrations of oxygen beginning at 1 to 5 minutes after birth.

Pulmonary function often changes during major surgery, particularly when the procedure tends to compress the lungs. This requires compensatory changes in assisted ventilation and inspired oxygen. Post-operatively, as this restriction of lung expansion is relieved, PaO_2 can rise rapidly. The most striking changes during surgery occur with ligation of a patent ductus arteriosus which has caused pulmonary edema and reduction of lung compliance. In many cases, the appearance of the lung changes from dark red to bright pink within moments after the ductus is ligated; compliance changes almost as rapidly.

The best solution to this problem is a system that measures arterial oxygenation (PaO_2 or SaO_2) continuously. Several such systems have been developed that are now

RETROLENTAL FIBROPLASIA: ANESTHETIC IMPLICATIONS

undergoing clinical testing and should be available in the near future. Figures 28.3 and 28.4 show data from one such system and illustrate the rapid changes in oxygenation that can occur.

4. **Hyperoxia while breathing room air.** In some very small premature infants, PaO_2 reaches potentially dangerous levels while breathing room air. This can occur during hyperventilation at an atmospheric pressure near that at sea level. A simplified version of the equation used to calculate alveolar partial pressure of oxygen (PA_{O_2}) is as follows:

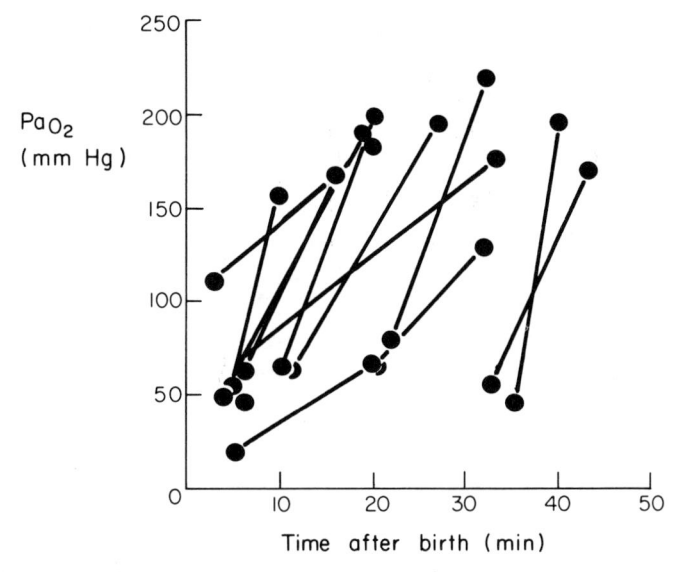

Figure 28.2. Changes in PaO_2 during the resuscitation of 12 premature infants who suffered intrapartum asphyxia. All weighed 1500 gm or less at birth. All were intubated and given assisted ventilation with an increased inspired oxygen at 1 to 5 minutes after birth. The descending aorta was catheterized via the umbilical artery, and blood was sampled through the catheter for measurements of PaO_2. Each *line* connects two measurements from the same infant. The first measurement was always made after the onset of assisted ventilation. At the time of the second measurement the inspired oxygen was always the same or lower than it was at the first measurement. Note that the PaO_2 rises to a dangerously high level in 11 of the 12 infants and that the time of this rise is quite variable.

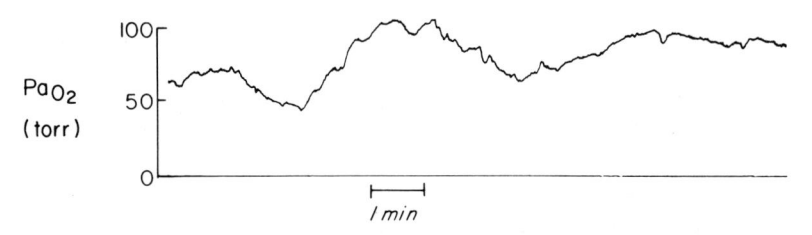

Figure 28.3. Continuously recorded intra-arterial PO_2 in a 2350-gm infant with mild hyaline membrane disease who is breathing 35 per cent O_2. Note the marked and rapid fluctuations in PaO_2 with spontaneous respiration.

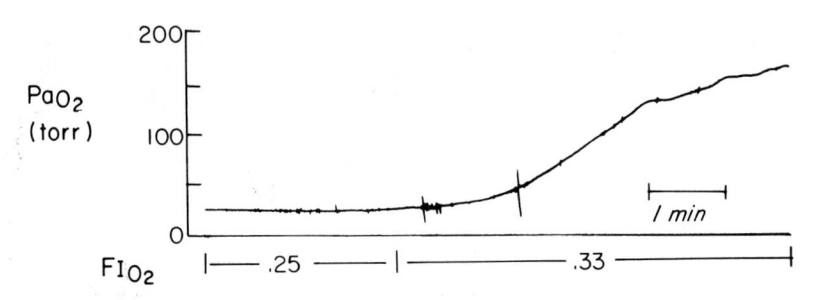

Figure 28.4. Continuously recorded intra-arterial PO₂ in a 2350-gm, 33-week gestation infant with hyaline membrane disease who was being treated with continuous positive airway pressure at 5 torr. Note the rapid rise in PaO₂ from a dangerously low to a dangerously high level when inspired oxygen ($F_{I_{O_2}}$) was raised from 25 to 33 per cent.

$PA_{O_2} = (P\ atmos - P_{H_2O}) \times (F_{I_{O_2}}) - (PA_{CO_2})$

P atmos = atmospheric pressure
P_{H_2O} = water vapor pressure
$F_{I_{O_2}}$ = fraction inspired oxygen (100% O₂ = $F_{I_{O_2}}$ of 1.0; room air = $F_{I_{O_2}}$ of 0.21)
PA_{CO_2} = partial pressure of CO₂ in the alveolus for which Pa_{CO_2} can be substituted.

For an infant who is breathing room air at sea level and has a normal Pa_{CO_2} of 40 torr, the equation becomes.

$PA_{O_2} = (760 - 47) \times 0.21 - 40 = 110\ torr$

Arterial P_{O_2} can be substantially less than PA_{O_2} if there is significant pulmonary disease. With effective ventilation and well matched ventilation and perfusion, it can approach or equal PA_{O_2}. If the same infant hyperventilates or is hyperventilated by manual or mechanical means so that PaCO₂ falls to 20 torr, PA_{O_2} will rise to 130 torr and PaO₂ may approach this. This occurs in very premature infants who have no significant lung disease but have poor control of respiration and apneic episodes that require mechanically assisted ventilation which has led to hypocarbia. The same thing can occur during surgery in a small premature infant with normal lungs during manual ventilation with an anesthesia bag.

5. Hyperoxia with cyanotic congenital heart disease. There used to be an axiom that hyperoxia could not occur if there was a cyanotic congenital heart lesion, and that a high PaO₂ while breathing 100 per cent oxygen ruled out such lesions. Recent experience has shown that this is not correct and that hyperoxia can occur in infants with certain cyanotic heart lesions when given 100 per cent oxygen.[12]

It has been thought that, except for patent ductus arteriosus, major congenital heart disease almost never occurs in prematures. This is incorrect. Premature infants who are small enough to be at significant risk for RLF can have major congenital heart lesions, including cyanotic lesions.[13] The rules about careful monitoring of PaO₂ apply equally to them, until there is certainty that the lesion is one in which hyperoxia is impossible.

6. Equipment for control of oxygen therapy. Many delivery and operating room resuscitation areas may need additional equipment and some reorganization to follow the guidelines of oxygen therapy for premature infants.[4] There must be an **oxygen-air blender** that can deliver any concentration of oxygen between room air and 100 per cent and deliver the mixture at a flow high enough so that there is no accumulation of exhaled CO₂ within the gas delivery system.[14] There must be an **oxygen analyzer** to check the concentration of oxygen actually delivered. If the infant is breathing spontaneously in a hood, this means sampling the gas near the infant's nose. If ventilation is assisted or controlled via an endotracheal tube, this means sampling as close to the tube connection as the system will allow. When in use, the accuracy of the analyzer must be checked in room air and 100 per cent oxygen every 8 hours.[4]

Measurements of pH, PO_2, and P_{CO_2} must be readily available. In neonatal intensive care units, the American Academy of Pediatrics recommends that it should take no more than 5 minutes from the time an arterial blood specimen is drawn until the measurements are made and the results are given to those caring for the infant.[4] The need for this rapid response should be obvious. This should also apply when oxygen therapy to a premature infant is undertaken in other areas of the hospital.

Given the extreme instability of PaO_2 in sick newborn infants and the extreme variability in sensitivity of the retinal vasculature to hyperoxia, prevention of RLF might seem to be a hopeless effort, but this is not true. During the past 10 years there has been increasingly precise control of oxygen therapy, in an attempt to maintain PaO_2 within the narrow range considered to be safe, and recent experience suggests that these measures are successful. Most infants who weigh less than 1500 gm now receive high concentrations of oxygen and/or ventilatory assistance at some time; however, in nurseries that employ strict control measures, only about 10 per cent have any permanent RLF when re-examined later in infancy. Furthermore, most of those who have been affected have a less severe form of the disease. This suggests permanent damage can be prevented completely in most premature infants and, among the most susceptible, damage can usually be kept to a minimum.

References

1. James LS, Lanman JT: History of oxygen therapy and retrolental fibroplasia. Pediatrics (Suppl) 57: 591, 1976.
2. Betts EK, Downes JJ, Schaffer DB, et al.: Retrolental fibroplasia and oxygen administration during general anesthesia. Anesthesiology. In press.
3. Kushner BJ, Essner D, Cohen IJ, et al.: Retrolental fibroplasia. II. Pathologic correlation. Arch Ophthalmol 95:29, 1977.
4. American Academy of Pediatrics: *Standards and Recommendations for the Hospital Care of Newborn Infants*, LS James, ed, ed 6. American Academy of Pediatrics, Evanston, Ill., 1977.
5. Akeson N: What is the current incidence of RLF? Pediatrics 58:627, 1976.
6. Kinsey VE, Arnold HJ, Kalina RE, et al.: PaO_2 levels and retrolental fibroplasia. Pediatrics 60: 655, 1977.
7. Kingham JD: Acute retrolental fibroplasia. Arch Ophthalmol 95:39, 1977.
8. Aranda J, Sweet A: Sustained hyperoxemia without cicatricial retrolental fibroplasia. Pediatrics 54:434, 1974.
9. Aranda JF, Saheb N, Stern L, et al.: Arterial oxygen tension and retinal vasoconstriction in newborn infants. Am J Dis Child 122:189, 1971.
10. Lechner D, Kalina RE, Hodson WA: Retrolental fibroplasia and factors influencing oxygen transport. Pediatrics 59:916, 1977.
11. Schlueter MA, Tooley WH: Right-to-left shunt through the ductus arteriosus in newborn infants. Pediatr Res 8:80, 1974.
12. Tooley WH, Stanger P: The blue baby—circulation or ventilation or both? N Engl J Med 287:983, 1972.
13. Levin DL, Stanger P, Kitterman JA, et al.: Congenital heart disease in low birth weight infants. Circulation 52:500, 1975.
14. Gale R, Redner-Carmi R, Gale J: Accumulation of carbon dioxide in oxygen hoods. Pediatrics 60: 453, 1977.

APPENDICES

APPENDIX A

Fetal and Neonatal Effects of Maternally Administered Drugs

Richard G. Wright, M.D.
Sol M. Shnider, M.D.

It has been estimated that an average of four of every five pregnant women take some form of medication during pregnancy. Hill et al.[60] have recently reported on the drug use of 231 women during pregnancy. If labor and delivery are excluded, the number of drug preparations taken per patient was reported as 9.6. Prescription drugs accounted for a mean of 6.4 drugs per patient, and over-the-counter medications represented the remaining 3.2 drugs per patient. In addition, many parturients receive some medication during labor and delivery to relieve pain or anxiety. When obstetric complications arise, patients may require substantial doses of several drugs to ensure a safe outcome.

It is probable that all maternally administered drugs cross the placenta to some extent. Movement is primarily by passive diffusion. Both a large transplacental drug gradient and a high diffusion constant facilitate movement across the placental membrane. Drugs with a high diffusion constant are those of low molecular weight and high lipid solubility which exist primarily in the non-ionized unbound form.

When administered during the first trimester, the period of organogenesis, certain drugs may modify development of fetal tissues with resultant congenital anomalies. However, drugs are not the sole factor which may have an adverse effect on fetal tissue organization and development. In fact, the cause of most malformations is not known. Only a small percentage are directly attributable to known hereditary and environmental factors (the latter including infection, irradiation and drug use). Organogenesis is complete by the end of the first trimester, with important exceptions being the teeth, or genital system and central nervous system. The vast majority of congenital malformations arise during the first trimester of pregnancy when organ systems are developing and embryonic cells are rapidly dividing. The teratogenic effects of a drug are both dose-related and time-related. The timing of a teratogenic influence is crucial in determining the system affected. In humans, for example, the period of greatest development and organization of the cardiovascular system is between 20 and 40 days after conception; that of the limbs is from 24 to 46 days, and that of the nervous system is from 15 to 25 days. Exposure to an appropriate teratogen between 15 and 25 days after conception may, for example, result in nervous system but not skeletal anomalies. It is possible for teratogenic drugs to exert their effects on development within the first 2 weeks of conception—before the woman knows that she is pregnant. However, from the time of fertilization until implantation of the blastocyst, most deleterious drugs abort the conception rather than deform it.

Only three types of drugs are definitely known to be teratogenic in humans: certain antimetabolites, thalidomide and steroid hormones with androgenic activity. Epidemiologic surveys have been undertaken to examine the possible association between congenital defects in the infant and maternal drug ingestion. Most studies are difficult to interpret. Associations are loose, and it is usually impossible to differentiate the effects of a drug from those of the maternal disease for which the medication was prescribed. From these studies it seems that many drugs are highly suspect for inducing fetal abnormalities but that the risk is often relatively low. Although considerable work has been done on teratogenicity in animals, it should be stressed that little, if any, parallel exists between the ability to induce abnormalities in a particular species of animal and in humans.

Drugs administered at any time during pregnancy or labor may modify fetal and newborn physiology. Such changes are usually of no clinical relevance, but, on occasion, they may be either detrimental or beneficial.

Analgesic or anesthetic drugs administered to the mother prior to delivery may depress the fetus and lessen the reserve of the newborn for adapting to extrauterine life. The most widely used method for evaluating the condition of the infant in the delivery room is the Apgar score. There are five signs: heart rate, respiratory effort, muscle tone, response to stimulation and skin color. A score of 0, 1 or 2 is assigned to the presence or absence of each sign. Apgar scoring quickly identifies those infants with significant depression of vital function. Maternally administered drugs may reduce neonatal vigor and subsequently result in lower Apgar scores. Such drug-induced depression is infrequent in uncomplicated well conducted obstetrics but may occur, for instance, with general anesthesia for cesarean section. When drug depression does occur, it is in the form of respiratory depression, and ventilation may require support for a short period of time.

Although the Apgar score is useful in identifying those infants requiring active resuscitation, it fails to detect both subtle drug effects as well as those extending past the immediate newborn period. Scanlon et al.[131] have developed a simple, rapid and reproducible technique of assessing certain aspects of behavior in the first few hours of life. The examination is an adaptation of standard neurological and behavioral testing of newborns as developed by Prechtal and Beintema[144a] Beintema,[8b] and Brazelton et al.[15c] Neonates who are vigorous as assessed by Apgar score may score low on the Scanlon neurobehavioral examination in the first hours of life. These neurobehavioral changes are transient, and their clinical significance, if any, is not known. Bupivacaine (Marcaine) and chloroprocaine (Nesacaine), the two local anesthetics most popular in obstetrics, produce minimal neurobehavioral changes in the newborn.

The following table lists some of the more frequently used drugs with their possible effects on the fetus and newborn. Comments and references are included where appropriate.

Fetal and Neonatal Effects of Maternally Administered Drugs

Drug	Effects	Comments	References
Anticonvulsants			
Diphenylhydantoin (Dilantin)	Suspicion of multiple congenital anomalies (fetal hydantoin syndrome)	Possible relationship exists independent of the epileptic state	9, 40, 50a, 52b, 59a, 59b, 84, 92, 96, 98, 99, 107, 154, 155, 170b, 178
Magnesium sulfate	Neonatal depression Hypotonia Hypotension	Effect of high blood levels associated with therapy of preeclampsia	1, 39, 83, 129
Trimethadione (Tridione)	Suspicion of teratogenicity		45a, 124a, 177
Anticoagulants (oral)			
Coumadin (Dicumarol)	Intracranial hemorrhage, fetal death	Most significant during the third trimester and labor	13, 41, 50b
	Suspicion of teratogenicity: Bony abnormalities including: stippling on x-ray, kyphoscoliosis, broad short hands and fingers, skull abnormalities, nasal hypoplasia. Ophthalmologic abnormalities including: optic atrophy, cataracts, microophthalmia. Mental retardation		8a, 25, 141, 142
(Heparin does not cross the placenta)			
Antihypertensives			
Reserpine (Serpasil)	Nasal obstruction Lethargy Anorexia Respiratory depression Impairment of nonshivering thermogenesis	Accompanies late pregnancy use	34, 175
Diazoxide (Hyperstat)	Hyperglycemia Alopecia, Hypertrichosis laruginosa Decreased bone age	May occur with acute intravenous use May follow weeks of oral use	97, 109

Drug	Effects	Comments	References
Propranolol (Inderal)	Possibly associated with intrauterine growth retardation Bradycardia Hypoglycemia	Associated with chronic use	46, 51a, 116, 166
	Abnormally long time to establish sustained respiration and low Apgar scores	Follows 1 mg intravenously minutes prior to delivery	164
Nitroprusside (Nipride)	Cyanide intoxication	Possibility suggested from animal study, no human data available	121
Ganglionic blockers, e.g. trimethaphan (Arfonad) pentolinium, trimethidinium, hexamethonium, mecamylamine	Neonatal ileus		51b
Diuretics			
Ethacrynic acid (Edecrin)	Neonatal deafness	Potential cited	42
Thiazides	Hyponatremia Thrombocytopenia		70, 123
Antithyroid medication			
Methimazole (Tapazole)	Suspicion of causing aplasia cutis		103a
Propylthiouracil	Goiter ± hypothyroidism	Goiter is not a common occurrence and when it does occur, the gland is not extremely large. Hypothyroidism is less common and not clearly related to drug therapy. The drug readily crosses the placenta. Presumably sufficient maternal thyroid hormone crosses to meet fetal needs in most instances.	18, 67
Iodide	Goiter ± hypothyroidism	A large goiter occasionally results in cephalo-pelvic disproportion.	18
Radioactive iodine	Hypoplastic or absent thyroid giving rise to hypothyroid state Carcinoma of the thyroid	Destruction of the fetal thyroid Potential carcinogenic effect with a long latent period	18, 43
Oral hypoglycemics Sulfonylureas			
Tolbutamide (Orinase)	Suspicion of multiple congenital anomalies	Anomalies are possibly unrelated to drug ingestion but to the diabetic state per se	78, 134

FETAL AND NEONATAL EFFECTS OF DRUGS

Drug	Effect	Comment	References
Chlorpropamide (Diabinese)	High combined perinatal mortality rate	In one study, high doses of chlorpropamide gave more than double the incidence of perinatal mortality than tolbutamide therapy.	64
Antimetabolites			
Chlorambucil, cyclophosphamide, busulfan	Suspicion of gross malformations		153, 157
Busulfan	Intrauterine growth retardation		15b
Folate antagonists, e.g. aminopterin, amethopterin (Methotrexate)	Teratogenic	Potential complication of third trimester use Proved	38, 161
Antimicrobial agents			
Aminoglycosides, e.g. streptomycin, gentamycin	Deafness	Potential exists throughout pregnancy, streptomycin is the only one extensively investigated	23, 26, 122, 171
Tetracycline	Dental discoloration Enamel hypoplasia Diminished growth of long bones	Mechanism is through the chelation of calcium	23, 24, 119, 163
	Cataracts	Possible association	53
Sulfonamides	Increased unbound bilirubin with increased risk of kernicterus	Drug competes with bilirubin for albumin binding, relevant when administered near delivery, especially when long-acting drug used	147
Chloramphenicol (Chloromycetin)	"Grey baby syndrome"	Risk when administered close to delivery, more likely when hepatic and renal function immature	17, 23, 73, 139
Novobiocin	Hyperbilirubinemia with increased risk of kernicterus Thrombocytopenia	Competes with bilirubin for conjugation, relevant when given near term	23, 37, 158
Antimalarial agents			32a
Quinine	Suspicion of congenital anomalies of the central nervous and skeletal systems Deafness Optic nerve hypoplasia Thrombocytopenia		60, 87, 167
Steroids			
Cortisone	Suspicion of cleft palate, abortion, fetal death	Effects due to drug or disease per se?	15a, 36, 54, 170a

Drug	Effects	Comments	References
Prednisone	Neonatal hypoadrenalism	Poor placental transfer makes the incidence low	15, 72, 175
Betamethasone	Lung maturation	Induces surfactant production	82
17-α-hydroxyprogesterone caproate	Possibility of strabismus, premature cranial suture closure	Isolated case reports, very possibly due to coincidence	117
Stilbesterol	Adenocarcinoma of vagina	Proved, transplacental carcinogen with a long latent period	57
Progestins, androgens	Masculization of the female fetus: labial fusion early, clitoral hypertrophy late		14, 65, 68b, 172, 174
Progestins, estrogens	Suspicion of increased incidence of cardiovascular defects		56
Tranquilizers			
Major			
Phenothiazines	Suspicion of congenital anomalies, especially cardiovascular and respiratory	More likely with the 3-carbon aliphatic side chain, e.g. chlorpromazine	29, 126, 150, 159, 168
Chlorpromazine (Thorazine)	Possible retinopathy	Due to affinity of the drug for melanin	58a
Minor			
Benzodiazepines, diazepam (Valium)	Suspicion of cleft lip and/or palate	The cause and effect relationship of minor tranquilizers and congenital anomalies is not proved but the Food and Drug Administration recommends that these drugs not be used in the first trimester.	128
	Neonatal withdrawal	Chronic exposure	88
	Decreased Apgar scores	Large doses in labor	44a
	Decreased neonatal muscle tone	Large doses in labor	30, 44a
	Decreased ability to withstand cold stress		30, 113a
	Decreased fetal heart rate beat-to-beat variability	Lessens diagnostic capabilities of fetal heart rate monitoring	133, 176
	Bilirubin displacement from albumin	Due to sodium benzoate preservative, unlikely of clinical significance unless administered directly to the neonate	105, 135
Chlordiazepoxide (Librium)	Suspicion of congenital anomalies	The cause and effect relationship of minor tranquilizers and congenital anomalies is not proved, but the Food and Drug Administration recommends that these drugs not be used in the first trimester.	55, 95

FETAL AND NEONATAL EFFECTS OF DRUGS

Antidepressants			
Tricyclics, e.g. imipramine (Tofranil)	Neonatal withdrawal syndrome	Chronic exposure	4, 10
Amphetamines	Suspicion of craniofacial and central nervous system anomalies		63
	Suspicion of congenital heart disease, congenital biliary atresia, oral clefts		80c, 94, 108
	Suspicion of cardiovascular anomalies		
Lithium	Bradycardia, arrhythmias		33, 93, 136, 137, 156a
	Goiter		
	Hypotonia		
Sedatives, hypnotics			
Glutethimide (Doriden)	Neonatal withdrawal syndrome	Possible association with chronic use	55, 95
Meprobamate (Miltown, Equanil)	Suspicion of congenital anomalies		
Barbiturates	Neonatal depression	Result of inappropriately large doses in labor or for induction-maintenance of general anesthesia for delivery	76, 125
	Decreased serum bilirubin	Chronic use induces hepatic enzymes	89, 115
	Hemorrhagic disease of the newborn	Rare case reports with decreased Stuart-Prower factor with chronic use	138
Bromide-containing sedatives	Neonatal withdrawal syndrome	Chronic exposure	12, 35
	Acneiform rash	Sporadic reports	60
	Lethargy		
	High-pitched cry		
	Feeding problems		
Thalidomide	Congenital limb defects (amelia, phocomelia), possible cardiovascular and uterovaginal anomalies	Proved, no longer available	61, 79, 90, 160a
Analgesics (non-narcotic)			
Salicylates	Suspicion of congenital anomalies	Low index of suspicion	106, 120, 149
	Possibly small for gestational age and increased incidence of stillbirths	Conflicting data in patients consuming large amounts	140, 165
	Possible increased incidence of post-date deliveries	Data conflicts; the postulated mechanism is via prostaglandin synthesis inhibition	81, 140
	Increased unbound bilirubin with increased risk of kernicterus	Competes with bilirubin for albumin	60
	Platelet dysfunction and decreased factor XII	Possibility of increased hemorrhagic phenomenon	11

Drug	Effects	Comments	References
Acetaminophen	Possible pulmonary hypertension in newborn period	Large doses, prostaglandin synthatase inhibition may allow ductus arterisosus constriction in utero	80a, 80b, 86a
Indomethacin	Possible interstitial nephritis	One case report	60
	Possible pulmonary hypertension in newborn period	Large doses, prostaglandin synthatase inhibition may allow ductus arteriosus constriction in utero	80a, 80b, 86a
Propoxyphene (Darvon)	Neonatal withdrawal syndrome	Chronic abuse	44b
Analgesics (narcotics)	Small for gestational age	With chronic abuse	69
	Lung maturation	Reported acceleration of appearance of mature L/S ratio in heroin addicts	47, 49
	Decreased incidence of neonatal jaundice	Heroin reported to induce fetal hepatic enzymes	3, 104, 180
	or		
	Increased incidence of neonatal jaundice	Reported with methadone only; mechanism unknown	179
	Intrauterine death	Associated with maternal narcotic withdrawal	20, 118
	Neonatal withdrawal syndrome	With chronic abuse	48, 58b, 71, 77, 124b, 179
	Neonatal depression	Inappropriate doses during labor, morphine most depressant	145
Inhalation anesthetics			
Halothane, cyclopropane, nitrous oxide	Dose-related neonatal depression		101
	Suspicion of spontaneous abortion, congenital anomalies	A possible effect of exposure, the only work is in animals	2, 5, 152
Operating room environment	Increased incidence of spontaneous abortion, congenital anomalies	A possible effect of chronic operating room exposure; potential sources include trace anesthetic gases, irradiation, stress, infection, etc.	21, 27, 28, 127
Local anesthetics			
Lidocaine, mepivacaine	Decreased neonatal Apgar scores	Rare with conventional uncomplicated anesthesia	100, 146
	Decreased Scanlon neurobehavioral scores	Significantly different from neonates not exposed to local anesthetics	131

FETAL AND NEONATAL EFFECTS OF DRUGS

Chloroprocaine, bupivacaine	Seizures, cardiovascular collapse	With high toxic levels such as follow direct injection into the fetus	110, 148
Vasopressors			
Ephedrine	No effect on Apgar or neurobehavioral scores	No difference from neonates not exposed to drugs	62, 114b, 132
Centrally acting pressors (ephedrine, mephentermine)	Increased fetal heart rate variability	Direct placental transfer	66, 144
Peripherally acting pressors (methoxamine, phenylephrine)	As therapy of spinal hypotension, prevents fetal asphyxia	Returns uterine blood flow toward control with correction of spinal hypotension	66
Skeletal muscle relaxants	As therapy of spinal hypotension, does not prevent fetal asphyxia	Uterine blood flow does not recover with correction of spinal hypotension	
Anticholinergics	No clinical effect	Quaternary ammonium compounds do not cross the placenta in clinically significant amounts, with the possible exception of gallamine	102
Atropine	Fetal tachycardia, decreased beat-to-beat variability, elimination of variable and early decelerations	Anticholinergic effect following placental transfer	
Oxytocics, myometrial depressants			
Oxytocin	Increased incidence of neonatal hyperbilirubinemia	Consensus of somewhat conflicting data	6, 7, 19, 31, 45b, 111, 162, 173
Isoxsuprine (Vasodilan), ritodrine	Asphyxia Tachycardia Hyperglycemia	Uterine hypertonus from overdose β-adrenergic effect following placental transfer	16, 143
Social drugs			
Alcohol	Fetal alcohol syndrome (includes small for gestational age with persisting growth lag, craniofacial, cardiovascular and possibly renal abnormalities, mental and psychomotor retardation)	Proved with chronic abuse	32b, 52a, 68a, 103b, 112, 113b, 156b, 160b
	Neonatal depression, hypoglycemia, increased heat loss	Acute overdose in prematurity	169
	Neonatal withdrawal syndrome	Chronic abuse	60

Drug	Effects	Comments	References
Tobacco	Small for gestational age	Chronic abuse	60
	Spontaneous abortion	Chronic abuse	74
	Decreased fetal breathing	Induced by two cigarettes, significance unknown	86b
	Lower neonatal bilirubin levels	Possible transplacental induction of hepatic enzymes with cyanide from tobacco	60
Lysergic acid diethylamide (LSD)	Chromosomal breaks, possibly skeletal malformations		22, 91, 151
Environmental toxins			
Lead	Small for gestational age		60
	Failure to thrive		
	Spasticity		
	Mental retardation		
Mercury	Cerebral palsy		60
	Mental retardation		
	Convulsions		
	Involuntary movements		
	Defective vision		
Vitamins			
Vitamin D	Congenital supravalvular aortic stenosis	Excessive intake	60
	Mental retardation		
	Hypercalcemia		
Vitamin K	Increased incidence of hyperbilirubinemia and risk of kernicterus	Water-soluble analogues with prematurity	85

References

1. Aldrete JA: In *The Anesthesiologist, Mother and Newborn.* Williams & Wilkins, Baltimore, 1974, p 133.
2. Andersen NB: Anesthesiology 29:113, 1968.
3. Annunziato D: Pediatrics 47:787, 1971.
4. Athinarayanan P, Pierog SH, Nigam SK, et al.: Am J Obstet Gynecol 124:212, 1976.
5. Basford AB, Fink BR: Anesthesiology 29:1167, 1968.
6. Beazley JM, Alderman B: Br J Obstet Gynecol 82:265, 1975.
7. Beazley JM, Alderman B: Lancet 1:45, 1975.
8a. Becker MH, Genieser NB, Finegold M: Am J Dis Child 129:356, 1975.
8b. Beintema DJ: Clin Dev Med 28: 1968.
9. Biale Y, Lewenthal H, Aderet NB: Obstet Gynecol 45:439, 1975.
10. Bitnum S: Can Med Assoc J 100:351, 1969.
11. Bleyer WA, Breckenridge RT: JAMA 213:2049, 1970.
12. Bleyer WA, Marshall RE: JAMA 221:185, 1972.
13. Bloomfield DK: Am J Obstet Gynecol 107:883, 1970.
14. Bongiovanni AM, Digorge AM, Grumach MM: J Clin Endocrinol 19:1004, 1959.
15a. Bongiovanni AM, McPadden AJ: Fertil Steril 11:181, 1960.
15b. Boros SJ, Reynolds JW: Am J Obstet Gynecol 129:111, 1977.
15c. Brazelton TB, Robey TS, Lother GA: Pediatrics 44:275, 1969.
16. Brettes JP, Renaud R, Gandar R: Am J Obstet Gynecol 124:164, 1976.
17. Burns LE, Hodgman JE, Cass AB: N Engl J Med 261:1318, 1959.
18. Burrow GN: N Engl J Med 298:150, 1978.
19. Chalmers I, Campbell H, Turnbull AC: Br Med J 2:116, 1975.
20. Chappel JN: JAMA 221:1516, 1972.
21. Cohen EN, Bellville JW, Brown BW: Anesthesiology 35:343, 1971.
22. Cohen MM, Hirschhorn K, Verbo S, et al.: Pediatr Res 2:486, 1968.
23. Cohlan SQ: N Y J Med 64:493, 1964.
24. Cohlan SQ, Bevelander G, Tiamsic T: Am J Dis Child 105:453, 1963.
25. Collins P, Olufs R, Kravitz H, et al.: Am J Obstet Gynecol 127:4, 1977.
26. Conway N, Birt BD: Br Med J 2:260, 1965.
27. Corbett TH, Cornell RG, Endres JL, et al.: Anesthesiology 41:341, 1974.
28. Corbett TH, Cornell RG, Lieding K: Anesthesiology 38:260, 1973.
29. Corner BD: Med J Southwest 77:284, 1962.
30. Cree JE, Meyer J, Hailey DM: Br Med J 4:251, 1973.
31. Davidson DC, Ford JA, McIntosh W: Br Med J 4:106, 1973.
32a. Day HJ, Conrad FG, Moore JE: Am J Med Sci 236:475, 1958.
32b. DeBeukelaer MM, Randall CL, Stroud DR: J Pediatr 91:759, 1977.
33. De La Torre R, Krompotic E: Teratology 13:131, 1976.
34. Desmond MM, Rogers SF, Lindley JE, et al.: Obstet Gynecol 10:140, 1957.
35. Desmond MM, Schwanecke RP, Wilson GS, et al: J Pediatr 80:190, 1972.
36. Doig RK, Coltman OM: Lancet 2:730, 1956.
37. Done AK: Clin Pharmacol Ther 5:432, 1964.
38. Emerson DJ: Am J Obstet Gynecol 84:356, 1962.
39. Engel RR, Elin RJ: J Pediatr 77:631, 1970.
40. Fedrick J: Br Med J 2:442, 1973.
41. Fillmore SJ, McDevitt E: Ann Intern Med 73:731, 1970.
42. Finnerty F: Clin Obstet Gynecol 18:145, 1975.
43. Fisher WD, Voorhess ML, Gardner LI: J Pediatr 62:132, 1963.
44a. Flowers CE, Rudolph AJ, Desmond MM: Obstet Gynecol 34:68, 1971.
44b. FDA Drug Bull 8:14, 1978.
45a. German J, Kowal A, Ehlers KH: Teratology 3:349, 1970.
45b. Ghosh A, Hudson FP: Br Med J 3:636, 1973.
46. Gladstone GR: J Pediatr 86:962, 1975.
47. Glass L, Rajegowda BK, Evans HE: Lancet 2:685, 1971.
48. Glass L, Rajegowda BK, Kahn EJ, et al.: N Engl J Med 286:746, 1972.
49. Gluck L, Kulovich MV: Am J Obstet Gynecol 115:539, 1973.
50a. Goodman RM, Katznelson MB, Hertz M, et al: Am J Dis Child 130:884, 1976.
50b. Gordon RR, Dean T: Br Med J 2:719, 1955.
51a. Habib A, McCarthy JS: J Pediatr 91:808, 1977.
51b. Hallum JL: Arch Dis Child 29:354, 1954.
52a. Hanson JW, Jones KL, Smith DW: JAMA 235:1458, 1976.
52b. Hanson JW, Myrianthopoulos NC, Harvey MAS, et al.: J Pediatr 89:662, 1976.
53. Harley JD, Farrar JF, Gray JB, et al.: Lancet 1:472, 1964.
54. Harris JWS, Ross IP: Lancet 1:1045, 1956.
55. Hartz SC, Heinonen OP, Shapiro S, et al.: N Engl J Med 292:726, 1975.
56. Heinonen OP, Slone D, Monson RR, et al.: N Engl J Med 296:67, 1977.
57. Herbst AL, Ulfelder H, Poskanzer DC: N Engl J Med 284:878, 1971.
58a. Herxheimer A: Lancet 1:448, 1971.
58b. Herzlinder RA, Kandall SR, Vaughan HG: J Pediatr 91:638, 1977.
59a. Hill RM: Am J Dis Child 130:923, 1976.
59b. Hill RM, Vernaiud WH: Am J Dis Child 127:645, 1974.
60. Hill RM, Craig JP, Chaney MD, et al.: Clin Obstet Gynecol 20:381, 1977.
61. Hoffmann W, Grospietsch G, Kuhn W: Lancet 2:794, 1976.
62. Hyman MD, Shnider SM: Anesthesiology 34:81, 1971.
63. Idanpaan-Heikkila J: Lancet 2:282, 1973.
64. Jackson WPU, Campbell GD, Notelovitz MB, et al.: Diabetes (Suppl) 11:98, 1962.
65. Jacobson BD: Am J Obstet Gynecol 84:962, 1962.

66. James FM, Greiss FC, Kemp RA: Anesthesiology 33:25, 1970.
67. Javett SN, Senior B, Braudo JL, et al.: Pediatrics 24:65, 1959.
68a. Jones KL, Smith DW: Teratology 12:1, 1975.
68b. Jost A: Harvey Lect 55:201, 1961.
69. Kandall SR, Albin S, Lowinson J, et al.: Pediatrics 58:681, 1976.
70. Kelly JV: Clin Obstet Gynecol 20:395, 1977.
71. Kendall SR, Gartner LM: Pediatr Res 7:92, 1973.
72. Kenny FM, Preeyasombat C, Spaulding JS, et al.: Pediatrics 37:960, 1966.
73. Kent SP, Wideman GL: JAMA 171:1199, 1959.
74. Kline J, Stein ZA, Susser M, et al.: N Engl J Med 297:793, 1977.
75. Kopelman AE, McCullar FW, Heggeness L: JAMA 231:62, 1975.
76. Kosaka Y, Takahashi T, Mark LC: Anesthesiology 31:489, 1969.
77. Kron RE, Litt M, Finnegan LP: Pediatr Res 7:64, 1973.
78. Larsson Y, Sterkey G: Lancet 2:1424, 1960.
79. Lenz W, Knapp K: Dtsch Med Wochenschr 87:1232, 1962.
80a. Levin D, Fixler D, Morriss F, et al.: J Pediatr. 92:478, 1978.
80b. Levin D, Hyman A, Heymann MA, et al.: J Pediatr 92:265, 1978.
80c. Levin JN: J Pediatr 79:130, 1971.
81. Lewis RM, Schulman JD: Lancet 2:338, 1975.
82. Liggins GC, Howie RN: Pediatrics 50:515, 1972.
83. Lipeltz PJ: Pediatrics 39:401, 1968.
84. Lowe CR: Lancet 1:9, 1973.
85. Lucey JF, Dolan RG: Pediatrics 23:553, 1959.
86a. Manchester D, Margolis HS, Sheldon RE: Am J Obstet Gynecol 126:467, 1976.
86b. Manning F, Winpugh E, Boddy K: Br Med J 1:552, 1975.
87. Matz GJ, Nauntan RF: Arch Otolaryngol 88:370, 1968.
88. Mazzi E: Am J Obstet Gynecol 129:586, 1977.
89. Mauer HM, Wolff JA, Finster M, et al.: Lancet 2:122, 1968.
90. McBride WG: Lancet 2:1358, 1961.
91. McGlothlin WH, Sparkes RS, Arnold DO: JAMA 212:1483, 1970.
92. Meadow SR: Proc R Soc Med 63:48, 1970.
93. Milkovich L, van den Berg BJ: Am J Dis Child 131:924, 1977.
94. Milkovich L, van den Berg BJ: Am J Obstet Gynecol 129:637, 1977.
95. Milkovich L, van den Berg BJ: N Engl J Med 291:1268, 1974.
96. Millar JHD, Nevin NC: Lancet 1:328, 1973.
97. Milner RD, Chouksey SK: Arch Dis Child 47:537, 1972.
98. Mirkin BL: J Pediatr 78:329, 1971.
99. Monson RR, Rosenberg L, Hartz SC, et al.: N Engl J Med 289:1049, 1973.
100. Morishima HO, Daniel SS, Finster M, et al: Anesthesiology 27:147, 1966.
101. Moya F: N Y J Med 62:2169, 1962.
102. Moya F, Thorndike V: Clin Pharmacol Ther 4:628, 1963.
103a. Mujtaba Q, Burrow GN: Obstet Gynecol 46:282, 1975.
103b. Mulvihill J, Klimas JT, Stokes DC: Am J Obstet Gynecol 125:937, 1976.
104. Nathenson G, Cohen MI, Litt IF: J Pediatr 81:899, 1972.
105. Nathenson G, Cohen MI, McNamara H: J Pediatr 86:799, 1975.
106. Nelson MM, Forfar JO: Br Med J 1:523, 1971.
107. Niswander JD, Wertelecki W: Lancet 2:1062, 1973.
108. Nora JJ, Vargo TA, Nora AH, et al.: Lancet 1:1290, 1970.
109. Nuwayhid B, Brinkman CR, Katchen B, et al.: Obstet Gynecol 46:197, 1975.
110. O'Meara OP, Brazie JV: N Engl J Med 278:1127, 1968.
111. Oski FA: Am J Dis Child 129:1139, 1975.
112. Ouellette EM, Rosett HL, Rosman NP, et al.: New Engl J Med 297:528, 1977.
113a. Owen JR, Irani SF, Blair AW: Arch Dis Child 47:107, 1972.
113b. Palmer RH, Ouellette EM, Warner L: Pediatrics 53:490, 1974.
114a. Prechtal HFR, Beintema D: Clin Dev Med 12: 1964.
114b. Ralston DH, Shnider SM: Anesthesiology 48:34, 1978.
115. Ramboer C, Thompson RPH, Williams R: Lancet 1:966, 1969.
116. Reed RL, Cheney CB, Fearon RE, et al.: Anesth Analg 53:214, 1974.
117. Reifenstein EC: Ann NY Acad Sci 71:762, 1958.
118. Rementeria JL, Nunag NN: Am J Obstet Gynecol 116:1152, 1973.
119. Rendle-Short TJ: Lancet 1:1188, 1962.
120. Richards ID: Br J Prev Soc Med 23:218, 1969.
121. Ring G, Krames E, Shnider S, et al.: Obstet Gynecol 50:598, 1977.
122. Robinson GC, Cambon KG: N Engl J Med 271:949, 1964.
123. Rodriguez SU, Leikin SL, Hiller MC: N Engl J Med 270:881, 1964.
124a. Rosen RC, Lightner ES: J Pediatr 92:240, 1978.
124b. Rothstein P, Gould JM: Pediatr Clin North Am 21:307, 1974.
125. Rucker E: J Med Assoc State Ala 23:59, 1953.
126. Rumeau-Rouquette C, Goujaro J, Huel G: Teratology 15:57, 1977.
127. Rushton DI: Lancet 2:141, 1976.
128. Safra MJ, Oakley GP: Lancet 2:478, 1975.
129. Savory J, Monif GRG: Am J Obstet Gynecol 110:556, 1971.
130. Scanlon JW: Bull N Y Acad Med 52:231, 1976.
131. Scanlon JW, Brown WU, Weiss JB, et al.: Anesthesiology 40:121, 1974.
132. Scanlon JW, Ostheimer GW, Lurie AO, et al.: Anesthesiology 45:400, 1976.
133. Scher J: J Obstet Gynecol Br Commonw 79:635, 1972.
134. Schiff D, Aranda JV, Stern L: J Pediatr 77:457, 1970.
135. Schiff D, Chan G, Stern L: Pediatrics 48:139, 1971.

136. Schou M: Acta Psychiatr Scand 54:193, 1976.
137. Schou M, Goldfield MD, Weinstein MR, et al.: Obstet Gynecol Surv 28:794, 1973.
138. Schulz J, van Creveld S: Etudes Neo-Natales 7:133, 1958.
139. Scott WC, Warner RF: JAMA 142:1331, 1950.
140. Shapiro S, Siskind V, Monson RR, et al.: Lancet 1:1375, 1976.
141. Shaul WL, Emery H, Hall JG: Am J Dis Child 129:360, 1975.
142. Shaul WL, Hall JG: Am J Obstet Gynecol 127:191, 1977.
143. Shenker L: Obstet Gynecol 26:104, 1965.
144. Shnider SM, deLorimier AA, Holl JW, et al.: Am J Obstet Gynecol 102:911, 1968.
145. Shnider SM, Moya F: Am J Obstet Gynecol 89:1009, 1964.
146. Shnider SM, Way EL: Anesthesiology 29:951, 1968.
147. Silverman WA, Anderson DH, Blank WA, et al.: Pediatrics 18:614, 1956.
148. Sinclair JC, Fox HA, Lentz JF: N Engl J Med 273:1173, 1965.
149. Slone D, Siskind V, Heinonen OP, et al.: Lancet 1:1373, 1976.
150. Slone D, Siskind V, Heinonen O, et al.: Am J Obstet Gynecol 128:486, 1977.
151. Smart RG, Bateman K: Can Med Assoc J 99:805, 1968.
152. Smith BE, Gaub ML, Moya F: Anesthesiology 26:260, 1965.
153. Sokal JE, Lessmann EM: JAMA 172:1765, 1960.
154. South J: Lancet 2:1154, 1972.
155. Speidel BD, Meadow SR: Lancet 2:839, 1972.
156a. Stevens D, Burman D, Midwinter A: Lancet 2:595, 1974.
156b. Streissguth AP, Herman CS, Smith DW: J Pediatr 92:363, 1978.
157. Stutzman L, Sokal JE: Clin Obstet Gynecol 11:416, 1968.
158. Sutherland JM, Keller WH: Am J Dis Child 101:447, 1961.
159. Szabo KT, Brent RL: Lancet 1:565, 1974.
160a. Taussig HB: JAMA 180:1106, 1962.
160b. Tenbrinck MS, Buchin SY: JAMA 232:1144, 1975.
161. Thiersch JB: Am J Obstet Gynecol 63:1298, 1952.
162. Thiery M, De Hemptinne D, Schuddinck L, et al.: Lancet 1:161, 1975.
163. Toaff R, Ravid R: In *Drug Induced Diseases*. Excerpta Medica Foundation, Amsterdam, 1968, p 113.
164. Tunstall ME: Br J Anaesth 41:792, 1969.
165. Turner G, Collins E: Lancet 2:338, 1975.
166. Turner GM, Oakley CM, Dixon HG: Br Med J 4:281, 1968.
167. Uhlig H: Arzenim Forsch 12:61, 1957.
168. Vince DJ: Can Med Assoc J 100:223, 1969.
169. Wagner L, Wagner G, Guerrero J: Am J Obstet Gynecol 108:308, 1970.
170a. Warrell DW, Taylor R: Lancet 1:117, 1968.
170b. Waziri M, Lonasescu V, Zellweger H: Am J Dis Child 130:1022, 1976.
171. Weinstein L, Dalton C: N Engl J Med 279:526, 1968.
172. Wilkins L: JAMA 172:1028, 1960.
173. Wynne J, Milner AD, Hodson AK: Arch Dis Child 50:331, 1975.
174. Yaffe SJ: Can Med Assoc J, 98:301 1968.
175. Yaffe SJ, Stern L: In *Perinatal Pharmacology and Therapeutics*. Academic Press, New York, 1976, p 355.
176. Yeh SY, Paul RH, Cordero L, et al.: Obstet Gynecol 43:363, 1974.
177. Zackai EH, Mellman WJ, Neiderer B, et al.: J Pediatr 87:280, 1975.
178. Zellweger H: Clin Pediatr 13:338, 1974.
179. Zelson C: N Engl J Med 288:1393, 1973.
180. Zelson C, Rubio E, Wasserman E: Pediatrics 48:178, 1971.

# APPENDIX B

Anesthesia Record—Obstetrics

University of California, San Francisco, Hospital and Clinics

ANESTHESIA RECORD—OBSTETRICS

AGE	B/P	P	HGB	HCF	BLOOD TYPE	WEIGHT	HEIGHT

UNIT NUMBER

OPERATION PROPOSED:

PT. NAME

PRE-OP EVALUATION: PARITY: DRUG ALLERGIES:

MATERNAL COMPLICATIONS:

BIRTHDATE

MEDICAL

OBSTETRICAL

ASA

LOCATION   DATE

Anesthesia & Possible Complications Discussed By _____
Signature

| PREMED | | TIME | | EFFECT | |

AGENTS | | | | | | | | | | | | | TOTALS

TIME

ANES. LEVEL

INPUT: Fluids, Blood 200

OUTPUT: EBL, Urine

Temperature

MONITORS 150
- Cuff
- BP Doppler
- Direct
- EKG Pulse
- PCS ES
- CVP PAP 100
- UO PNS
- F_1O_2 UC
- FHR

Endot. Intub. 50

Systolic Blood Pressure Respiration
Diastolic
Pulse
> < ●

Anesthesia Operation
X ⊙
X——⊙
X ⊙

CERVICAL DILATION

FSS

FHR

SURGEONS   OPERATION   ANESTHETIST

INTAKE				ANESTHESIA START	D.A.P.P.	T.A.T.	B. TIME	B. WT.
Time Started	Type, Number	Time Completed	Amount Absorbed	Time of Skin Incision			APGAR Score	1 Min.	5 Min.

Time of Uterine Insicion — HT. Rate
Analgesic Score M.D.   Pt. — Rhythm. Resp.
Amnesia — Reflexes
Comments: — Muscle Tone
— Color
— TOTAL

BLOCK TECHNIQUE

Type of Block — Time Sust. Resp.
Pt. Position — Resuscitation
Prep Solution — Gastric Aspriate   ML.
Needle
Interspace
Paresthesias
CSF

University of California, San Francisco
Hospitals and Clinics
San Francisco, CA 94143

DEPARTMENT OF ANESTHESIA
ANESTHESIA RECORD — OBSTETRICS

APPENDIX C

Obstetric Anesthesia Code Sheet

University of California, San Francisco

OBSTETRIC ANESTHESIA CODE SHEET

University of California San Francisco – **OBSTETRICAL ANESTHESIA CODE SHEET**

Unit Number ☐☐ ☐☐ ☐☐ ☐

Resident Number ☐☐☐☐

Patient Name ☐☐☐☐☐☐☐☐☐☐☐☐☐☐☐☐☐☐☐☐☐☐☐☐☐☐☐☐☐☐

Age ☐☐☐   Infant Number ☐☐ ☐☐ ☐☐ ☐

Date ☐☐ ☐☐ ☐☐
     Month Day Year

A Parity
- ☐ Primip
- ☐ Multip
- ☐ Grand multip (5 or more)

Gestation
- ☐ Single
- ☐ Twin
- ☐ Triplet
- ☐ Other

ANTEPARTUM MEDICAL COMPLICATIONS
- ☐ None
  - ☐ rheumatic heart disease
  - ☐ congenital heart disease
  - ☐ chronic hypertensive disease
  - ☐ other cardiac disease (specify) _____
  - ☐ post open heart surgery
  - Diabetes Mellitus
    - ☐ gestational only
    - ☐ non-insulin dependent prior to pregnancy
    - ☐ insulin dependent prior to pregnancy
  - ☐ other endocrine disease (specify) _____
  - ☐ anemia (< 10 gm)
  - ☐ hemoglobinopathy   ☐ sickle
    - ☐ thalassemia   ☐ Other (specify) _____
  - ☐ coagulopathy   ☐ DIC   ☐ ITP
    - ☐ Mini Heparin   ☐ Heparin
    - ☐ Other (specify) _____
  - ☐ other hematological disease (specify) _____
  - ☐ pulmonary disease (specify) _____   ☐ pneumonia
    - ☐ asthma   ☐ other (specify) _____
  - ☐ renal or urogenital disease (specify) _____
  - ☐ psychiatric disease (specify) _____
  - ☐ hepatic disease (specify) _____
  - ☐ musculo-skeletal disease (specify) _____
  - ☐ infectious disease (other than chorioamnionitis) (specify) _____
  - ☐ rubella (first trimester)
  - ☐ fever of unknown origin
  - ☐ carcinoma of cervix
  - ☐ other carcinoma (specify) _____

Chronic drug abuser
- ☐ narcotic   ☐ barbiturates
- ☐ ethanol   ☐ other (specify) _____

- ☐ surgery during pregnancy
- ☐ other medical (specify) _____

A ANTEPARTUM OBSTETRICAL COMPLICATIONS
- ☐ None
  - ☐ polyhydramnios
  - ☐ premature labor (< 38 weeks)
  - Toxemia
    - ☐ mild pre-eclampsia
    - ☐ severe pre-eclampsia
    - ☐ eclampsia (antepartum)
  - Rh Sensitized
    - ☐ no intrauterine transfusion
    - ☐ intrauterine transfusion
  - Premature rupture of membranes > 24 hrs
    - ☐ no fever
    - ☐ with fever
    - ☐ chorioamnionitis
    - ☐ Other

☐☐ ☐ WEEKS GESTATION

B Labor
- ☐ No oxytocin
- ☐ Elective induction
- ☐ Oxytocin augmentation
- ☐ Indicated induction:
  - ☐ Post maturity   ☐ Abnormal OCT
  - ☐ PROM
  - ☐ Toxemia
  - ☐ Isoimmunization
  - ☐ Diabetes Mellitus
  - ☐ Falling estriols
  - ☐ Other (specify) _____

Presentation (check one)

Vertex	☐ Occiput Ant	☐ Sinciput
	☐ Occiput Post	☐ Brow
	☐ Occiput Trans	☐ Face
Breech	☐ Frank	
	☐ Footling	
	☐ Complete	
☐ Transverse lie		
☐ Compound		

Delivery
- ☐ Spontaneous
- ☐ Manual rotation
- ☐ Low forceps
- ☐ Piper forceps
- ☐ Mid forceps—no rotation
- ☐ Mid forceps—rotation
- ☐ Vacuum extraction
- ☐ **Cesarean section**

Breech (one only)
- ☐ Spontaneous
- ☐ Assisted breech extraction
- ☐ Total breech extraction
- ☐ Internal podalic extraction

C ANESTHESIA: BEFORE BIRTH OF BABY
☐ No Anesthesia
    ☐ Lamaze (or other)

Systemic medication (3 most recent)

Drug$_{xx}$	Dose$_{xxx}$	Route$_x$	Hours before birth$_x$
1.			
2.			
3.			

☐ Inhalation analgesia

	Self Adm.	Contin.	Intermitt.	Complications of analgesia	
N_2O	☐	☐	☐	☐ None	☐ Low dose Ketamine
MOF	☐	☐	☐	☐ Unconsciousness	
Enflurane	☐	☐	☐	☐ Vomit or regurgitate	
Other (____)	☐	☐	☐	☐ Aspiration	
				☐ Other _____	

☐ General Anesthesia

Induction	Intubation	Maintenance (before delivery)
☐ Thiopental	☐ after relaxation	☐ N_2O
☐ Ketamine	☐ awake	☐ Halothane
☐ Other _____	☐ not done	☐ Enflurane
_____	☐ Other _____	☐ Other _____

Complications of General Anesthesia
☐ None
    ☐ hypotension   ☐ difficult intubation
    ☐ aspiration   ☐ arrhythmia
    ☐ hypoxia   ☐ recall
    ☐ Other _____   ☐ prolonged paralysis

☐ Regional
    ☐ Epidural   ☐ Caudal   ☐ Spinal

Drug   Dose (mg) Antepartum

☐ Chloroprocaine   ____ ____ ____
☐ Bupivacaine   ____ ____ ____
☐ Lidocaine   ____ ____ ____
☐ Tetracaine   ____ ____ ____
☐ Etidocaine   ____ ____ ____
☐ Other _____   ____ ____ ____

Supplementation after Delivery
☐ None
    ☐ Systemic medication
    ☐ Inhalation analgesia
    ☐ General anesthesia
    ☐ Local infiltration

Complications of Regional Anesthesia
☐ None
☐ hypotension
☐ CNS reaction
☐ paresthesia
☐ wet tap
☐ total spinal
☐ respiratory insufficiency
☐ failed block
☐ spinal headache
    ☐ Other (specify)_____

Therapy of headache
    ☐ conservative
    ☐ saline epidural
    ☐ blood patch

Hypotension
☐ Yes   ☐ No
    Prophylaxis
    ☐ None
        ☐ LUD
        ☐ fluids
        ☐ vasopressor
        ☐ Other _____
    Therapy
    ☐ None
        ☐ Oxygen
        ☐ spontaneous recovery
        ☐ fluids
        ☐ LUD
        ☐ vasopressor

OBSTETRIC ANESTHESIA CODE SHEET

☐ Paracervical block

Drug$_{xx}$	Dose$_{xxxx}$

☐ Pudendal block or local infiltration

Drug$_{xx}$	Dose$_{xxxx}$

Complications of paracervical or pudendal block
☐ None
    ☐ fetal bradycardia
    ☐ maternal toxic reaction
    ☐ Other _____

Analgesia Score (delivery)
    for epidural, spinal, inhalation analgesia

Doctor		Mother	
☐	None — 0	☐	☐ Epidural allowed to wear off
☐	Poor — 1+	☐	
☐	Fair — 2+	☐	
☐	Good — 3+	☐	
☐	Excellent — 4+	☐	
☐	Unable to obtain	☐	

Amnesia   ☐ Total   ☐ Partial   ☐ None   ☐ Unable to obtain

Duration of Anesthesia Antepartum (DAPP)		Total Anesthesia Time	
Hours	Minutes	Hours	Minutes

Uterine incision to delivery time (C-section) _____ _____ _____ seconds.

D **COMPLICATIONS**

Prolonged Labor	Etiology	Relation to Epidural
☐ Nil	☐ CPD	☐ None
☐ slow latent	☐ ineffective uterine force	☐ caused by
☐ active phase arrest	☐ abnormal presentation	☐ worsened
☐ slow slope active	☐ unknown	☐ improved
☐ arrest of descent		☐ unknown
☐ prolonged second stage		
☐ Other (specify) _____		

Vaginal Bleeding
☐ Nil
    ☐ placenta previa   ☐ marginal separation
    ☐ abruptio placenta   ☐ Other (specify) _____
    _____

ANESTHESIA FOR OBSTETRICS

D Other Labor Problems
- ☐ Nil
  - ☐ hypertonic uterus
  - ☐ rupture of uterus
  - ☐ cardiac
  - ☐ pulmonary embolus
  - ☐ D.I.C.
  - ☐ postpartum hemorrhage
  - ☐ Other _____

Obstetrical Medications
- ☐ Nil
  - ☐ MgSO$_4$
  - ☐ Antihypertensives (specify) _____
  - ☐ Barbiturates
  - ☐ Diuretics
  - ☐ Other (specify)
  - ☐ Betamimetics
  - ☐ Intravenous Etoh
  - ☐ Steroids
  - ☐ Diazepam
  - ☐ Other (specify) _____

Delivery Complications
- ☐ Nil
  - Cord
    - ☐ Nuchal cord—loose
    - ☐ Nuchal cord—tight
    - ☐ Prolapsed cord
    - ☐ Other (specify) _____
  - ☐ Precipitous Labor
  - ☐ B.O.A.
  - ☐ Should dystocia
  - ☐ Manual removal of placenta

D IF Cesarean Section (check one)
- ☐ Elective repeat — no labor
- ☐ Previous section — in labor
- ☐ Elective — primary — no labor
- ☐ Emergency — no labor
- ☐ Emergency — in labor

Indications for Section
- ☐ Previous section
- ☐ Failure to progress
- ☐ Placenta previa
- ☐ Chorioamnionitis
- ☐ Toxemia
- ☐ Chronic UPI from other causes
- ☐ Failure of induction
- ☐ Other (specify) _____
- ☐ Active bleeding
- ☐ Fetal distress
- ☐ CPD
- ☐ Prolapsed cord
- ☐ Tetanic contraction
- ☐ Malpresentation
- ☐ Breech
- ☐ Failed forceps
- ☐ Rh problem
- ☐ Herpes

E Fetal Distress
- ☐ None or undetected
  - ☐ Meconium
  - ☐ Fetal heart rate pattern abnormality
  - ☐ Increased fetal activity
  - ☐ Decreased fetal activity
  - ☐ Other (specify) _____

Fetal Distress — Relative to Anesthesia
- ☐ No distress
- ☐ Caused by anesthesia
- ☐ Worsened by anesthesia
- ☐ Improved by anesthesia
- ☐ No relation to anesthesia
- ☐ Unknown

E Special Studies
- ☐ None
  - ☐ Continuous FHR monitoring
  - ☐ Cord bloods
  - ☐ Fetal scalp samples _____
  - ☐ Local anesthetic levels
  - ☐ Catecholamines
  - ☐ Neurobehavior Exam
  - ☐ Other (specify) _____

F FETAL HEART RATE PATTERN ABNORMALITY
- ☐ No continuous FHR monitoring
- ☐ Normal record
- ☐ Abnormal record
  - Baseline Abnormalities
    - **Bradycardia**
      - ☐ moderate 119-100 min
      - ☐ marked < 100/min
    - **Tachycardia**
      - ☐ moderate 161-180/min
      - ☐ marked > 180/min
    - **Baseline Variability**
      - ☐ decreased
      - ☐ increased
      - ☐ sinusoidal
      - ☐ saltatory
  - **Early Deceleration**
    - ☐ mild
    - ☐ moderate
    - ☐ severe
  - **Late Deceleration**
    - ☐ mild
    - ☐ moderate
    - ☐ severe
  - **Variable Deceleration**
    - ☐ mild
    - ☐ moderate
    - ☐ severe
  - ☐ acceleration
  - ☐ unable to classify

F Treatment of Fetal Distress
- ☐ No distress
- ☐ No treatment
- ☐ Positional change
- ☐ Correction of hypotension
- ☐ Glucose to mother
- ☐ Spontaneous recovery
- ☐ Oxygen administration
- ☐ NaHCO$_3$ to mother
- ☐ Delivery of fetus
- ☐ Other

OBSTETRIC ANESTHESIA CODE SHEET

F

Fetal Scalp Blood ☐ Nil

	pH	Minutes before birth
Last sample	___•___ ___	___ ___ ___
Next to last	___•___ ___	___ ___ ___
First sample	___•___ ___	___ ___ ___

Umbilical Vein ☐ NIL   Umbilical Artery ☐ NIL

	pH	pO_2	pCO_2	BE
UV	___•___ ___	___ ___	___ ___ ___	___ ___ •___
UA	___•___ ___	___ ___	___ ___ ___	___ ___ •___

Maternal Artery (before anesthetic) ☐ NIL   Maternal Artery (at time of delivery) ☐ NIL

	pH	pO_2	pCO_2	BE
MA before	___•___ ___	___ ___ ___	___ ___ ___	___ ___ ___•___
MA at time	___•___ ___	___ ___ ___	___ ___ ___	___ ___ ___•___

Time Until Sustained Respirations (TSR)
☐ stillborn
☐ less than 90 sec.
☐ more than 90 sec.
☐ DNS

Resuscitation — Ventilation (list all that apply)
☐ none
☐ laryngoscopy
☐ oxygen-mask positive pressure
☐ oxygen over face
☐ endotracheal suction
☐ oxygen-endotracheal tube, positive pressure

Resuscitation — Drugs (within one hour of birth)
☐ none
☐ narcotic antagonists
☐ Other (specify) _____
☐ sodium bicarbonate
☐ volume expander

Congenital Anomalies
☐ none
☐ infant (specify) _____
☐ placental abnormalities (specify) _____
☐ cord abnormalities (specify) _____

Apgar Score 1 Minute		
☐ 0	☐ 4	☐ 8
☐ 1	☐ 5	☐ 9
☐ 2	☐ 6	☐ 10
☐ 3	☐ 7	☐ DNS

Apgar Score 5 Minutes		
☐ 0	☐ 4	☐ 8
☐ 1	☐ 5	☐ 9
☐ 2	☐ 6	☐ 10
☐ 3	☐ 7	☐ DNS

BIRTH WEIGHT ___ ___ ___ ___ gms

☐ Family Centered Birth Program
  ☐ delivered in bed

SPECIAL NEWBORN PROBLEMS
☐ Specify _____

442 ANESTHESIA FOR OBSTETRICS

Baby Unit Number _____

Last Name _____

Maternal Unit Number _____

NEONATAL COMPLICATIONS

☐ Pedi Set-up

Air Leaks
- ☐ pneumothorax
- ☐ pneumomediastinum
- ☐ pneumopericardium
- ☐ air embolus
- ☐ pneumoperitoneum
- ☐ interstitial air leak
- ☐ subcutaneous air

☐ Apnea

☐ Asphyxia

Birth Trauma
- ☐ laceration
- ☐ fractured clavicle
- ☐ fractured skull
- ☐ cephalohematoma
- ☐ other — (specify) _____

Catheters
- ☐ UA
- ☐ UV
- ☐ other
- ☐ complications — (specify) _____

Intravenous Nutrition
- ☐ JV
- ☐ saphenous
- ☐ brachial
- / _____ = days
- ☐ complications (specify) _____

☐ Congenital Anomalies (specify) _____
☐ Congenital Heart Disease (specify) _____
☐ Death
    age _____ (days)
☐ Delayed absorption of lung fluid
☐ HDN
  G29 ☐ hydrops
  V23/exchange transfusion no. _____
☐ HMD
- ☐ CPAP
- ☐ IMV
- ☐ paralysis

☐ Hydrocephalus
- ☐ Rx. with lumbar puncture
- ☐ Rx. with diuretics
- ☐ shunt

☐ Hypotension

☐ Infection
- ☐ pneumonia
- ☐ meningitis
- ☐ organism (specify) _____
- ☐ positive culture from (specify) _____

☐ Intracranial Hemorrhage
- ☐ LP fetal hemoglobin
- ☐ CT scan

☐ Meconium Aspiration Pneumonitis
- ☐ meconium below cords
-   amount _____ cc

☐ Necrotizing Enterocolitis
☐ PDA
☐ Pulmonary Edema
☐ Persistent Pulmonary Hypertension
☐ ph < 7.10
☐ Polycythemia, Rx with exchange transfusion
☐ Pulmonary Hemorrhage
☐ RLF
- ☐ vascular with tortuosity
- ☐ vascular with neovascularization
- ☐ vascular with hemorrhage
- ☐ cicatricial without detached retina
- ☐ cicatricial with detached retina

☐ Seizures
☐ Other (specify) _____
☐ Unusual case (specify) _____

Index

Abdominometry, 142
Abruptio placentae, 248-250
  anesthetic management of, 249
  blood transfusions, 249-250
  clotting abnormalities, 248-249
  concealed hemorrhage, 248
  etiology of, 248
  hemorrhage in, 248
  iliac artery ligation, 249
  obstetric management of, 249
Abscess, epidural, 306
Acetylcholine, effect of magnesium, 227
Accelerations, with contractions, 362-363
Accidents, neurologic, 307
Acid aspiration syndrome, 123, 291-294
  symptoms of, 291
  therapy, 293
Acid-base balance and carbon dioxide, 20, 21
Acid-base status
  general versus epidural anesthesia, 271
  general versus spinal anesthesia, 271
Acidosis
  metabolic, maternal, 147
  neonatal, correction of, 396
Active transport, 14
Acupuncture, 68
Adenyl cyclase, 148
Adrenergic agents, beta, 142-149
  elimination half-life of, 148
  methanesulfonamide, 143
  nylidrine hydrochloride, 143
  orciprenaline (Alupent), 147
  p-hydroxy phenyl isopropylaterenol, 143
  placental transfer of, 148
  side effects of, 145
Adrenergic blockers, 148
Adrenergic receptors, 31, 143
  beta stimulants effects of, 146
  in uterine muscle, 48
  stimulation of, 146
Afterload reduction
  therapy for
    aortic insufficiency, 191
    mitral insufficiency, 189
Airway, establishment of, newborn, 389-390
Albumin
  levels in pregnancy and preeclampsia, 226
  to globulin ratio, 10
Aldosterone, 224
Alkalemia, maternal
  during labor, 4
  effect on uterine blood flow, 37
Alkaline phosphatase, 10
Alkalosis, maternal
  metabolic, 36-37, 323
  respiratory, 323
Alphaprodine, 78, 83
  effect on uterine activity, 45
Alveolar-capillary membrane, 292
Alveolar cells, type II, 349
Alveolar ventilation, 312
Amide-linked local anesthetics, 111
  protein binding of, 258
Aminophylline, maternal and fetal effects, 150
Amniocentesis, 243, 349
Amniotic cell culture, 351-352
Amniotic fluid
  analysis of, 349
  Δ O.D. 450 in, 353
  surfactant determination, 349
Amobarbital, 75
Amphetamines, 314
Analgesia
  caudal block, 101-103
  in cesarean section with conduction anesthesia, 254, 259
  inhalation, 121
  intrathecal, continuous, 304
  local perineal infiltration, 107
  lumbar epidural block, 99-101, 114
  lumbar sympathetic block, 106
  paracervical block, 105
  pudendal block, 107
  saddle block, 104
  supplementary drugs for, 259
  systemic medication, 75
Anectine (see Succinylcholine)
Anemia, in preeclampsia, eclampsia, 225
Anesthesia, (see also specific agents and methods)
  for cesarean section, 254-272
  for toxemic patient, 230-233
  inhalation (see Inhalation anesthesia)
  local (see Regional anesthesia)
  maternal safety, 122-123
  psychological, 65-70
Anesthesiologists and teratogenicity, 318-319
Anesthetic agents
  effects of
    on mother and fetus, 75, 93, 121, 254, 263-268
    on neonate, 75, 93, 121, 370
  teratogenicity of, 314
Anesthetic management of surgery during pregnancy
  elective surgery, 326
  emergency surgery, 326
  urgent surgery, 326
Anesthetic requirements in pregnancy, 9, 121, 261, 312-314
Anesthetics
  inhalation (see Inhalation agents)
  local (see Regional anesthesia, drugs for, and specific drugs)
Angiotensin, 224
  effect of
    on toxemic patient, 206
    of uterine blood flow, 32, 217
Animal preparations, chronic maternal-fetal, 23
Animal studies and teratogenicity
  anesthetics, 317-319
  systemic medications, 314-315
Anomalies of the upper airway, 403
Antacids, oral, 123
  administration of
    before general anesthesia, 261
    before regional anesthesia, 256
  therapy for acid aspiration, 296-297
Antagonists, 75, 88
Antepartum fetal evaluation, 357
Antibiotics, 391
  for aspiration of fecal or bacterial matter, 291
  therapy for acid aspiration, 296
Antiarrhythmic drugs, 217
Anticholinergics
  effect on gastric emptying, 288
  therapy, 297
Anticoagulated patient, 241
Anticonvulsives, 229
Antihypertensive agents, 34-35
  in treatment of preeclampsia, 229
Anxiety
  maternal, 320
  supplementary drugs for, 259
Aorta
  coarctation of, maternal, 200
    and dissecting aneurysm, 209
    and hypertension, 206
    anesthetic considerations of, 201
    pathophysiology of, 201
    prognosis of, 200
    symptoms of, 200
  dissecting aneurysm of, 209
    anesthetic considerations of, 209
    etiology of, 209
    pathophysiology of, 209
    symptoms of, 209
Aortic regurgitation, 190
Aortic valve

INDEX

Aortic valve—*continued*
  congenital malformation (bicuspid), 202
  insufficiency of, 190-191
    anesthetic considerations of, 191
    pathophysiology of, 190-191
    prognosis of, 190
    symptoms of, 190
  replacement of, 214
    anesthetic considerations of, 214
    complications of, 214
  stenosis of, 191-193
    anesthetic considerations of, 192
    pathophysiology of, 192
    prognosis of, 191-192
    symptoms of, 192
Aortocaval compression syndrome, 8-9
  effect on fetus, 270
  etiology of, 279
  left uterine displacement for, 256
Apgar score
  after maternal hypotension, 281
  and resuscitation, 372
  duration of epidural anesthesia, 270
  duration of general anesthesia, 266
  evaluation of neonate, 268, 371, 391-395
  limitations, 374-375
  percentage distribution of, 373
  prognostic value, 373
Apnea, in prematurity, 150
Apomorphine, 297
Arachnoiditis, chronic adhesive, 306
Arterial blood gases
  determination of
    following gastric aspiration, 290
    in acid aspiration syndrome, 292
Arteriosclerosis, 209
Asphyxia
  intrapartum and shock, 396
  intrauterine, 357
  pathophysiology of neonate, 385
  perinatal pharmacology, 157
Aspiration, 123
  of airway in newborn, 390
  of gastric contents, 260-261, 288-299
  of meconium, 407-409
  prevention of, 260-261, 296
Aspiration syndromes, 407-410
  acid, 291-294

Aspiration pneumonitis, meconium, 390
Aspirin, 154
Asymmetric septal hypertrophy (ASH), 210-212
  anesthetic considerations of, 211
  pathophysiology of, 210-211
  prognosis of, 210
  symptoms of, 210
Atelectasis, 291
Atony, uterine, 252
Atrial, maternal, 194-196
  septal defects in, 194-195
    anesthetic considerations of, 195
    pathophysiology of, 195
    prognosis of, 194-195
    symptoms of, 195
Atrial fibrillation
  and asymmetric septal hypertrophy, 211
  and mitral insufficiency, 189
  and mitral stenosis, 186
  treatment of, 215-216
Atrial flutter
  and asymmetric septal hypertrophy, 211
  treatment of, 216
Atropine, 261, 297
Autotransfusion during labor, 181
Awareness, maternal, 266-267
Azygos flow, 304

Backache, regional anesthesia complications, 302
Barbiturates
  behavioral teratology, 320
  effects of
    on newborn, 75
    on uterine blood flow, 23-25
    for labor and delivery, 75-76
    for preeclampsia-eclampsia, 229
Baroreceptor influence of uterine contractions, 361
Baseline rate, fetal, 360
Baseline variability, fetal, 360
Beat-to-beat variability, fetal, 77, 360
Behavioral teratology, 320
Benzyl alcohol, 307
Betamimetic therapy, 327
Bicarbonate
  and intracranial hemorrhage, 396
  correction of acidosis, 396
  effect of uterine blood flow, 37-38
Bilirubin, in amniotic fluid, 352
Biparietal diameter (BPD), 347
Birthing room, 71

Birth weight, 374
Bladder dysfunction, regional anesthesia complication, 302
Bleeding time, 237
Blood coagulation, laboratory methods for study, 237-238
Blood loss, 6
  at cesarean section, 252
  influence of anesthesia, 267
Blood patch epidural, 260, 302
Blood pressure
  aortic, in neonate, 397
  in labor, 7-9
  in pregnancy, 7-9
  supine hypotensive syndrome, 7
Blood volume, maternal, 6
  central and mitral stenosis, 187
  central, after delivery, 181
Bohr effect, 262
Bowel obstruction, 393
Bradycardia
  fetal, 360
    from paracervical block, 105
    with maternal hypotension, 279
  maternal
    and aortic insufficiency, 191
    and aortic stenosis, 192
    and mitral insufficiency, 189
Brazelton Neonatal Behavioral assessment scale, 380
Breaks, villi, 14
Breathing
  capacity, 315
  fetal, 348
  frequency, of newborn, 386
  time, 370
Breech presentation, 171-174
  anesthetic considerations, 173-174
  decomposition, 173
  etiology, 171
  extraction, 172
  indications for cesarean section, 172
  internal podalic version, 175
  methods of delivery
    assisted delivery, 172
    partial extraction, 172
    spontaneous delivery, 172
    total extraction, 172-173
  obstetrical management, 171-172
  regional anesthesia for, 174
Bromides, behavioral teratology, 320
Bromsulphalein excretion, 10
Bronchitis, 292
Bronchospasm, 292
Brow position
  anesthetic management, 175
  obstetric management, 175

INDEX

B-scan ultrasonography, 243
Bundle branch block, 216-217
Bulk flow, 14
BUN, 10
Bupivacaine
  effect of
    on neurobehavioral examination, 61
    on uterine activity, 46, 49
    on uterine blood flow, 28-29
  for cesarean section, 115-116
  for lumbar epidural block, 101
  for lumbar sympathetic block, 107
  in labor, 117-118
  in obstetrics, 113
  prolonged neural blockade, 301
  protein binding of, 258
  teratogenicity of, 318
  with epinephrine, 49, 54, 258

Calcium, 46
Capillary engorgement, in pregnancy, 3
Carbocaine (see Mepivacaine)
Carbon dioxide
  acid-base balance, 20-21
  maternal, 323-324
  narcosis, 366
  teratogenicity, 319
Cardiac arrest, treatment of, 97, 398-399
Cardiac disease in pregnancy
  aortic insufficiency, 190-191
  aortic stenosis, 191-192
  asymmetric septal hypertrophy, 210-211
  atrial fibrillation, 215-216
  atrial septal defect, 194-195
  cardiomyopathy of pregnancy, 207-208
  coarctation of the aorta, 200-201
  congenital heart disease, 193-204
  coronary artery disease, 212
  dissecting aneurysms of the aorta, 209-210
  mitral stenosis, 183-188
  mitral valvulotomy, 212-213
  patent ductus arteriosus, 196-197
  pulmonary hypertension, 204-206
  pulmonic stenosis, 202-204
  rheumatic heart disease, 183
  surgery
    aortic valve replacement, 214
    open heart surgery, 215
  tetralogy of Fallot, 197-199
  ventricular septal defect, 193-194
Cardiac drugs, inotropic, 290

Cardiac dysrhythmias, 215-217
Cardiac massage of newborn, 398-399
Cardiac output
  during labor and delivery, 7, 181
  during puerperium, 7
  in pregnancy, 7
Cardiac patient during pregnancy, 180
Cardiac sounds, 358
Cardiomyopathy of pregnancy
  anesthetic considerations of, 208
  pathophysiology of, 208
  prognosis of, 208
  symptoms of, 208
Cardiotachometer, 358
Cardiovascular changes
  during pregnancy, 5-9, 180, 313
  during pregnancy and parturition, 180-181
Cardioversion
  direct current, 218
  mitral stenosis, 186
Catecholamines
  and stress, effect on uterine blood flow, 31-32
  effect on toxemic patient, 206
  endogenous secretion of, 231
  placental transfer of, 148
Catheterization of umbilical vessels, 395
Caudal anesthesia
  contraindications, 105
  for toxemic patient, 232
  technique, 101-102
Central nervous system
  changes during pregnancy, 9
  susceptibility to teratogens, 320
Central venous pressure (CVP)
  in acid aspiration syndrome, 292
  monitoring
    for fluid management, 290
    for severe heart disease, 182
    in toxemic patient, 230
  response to fluids, 284
Cephalopelvic disproportion, 42
Cerebral ischemic attacks, transient, 207
Cerebrospinal fluid (CSF)
  in pregnancy, 9
  pressure, 9
Cervical spine fracture, 364
Cesarean section
  anesthesia for, 254-272
  blood loss from, 252, 268
  choice of anesthesia for, 254-255
  choice of local anesthetics for, 113-114, 257
  effect of anesthesia on blood

loss, 268
elective
  clinical condition of newborn, 269
  hypotension and condition of newborn, 270
emergency, 272
for eclampsia, 232
for multiple births, 178
for placenta praevia, 243, 245-246
general anesthesia for, 260
  technique, 261
indications for, 255
maternal analgesia with conduction anesthesia, 259
maternal awareness during, 266
regional anesthesia for, 255
  technique, 256
  management of complications, 256
Chemoreceptor influence of uterine contraction, 361
Chest physiotherapy, 391
Chlordiazepoxide, 315
Chlormethiazole, 229
Chloroform, carcinogenicity of, 320
Chloroprocaine
  effect of
    on neurobehavioral examination, 61, 382
    on uterine blood flow, 30
  for cesarean section, 114-115
  for lumbar epidural block, 101
  for paracervical block, 105
  half-life of, 110
  in labor, 118-119
  in obstetrics, 110
  placental transfer of, 258
  with epinephrine, 49-50, 258
Chlorpromazine, 77
  behavioral teratology, 320
  teratogenicity of, 314
Choanal atresia, 390
  bilateral, 402
  functional, 403
Choanal stenosis, 402
Cholesterol, 10
Cholinesterase, atypical, 265
Chromosomal abnormalities, 351-352, 377
Chronic hypertension, 224
Chronic hypoxemia, 319
Cicatricial phase, 411-412
Circulation, fetal, 59-60
Citanest (see Prilocaine)
Cleft palate, 317
Closing volume, 4
Clot observation test, 249
Clot retraction, 238
Coagulation

INDEX

Coagulation—*continued*
  disorders
    treatment of, 238
    screening tests for, 238
  factors, 235
  mechanism, 235
Colloid, 295
Colon-Morales device, 256
Coronary artery disease
  anesthetic considerations, 212
  occurrence of, 212
Common pathway, 236
Comparative negligence doctrine, 335
Complications of anesthesia
  aspiration, 123, 260, 288
  bladder dysfunction, 302
  convulsions, 95-97
  headache, 259-260
  hypertension, 98-99
  hypotension, 94-95, 256, 284
  total spinals, 97-98, 257
Concentration gradient, 14-16
Conduction anesthesia
  effects of
    on course of labor, 46-48
    for cesarean section, 254, 259
    for toxemic patient, 231
Congenital anomalies, 347
  and chromosomal abnormalities, 377
  from teratogenic medications, 315-317
  in offspring of operating room personnel, 318
Congenital bronchial stenosis, 406-407
Congenital heart disease
  maternal
    incidence of, 180
    mortality, 180
    types of
      aortic stenosis, 202
      atrial septal defect, 194-195
      coarctation of the aorta, 200
      Eisenmenger's syndrome, 199-200
      patent ductus arteriosus, 196-197
      pulmonary stenosis, 202-204
      tetralogy of Fallot, 197-199
      ventricular septal defect, 193-194
Congenital tracheal rings, 406
Congestive heart failure due to eclampsia, 226
Contractility
  myocardial
    in asymmetric septal hypertrophy, 211
  right ventricular
    in pulmonary hypertension, 205
Convulsions, maternal
  grand mal, 225
    control of, 229
  lidocaine-induced, 29
  local anesthesia, 95-97
    intravenous injection of, 303
    treatment of, 304
Cord lesions and vascular anomalies, 307-308
Corpus luteum, 343
Cortisone, 295-296
Creatinine, 10
Cretinism, 376
Cricoid pressure, 261, 298
Crying time, 370
Cryoprecipitate, 250
Curare
  placental transfer of, 57, 265
  prevention of fasciculations, 265
  teratogenicity of, 317
  with magnesium, 232
Cyanide toxicity, fetal, 35
Cyanosis in acid aspiration syndrome, 292
Cyclic adenosine monophosphate, 148
Cyclic nucleotide phosphodiesterase, 150
Cyclopropane
  effect of
    on the newborn, 127
    on uterine activity, 43
  teratogenicity of, 317
  use in obstetrics, 136
Cyprane inhaler, 128
Cytochrome P-450, 61, 155

Death, causes of (*see* Mortality)
Decamethonium, 228
Decelerations (*see also* early, late, and variable decelerations)
  fetal heart rate
    early, 361
    late, 361
    mild, 361
    moderate, 361
    severe, 361
    variable, 361
  grading of, 362
Decreased variability of fetal heart rate, non-asphyxic causes of, 359
Dehydroisoandrosterone sulfate (DS), 343
DeLee trap, 390
Demerol (*see* Meperidine)
Depression of newborn
  from barbiturates, 76
  from inhalation agents, 123-124
  from narcotics, 79
  measured by Apgar score, 267, 393
  respiratory causes, 387

Detoxification pathways in fetus, 60-61
Dexamethasone, 229
  for aspiration of gastric contents, 295
  in eclampsia, 229-230
Diabetes, 309
  and large birth weight infants, 377
  and use of adrenergic agents, 148
  treatment of hypoglycemia, 398
Diacetylmorphine (heroin), 314
Diaphragmatic hernia, 376, 392, 410
  with hypoplastic lungs, 414
Diazepam
  effects of
    on fetus, 77
    on neonate, 77
    on uterine blood flow, 25
  for treatment of preeclampsia-eclampsia, 229
  placental transfer of, 77
  teratogenicity of, 316
  use in obstetrics, 77
Diazoxide, 149-150, 229
  half-life of, 150
  placental transfer of, 149-150
Dibucaine, 110-111
Diethyl ether
  effect on uterine activity, 43-44
  teratogenicity of, 317
Diethylstilbesterol, 53
Diffusion, 14-17
  distance, 17
  hypoxia, 133
Digoxin
  and mitral stenosis, 186
  placental transfer of, 218
Dissociative anesthesia, 75, 85
Dissociative or amnesia drugs, 85
Diuretics, 227
Dopamine
  effect of
    on maternal blood pressure, 218
    on uterine blood flow, 33, 218, 325
  therapy for mitral stenosis, 187
Doppler principle, 358
Double catheter technique
  for epidural anesthesia, 103
Double set-up, 244-248
Drug(s)
  absorption of, 53
  biotransformation of, 53
  distribution of
    maternal, 53-57
    fetal, 59-60
  excretion by fetus, 60-61
  fetal uptake of, 58-59
  metabolism by fetus, 60-61

INDEX

protein dissociation, 55-56
supplementary, for anxiety and analgesia, 259
Drug overdose, regional anesthesia complication, 303
Dubowitz score, 378
Ductus arteriosus, mechanism of, 154, 385
Duranest (see Etidocaine)
Dyspnea, 292
Dysrhythmias, supraventricular, 195

Early decelerations, fetal heart rate, 361
Eclampsia, postpartum, 233
Edema
  generalized, 225
  interstitial, 292
  intra-alveolar, 292
  pulmonary, 226, 292, 295
Eisenmenger's syndrome, maternal, 199
  anesthetic considerations of, 200
  pathophysiology of, 199-200
  prognosis of, 199
  symptoms of, 199
Electromyography, 309
Embryology of the upper airway, 402
Emetics, 297
Emptying the stomach, 297
Endocarditis
  bacterial, 193
  infective, 183
Endotracheal intubation, 123, 297-298
  for general anesthesia, 261
  for meconium, 390
Enflurane
  and oxytocic agents, 44
  effect of
    on maternal bleeding, 44
    on uterine activity, 43
    on uterine blood flow, 27
  for cesarean section, 135
  for toxemic patient, 232
  for vaginal delivery, 135
Entonox, 128
Environmental pollution, 125-126, 318-319
Ephedrine
  and hypertension, 207
  effects of
    on fetal oxygen, 285
    on uterine activity, 48
    on uterine blood flow, 32, 217, 257, 286
  for treatment of hypotension, 232, 257, 285
  prophylaxis for hypotension, 256, 282
Epidural

block (see Lumbar epidural block)
  catheters, 304
  hematoma, 305, 308
  saline infusion, 302
  space contamination, 306
  veins
    cannulation of, 304
    engorgement of, 9
    rupture of, 302, 308
Epinephrine
  as a vasoconstrictive adjuvant, 113
  effect of
    on local anesthetic concentration, 54
    on uterine activity, 48-50
    on uterine blood flow, 217
  local anesthesia and
    effect on uterus, 325
    for cesarean section, 258
    in toxemic patient, 232
Erdheim's medial necrosis, 209
Esophageal
  atresia, 392-393, 406
  reflux, 313
Esophagitis, 9
Ester-linked local anesthetics, 109-110, 258
  placental transfer of, 258
Estradiol (E_2), 343
Estriol (E_3)
  fetal adrenal disorders, 344
  fetal CNS abnormalities, 344
  fetal liver dysfunction, 344
  hepatointestinal circulation interruption of, 344
  maternal renal disease, 344
  placental abnormalities, 344
Estrone (E_1), 343
Ethanol, 152-154
  effects on uterine contractility, 153
  placental transfer of, 153
  side effects, 154
Ethrane (see Enflurane)
Etidocaine
  effect of
    on neurobehavioral examination, 61
  for cesarean section, 113
  in obstetrics, 112
  prolonged neural blockade, 302
  protein binding of, 258
  teratogenicity of, 318
  with epinephrine, 54
Euglobin clot lysis time, 238
Evaluation of the neonate, 370-384
Extramural lesions of the trachea
  tumors, 406
  vascular rings, 406
Extrinsic pathway, 236
Extubation, awake, 299

Face position
  anesthetic management of, 175
  obstetric management of, 176
Factor XI deficiency, 240
Family-centered maternity care, 70
Fasciculations
  effect of magnesium, 232
  prevention of, 265, 298
Femoral venous pressure, 313
Fenoprofen, 155
Fenoterol (Partusisten), 143
Fentanyl, 78, 85
Ferguson's reflex, 47
Fetal
  acidosis
    causes of, 270
    from maternal hypotension, 281
  age, determination of, 347
  alcohol syndrome, 154
  antepartum evaluation, 357
  asphyxia
    decrease in placental function, 14
    diagnosis of, 357-369
    etiologic factors, 270, 279
    stress as a cause of, 31
  breathing, 348-349
  circulation, 59-60
  congenital anomalies, 347
  distribution of drugs, 59-60
  electrode, 358
  growth, 347
  hemolytic anemia, 352
    increase of bilirubin, 352
    intrauterine transfusion, 352
  hepatic enzyme, 60-61
  hypoxia, etiologic factors, 270
  metabolism and excretion of drugs, 60-61
  scalp sampling, 357, 359-360
  uptake of drugs, 58-59
  weight, estimation of, 347
α-Fetoprotein, 352
Fetus
  evaluation of, 343-355
  treatment in utero, 360
Fibrin-fibrinogen degradation products, 238
Fibrinogen, 237, 250
Fibrinolysis, 237
Fick's diffusion equation, 14, 57
Filters, micropore, 306
Finnish Register of Congenital Malformations, 316
Flow volume loops, 5
Fluids, intravenous, in hypotension of regional blockade, 95, 256, 285
Fluroxene
  carcinogenicity of, 320
  effect of
    on uterine blood flow, 28

INDEX

Fluroxene—continued
  teratogenicity of, 317
Foam test, 142, 349
Foot drop, 308
Forane (see, Isoflurane)
Frankenhausen's ganglion, 105
Functional residual capacity, 3, 261, 312
  of newborn, 386
Furosemide
  in aspiration of gastric contents, 295
  in eclampsia, 229

Gallamine, placental transfer of, 265
Gastric
  acid secretion, 289
  contents, volume of, 393
  distension, prevention of, 393
  emptying, delay in, 288
  motility
    after narcotics, 79
    after scopolamine, 86
    in pregnancy, 9
  reflux, 9
Gastrin, 9, 289
  plasma levels of, 313
Gastroesophageal junction, 9
Gastrointestinal changes during pregnancy, 9
General anesthesia (see Inhalation anesthesia)
Gestational age, 142
  assessment of weight and, 378
  assessment of (table), 379
  methods of assessment, 378
Gestational hypertension, 224
Glomerular filtration rate, 10
Glucocorticoids, 145
Glycopyrrolate, 261, 297, 326
Grunting, form of respiration, 409

Halogenated agents for cesarean section, 266
Halothane
  and oxytocic agents, 44
  behavioral teratology, 320
  carcinogenesis of, 320
  effect of
    on fetus and neonate, 123
    on maternal bleeding, 44
    on uterine activity, 43
    on uterine blood flow, 26, 324
  for cesarean section, 135
  for toxemic patient, 232
  for vaginal delivery, 135
  technique for uterine relaxation, 130-131
  teratogenicity of, 317
  uterine relaxant, 26, 43-44
Heartburn, 288
Heat loss in newborn, prevention of, 391

Heart block, 216
Heart disease in pregnancy (see Cardiac disease)
Heart rate
  fetal
    monitoring of, 230, 357
  maternal
    with coarctation of the aorta, 201
    with pulmonary stenosis, 203
    with ventricle septal defect, 194
Heart rate monitor(s)
  cardiotachometer, 358
  Doppler ultrasound device, 358
  fetal electrode, 358
  intra-amniotic catheter, 358
  tokodynamometer, 358
Heart rate patterns, fetal
  abnormal, 364-369
    characteristics of, 366
    ominous, 364
      acute stress pattern, 365
      chronic stress pattern, 367
      sinister pattern, 365, 368
      stress pattern, 365
  baseline rate
    tachycardia, 360
    bradycardia, 360
  baseline variability
    beat-to-beat, 360
    long term, 360
  decrease in beat-to-beat variability, 77, 359
  normal, 363-364
    characteristics of, 363
    variability, 358-360
Hematocrit
  in preeclampsia, 226
  in pregnancy, 6
Hematoma, epidural, 305
Hemoglobin, in pregnancy, 6
Hemorrhage
  acute, effects of, 247
  antepartum, 243-251
    in abruptio placenta, 248-250
    in placenta praevia, 243-248
    other causes of, 250-251
  concealed, 248
  intra-alveolar, 292
  intracranial, 377, 396
  postpartum, retained placenta, 251-252
    anesthetic management of, 251-252
Hemorrhagic shock, 246
Henderson-Hasselbalch equation, 359
Heparin, fibrinogen deficiency, 250
Hepatic
  blood flow, 10
  changes during pregnancy, 10
  neoplasms, 321

Hexoprenaline, 143
High-risk fetus, identification of, 388
Horner's syndrome, 303
Human studies and teratogenicity
  anesthetics, 318
  systemic medications, 315
Hydralazine (apresoline), 34, 76, 218, 229
  cardiovascular effects of, 218
Hydration, intravenous, 94-95, 256, 282
Hydrocortisone in aspiration of gastric contents, 296
p-Hydroxy phenyl isopropyl-arterenol, 143
Hydroxyzine during labor, 77
Hyperbaric oxygen, 319
Hyperbilirubinemia, 150
Hypercapnia
  effects on uterine blood flow, 35-36
  maternal, 324
Hyperglycemia, maternal and fetal, and adrenergic agents, 148
Hyperoxia
  maternal, 261, 267, 323
  neonatal, 415
    while breathing room air, 415
    with cyanotic congenital heart disease, 416
Hyper-reflexia, 226
Hypertension
  antihypertensive therapy in toxemia, 229
  chronic maternal, 376
  classification of, 224
  essential, 206
  in pregnancy, 7
  in pulmonary disease, 204
  malignant, 207
  vasopressor-induced, 98
  with ventrical septal defect, 194
Hypertensive disorders
  anesthetic considerations of, 206-207
  incidence of, 206
  pathophysiology of, 207
  prognosis of, 206
  symptoms of, 206-207
Hyperventilation
  and hypovolemic shock, 396
  causing hyperoxia, 415
  during pregnancy, 3, 34
  effect of
    on fetus, 270
    on uterine blood flow, 36
  maternal, 262
Hypnosis, 65-66
Hypocapnia

INDEX

effect on uterine blood flow, 35-36
  maternal, 36, 323
Hypoglycemia, treatment of, 398
Hypoplastic lungs with diaphragmatic hernia, 414
Hypotension
  and hypovolemic shock, 397
  arterial, 279-286
  cause of fetal acidosis, 270
  condition of infant, 270
  etiology of, 279
  from regional anesthesia, 17, 94, 256
  from segmental lumbar epidural block, 177
  hypovolemic, 396
  in pregnancy, 7-9
  in toxemic patient, 232
    treatment of, 232
  maternal, and fetal asphyxia, 324
  orthostatic, 79
  prevention and therapy, 18, 256, 282, 285-286
  safety of prophylaxis, 284-285
  systemic, 29-31
Hypotensive syndrome, supine, 7-9
Hypothermia, 377
Hypovolemia
  diagnosis of, 396
  treatment of, 397
Hypoxia
  complication of general and regional anesthesia, 321
  diffusion, 133
  effect of
    on fetus, 270
    on uterine blood flow, 35
  fetal, 270
  maternal, 261, 270
  teratogenicity of, 315

Idiopathic thrombocytopenic purpura, 239
Iliac artery ligation, 249
Imipramine, 314
Indomethacin, 154
Induction agents, intravenous (see also specific agents)
  effects on uterine blood flow, 23-26
Infant
  low birth weight, 142
  preterm, 142
  problems of, 376
Induction, position during, 298
Infection
  chemical contamination, 306-307
  epidural abscess, 306
  micropore filters, 306
  spinal canal, 306

subarachnoid, 306
upper respiratory, 3
Inferior vena cava
  compression of, 7-9, 46, 279
  obstruction of, 7-9
  occlusion of, 313
Informed consent, 336-338
Infundibular stenosis, 202
Inhalation agents (see also specific agents)
  anesthetic requirement, 9
  effect on uterine activity, 42-44
  placental transfer, 123
Inhalation analgesia, 121-137
  apparatus for, 126-128
  effects of
    on fetus and neonate, 123
    on labor, 125
    on uterine activity, 44
  indications for, 121-122
  risks, 123
  techniques of, 129-130
Inhalation anesthesia, 121-137
  effects of
    on fetus and neonate, 123
    on labor, 125
  environmental pollution from, 125-126, 318-319
  for cesarean section, 254, 260-261
    advantages of, 260
    management of, 260
    suggested technique, 261
  for multiple births, 177
  for placenta praevia, bleeding, 246
  indications for, 122
  maternal hypoxia, 321-322
  risks, 123
  techniques, 130-131
Injection, massive misplaced from regional anesthesia, 303
Innovar, 88
Inotropes and vasopressors, 217
Internal podalic version, 175
Intervertebral disc, prolapsed, 308
Intra-amniotic catheter, 358
Intracranial hemorrhage and sodium bicarbonate administration, 396
Intrapartum asphyxia
  and shock, 396
  treatment of hypoglycemia, 398
Intrathecal analgesia, continuous, 304
Intrathoracic pressure, 387
Intrauterine
  asphyxia, 357
    avoidance of, 321
  death, 319
  fetal transfusion, 352

growth retardation, 142, 376
  pathology of, 376
  treatment of hypoglycemia, 398
  growth standards, 376
Intravascular coagulation, 226
  disseminated, 240
Intravascular coagulopathy, 224
Intravenous hydration, 256
Intravenous injection, 303-304
  prevention of, 304
  regional anesthesia complication, 301
    convulsions, 304
    epidural vein cannulation, 304
Intrinsic pathway, 236
Intubation, 297-298
  awake, 298
  for severely depressed neonates, 394-395
  tracheal, for aspiration, 390
Ion-trapping, 58
Isoflurane, 135
  carcinogenicity of, 320
  effect
    on uterine activity, 43
    on uterine blood flow, 27
Isoproterenol, 218
Isoxsuprine (Vasodilan), 142
  effect on uterine blood flow, 33

Jaundice, 377

Kennedy device, 256
Kernicterus, 78
Ketamine, 85
  contraindicated for eclampsia, 232
  dissociative anesthesia, 85
  effects of
    on newborn, 85
    on uterine activity, 45
    on uterine tone, 86, 325
  for placenta praevia, 174, 246
    nitrous oxide anesthesia, effect on ENNS, 382
  respiratory depression from, 85

Labor
  abnormal progress of, 42
  effect of anesthesia, 42-50
Lacerations
  cervical, 252
  vaginal, 252
Lactate, 21
Lamaze, 66
Laryngeal anomalies, 405
Laryngoscopy, neonatal, technique for, 394
Laryngospasm, neonatal, 390
Late deceleration, fetal heart rate and fetal pH, 361, 365
  grading of, 362

Latency of analgesia, 129
Lawsuits, malpractice, 331
  prevention, 335
LeBoyer technique, 69
LDH, 10
Lecithin, 349
  and sphingomyelin (L/S ratio), 142, 349-350
Left uterine displacement (LUD), 8-9
  mechanical devices for, 256
  prevention of hypotension, 282
Lesions
  cord, 307
  nerve, 308
  root, 308
  trunk, 308
Lidocaine
  antiarrhythmic drug, 217-218
  carbonated, 112, 116
  effect of
    on neurobehavioral examination, 61, 382
    on uterine activity, 46
    on uterine blood flow, 28-29
  for spinal anesthesia, 104, 257
  in obstetrics, 112
  with epinephrine, 49, 54
Liver disease, hemostatic function in, 240
Local anesthetic agents (see also specific drugs)
  basic requirements, 109
  convulsions, 95
  doses in pregnancy, 313
  effect of
    on uterine activity, 45-48
    on uterine blood flow, 28-29
  teratogenicity, 318
  toxicity, 400
  use in convulsive disorders, 231
  with epinephrine, 258
Local perineal infiltration anesthesia, 107
  for multiple births, 177
  for toxemic patient, 231
Long-term variability, fetal, 360
Lumbar epidural block, 99-101
  continuous, for labor and vaginal delivery, 116
  contraindications to, 105
  dose requirements, 257-258
  double catheter technique, 103
  effect of
    on early neonatal behavioral scale, 382
    on newborn, 382
    on uterine activity, 47-48
  for cesarean section, 255-258, 270
  for patient with mitral insufficiency, 189-190
  primary advantages, 231
  segmental, 171
    for multiple births, 171
    for patient with mitral stenosis, 187
  hypotension from, 177
  technique, 99-103
  toxic reactions, 257
  total spinals, 257
Lumbar sympathetic block, 106
  technique, 106-107
Lumbosacral trunk injury, 308
Lung
  compartments, 315
  compliance, 386
  fluid, 386
  volumes and capacities, 3-5

MAC, 121, 124, 261-262
Magnesium and aluminum hydroxide, 297
Magnesium intoxication, 400
Magnesium sulfate
  for treatment of toxemia, 227
  potentiation of muscle relaxants, 228
Magnesium trisilicate, 296
Malpractice lawsuits, 331
Malpractice litigation, 333
Marcaine (See Bupivacaine)
Marfan's syndrome, 209
Maternal-infant bonding, 383
Maturity, fetal, 142
  pulmonary, 146
Meconium
  appearance in amniotic fluid, 407
  aspiration, 390, 407
    treatment of 408
  pneumonitis, 390
    treatment of, 390
  removal from airway, 408
Medical records, 338-339
Mefenamic acid, 155
Mendelson's syndrome, 291-294
Meperidine
  effects of
    on fetus, 81
    on neonate, 76, 78
    on uterine activity, 44
  neurobehavioral changes from, 83
  placental transfer of, 81
  teratogenicity of, 314
Mephentermine (Wyamine)
  effect on uterine blood flow, 32, 257
  prophylactic use of, 285
Mepivacaine
  effect of
    on neurobehavioral examination, 61, 382
    on uterine blood flow, 28-30
  for paracervical block, 106
  in obstetrics, 112
  with epinephrine, 54
Meprobamate, 316
  behavioral teratology, 320
Metabolic alkalosis, effect on uterine blood flow, 36-37
Metaraminol, effect on uterine blood flow, 32, 217
Methadone, 314
Methanesulfonamide, 143
Methemoglobinemia, 112
Methohexital, effect on uterine blood flow, 24-25
Methoxamine (Vasoxyl), effect of
  on fetus, 286
  on uterine activity, 48
  on uterine blood flow, 32, 217, 257, 325
Methoxyflurane
  and high inspired oxygen effect on ENNS, 382
  blood solubility of 134
  carcinogenicity of, 320
  effects of
    on neonate, 135
    on uterine blood flow, 27
  for toxemic patient, 231
  renal effects of, 134-135
  serum inorganic fluoride level, 134
  techniques of administration, 134
  teratogenicity of, 317
  vaporizers for, 127-128
Methyldopa, 229
Methylprednisolone for aspiration of gastric contents, 296
Methylxanthines, 150
Metoprolol, 149
Micrognathia, 376
Microphthalmia, 319
Mid-forceps rotation, 171
  analgesia for, 171
Mid-vacuum extraction, 171
Minute ventilation, 3-4
  for newborn, 386
Mitral valve
  insufficiency of, 188-193
    anesthetic considerations of, 189
    pathophysiology of, 188
    prognosis of, 188
    symptoms of, 188
  replacement, 213
    anesthetic considerations, 214
    complications of, 213
  stenosis of, 183-188
    anesthetic considerations of, 186
    pathophysiology of, 186

INDEX

prognosis of, 185
symptoms of, 185
Mitral valvulotomy
  anesthetic considerations, 213
  complications of, 213
Montevideo units, 42, 363
Morbidity
  fetal, and maternal cardiac care during anesthesia, 182
  maternal, from aspiration of gastric content, 288, 290
Morphine, 78, 84
  teratogenicity of, 314
Morphogenesis of organs, 318
Mortality, maternal
  abnormal positions and multiple births, 175
  due to aspiration of gastric contents, 288, 290
  due to eclampsia, 226
  due to rheumatic heart disease, 182
  from uterine rupture, 250–251
Mortality, neonatal, 387
  from abnormal positions and multiple births, 176
  from low birth weight, 376
  from meconium aspiration, 390, 408
Multiple gestations, 175
  anesthetic considerations, 177
Multivillous stream system, 16
Muscle relaxants
  effect of magnesium, 228
  effects on neonatal respiration, 264
  placental transfer of, 57, 264–265
  prevention of fasciculations, 265
Myelitis, 307
Myelography, 309
Myelomeningocele, 376

Nalorphine, 315
Naloxone, 89, 230, 399
  teratogenicity of, 315
Narcotics (see also specific drugs)
  depression from, 399
  effects of
    on gastric emptying, 288
    on gastric motility, 79
    on infant, 76
    on labor, 75
  hypoventilation from, 79
  nausea and vomiting from, 79
  neonatal addiction, 399
  orthostatic hypotension from, 79
  placental transfer of, 81
  preeclampsia-eclampsia, 229
  respiratory depression from, 79

Nasal obstruction, 403
National Collaborative Study, 319
Natural childbirth, 66
Neosynephrine (see Phenylephrine)
Nervous system
  developmental anomalies of, 376
  maturation of, 378
Nesacaine (see Chloroprocaine)
Neurobehavioral examination
  after cesarean section, 271
  Brazelton neonatal behavioral assessment scale, 380
  early neonatal neurobehavioral scale (ENNS), 381
  effect of
    ketamine-nitrous oxide anesthesia, 382
    lumbar epidural anesthesia, 382
    methoxyflurane with high inspired oxygen, 382
    nitrous oxide with low inspired oxygen, 382
    thiopental-nitrous oxide anesthesia, 382
  effects of local anesthetics, 61
  evaluation of the neonate, 376
  Prechtl and Beintema neurological examination, 381
  Scanlon method, 258
Neuroleptanalgesia, 75, 88
Neurologic accidents, 307
Neurologic complications of regional anesthesia, 301–311
  backache, 302
  bladder dysfunction, 302
  chemical contamination, 306–307
  of epidural space, 306
  of subarachnoid space, 306
  drug overdose, 303
  epidural hematoma, 305
  Horner's syndrome, 303
  intravenous injection, 303
  massive misplaced injection, 303
  post-puncture headache, 302
  prolonged neural blockade, 301–302
  shivering, 302–303
  spinal artery syndrome, anterior, 305
  subarachnoid injection, 303
  subdural injection, 303
  trauma, 304–305
Neurologic deficits postpartum
  diagnosis of, 308–309
  tests for, 309
Newborn
  acidosis, correction of, 396

Apgar score, 371–375
assessment of
  gestational age and weight, 376, 379
body temperature, 391
breathing frequency, 386
changes at birth, 385
circulation 385
condition of
  effect of duration of prepartum anesthesia, 263
  elective cesarean section, 269
  regional vs. general anesthesia, 268
depression of
  from barbiturates, 76
  from inhalation agents, 123, 267–268
  from narcotics, 79
  measured by Apgar score, 371, 393
  respiratory causes, 387
developmental anomalies of nervous system, 376
effect of magnesium, 227
effect of succinylcholine, 264
Electroencephalographic records, 381
evaluation of, 268, 370–383
functional residual capacity, 386
general examination of, 376
kernicterus, 78
lung compliance, 386
lung fluid, 386
maturation of nervous system, 378–379
minute ventilation, 386
neurobehavioral changes, 83
neurobehavioral testing, 379–383
  decrement behavior, 382
  muscle tone, 382
  reflex responses, 382
  response to stimulation, 382
  state of wakefulness, 382
of toxemic mother, 233
resuscitation of (see Resuscitation of the newborn)
tidal volume, 386
Nisentil (see Alphaprodine)
Nitroprusside, 34–35, 187, 229
Nitrous oxide
  administration of, 131–133
  effects of
    on fetus and neonate, 123–124, 133, 266
    on plasma norepinephrine, 133
    on uterine activity, 43
  for toxemic patient, 231
  placental transfer of, 266
  teratogenicity of, 317

Nitrous oxide—*continued*
  with low inspired oxygen, effect on ENNS, 382
Non-stress test, scoring, 354
Norepinephrine
  effects of on uterine blood flow, 32, 217
  plasma, 67, 267
Normeperidine, 82
Nylidrin hydrochloride, 143

Ominous heart rate pattern, 364
Open-heart surgery during pregnancy
  anesthetic considerations, 215
  fetal mortality, 215
Opiates, 316
Oral clefts, 316
Orciprenaline (Alupent), 143
Orthostatic hypotension, 79
Ovarian cystectomy, 325
Oxygen
  affinity, 20
  air blender, 416
  analyzer, 416
  capacity, 20
  changing PaO_2, 414
  consumption, 3, 261, 312, 391
    and skin temperature, 391
  lack of, 21
  measurement of PaO_2, 413
  supplementary, 259
  teratogenicity of, 319
  therapy for newborn depression, 388
  transfer to the fetus, 19-21
  uptake, 4
Oxygenation maternal, 321
Oxyhemoglobin dissociation curve, 324
Oxytocics, effect on uterus, 44, 267
Oxytocin
  augmentation, 363
  challenge test, 353

Pain, of labor, 93, 181
  effects of gastric emptying, 288
Pancuronium
  effect on neonate, 265
  prevention of fasciculations, 265
  with magnesium, 232
Paraaminobenzoic acid, 110
Paracervical block
  effect on uterine activity, 45-46
  fetal bradycardia, 105
  Frankenhauser's ganglion, 105
  neonatal depression from, 105
  technique, 105
Paracetamol, 155
Paroxysmal atrial tachycardia (PAT), 216
Partial thromboplastin time, 237

Particulate matter, aspiration of
  atelectasis from, 291
  treatment of, 291
Patent ductus arteriosus, maternal, 196
  anesthetic considerations of, 197
  pathophysiology of, 196
  prognosis of, 196
  symptoms of, 196
Pentazocine, 78, 84
  effect of on uterine activity, 44
  teratogenicity of, 314
Penthrane (*see* Methoxyflurane)
Penthrane analgizer, 127-128
Pentobarbital, 75, 314
Pentothal (*see* Thiopental)
Peridural block (*see* Lumbar epidural block)
Perinatal
  morbidity, 141
  mortality, 70, 141
  pharmacology, 53-61
  and asphyxia, 157
Peripartum cardiopathy, 207-208
Persistent occiput posterior, analgesia for, 170-171
Pharmacology, perinatal, 53-61
Phenazocine, 314
Phenobarbital, 314
Phenothiazine derivatives, during labor, 76
Phenylephrine
  effect of
    on fetus, 286
    on uterine blood flow, 32, 217, 257, 325
Pheochromocytoma, 206
Phospholipids
  in amniotic fluid, 350
  phosphatidylglycerol (PG), 349
  phosphatidylinositol (PI), 349
Physician-patient relationship, 331
Physiologic changes during pregnancy, 3-10, 312
Physostigmine, 88
Pierre-Robin syndrome, 27, 376, 403-405
Pinocytosis, 14
Piper forceps, 173
Piperocaine, 110
Pitocin (*see* Oxytocin)
pKa, 56, 58
Placenta, 12, 243
  abruption of (*see* Abruptio placentae)
  area of, 16
  circumvallate, 250
  immunologic injury of, 224
  mechanisms of exchange, 13-14
  praevia, 243-248
    anesthetic management of,
      244-248
    antepartum hemorrhage, 243
    cesarean section in, 243
    diagnosis of, 243
    double set-up, 244-245
    incidence of, 243
    permeability of membrane, 16-17
    production of estrogens, 343
    retained, 251
Placental
  anatomy and circulation, 12-13
    fetal circulation, 12
    maternal circulation, 12
  insufficiency, 376
  lactogen, 142
    human (HPL), 345
  localization, 347
  respiratory function, 360
  syncytiotrophoblast, 345
  transfer
    determinants of, 53-61
    diazepam, 77
    of catecholamines, 148
    of ethanol, 153
    local anesthetics, 258
  vasculitis, 224
Plasma
  norepinephrine, 67, 267
  pseudocholinesterase, 10, 110
    reduced in parturients, 264
  volume
    in preeclampsia, 226
    in pregnancy, 6
Plasminogen, 237
Platelet
  adhesiveness, 238
  aggregation, 235, 238
    study, 238
  count, 237
  disorders, 238
  transfusions
    antiplatelet antibodies, 239
    complications of, 239
Platypelloid pelves, 308
Pneumothorax, 400
Polyps, 250
Pontocaine (*see* Tetracaine)
Porphyria, 309
Position, abnormal, 170-175
  persistent occiput posterior, 170-171
Positive end expired pressure (PEEP), 290
Positive pressure ventilation
  maternal, 262
  therapy for acid aspiration syndrome, 294-295
Post-dural puncture headache
  blood patch epidural for, 260, 302
  complication of regional anesthesia, 259, 302
  complication of spinal anesthe-

INDEX

sia, 259
  incidence of, 302
  influence of needle size and bevel on, 259
  management of, 302
  therapy for, 260
Post-maturity, 377
Postpartal heart disease, 208
Practolol, effects of, 149
Preeclampsia-eclampsia, 224
  anesthesia for, 230
  cardiovascular changes, 206
  effect of on fetal and neonatal parameters, 233
  etiology of, 224
  hypertension, 224
  intrauterine growth retardation, 376
  pathophysiology of, 224
  plasma volume, albumin and hematocrit in, 226
  therapy for, 227
Pregnancy
  after valvular surgery, 212
  open-heart surgery during, 215
  physiologic changes in, 3-10
Preload, in asymmetric septal hypertrophy, 211
Premature infant (see Infant, Low birth weight or Preterm infant)
Premature labor (see Preterm labor)
Prenatal anesthesia clinics, 71
Presentation, 170
  abnormal, 170
  breech, 171
    extraction, 172
    methods of delivery, 172
    types of, 172
Preterm infant, 142
  anesthetic management of, 155-158
  problems of, 377
Preterm labor, 142
  causes of, 325
  pharmacologic therapy for, 141-155, 325
  prevention of, 325
Prilocaine
  in obstetrics, 112
  teratogenicity of, 318
Procaine, effect of on uterine blood flow, 28-29
Prochlorperazine, 77, 314
Progesterone, 9
Progress of labor, 42
Prolapse of umbilical cord, in breech presentation, 173
Prolonged neural blockade, regional anesthesia complication, 301
Promazine, 77
Promethazine, 76

Pronethanol, 148
Prophylactic measures, for hypotension, 256
Propiomazine, 76
Propitocaine, effect of on uterine activity, 46
Propoxyphene, 314
Propranolol, 146
  antiarrhythmic drug, 217
  fetal acidosis, 149
  treatment for sinus tachycardia, 186
Prostaglandins, 224
  inhibitors, 154
    side effects of, 154
Protective airway reflexes obtundation of, 76
Protein binding
  differential, by fetal and maternal blood, 60
  of local anesthetics, 55, 112
Proteinuria, 225
Prothrombin, 237
  time (PT), 237
Pseudocholinesterase, plasma, 10, 110, 264
Psychoactive compounds, subteratogenic doses, 320
Psychological anesthesia for obstetrics, 65-70
Psychological stress, 67
Psychoprophylaxis, 66-67
Pudendal block
  effect of on uterine activity, 47-48
  for multiple births, 177
  for toxemic patient, 231
  technique, 107
Puerperal cardiomyopathy, 208
Pulmonary
  aspiration of gastric contents, 9, 288-299
    acid aspiration syndrome, 123, 291-294
    fecal or bacterial material, 290-291
    morbidity and mortality, 288, 290
    particulate matter, 291
    pathophysiology of, 290
    prevention of, 296
    therapeutic considerations of, 290
    signs and symptoms of, 288
  capillary wedge pressure (PCW) 182
    and aortic insufficiency, 191
    and mitral insufficiency, 189
  compliance
    in acid aspiration syndrome, 292
  congestion and mitral insufficiency, 188
  edema 226, 292

  in acid aspiration syndrome, 292
  hypertension, primary, 204
    maternal
      anesthetic considerations of, 205
      pathophysiology of, 204
      prognosis of, 204
      symptoms of, 204
    mitral stenosis, 183
  mixing index, 315
Pulmonary surfactant, 146
Pulmonic stenosis, maternal
  anesthetic considerations of, 203
  pathophysiology of, 203
  prognosis of, 202
  symptoms of, 202

Radial arterial line, 181
Radioisotope scanning, 243
Receptors, adrenergic
  beta receptors β_2, 143
  beta stimulants, 146
    effects of, 146
    elimination half-life, 148
  in uterine muscle, 48
  stimulation of, 148
Red blood cell volume in pregnancy, 6
Regional anesthesia (see also Lumbar epidural block)
  complications of
    convulsions, 95-257
    hypertension, 93
    hypotension, 93, 256, 279
    maternal hypoxia, 321
    neurologic, 301-311
    post dural puncture headache, 259
    shivering, 302
    total spinal anesthesia, 97, 257
  drugs for, 114-116
  effects of
    on course of labor, 46-48
    on newborn, 382
    on uterine activity, 45-48
    on uterine blood flow, 29-31
  for cesarean section, 255-256
  for labor and vaginal delivery, 93
  for multiple births, 177
  for toxemic patient, 231
  management of complications, 93, 256
  techniques of
    caudal block, 101
    double catheter, 103
    for cesarean section, 255-256
    lumbar epidural block, 99
    lumbar sympathetic block, 106
    paracervical block, 105

Regional Anesthesia—*continued*
  pudendal block, 107
  spinal block, 104
Regurgitation, 313
Renal changes during pregnancy, 10
Renal disease
  effect of on estriol values, 344
  hypertensive disorders, 206
Renal plasma flow (RPF), 10
Reserpine, behavioral teratology, 320
Respiratory changes during pregnancy, 3-5, 312
Respiratory depression
  from barbiturates, 76
  from ketamine, 85
  from narcotics, 79
Respiratory distress syndrome (RDS)
  in premature infants, 376
  prevention of, 142, 145
Respiratory failure, neonatal
  causes of, 403
Respiratory failure, neonatal—*continued*
  recognition of, 402
Respiratory system, neonatal
  anomalies of the upper airway, 403
  chonal atresia, 402
  choanal stenosis, 402
  congenital bronchial stenosis, 406-407
  congenital defects of, 402
  congenital tracheal rings, 406
  embryology of the upper airway, 402
  esophageal atresia, 406
  extramural lesions of the trachea, 406
  laryngeal anomalies, 405
  nasal obstruction, 403
  subglottic stenosis, 405
  subglottic tracheal hemangiomas and webs, 406
  tracheal agenesis syndrome, 406
  tracheoesophageal fistula, 406
Resuscitation cart, 94, 99
Resuscitation of newborn
  Apgar score, 371
  asphyxia and, 385
  cardiac drug therapy, 400
  cardiac massage, 399
  correction of acidosis, 396
  equipment for, 388
  establishment of ventilation, 386
  intubation of severely depressed, 394
  special problems in
    local anesthetic toxicity, 400

magnesium intoxication, 400
narcotic depression, 399
pneumothorax, 400
vaginal squeeze, 386
Retinal detachment, 319
Retrolental fibroplasia
  anesthetic implications, 411
  changing PaO_2, 414
  from hyperbaric oxygen, 319
  hyperoxia, 412
  in premature infants, 377
  measurement of PaO_2, 413
  pathogenesis of, 411
Rheumatic heart disease and pregnancy
  incidence of, 180
  infective endocarditis, 183
  maternal mortality, 182
  types of
    aortic insufficiency, 190
    aortic stenosis, 191
    mitral insufficiency, 188
    mitral stenosis, 183
Ritodrine, effect of
  on acid-base status, 147
  on cardiovascular function, 147
  on uterine blood flow, 33
  on uterine contractions, 147
Rubella syndrome, maternal, 202
Rumpel-Leede test, 238
Rupture of uterus
  anesthetic management of, 250-251
  causes, 250
  incidence of, 250-251
  symptoms of, 251
Ruptured placenta, 396

Saddle block, (*see* Subarachnoid block)
Salbutamol, 143
Salicylates, behavioral teratology, 320
Saline, epidural injection of, for headache, 302
Scanlon method for neurobehavioral assessment, 258
  protocol for, 381
Scavenging systems, 318
Scopolamine, 86, 297
Secobarbital, 75
  effect on newborn, 380
Seconal (*see* Pentobarbital)
Sedatives and hypnotics (*see* specific drugs)
Sedative-tranquilizers, 75
Sedation, treatment for preeclampsia-eclampsia, 229
Segmental lumbar epidural block
  for multiple births, 171
  hypotension, 171
Self administration

methoxyflurane, 134
nitrous oxide, 131-132
Sellick Maneuver, 261
Serum
  estriol, 142
  inorganic fluoride
    after methoxyflurane, 134
    neonatal levels, 135
SGOT, 10
Shake test, 142, 349
  risk of IRDS, 351
  technique, 350
Shirodkar procedure, 325
Shivering, regional anesthesia complication, 302
Shock
  hemorrhagic, 246
  hypovolemic, in newborn, 396
    diagnosis of, 396
    treatment of, 396
Shoulder presentation
  anesthetic management of, 175
  obstetric management of, 175
Sinister pattern, 365
  abnormal, of fetal heart rate, 364
  and heart rate variability, 365
Sinus tachycardia, and mitral stenosis, 186
Skeletal malformations, 317
Sodium benzoate, a bilirubin-albumin uncoupler, 77
Sodium citrate, 297
Sphingomyelin, 349-350
Spina bifida, 376
Spinal anesthesia (*see* Subarachnoid block)
Spinal
  artery syndrome, anterior, 305
  cord termination, 305
  headache, 259, 302
    influence of needle size and bevel, 259, 302
    therapy, 260
  roots, 304
Spiral arteries, 13
Spontaneous abortions and teratogenicity, 318
Standards
  of care, 333
  of practice, 334
Stenosis
  aortic, 191, 202
  idiopathic hypertrophic subvalvular, 210
  infundibular, 202
  mitral, 183
  pulmonic, 202
Steroids
  intravenous, for treatment of aspiration, 290
  use of cortisone, 295
    dexamethasone, 295

INDEX

hydrocortisone, 296
methylprednisolone, 296
Stillbirth, 319
Stomach emptying, 297
Stress
  cause of fetal asphyxia, 31-32
  on cardiovascular system during labor and delivery, 181
  maternal emotional, 320
  pattern, abnormal, of fetal heart rate
    acute, 365
    chronic, 365
  tests
    non-stress test, 354-355
    oxytocin challenge test (OCT), 353
Stroke volume, during labor, 181
Subarachnoid
  infection, 306
  injection
    complication of regional anesthesia, 303
  space contamination, 306
    detergents, 307
    myelitis, 307
Subarachnoid block
  choice of local anesthetics, 257
  complications from
    headache, 259-260
    hypotension, 237, 256-257
    infection, 305-306
    total spinal, 97, 257, 303
    toxic reaction, 257, 303
  contraindications, 105
  dose requirements, 257
  effect on uterine activity, 44, 47-48
  for cesarean section, 114, 255-256
    technique, 256
  for eclamptic patient, 231
  for vaginal delivery, 114
  management of complications, 256
  technique, 105
  therapy for headache, 260
Subglottic
  stenosis, 405
  tracheal hemangiomas, 406
Sublimaze (see Fentanyl)
Succinylcholine
  dose response curve, 228
  effect of
    magnesium, 227
    on neonatal respiration, 264
    placental transfer of, 57
Suction
  mouth-to-tube, 390
    technique for, 390
  of trachea, 390
    for meconium, 390
Supine hypotension syndrome, 7-9

Supraventricular tachycardia, in asymmetric septal hypertrophy, 211
Surgery during pregnancy, 326
  anesthetic management, 326
  elective, 326
  emergency, 326
  open-heart, 215
  urgent, 326
Suxamethonium (see Succinylcholine)
Sympathomimetics, effect on uterine vasoconstriction, 325
Syntocinon (see Oxytocin)
Systemic medications, 75
  teratogenicity of, 314

Tachycardia (see also Heart rate patterns, fetal
  fetal, 360
Tachypnea, 292
Talwin (see Pentozacine)
Temperature of body in newborn, maintenance of, 391
Teratogenicity of anesthetics, 314
  behavioral, 320
  biochemical, 314
  morphologic, 314
  and operating room personnel, 318
Terbutaline (Brethine), 143
Tetracaine, 104, 110, 257
  for spinal anesthesia, 110
  prolonged neural blockade, 301
Tetralogy of Fallot, maternal anesthetic considerations of, 198
  pathophysiology of, 198
  prognosis of, 197
  symptoms of, 198
Thalidomide, 314
Theophylline, 150
Thermal sensory information, 303
Thermodilution pulmonary artery catheter, 181
Thiamylal
  effect on uterine blood flow, 24-25
  teratogenicity of, 314
Thiopental
  effect of
    on fetus and neonate, 263
    on uterine blood flow, 24-25
    placental transfer of, 263
      nitrous oxide anesthesia, effect of on ENNS, 382
Thrombin, 237
Thrombin time, 237
Thrombocytopenia, 238
Tidal volume of newborn, 386
Timed forced expiratory volume, 5
Time to sustained respiration, 370
Tocodynamometer, 42, 358
Torr-minutes, 42
Total protein concentration, 10
Toxemia of pregnancy, (see Preeclampsia-eclampsia), 224
Toxemic coma, 226
Tracheal
  agenesis syndromes, 406
  intubation (see Intubation, tracheal)
  lavage for aspiration of gastric contents, 290
  suctioning
    for acid aspiration syndrome, 293
    for meconium, 390
    techniques of, 390
Tracheo-esophageal fistula, 376
  with polyhydramnios, 406
Tranquilizing agents
  effects of on uterine activity, 45
  for the toxemic patient, 230
  teratogenicity of, 315
Transplacental carcinogenesis, 320
Trauma
  mechanical, 320
  regional anesthesia complication, 304
  teratogenicity of, 320
Trendelenburg position, 256
  therapy for hypotension, 285
Trichloroethylene, 133
  carcinogenicity of, 320
  compared to methoxyflurane, 133-134
  for cesarean section, 136
Tri-hydroxymethylaminomethane (THAM), effect of on uterine blood flow, 37
Trimethaphan (Arfonad), 209, 229
d-Tubocurarine, 228
Twilight sleep, 87

Ultrasonic cephalometry, 142
Ultrasonic mist, 391
Ultrasonography, 243, 346
  real-time device, 347
Ultrasound, 358
Umbilical blood flow, 18-19, 59
Umbilical cord blood sampling
  for acid-base status and oxygenation, 387
  normal values (table), 388
  technique of, 387
Umbilical vessel catheterization, 395
  rupture and shock, 396

INDEX

Upper airway reflexes, 288
Uric acid levels, 226
Urinary estriol, 142
Urine output, acid in fluid management, 290
Uterine activity, 363
　effect of
　　anesthesia, 42-50
　　　inhalation agents, 42-44
　　　parenteral agents, 44-45
　　　regional anesthesia, 45-48
　　　vasopressors, 48-50
　　measurement of, 42, 363
Uterine atony, 252
　maternal resuscitation, 252
Uterine bleeding, 267
Uterine blood flow, 17-18, 23-41
　effects of
　　anesthetic agents, 267
　　antihypertensive agents, 34-35
　　barbiturates, 23-25
　　catecholamines and stress, 31-32
　　diazepam, 25
　　enflurane, 27
　　fluroxene, 28
　　halothane, 26, 324-325
　　hypotension, 279, 324
　　isoflurane, 27
　　ketamine, 25-26
　　local anesthetics, 28-29
　　magnesium sulfate, 35
　　methoxyflurane, 27
　　regional anesthesia, 29-31
　　respiratory gases, 35-38
　　vasopressors, 32-34
　factors causing a decrease in, 18, 279
　humans, 53
　measurement of, 23
　sheep, 53
　with hypotension, 285
　with stress, 67
Uterine contractions
　monitoring of, 230, 363
　patterns of, 361
　　early decelerations, 361
　　late decelerations, 361
　　variable decelerations, 361
Uterine hypotonus, 325
Uterine ischemia, 224
Uterine relaxation, 42
　general anesthesia for multiple births, 177
　halothane for, 26, 43-44
Uterine rupture, 250-251
Uterine vascular resistance, 325
Uterine vasoconstriction
　caused by
　　vasopressors, 286
　　sympathomimetics, 325
Utero-placental circulation, 12-22, 23
Utero-placental insufficiency, cord blood sampling diagnosis, 387

Vaginal adenosis, 53
Vaginal delivery
　choice of local anesthetic for, 116
　psychological anesthesia for, 65-70
　regional anesthesia for, 93
　systemic medication for, 75
Vaginal squeeze, 386
Valium (see Diazepam)
Valvular surgery, pregnancy after, 212
Vaporizers, 126-128
Variable decelerations
　grading of, 362
　of fetal heart rate, 361
　severe, 21, 361
Varicosities
　vaginal, 250
　vulvar, 250
Vascular resistance
　pulmonary, 385
　　and atrial septal defect, 195
　　and Eisenmenger's syndrome, 200
　　and pulmonary hypertension, 205
　　and ventricle septal defect, 194
　systemic, 385
　　and aortic insufficiency, 191
　　and aortic stenosis, 192
　　and asymmetric septal hypertrophy, 211
　　and atrial septal defect, 195
　　and coarctation of the aorta, 201
　　and Eisenmenger's syndrome, 200
　　and mitral insufficiency, 189
　　and mitral stenosis, 187
　　and pulmonary hypertension, 205
　　and pulmonary stenosis, 203
　　and tetralogy of Fallot, 198
　　and ventricle septal defect, 194
Vasodilators, 218
Vasopraevia, 250
Vasopressin, 206
Vasopressors (see also specific drugs)
　and inotropes, 217
　effect of
　　on uterine activity, 48-50
　　on uterine blood flow, 32-34
　prophylactic use of, 257, 284-285
　therapy for hypotension, 285
Vasoxyl (see Methoxamine)
Vena caval compresion (see Inferior vena cava)
Venous return
　of Eisenmenger's syndrome, 200
　of tetralogy of Fallot, 198
Ventilation, maternal, 262
　intermittent mandatory, 295
　positive and expired pressure, 295
Ventilation, newborn
　breathing frequency, 386
　establishment of, 386
　functional residual capacity, 386
　lung compliance, 386
　minute ventilation, 386
　tidal volume, 386
Ventricles, cardiac, maternal septal defects in
　anesthetic considerations of, 194
　pathophysiology of, 193
　prognosis of, 193
　symptoms of, 193
Ventricle compromise, right, 194
Ventricular dysrhythmias, 216
Ventricular failure
　left and mitral insufficiency, 188
　right, and mitral stenosis, 187
　with ASD, treatment of, 195
Ventricular filling pressure
　left, 201
　right, 203
Ventricular volume, right and pulmonary hypertension, 205
Versions, internal podalic, 175
Vital capacity, maternal, 4
Vitamin K, 236
Von Willebrand's disease, 239
Vulvar varicosities, 250
V-wave, in mitral insufficiency, 189

Wheezing, expiratory, 292
Whole blood prothrombin activation rate, 238
Wolff-Parkinson-White syndrome, 210

Xenon-133 clearance technique, 31
X-rays, chest,
　acid aspiration syndrome, 290-292
　meconium aspiration pneumonitis, 391
Xylocaine (see Lidocaine)